AF327163

Dynamic Reconstruction of the Spine

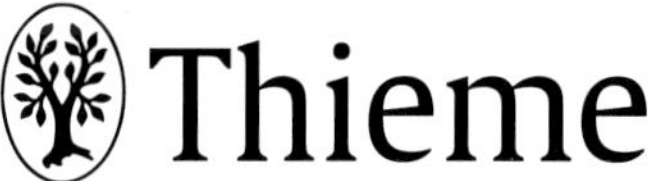

Dynamic Reconstruction of the Spine

Daniel H. Kim, M.D., F.A.C.S.
Professor
Department of Neurosurgery
Director, Spinal Neurosurgery and Reconstructive Peripheral Nerve Surgery
Stanford University Medical Center
Stanford, California

Frank P. Cammisa Jr., M.D., F.A.C.S.
Associate Professor of Clinical Surgery
Weill Medical College of Cornell University
Chief, Spinal Surgical Service
Associate Attending Surgeon
The Hospital for Special Surgery
New York, New York

Richard G. Fessler, M.D., Ph.D.
John Harper Seeley Professor and Chief
Section of Neurosurgery
Department of Surgery
The University of Chicago Hospitals
Chicago, Illinois

Thieme
New York • Stuttgart

Thieme Medical Publishers, Inc.
333 Seventh Ave.
New York, NY 10001

Executive Editor: Timothy Hiscock
Associate Editor: Birgitta Brandenburg
Assistant Editor: Ivy Ip
Editorial Assistant: Judith Tomat
Vice President, Production and Electronic Publishing: Anne T. Vinnicombe
Production Editor: Print Matters, Inc.
Sales Director: Ross Lumpkin
Associate Marketing Director: Verena Diem
Chief Financial Officer: Peter van Woerden
President: Brian D. Scanlan
Compositor: Compset
Printer: Everbest

Library of Congress Cataloging-in-Publication Data

Dynamic reconstruction of the spine / [edited by] Daniel H. Kim, Frank P. Cammisa, Richard G. Fessler.
    p. ; cm.
  Includes bibliographical references and index.
  ISBN 1-58890-484-9 (US : HC) -- ISBN 3-13-142681-0 (GTV : HC) 1. Spine--Surgery. 2.
Arthroplasty. 3. Intervertebral disk prostheses. I. Kim, Daniel H. II. Cammisa, Frank P.
III. Fessler, Richard G.
  [DNLM: 1. Spine--surgery. 2. Arthroplasty, Replacement--methods. 3. Prostheses and Implants.
WE 725 D997 2006]
  RD768.D96 2006
  617.5'6059--dc22
                                                                          200604387

Important note: Medical knowledge is ever-changing. As new research and clinical experience broaden
our knowledge, changes in treatment and drug therapy may be required. The authors and editors of the
material herein have consulted sources believed to be reliable in their efforts to provide information
that is complete and in accord with the standards accepted at the time of publication. However, in view
of the possibility of human error by the authors, editors, or publisher of the work herein or changes in
medical knowledge, neither the authors, editors, or publisher, nor any other party who has been
involved in the preparation of this work, warrants that the information contained herein is in every respect accurate or complete, and they are not responsible for any errors or omissions or for the results
obtained from use of such information. Readers are encouraged to confirm the information contained
herein with other sources. For example, readers are advised to check the product information sheet
included in the package of each drug they plan to administer to be certain that the information
contained in this publication is accurate and that changes have not been made in the recommended
dose or in the contraindications for administration. This recommendation is of particular importance
in connection with new or infrequently used drugs.

Some of the product names, patents, and registered designs referred to in this book are in fact registered
trademarks or proprietary names even though specific reference to this fact is not always made in the
text. Therefore, the appearance of a name without designation as proprietary is not to be construed as
a representation by the publisher that it is in the public domain.

Printed in China

5 4 3 2 1

TMP ISBN 1-58890-484-9
          978-1-58890-484-3
GTV ISBN 3-13-142681-0
          978-3-13-142681-9

Dedication

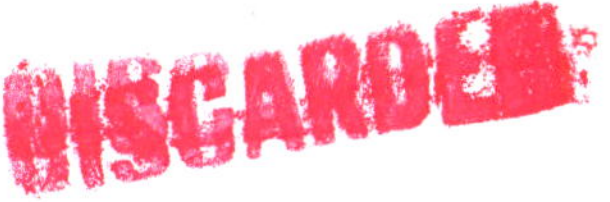

To Jane and John Evans for their passionate endorsement of surgical innovation and whose gracious support has contributed to the well-being of patients.

—Daniel H. Kim

I dedicate this volume to my wife Gail and our children Annie, Trey, and Jack. I will always appreciate their support throughout this endeavor.

—Frank P. Cammisa Jr.

To my teachers and mentors Sean Mullan, Al Rhoton, Fred Brown, and Javad Hekmatpanah, for giving me the opportunity to utilize the knowledge, skills, and advice that they so generously gave to me for the benefit of the many patients for whom I have had the privilege to care.

—Richard G. Fessler

Contents

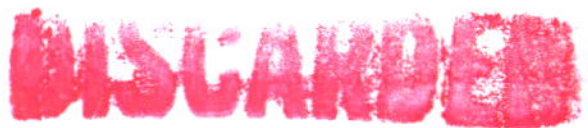

Preface . . . . **xi**

Acknowledgments . . . . **xiii**

Contributors . . . . **xv**

Section I. Motion Preservation of the Spine

Chapter 1.   Historical Review of Spinal Arthroplasty and Dynamic Stabilizations 1
Karen M. Shibata and Daniel H. Kim

Chapter 2.   Current Concepts in Spinal Fusion versus Nonfusion 16
David H. Walker and Praveen V. Mummaneni

Section II. Restoration of Cervical Motion Segment

Chapter 3.   Biomechanical Aspects Associated with Cervical Disk Arthroplasty 27
Denis J. DiAngelo and Christian M. Puttlitz

Chapter 4.   Biomechanical Testing Protocol for Evaluating Disk Arthroplasty 33
Denis J. DiAngelo and Kevin T. Foley

Chapter 5.   Cervical Disk Arthroplasty: Rationale, Indications, and Clinical Experience 42
Moe R. Lim, Joon Y. Lee, and Alexander R. Vaccaro

Chapter 6.   Spinal Kinetics Cervical Disc 52
Daniel H. Kim, Michael L. Reo, Janine Robinson, and Steve Moscaret

Chapter 7.   Bryan Cervical Disc Device 59
Robert Hacker

Chapter 8.   Prestige Cervical Artificial Disk 67
James T. Robertson

Chapter 9.   ProDisc-C Cervical Artificial Disk 72
Gerard K. Jeong, Frank P. Cammisa Jr., and Federico P. Girardi

Chapter 10. PCM (Porous Coated Motion) Artificial Cervical Disc 78
Luiz Pimenta, Roberto C. Díaz, Paul C. McAfee, and Andy Cappuccino

Chapter 11. Cervidisc Concept, Six Years Follow-Up and Introducing Cervidisc II: DISCOVERY . . . 86
Aymen S. Ramadan, Véronique Maindron-Perly, and Peggy Schmitt

Chapter 12. CerviCore Cervical Intervertebral Disk Replacement 92
Steven S. Lee, Kenneth J. H. Lee, Jean-Jacques Abitbol, and Jeffrey C. Wang

Section III.   Restoration of Lumbar Motion Segment

Part A. Lumbar Nucleus Replacement

Chapter 13. Prosthetic Disk Nucleus Partial Disk Replacement: Pathobiological
and Biomechanical Rationale for Design and Function 99
Charles Dean Ray, Joseph E. Hale, and Britt K. Norton

Chapter 14. The Raymedica Prosthetic Disk Nucleus (PDN): Stabilizing the Degenerated
Lumbar Vertebral Segment without Fusion or Total Disk Replacement 105
Charles Dean Ray

Chapter 15. Functional Lumbar Artificial Nucleus Replacement: The DASCOR System 114
John Emery Sherman and Bruce Randall Bowman

Chapter 16. NeuDisc 122
Rudolf Bertagnoli, Ann Prewett, James J. Yue, and Christopher Sabatino

Chapter 17. Pioneer Surgical Technology NUBAC Artificial Nucleus 128
Qi-Bin Bao, Hansen A. Yuan, and Matthew N. Songer

Chapter 18. SINUX (Sinitec) 137
Jan Zoellner

Chapter 19. NuCore Injectable Disk Nucleus 142
Scott H. Kitchel, Lawrence M. Boyd, and Andrew J. Carter

Part B. Lumbar Total Disk Replacement

Chapter 20. Biomechanical Considerations for Total Lumbar Disk Replacement 149
Jean-Charles Le Huec, S. Aunoble, Y. Basso, C. Tournier, and K. Yamada

Chapter 21. Indications for Total Lumbar Disk Replacement 154
Rudolf Bertagnoli

Chapter 22. CHARITÉ Artificial Disc 160
Fred H. Geisler

Chapter 23. ProDisc Lumbar Artificial Disk 179
Jack E. Zigler and Matthew T. Bennett

Chapter 24. MAVERICK Total Disc Replacement 186
Matthew F. Gornet

Chapter 25. The Mobidisc Prosthesis 196
Jean-Paul Steib, J. Beaurain, J. Delecrin, and the Mobidisc group (J. Allain,
M. Ameil, H. Chataigner, M. Gau, J. Huppert, M. Onimus, and W. Zeegers)

Chapter 26. Activ-L Lumbar (Aesculap) Total Disk Arthroplasty 204
James J. Yue and Rolando Garcia

Chapter 27. The Flexicore Disk 212
    Alok D. Sharan and Thomas Errico

Chapter 28. Management of Vascular and Surgical Approach–Related Complications for Lumbar
    Total Disk Replacement 221
    Sang-Ho Lee and Sang Hyeop Jeon

Chapter 29. Complications of Lumbar Disk Arthroplasty 227
    Sang-Ho Lee and Chan Shik Shim

Part C. Dynamic Posterior Stabilization

Chapter 30. Rationale for Dynamic Stabilization 237
    Donal S. McNally

Chapter 31. Rationale for Dynamic Stabilization II—SoftFlex System 244
    Dilip K. Sengupta

Interspinous Process Spacers

Chapter 32. The X STOP Interspinous Process Decompression System for the
    Treatment of Lumbar Neurogenic Claudication 251
    Richard M. Thunder, Ken Y. Hsu, and James F. Zucherman

Chapter 33. Dynamic Lumbar Stabilization with the Wallis Interspinous Implant 258
    Jacques Sénégas

Chapter 34. Coflex 268
    Eun-Sang Kim and Doo-Sik Kong

Chapter 35. DIAM (Device for Intervertebral Assisted Motion) Spinal Stabilization System . . . 274
    Kern Singh and Frank M. Phillips

Chapter 36. Tension Band System 284
    Sang-Ho Lee, Ewy Ryong Chung, and Dong Yeob Lee

Chapter 37. Shape Memory Implant (KIMPF-DI Fixing) System 292
    Young-Soo Kim and Ho-Yeol Zhang

Pedicle Screw–Based Systems

Chapter 38. Treatment of Mobile Vertebral Instability with Dynesys 299
    Gilles Dubois, O. Schwarzenbach, N. Specchia, and T. M. Stoll

Chapter 39. Graf Soft Stabilization: Graf Ligamentoplasty 305
    Young-Soo Kim and Dong-Kyu Chin

Chapter 40. Isobar TTL Dynamic Instrumentation 312
    Antonio E. Castellvi, James J. Paraiso, and David Pienkowski

Chapter 41. Minimally Invasive Posterior Dynamic Stabilization System 323
    Luiz Pimenta, Roberto Díaz, and Dilip K. Sengupta

Chapter 42. Nonfusion Stabilization of the Degenerated Lumbar Spine with Cosmic 330
    Archibald von Strempel

Chapter 43. BioFlex Spring Rod Pedicle Screw System 340
    Young-Soo Kim and Byung-Jin Moon

Part D. Facet Replacement

Chapter 44. Facet Replacement Technologies 347
    Moe R. Lim, Joon Y. Lee, and Todd James Albert

Chapter 45. TOPS—Total Posterior Facet Replacement and Dynamic Motion Segment
    Stabilization System 354
    Larry T. Khoo, Luiz Pimenta, and Roberto C. Díaz

Chapter 46. Total Facet Arthroplasty System (TFAS) 364
    Scott Webb

Part E. Annular Repair

Chapter 47. Indications and Techniques in Annuloplasty 375
    Michael Y. Wang

Section IV. Future Biological Approaches to Disk Repair

Chapter 48. Molecular Therapy of the Intervertebral Disk 383
    S. Tim Yoon

Index 389

Preface

Imitation is the sincerest form of flattery. It's also the basis of a considerable amount of research and development into the use of artificial disks to treat degenerative and damaged disks and associated spinal conditions by maintaining or recreating the natural biomechanics of the spine.

While traditional fusion methods help to eliminate certain types of spinal pain, these procedures have been shown to decrease function by impairing the natural range of motion for patients in flexion, extension, rotation, and lateral bending. The innovative technologies of spinal arthroplasty and dynamic stabilization aim to provide stabilization via motion and spine preservation techniques. Significant efforts are being made in the use of implantable artificial intervertebral disks, which are intended to restore articulation between vertebral bodies so as to recreate the full range of motion normally allowed by the elastic properties of the natural disk. In addition, dynamic posterior stabilization techniques have been explored to mimic the posterior elements.

With a thorough review of the cervical and lumbar spine, the text incorporates both anterior and posterior approaches to dynamic stabilization. Divided into four main sections, this text discusses nucleus replacement, total disk replacement, and dynamic stabilization using interspinous process spacers, pedicle screw–based systems, facet replacement, and annular repair. Within each section, the chapters provide an exhaustive review of systems that have been proposed and/or that are being produced. In addition, a system's inventor(s) or surgeon(s) with expertise with that particular system authored each chapter, allowing for specific insight into each system.

The advances in dynamic reconstruction of the spine have been immense. This book covers those advances and current technology in dynamic reconstruction of the spine, and summarizes the vast literature and equipment currently being investigated not only to compare the instrumentation systems but also to provide insight into further research and development coming in this field.

This text will prove useful for those who specialize in spine surgery and as the use of artificial disks increases will broaden to include neurosurgeons, orthopedic surgeons, radiologists, fellow, residents, medical students, nurses, and physician assistants.

Showcasing the range of possibilities that are or will soon be within reach to treat spinal conditions now commonly treated with fusion procedures, this text presents a sneak preview into what might serve as the new gold standard in the treatment of spinal pain.

Acknowledgments

A tremendous amount of energy and teamwork accompanied the production of this book, and I am grateful to the many dedicated individuals and companies that contributed their time, talents, and resources. I would like to acknowledge the valuable input of the editors Frank P. Cammisa Jr., M.D., and Richard G. Fessler, M.D., the expertise and insight of all the authors, and the following individuals whose efforts and resolve made this book possible: Thelma Prescott, Karen Shibata, Christine Field, Kwon Soo Chun, Won Jae Lee, Dong Suk Shin, and Sung Ho Park.

Daniel H. Kim

Contributors

Jean-Jacques Abitbol, M.D., F.R.C.S.
Orthopaedic Surgeon
California Spine Group
San Diego, California

Todd James Albert, M.D.
Professor and Vice Chairman
Department of Orthopedics
Thomas Jefferson University
  Medical College
Philadelphia, Pennsylvania

S. Aunoble, M.D.
Département Orthopédie Pr Chauveaux
Spine Unit Pr Le Huec, CHU Pellegrin
Université Bordeaux
Bordeaux, France

Qi-Bin Bao, Ph.D.
Vice President, Spine Development
Pioneer Surgical Technologies
Marquette, Michigan

Y. Basso, M.D.
Département Orthopédie Pr Chauveaux
Spine Unit Pr Le Huec, CHU Pellegrin
Université Bordeaux
Bordeaux, France

J. Beaurain, M.D.
Service de Neurochirurgie
Hôpital Universitaire de Dijon
Dijon, France

Matthew T. Bennett, M.D.
Tier Orthopedic Associates
Vestal, New York

Rudolf Bertagnoli, M.D.
Chief of Spine Center
St.-Elisabeth-Klinikum
Straubing, Germany

Bruce Randall Bowman, Sc.D.
Eden Prairie, Minnesota

Lawrence M. Boyd, M.S., M.E.M.
Department of Biomedical Engineering
Duke University
Durham, North Carolina

Frank P. Cammisa Jr., M.D.
Associate Professor of Clinical Surgery
Weill Medical College of Cornell University
Chief, Spinal Surgical Service
The Hospital for Special Surgery
New York, New York

Andy Cappuccino, M.D.
Orthopedic and Spine Surgeon
Buffalo Spine Surgery
Lockport, New York

Andrew J. Carter, Ph.D.
Vice President, Research and Development and
  Polymer Operations
SpineWave, Inc.
Shelton, Connecticut

Antonio E. Castellvi, M.D.
Florida Orthopaedic Institute
Center for Spinal Disorders
Tampa, Florida

Dong-Kyu Chin, M.D., Ph.D.
Associate Professor
Department of Neurosurgery
Yonsei University College of Medicine
Yongdong Severance Hospital
Seoul, South Korea

Ewy Ryong Chung, M.D.
Wooridul Spine Hospital
Department of Orthopedic Surgery
Seoul, South Korea

J. Delecrin, M.D.
Service de Chirurgie Orthopédique
Hôpital Universitaire de Nantes
Nantes, France

Denis J. DiAngelo, Ph.D.
Associate Professor
Department of Biomedical Engineering
The University of Tennessee Health Science Center
Memphis, Tennessee

Roberto C. Díaz, M.D.
NeuroSpine Surgery
Minimally Invasive and Reconstructive Spine Surgery
Santa Rita Hospital
São Paulo, Brazil

Gilles Dubois, M.D.
Neurosurgeon
Clinique de l'Union
Saint Jean, France

Thomas Errico, M.D.
Chief of Spine Service
New York University Hospital for Joint Diseases
New York, New York

Richard G. Fessler, M.D., Ph.D.
John Harper Seeley Professor and Chief
Section of Neurosurgery
Department of Surgery
The University of Chicago Hospitals
Chicago, Illinois

Kevin T. Foley, M.D.
Professor
Department of Neurosurgery
The University of Tennessee Health Science Center
Memphis, Tennessee

Rolando Garcia, M.D.
Aventura Hospital and Medical Center
Aventura, Florida

Fred H. Geisler, M.D., Ph.D.
Founder
Illinois Neuro-Spine Center
Rush-Copley Medical Center
Aurora, Illinois

Federico P. Girardi, M.D.
Assistant Professor
Department of Orthopaedic Surgery
Weill Medical College of Cornell University
Hospital for Special Surgery
New York, New York

Matthew F. Gornet, M.D.
Staff Physician
The Orthopedic Center of St. Louis
Saint Louis, Missouri

Robert Hacker, M.D.
Oregon Neurosurgery Specialists
Eugene, Oregon

Joseph E. Hale, Ph.D.
Applied Research Manager
Senior Scientist
Spineology, Inc.
Saint Paul, Minnesota

Ken Y. Hsu, M.D.
St. Mary's Spine Center
San Francisco, California

Sang Hyeop Jeon, M.D.
Wooridul Spine Hospital
Department of General Surgery
Seoul, South Korea

Gerard K. Jeong, M.D.
Spine and Scoliosis Fellow
The Hospital for Special Surgery
New York, New York

Larry T. Khoo, M.D.
Codirector, Comprehensive Spine Center
Neurological and Orthopedic Spinal Surgery
University of California Los Angeles Medical Center
Santa Monica, California

Daniel H. Kim, M.D., F.A.C.S.
Professor
Department of Neurosurgery
Director, Spinal Neurosurgery and Reconstructive Peripheral
   Nerve Surgery
Stanford University Medical Center
Stanford, California

Eun-Sang Kim, M.D.
Clinical Professor
Department of Neurosurgery
Samsung Medical Center
Sungkyunkwan University School of Medicine
Seoul, South Korea

Young-Soo Kim, M.D., Ph.D.
Professor Emeritus
Department of Neurosurgery
Yonsei University College of Medicine
Yongdong Severance Hospital
Seoul, South Korea

Scott H. Kitchel, M.D.
Orthopedic Spine Associates
Eugene, Oregon

Doo-Sik Kong, M.D.
Neurosurgical Fellow
Department of Neurosurgery
Samsung Medical Center
Sungkyunkwan University
Seoul, South Korea

Jean-Charles Le Huec, M.D., Ph.D.
Professor
Department Orthopédie Pr Chauveaux
Spine Unit Pr Le Huec, CHU Pellegrin
Université Bordeaux
Bordeaux, France

Dong Yeob Lee, M.D.
Gimpo Airport Worridul Spine Hospital
Department of Neurosurgery
Seoul, South Korea

Joon Y. Lee, M.D.
Assistant Professor
Department of Orthopaedics
University of Pittsburgh Medical Center
Pittsburgh, Pennsylvania

Kenneth J. H. Lee, M.D.
Spine Care
Houston, Texas

Sang-Ho Lee, M.D., Ph.D.
Department of Neurosurgery
Wooridul Spine Hospital
Seoul, South Korea

Steven S. Lee, M.D.
Muir Orthopaedic Specialists
Walnut Creek, California

Moe R. Lim, M.D.
Assistant Professor
Department of Orthopaedics
University of North Carolina–Chapel Hill
Chapel Hill, North Carolina

Véronique Maindron-Perly
Clinical Research Manager
Scient'x
Paris, France

Paul C. McAfee, M.D.
Chief of Scoliosis and Spine Center
Orthopedic Spine Surgery
St. Joseph Medical Center
Baltimore, Maryland

Donal S. McNally, Ph.D., B.Sc.
Institute of Biomechanics
University of Nottingham
University Park
Nottingham, United Kingdom

Byung-Jin Moon, M.D.
Department of Neurosurgery
Kwang-Hye Spine Hospital
Seoul, South Korea

Steve Moscaret
Vice President, Marketing and New Business Development
Spinal Kinetics, Inc.
Redwood City, California

Praveen V. Mummaneni, M.D.
Assistant Professor of Neurosurgery
Emory Clinic
Atlanta, Georgia

Britt K. Norton, B.S., Ch.E., M.B.A.
CoreSpine Technologies, LLC
Eden Prairie, Minnesota

James J. Paraiso, D.O.
Orthopaedic Spine Fellow
Florida Orthopaedic Institute
Tampa, Florida

Frank M. Phillips, M.D.
Department of Orthopaedic Surgery
Rush University Medical Center
Chicago, Illinois

David Pienkowski, Ph.D.
Associate Professor
Departments of Biomedical Engineering and
    Orthopaedic Surgery
University of Kentucky
Lexington, Kentucky

Luiz Pimenta, M.D., Ph.D.
Professor
Chief of Minimally Invasive and Reconstructive
    Spine Surgery
Neurospine Surgery
Santa Rita Hospital
São Paulo, Brazil

Ann Prewett, Ph.D.
President
Replication Medical, Inc.
Cranbury, New Jersey

Christian M. Puttlitz, Ph.D.
Assistant Professor
Department of Mechanical Engineering
Orthopaedic Bioengineering Research Laboratory
Colorado State University
Fort Collins, Colorado

Aymen S. Ramadan, M.D.
Professor
Department of Neurosurgery
Neelain University
Geneva University Hospital
Geneva, Switzerland

Charles Dean Ray, M.S., M.D., F.A.C.S., F.R.S.H. (Lond.)
Past President, American College of Spine Surgery
Past President, International Spine Arthroplasty Society
Past President, North American Spine Society
Santa Barbara, California

Michael L. Reo
Director, Engineering
Spinal Kinetics, Inc.
Redwood City, California

James T. Robertson, M.D.
Professor
Department of Neurosurgery
University of Tennessee, Health Service Center
Memphis, Tennessee

Janine Robinson
Vice President, Engineering
Spinal Kinetics, Inc.
Redwood City, California

Christopher Sabatino, Ph.D.
Replication Medical, Inc.
Cranbury, New Jersey

Peggy Schmitt
Clinical Research Associate
Scient'x
Paris, France

O. Schwarzenbach, M.D.
Regionalspital Thun
Thun, Switzerland

Jacques Sénégas, M.D.
Professor
Centre Aquitain du Dos
Clinique Saint Martin
Pessac, France

Dilip K. Sengupta, M.D.
Associate Professor
Department of Orthopaedics
Dartmouth–Hitchcock Medical Center
Lebanon, New Hampshire

Alok D. Sharan, M.D.
Spine Surgery Fellow
NYU Hospital for Joint Diseases
New York, New York

John Emery Sherman, M.D.
Clinical Instructor
Department of Orthopedics
University of Minnesota
Minneapolis, Minnesota

Karen M. Shibata, B.A.
Department of Neurosurgery
Stanford University Medical Center
Stanford, California

Chan Shik Shim, M.D., Ph.D
Department of Neurosurgery
Wooridul Spine Hospital
Seoul, South Korea

Kern Singh, M.D.
Assistant Professor
Department of Orthopaedic Surgery
Rush University Medical Center
Chicago, Illinois

Matthew N. Songer, M.D.
Adjunct Professor Michigan Technological
   University
Assistant Clinical Professor
College of Human Medicine
Michigan State University
Marquette, Michigan

N. Specchia, M.D.
Clinica Ortopedica Università Politecnica
   delle Marche
Ancona, Italy

Jean-Paul Steib, M.D.
Service de Chirurgie Orthopédique du Rachis et de
Traumatologie du Sport
Hôpitaux Universitaires de Strasbourg
Strasbourg, France

Thomas M. Stoll, M.D.
Bethesda Spital
Basel, Switzerland

Archibald von Strempel, M.D., D.Eng., Prof.
Landeskrankenhaus Feldkirch
Orthopädische Abteilung
Feldkirch, Austria

Richard M. Thunder, M.D.
St. Mary's Spine Center
San Francisco, California

C. Tournier, M.D.
Département Orthopédie
Spine Unit
Université Bordeaux
Bordeaux, France

Alexander R. Vaccaro, M.D.
Professor
Department of Orthopaedic Surgery
Thomas Jefferson University Hospital
Rothman Institute
Philadelphia, Pennsylvania

David H. Walker, M.D.
Spine Surgeon
Medford, Oregon

Jeffrey C. Wang, M.D.
Associate Professor
Department of Orthopaedic and Neurosurgery
University of California–Los Angeles
Chief, Orthopaedic Spine Service
UCLA Comprehensive Spine Center
Santa Monica, California

Michael Y. Wang, M.D.
Assistant Professor
Spine Director
Department of Neurological Surgery
Keck School of Medicine
University of Southern California
Los Angeles, California

Scott Webb, D.O.
Orthopedic, Spine Surgeon
Florida Spine Institute
Clearwater, Florida

K. Yamada, M.D.
Département Orthopédie
Spine Unit
Université Bordeaux
Bordeaux, France

S. Tim Yoon, M.D., Ph.D.
Assistant Professor
Emory University
Department of Orthopaedic Surgery
Atlanta, Georgia

Hansen A. Yuan, M.D.
Professor
Department of Orthopedic and Neurological
  Surgery
Upstate Medical University
State University of New York
Syracuse, New York

James J. Yue, M.D.
Assistant Professor
Department of Orthopaedic Surgery
Chief Spine Surgery
Yale University School of Medicine
New Haven, Connecticutt

Ho-Yeol Zhang, M.D., Ph.D.
Clinical Associate Professor
Department of Neurosurgery
Yonsei University College of Medicine
Chief, Department of Neurosurgery
National Health Insurance Corporation
Ilsan Hospital
Seoul, South Korea

Jack E. Zigler, M.D.
Clinical Associate Professor
Department of Orthopaedic Surgery
Codirector Fellowship Program
University of Texas–Southwestern
  School of Medicine
Texas Back Institute
Plano, Texas

Jan Zoellner, M.D.
Associate Professor
Department of Orthopaedic Surgery
Mainz, Germany

James F. Zucherman, M.D.
St. Mary's Spine Center
San Francisco, California

Section I

Motion Preservation of the Spine

1

Historical Review of Spinal Arthroplasty and Dynamic Stabilizations

Karen M. Shibata and Daniel H. Kim

◆ **Overview**

◆ **Spinal Arthroplasty**
Nucleus Replacement
Total Disk Replacement

◆ **Dynamic Stabilization**
Interspinous Process Spacers
Pedicle Screw–Based Systems
Facet Replacement

◆ **Summary**

Advancements in nonfusion technology for the treatment of degenerative and damaged spinal disks and associated conditions have ushered in a new era of spine care. Commonly referred to as spinal arthroplasty and dynamic stabilization, this new technology is unlike traditional fusion methods (spinal diskectomy and arthrodesis), which purposely impair normal motion by disrupting articular surfaces and locking two or more spinal vertebrae to function as a single unit. Nonfusion techniques aim to provide stabilization while maintaining the mobility and function of the spine and eliminating the pain caused by the damaged spinal disks. Current research efforts and increasing interest in new motion and spine preservation technologies are certainly indications that the traditional spinal fusion approach will perhaps one day no longer be the gold standard for treatment.

The traditional fusion methods for treating symptomatic segmental disk disease, which include diskectomies (decompression) and arthrodesis (with or without decompression), are considered the standard of care in many instances. However, there are numerous problems and disadvantages generated from such procedures. Among these issues are loss of spinal mobility and flexibility, permanently altered motion characteristics and biomechanics, grafting collapse resulting in suboptimal sagittal balance, and autograft harvest site pain. In addition, one of the most prevalent concerns following fusion at one or more levels is the transference of stress to the adjacent levels, which often results in repeat surgeries, other complications, and more pain.[1–3]

The new motion preservation technologies of spinal arthroplasty and dynamic stabilization offer significant advantages, including the maintenance of range of motion and mechanical characteristics, restoration of natural disk height and spinal alignment, significant pain reduction, and prevention of adjacent segment degeneration.

The concept of motion and preservation of the spine has been around for more than 50 years. However, the most significant advances have been made within the last 2 decades.

Artificial disks have been in clinical use in Europe since the late 1980s and rapidly became a feasible treatment option during the 1990s. Since 2000, arthroplasty for both lumbar and cervical degenerative disk disease has been introduced in the United States for clinical trials. Efforts in dynamic stabilization technologies are quickly advancing, and in 2004 the U.S. Food and Drug Administration (FDA) approved the first lumbar arthroplasty device (SB Charité III, DePuy Spine, Raynham, MA) for use in the United States[4] (**Fig. 1–1**).

This chapter reviews the historical development of spinal arthroplasty and dynamic stabilization to provide some understanding of its evolution. Due to the overwhelming number of reports and studies conducted over the decades, this chapter does not attempt to list all of them but rather to highlight a handful and summarize the rest.

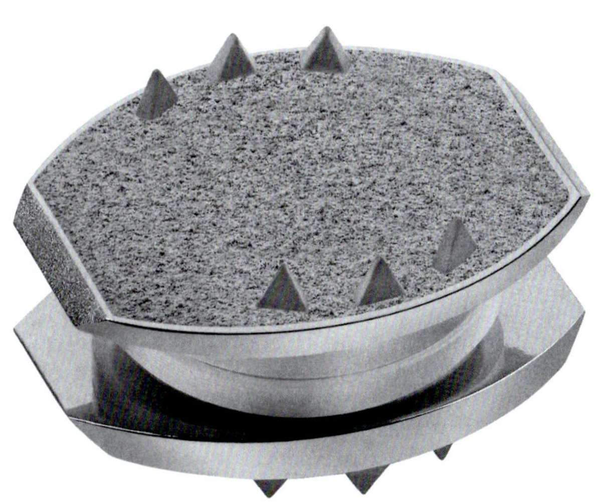

Figure 1–1 Charité Artificial Disk.

◆ Overview

Nonfusion spinal technology encompasses spinal arthroplasty devices (which replace part or the entire disk with an implant that imitates the functions of a normal disk and allows natural motion), and dynamic stabilization devices (which preserve the intervertebral disk and vertebral structure by attaching a device to the back of the spine to help stabilize the motion segment while leaving the intervertebral disks intact).

◆ Spinal Arthroplasty

Numerous attempts have been made over the last several decades to design effective spinal disk replacement devices. The progress of development in artificial disk technology may seem slow in comparison with other artificial joint technologies for the knee and hip. However, the distinction is not rooted in a lack of need, initiative, or effort, but rather in the complexities involved with the research and development process such as the design, surgical approaches and techniques, and patient selection, as well as the complexity of the structure and function of the spine itself.[2,5]

The intervertebral disk is considerably more complex because it is composed of three distinctively different tissues—annulus, nucleus, and end plate—and performs a dual function in maintaining spinal column stability while also providing the column with necessary flexibility. Therefore, much more consideration is required in designing an effective and reliable artificial disk that will maintain proper intervertebral spacing, allow for motion, provide stability, and bear loads.

In general, there are two types of spinal arthroplasty devices: nucleus replacement (replacing the nucleus only) and total disk replacement (replacing the entire disk).

In a nucleus replacement, only the inner portion of the disk (the nucleus) is removed and replaced with an implant. Ongoing research into various designs for replacements has incorporated the use of metal, ceramic, hydrogel, elastic coils, and other similar materials. Another promising replacement design consists of injectable polymers that are cured in situ to form a nucleus prosthesis, which has the desirable element of delivery via a minimally invasive, outpatient procedure. In comparison with total disk replacement, the primary advantage to this option is that it preserves the annulus and end plates while replacing only the defective portion of the nucleus.[6]

In a total disk replacement procedure, all or most of the disk tissue is removed and an entirely new device is implanted into the space between the vertebra. The many designs being studied for artificial disks incorporate metal, polyethylene, polyurethane, and other biomaterials or combinations of materials. The most commonly used design incorporates two plates that are anchored to the top and bottom surfaces of the vertebrae, above and below the disk being replaced, along with some type of compressible plastic-like piece between the plates. A total disk replacement would be used when all elements must be removed, including the nucleus and annulus, to remove the pain and treat the defective area.[7]

Nucleus Replacement

In the late 1950s, initial attempts at replacing the nucleus pulposus space involved implanting polymethyl methacrylate (PMMA), silicone, or stainless steel ball bearings.[8–10] Fernström attempted to preserve motion by inserting stainless steel ball bearings into the intervertebral disk space areas of the cervical and lumbar spine in an effort to reproduce the "ball joint" mechanism of the disk.[10] Unfortunately, the results were not very promising. McKenzie also published preliminary and long-term clinical study reports of this device reporting reasonably good results; however, its use has been discontinued because of concerns regarding subsidence and migration.[2,11,12] During this same period, Nachemson[13] performed biomechanical testing to demonstrate the relative restoration of some disk properties by injecting self-hardening silicone rubber into cadaver disks. He also tried silicon testicular prostheses but found that the implants rapidly dissolved after 20 to 30 thousand cycles of walking load.[9,13,14] Similarly, Hamby and Glaser tried injecting PMMA into the disk, which resulted in flow control problems.[8]

In 1973, Urbaniak et al used an injectable mixed silicon Dacron device in nonhuman primates and reported bone resorption along with aberrant bone formation.[15] In 1974, Schneider and Oyen performed experimental work on silicon nucleus replacement that was similar to Nachemson's work in the 1960s.[17] In an effort to replicate the natural properties of the nucleus, in 1975 Froning developed a discoid device with a central, collapsible bladder to be fixated to the vertebrae with a spike.[18] In 1977, Roy-Camille et al tried to contain medical grade silicone in a latex bag while injecting into a human cadaveric disk.[19]

Fassio and Ginestie designed and patented an elastic disk that had a Silastic central sphere and was bordered by a lateral plateau in an uncompressible synthetic resin.[20] They subsequently reported the first clinical study of the silicon nucleus using a monkey model, followed by human implantation into three patients in 1977. Follow-up reports showed a marked disk narrowing and absence of motion in all patients because the device had subsided and migrated into the vertebral body of all patients.[21] Later, Horst improved the design of the device, which had better positive locking and more uniform stress distribution.[22]

In the early 1980s, research efforts continued. Hou conducted biomechanical and animal studies in a monkey model and subsequently implanted a silicone prosthesis in more than 30 patients.[23] The results from this study were not published. In 1981, Edeland suggested that the principle of hydrophilic-hydroelastic intervertebral interposium be used as a nucleus replacement after diskectomy surgery. He described a disk containing a hydroscopic agent, which would be used to expand the disk after introduction.[24] In 1982, a nucleus replacement device was developed and patented by Kunze.[25] He designed a fish-shaped device with a fin-type tail with transverse grooves to provide a friction fit in concert with the broadened tail.

Research into reproducing both the mechanical and the physiological properties of the nucleus was accomplished by Bao and Highman, who subsequently developed a hydrogel intervertebral nucleus that contained ~70% water content

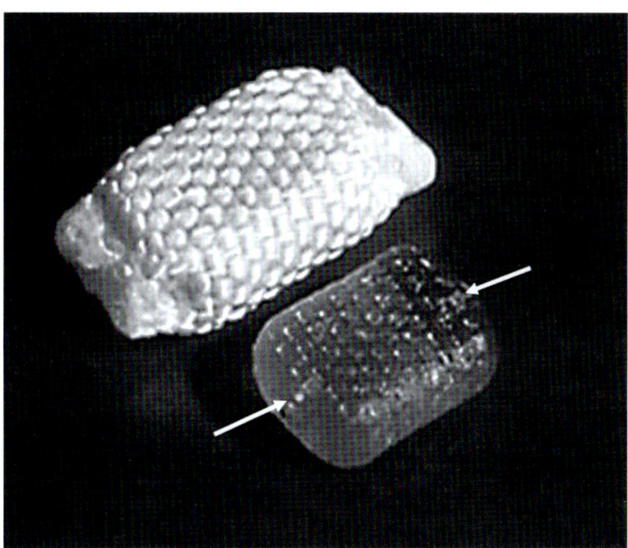

Figure 1–2 Photograph of the PDN-SOLO implant showing the internal copolymeric pellet (lower figure) and the intact implant with its woven jacket of high molecular weight polyethylene (HMWPE). The arrows at the ends of the pellet indicate the internal location of the x-ray visible Pt-Ir wire stubs.

under physiological loading conditions. Similar to natural nucleus material, the hydrogel contained the required mechanical properties and the ability to absorb and release water with changes in the applied load. Biomechanical studies have confirmed the restoration of disk anatomy after the implantation of this device.[26,27]

In 1988, Ray developed a nucleus replacement composed of dual-threaded cylinders with an ingrowth fiber capsule, an injectable thixotropic gel that would swell from a collapsed state.[28] However, technical problems in manufacturing and development led to concept changes. Subsequently, in 1990, Ray developed the Prosthetic Nucleus Device (PDN) (Raymedica, Inc., Bloomington, MN), which consisted of a hydrogel core enclosed in a woven polyethylene jacket resembling a pillow[29,30] (**Fig. 1–2**). The hydrogel contained hydrophilic properties to imitate the behavior of the nucleus pulposus. After several device migrations, additional design modifications were made.[31]

Recent Developments

The PDN device marked a new era in the development of nucleus replacement devices. Since 1996, the device has experienced widespread use in humans, with more than 4000 patients implanted internationally to date (with the PDN or the most recent PDN-SOLO device).[32] Clinical results from the beginning have been encouraging.[33] The first 10 PDN devices implanted in Germany in 1996 reported only one extrusion. By 2002, there were 480 procedures recorded with a removal rate of 5%.[34] The most recently updated version, the single PDN-SOLO device, shows considerable improvement over the initial paired PDN devices, and its methods of implantation have had good to excellent results.[32]

Newcleus (Centerpulse Spine-Tech, Minneapolis, MN), another nucleus replacement device implanted into humans, is a stand-alone device made of polycarbonate urethane curled into a preformed spiral and inserted via an open technique. This device was implanted into five patients in a pilot study.[35] The follow-up reports indicated no failures, migration, or complications, and retained disk motion was documented on plain x-rays with facet function monitored using a computed tomography scan.[36,37]

The Aquarelle (Stryker Spine, Allendale, NJ) is another hydrogel-based nuclear replacement that is composed of a polyvinyl alcohol, which is hydrated to a physiological water content of ~80% prior to implantation.[1,15] Once it reaches physiological equilibrium, the implant expands and contracts freely in situ. Testing indicated that extrusion occurred during in vitro testing only under loads well in excess of those expected in vivo.[38]

The NeuDisc SNI Hydrogel Polymer (Replication Medical, Inc., New Brunswick, NJ) has recently been reported as a hydrogel that imbibes water and expands preferentially in the axial direction[39] (**Fig. 1–3**).

The Prosthetic Intervertebral Nucleus (PIN) (Raymedica, Inc., Bloomington, MN) is an in situ curable polyurethane that is injected into a balloon catheter delivery system.[40] The curable protein hydrogel cures within minutes in the disk space, after which the catheter is removed.

The BioDisc (Cryolife, Kennesaw, GA) is an injectable protein hydrogel device based on Cryolife's surgical adhesive product. Early bench work fatigue testing at 10 million cycles indicated a 10% loss of disk height, which later recovers.[37]

The Injectable Disc Nucleus (IDN) (Spine Wave, Shelton, CT), is a hydrogel composed of synthetic silk-elastic copolymer produced through DNA bacterial synthesis fermentation, which cures within a few minutes. Early test results

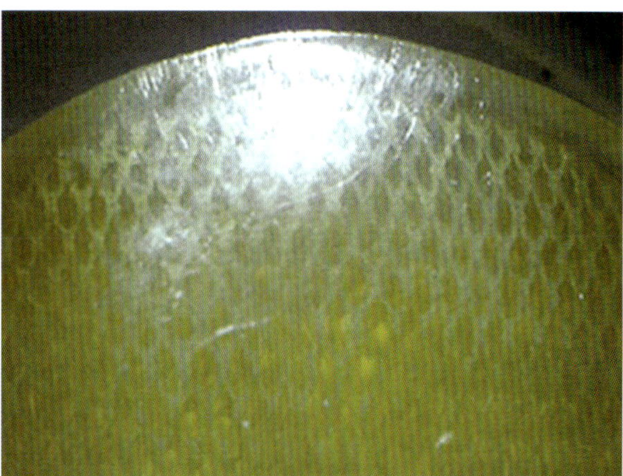

Figure 1–3 Flexion and extension motions about the major axis of the NeuDisc were performed to a simulated life of 10 years. Three of the flexion-extension samples were removed from endurance testing to be evaluated against controls. The remaining three samples proceeded to lateral bending testing. The three flexion-extension endurance samples removed for evaluation showed no signs of delaminations, tears, cracks, or major surface defects. All three samples had small wear lines oriented radially from the major axis.

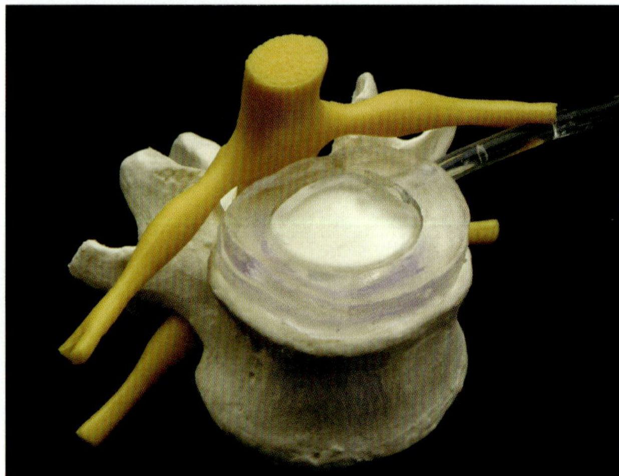

Figure 1–4   DASCOR Disc Arthroplasty Nucleus Replacement Device shown in a spine model. The in situ curable polymer is injected into a polyurethane balloon placed in the disk space. The balloon expands to fill any void that has been created during the diskectomy. The polymer cures in a matter of minutes from a liquid to a firm but pliable state.

indicate that disk height is restored under load, and the material resisted extrusion during cadaveric mechanical testing.[37]

The DASCOR (Disc Dynamics, Eden Prairie, MN) is an injectable cool polyurethane polymer that cures in situ within 12 to 15 minutes using a balloon, which is utilized to create space in the disk for the delivered material[6] (**Fig. 1–4**).

There are numerous other ongoing development studies under way, with new research efforts that will undoubtedly continue on in the future. Among these are a one-piece ceramic or metal implant that anchors to the inferior vertebral body as a hemiarthroplasty (being developed by Interpore Cross International, Irvine, CA); a hydrogel memory coiling material that imbibes fluid to restore disk height (by Mathys Medical in Switzerland); and a chemonucleolysis product to identify a formulation and dose to initiate the regeneration process of the nucleus pulposus (by NuVasive, Inc., San Diego, CA).

Total Disk Replacement

Total disk replacements can generally be categorized into two types: lumbar and cervical.

Lumbar Total Disk Replacement

Although initial efforts by Fernström in the late 1950s were not promising, much has been learned since then. During the 1980s, a renewed resurgence of interest in spinal arthroplasty brought about a flood of studies and research efforts. Steffee, who had been involved in designing artificial disks since the mid-1970s, made substantial advancements with the development of high-density polyethylene (PE)/CoCr prosthesis. This led to the development of the AcroFlex (DePuy Spine, Raynham, MA) device in the mid-1980s, which was composed of a polyolefin-based rubber

core sandwiched between titanium end plates and was subsequently used in six patients between 1988 and 1989.[41] However, because of disintegration of the rubber core in the preliminary clinical trials, further efforts were suspended.

In the 1990s, Steffee developed the second-generation version of the AcroFlex (DePuy Spine) that was similar to the first, except that now it consisted of silicone instead of rubber.[42–44] A 3-year follow-up published in 1993 on six patients who were implanted with the device indicated average results.[41,45] An improved design using HP-100 silicon elastomer developed by Steffee et al resulted in the third-generation AcroFlex artificial disk.[46,47] However, after the first 40 implantations, the elastomer developed minor defects in several cases, which were evident in a computed tomographic scan after 1 to 2 years. Similarly, later animal studies also indicated poor maintenance of sagittal and lateral flexion ranges of motion.[48]

A significant advancement in total disk replacement devices was made with the development of the SB Charité (DePuy Spine) prosthesis, which was designed by Schellnac and Büttner-Jans in 1982 and first implanted by Zippel in 1984. (For more details, see related chapter in this book.) The sliding core of this device consisted of ultra high molecular weight polyethylene (UHMWPE) interposed between metallic end plates. However, there were problems with migration and metal fatigue, which led to a second-generation (SB Charité II) device that featured flat extensions on both sides of the end plates. Although this version was an improvement over the previous device, fatigue fractures still led to early failures. Then a third and current version (SB Charité III; DePuy Spine) of the device was developed in 1987, which featured broader, flat end plates. Numerous

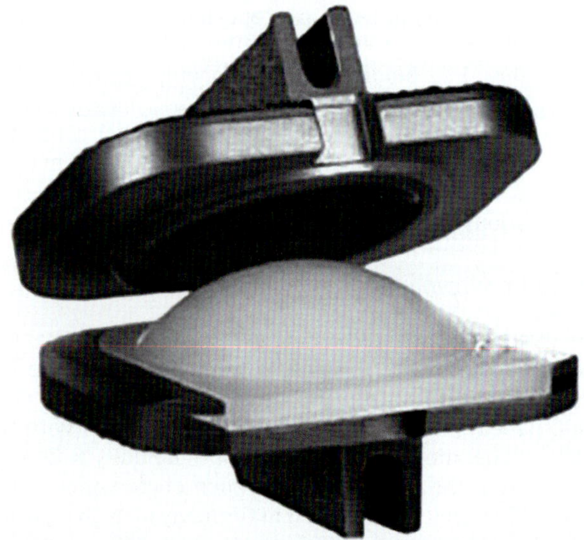

Figure 1–5   ProDisc-C cervical prosthesis is a semiconstrained, ball-and-socket design with fixed axis of rotation. It consists of two forged cobalt-chromium-molybdenum (CoCrMo) alloy end plates and an ultra high molecular weight polyethylene inlay element, which is fixed to the inferior prosthetic end plate. The metal end plates have two vertical fins for immediate fixation in the end plates and are plasma sprayed with titanium for long-term fixation through osseointegration.

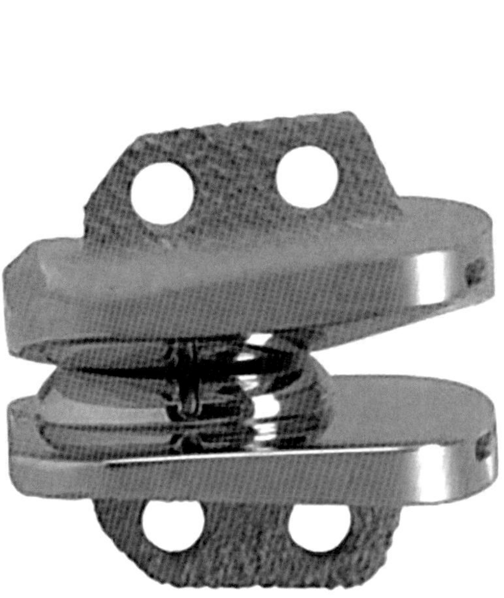

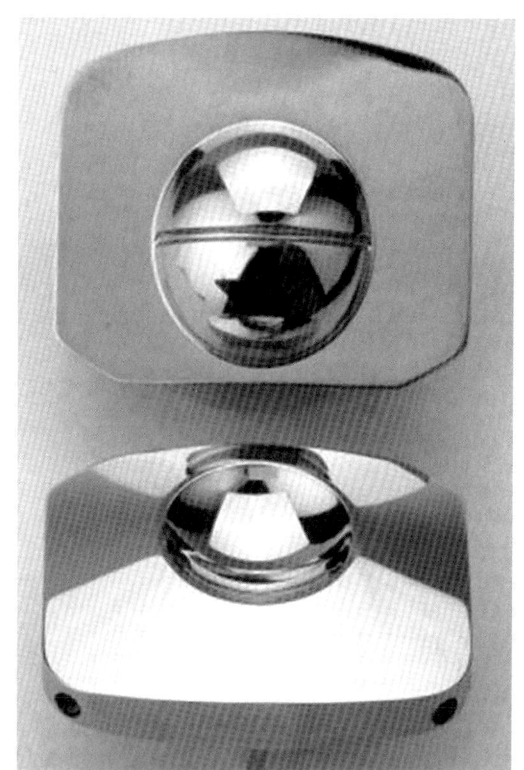

A   **B**

Figure 1–6   (A) Maverick Total Disk Arthroplasty two-piece ball-and-joint prosthesis. **(B)** Maverick metal-on-metal end plates (cobalt-chromium-molybdenum alloy).

studies worldwide since 1987 have indicated encouraging and promising results.[49] Among these are Griffith et al in 1994,[50] Lemaire et al in 1997,[51] Cinotti et al in 1996,[52] Zeegers et al in 1999,[53] McAfee et al in 2003,[54] and David in 2005.[55] The SB Charité III is currently the most widely implanted total disk replacement system, with more than 7000 implants worldwide.[36,52,56,57]

The ProDisc (Aesculap AG & Co., Tuttlingen, Germany), a total disk replacement device developed by Marnay[58] in the late 1980s, consisted of two cobalt-chromium-molybdenum (CoCrMo) alloy end plates coated with a titanium Plasmapore surface to improve osteointegration (**Fig. 1–5**). Unlike the free-floating core of the SB Charité III, the ProDisc implant relied on a single articulating interface between the core fixed to the inferior end plate and the superior metallic end plate. Initially, Marnay implanted the device into 64 patients between 1990 and 1993. In 1999, a long-term follow-up study indicated promising results.[59] After several design modifications, the second-generation design, the ProDisc II (Aesculap AG & Co.) was released in Europe in 1999. Favorable results were also reported by Mayer et al and Bertagnoli and Kumar on this improved device, which was implanted into 108 patients.[60,61] In 2001, the FDA allowed the first ProDisc implantations under an investigational device exemption. By early 2003, Sythes-Stratec Inc. (Oberdorf, Switzerland) acquired ProDisc. Recent studies continue to show positive results using this disk.[62]

The Maverick artificial disk (Medtronic Sofamor Danek, Memphis, TN) is a two-piece metal-on-metal design utilizing a polished, CoCrMo ball and socket that incorporates

a more posterior center of rotation (**Fig. 1–6**). It was first clinically used in January 2002 and early clinical results are encouraging.[63,64] Maverick FDA multicenter has completed its randomized portion of the study and is now in the continued access mode of the FDA approval process clinical trials, which began in the United States in May 2003 and span a 2-year follow-up period on the enrolled patients.

The FlexiCore (Stryker Spine, Kalamazoo, MI) intervertebral disk replacement device is another metal-on-metal design that is inserted as a single unit (**Fig. 1–7**). The dome-shaped end plates are shaped to approximate the concavities

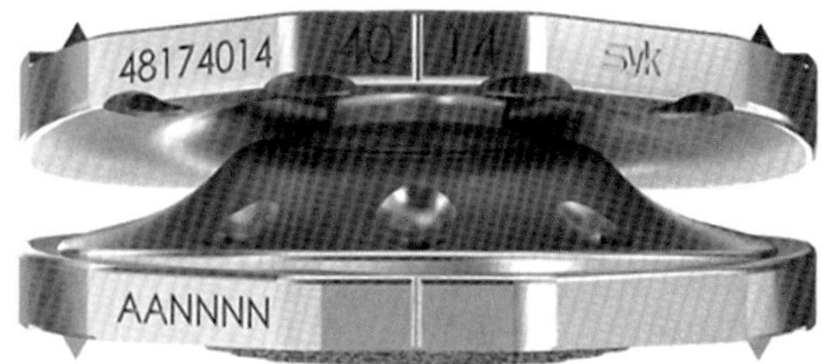

Figure 1–7   FlexiCore Intervertebral Disk (anterior view lordosed).

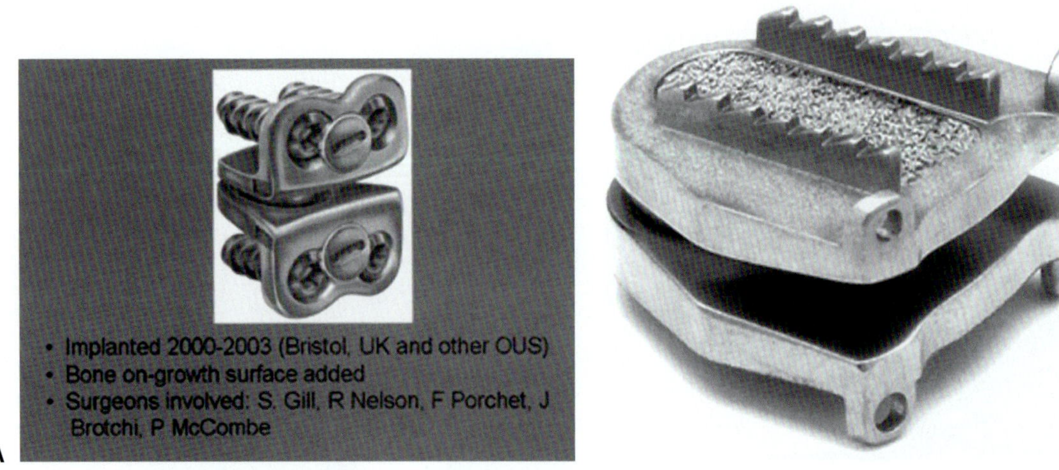

Figure 1–8 **(A)** Prestige II. **(B)** Prestige LP.

of the vertebral body end plates and can be inserted via multiple angles.[65] U.S. clinical trials through an Investigational Device Exemption (IDE) grant by the FDA for this device began in August 2003 with a 2-year follow-up period. The randomized study has been completed and is currently in continued access mode.

Cervical Total Disk Replacement

Subsequent to the first cervical disk arthroplasty attempt using Fernström's ball implantations during the 1950s, similar attempts were made by McKenzie beginning in 1969 (using Fernström balls) and by Harmon in 1957 (using Vitallium spheres).[11,66] Reitz and Joubert, from South Africa, also reported use of the Fernström prostheses for the treatment of intractable headaches and cervicobrachialgia, although no long-term follow-up is available.[67]

The next major advancement in cervical disk devices was made in 1989 by Cummins in Bristol, England, at Frenchay Hospital. The device, known today as the Prestige artificial disk (Medtronic Sofamor Danek, Memphis, TN), was initially constructed of stainless steel and secured to the vertebral bodies with solid screws. It allowed for unconstrained motion across the segments (**Fig. 1–8**).

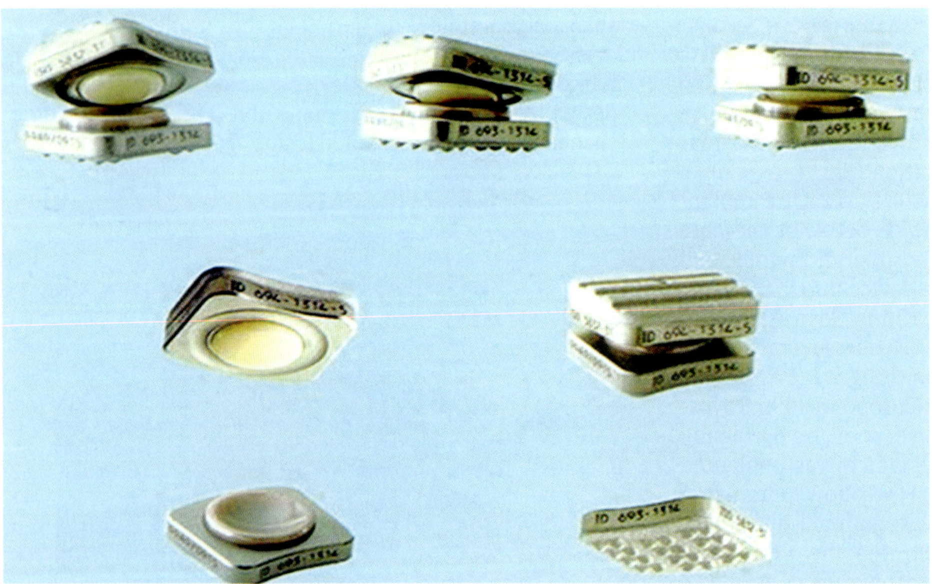

Figure 1–10 The Cervidisc is made of ceramic mobile interface, surrounded by titanium, zirconium, and hydroxyapatite coating.

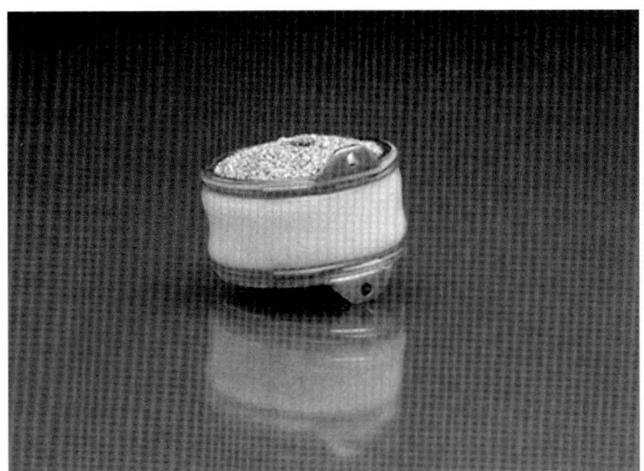

Figure 1–9 The Bryan disk device has porous titanium end plates that promote bony ingrowth. Device diameters range from 14 to 18 mm with one height. The metal tabs on the right side of the figure attach to the insertion instrument and also eliminate the risk of device migration into the central canal.

Initial clinical trials implanted this new prosthesis in 20 patients between 1991 and 1996 and the results were promising and encouraging.[68] The original Bristol/Cummins disk was modified in 1998 into the second-generation design, the Prestige I (Medtronic Sofamor Danek, Memphis, TN), which was designed to allow more physiological cervical motion that would otherwise be restrained by the facet joints and surrounding tissues. A 2-year follow-up study on 15 patients continues to show promise because cervical motion across the implanted site was preserved in all patients but one.[69] In 1999, the Prestige II (Medtronic Sofamor Danek, Memphis, TN) was developed, which featured a more anatomical end plate design. Subsequent clinical studies continued to show improved and encouraging results.[70] In 2002, further modifications led to the current design, the Prestige ST disk (Medtronic Sofamor Danek, Memphis, TN).

In 1999, Pointillart developed and implanted a spacer-type artificial disk. However, eight of the 10 patients who received the implant had spontaneous fusions after 2 years and efforts were subsequently discontinued.[71] Similarly in 1999, Ramadan began implantation of the Cervidisc, (Scient'x, Guyancourt, France) which consisted of titanium end plates bearing zirconia ceramic gliding surfaces (**Fig. 1–9**). (For more details on the Cervidisc, see related chapter in this book.)

The Bryan Cervical Disc (Medtronic Sofamor Danek, Memphis, TN) is a one-piece composite-type metal-on-polymer device composed of a wear resistant, elastic polymer nucleus with a fully variable instantaneous axis of rotation that is not dependent on supplemental fixation[71] (**Fig. 1–10**). This device, developed in the late 1990s, has undergone considerable research and numerous studies worldwide with satisfactory to promising results.[72–78] In 2002, clinical trials began in the United States under an IDE regulated by the U.S. FDA. (For more details on the Bryan disk, see related chapter in this book.)

The Porous Coated Motion (PCM) cervical disk (Cervitech, Inc., Rockaway, NJ), originally developed by Dr. McAfee, features a unique large layer radius UHMW polyethylene bearing surface attached to the lower end plate that allows translational motion in an arc consistent with the natural motion of the cervical spine segment[79] (**Fig. 1–11**). Human implantations were first performed in December 2002 in São Paulo, Brazil.[80] The results from a pilot study reported in 2004 indicated promising results.[79] Clinical trials in the United States are expected to begin soon. (For more details, see related chapter in this book.)

The ProDisc-C (Synthes, Inc., West Chester, PA), the cervical version designed based upon the lumbar ProDisc (Aesculap), is an articulating disk with a polyethylene core and metal end plates sprayed with titanium and two vertical fins for fixation in the end plates. Although research is still ongoing, initial investigative reports are encouraging.[81,82] The first im-

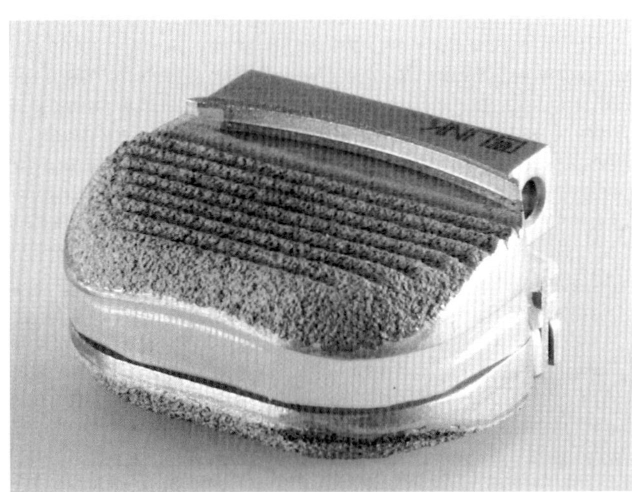

Figure 1–11 PCM (Porous Coated Motion) Artificial Disc.

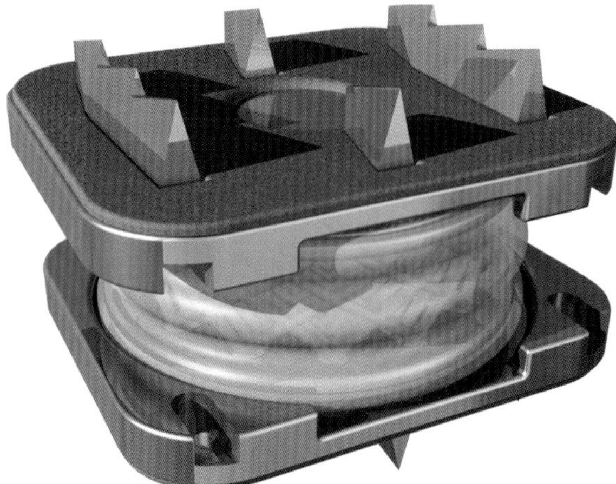

Figure 1–12 The Spinal Kinetics Cervical Disc's core construct is made of an elastomeric material surrounded by a redundant polymer fiber construct.

plantation in a human took place in December 2002,[83] and clinical trials in the United States are in progress.

The Spinal Kinetics Cervical Disc (Spinal Kinetics, Inc., Redwood City, CA) has a core construct made of an elastomeric material surrounded by a redundant polymer fiber construct that is crucial in its replication of natural motion and resistance (**Fig. 1–12**). In 2005, Spinal Kinetics initiated a nonrandomized clinical feasibility trial outside the United States with a follow-up at 6 weeks and 3 months postprocedure. The primary objective of this study was to determine the preliminary safety and feasibility of the Spinal Kinetics Cervical Disc for use with patients undergoing single-level or two-level cervical spinal procedures, as measured by overall patient success. At the time of this writing, preliminary results were being gathered for the 6-week and 3-month follow-up on these initial patients. Also at the time of this writing, a prospective randomized clinical trial protocol for the Spinal Kinetics Cervical Disc was under review by the U.S. FDA.

◆ Dynamic Stabilization

Dynamic stabilization describes the treatment method of achieving stabilization by maintaining the disk with a controlled motion of the segment.[84–86] Also referred to as "soft or flexible stabilization" or "dynamic neutralization," this method opts to preserve the intervertebral disk and vertebral structure while leaving the intervertebral disks intact. The three general categories of devices include interspinous process spacers, pedicle screw–based systems, and facet replacement systems. The effectiveness and safety of many of these devices and systems are still at the beginning stages of development and have yet to be approved for use in the United States.

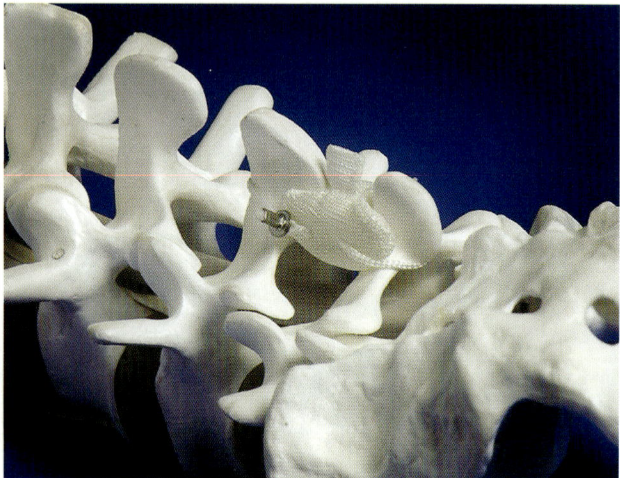

Figure 1–13   Device for Intervertebral Assisted Motion (DIAM) Spinal Stabilization System is a silicone "bumper" that is inserted between the spinous processes.

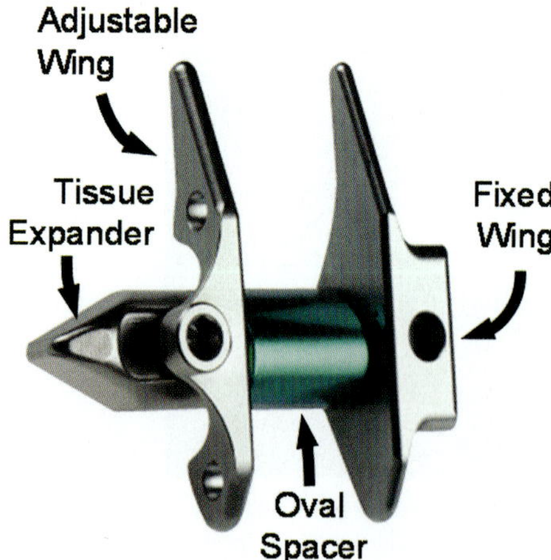

Figure 1–14   An image of the X STOP depicting the adjustable universal wing, tissue expander, fixed wing, and spacer. The tapered tissue expander allows for easier insertion between the spinous processes. The universal and fixed wings limit anterior and lateral migration. The spacer limits extension of the treated spinous processes.

Interspinous Process Spacers

In 1986, one of the first interspinous process implants for lumbar stabilization was developed. It consisted of a titanium interspinous blocker and an artificial ligament.[87] An initial observational study was subsequently completed, followed by a prospective controlled study from 1988 to 1993.[88,89] This was followed by additional design improvements that resulted in a second-generation device—the "Wallis" implant. Since then, several different designs have been developed by researchers.

The Device for Intervertebral Assisted Motion (DIAM) (Medtronic Sofamor Danek, Memphis, TN) was designed to dynamically support the vertebrae while at the same time maintaining distraction of the foramina. Because there are few long-term studies currently available on this device, clinical indications are still not firmly conclusive.[90–94] Regardless, the device has been gaining popularity since its European launch by Medtronic, Inc., in 2003 (**Fig. 1–13**).

The Fulcrum-Assisted Soft Stabilization (FASS) system was designed as an improvement over the Graf system.[95,96] In the FASS, a fulcrum is inserted between the pedicle screws in front of the ligament, which distracts the posterior annulus. The results of a recent evaluation study of this system were reported in 2005 by Sengupta and Mulholland, who indicated favorable results on the biomechanical properties of the fulcrum and ligament for future development of an applicable prototype.[95]

Other recently developed dynamic stabilization systems include the X STOP Interspinsous Process Decompression system (**Fig. 1–14**) (St. Francis Medical Technologies, Inc. Alameda, CA), Coflex (Paradign Spine, New York, NY) (**Fig. 1–15**), Tension Band system (**Fig. 1–16**), and the Abbott Spine Wallis Interspinous implant (Abbott Spine, Austin, TX).

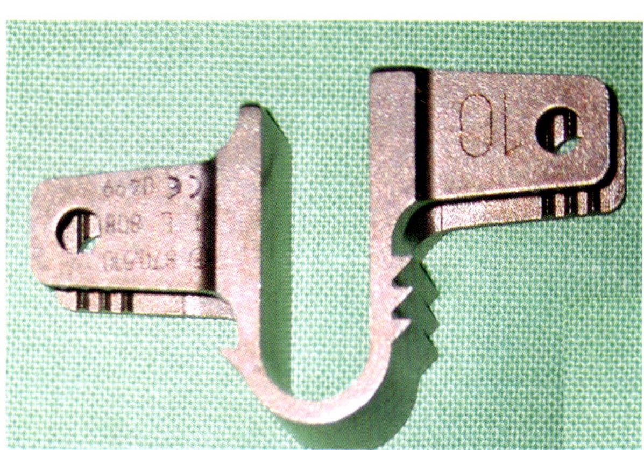
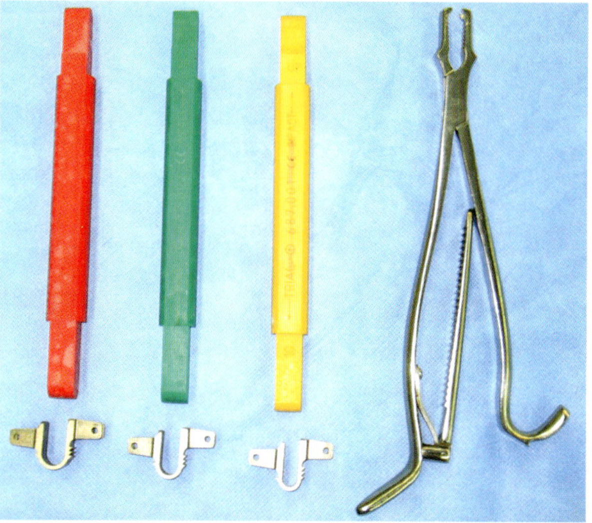

Figure 1–15 **(A)** The sagittal view of the Coflex. This device is designed to be placed between two adjacent spinous processes. Implant migration is prevented by the clamping of the lateral wings. **(B)** Sizes of Coflex and its template.

Pedicle Screw–Based Systems

The Graf ligament system (Neoligaments, Leeds, United Kingdom) consists of a nonelastic band as a ligament to connect pedicle screws across the segment to be stabilized, to lock the segment in full lordosis. An early study at the Centre for Spinal Studies and Surgery in Nottingham reported results in 1995 that indicated significant clinical success with outcomes similar to fusion.[84] Similarly, in a study between 1991 and 2001 that involved 41 patients, Markwalder et al reported favorable long-term results in a highly selected patient population.[97,98] Although numerous studies reported positive outcomes,[96,99–102] there were other studies that did not yield very impressive results.[103–106]

Similarly, the Dynesys Dynamic Stabilization System (DSS) (Zimmer Spine, Warsaw, IN) developed by Dubois is a nonfusion pedicle screw system for stabilization of the lumbar spine[86] (**Fig. 1–17**). The device was first implanted in Europe in 1994 and it has since been used to treat more than 9000 patients.[86] Although initial studies were encouraging,[86,107] some studies since then have reported lordosis and load-sharing problems with this system.[95,107,108] This device is

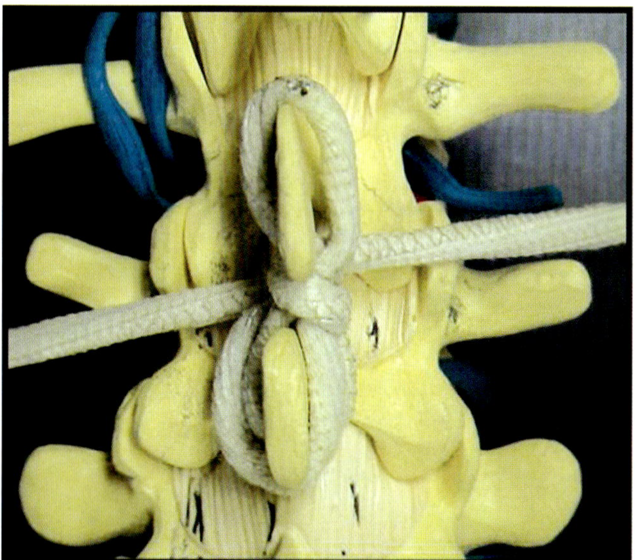
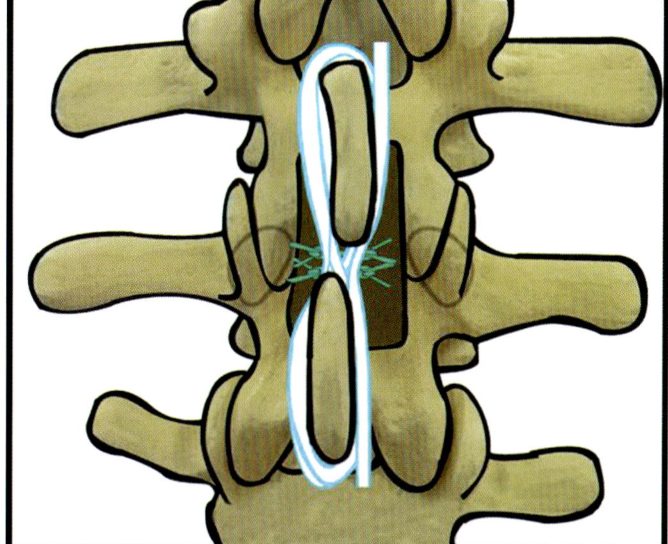

Figure 1–16 Tension Band System. **(A)** Both upper and lower spinous processes are surrounded with an artificial ligament as a figure 8 at the base of each spinous process. **(B)** The waist of the figure 8 is sutured several times at just inferior to the upper spinous process and just superior to the lower spinous process with traction of the artificial ligament. This multiple-sutured waist acts as an interspinous spacer.

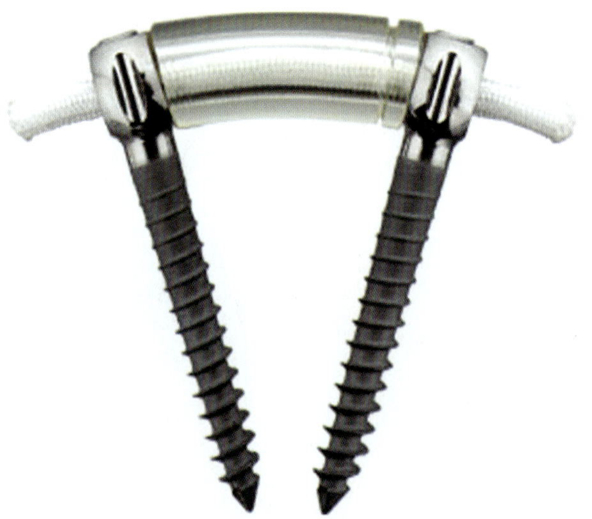

Figure 1–17   Functional model of Dynesys.

currently in the process of undergoing clinical trials in the United States.

The Leeds-Keio artificial ligament was designed as a non-rigid implant to stop movement in degenerative spondylolisthesis.[109,110] Mochida et al reported that this innovative method utilized fabric ligament, originally developed for reconstruction of the anterior cruciate ligament. Subsequent studies using this method indicated that nonrigid stabilization can produce equally good results as compared with fusion in patients with degenerative spondylolisthesis.[110,111]

Other recently developed dynamic stabilization systems include the Isobar TTL Semi-Rigid Spinal System (Scient'x USA, Maitland, FL) (**Fig. 1–18**) and DSS (**Fig. 1–19**).

Facet Replacement

Facet replacement devices, which are designed to replace degenerative facet joints with a prosthetic implant, are currently in the early stages of research and development. At the forefront of this new technology is the Total Facet Arthroplasty System (TFAS) (Archus Orthopedic, Redmond, WA). In March 2005, the TFAS received the CE Mark (See www.cemarking.net) to begin marketing in the European Union and received conditional IDE approval from the U.S. FDA to begin clinical trials. The first TFAS was successfully implanted in Europe in May 2005. Other device designs are currently under development by Facet Solutions (Logan, UT), Impliant (Netanya, Israel), and the Zyre by Quantum Orthopedics (Carlsbad, CA).

◆ Summary

Over the last half-century, understanding of the complexities and origins of spinal disorders and back pain has advanced remarkably. Alongside the influx of new knowledge, surgical approaches and devices have also continued to advance to now include spinal arthroplasty and dynamic stabilization, which represent a new era of treatment options. The continuing progression of new treatment approaches will depend upon the clinical outcomes of the continuing research studies and efforts by a multitude of researchers worldwide. Because the development of this new area of technology is still in its infancy, it may be a considerable amount of time before spinal fusion will no longer be considered the standard treatment method. In the interim, current research efforts to assess the efficacy of nonfusion approaches continue to gain momentum and generate interest as new technology unfolds in motion preservation.

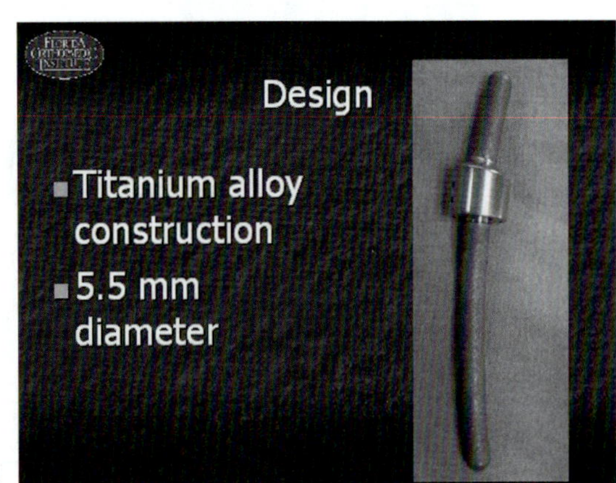

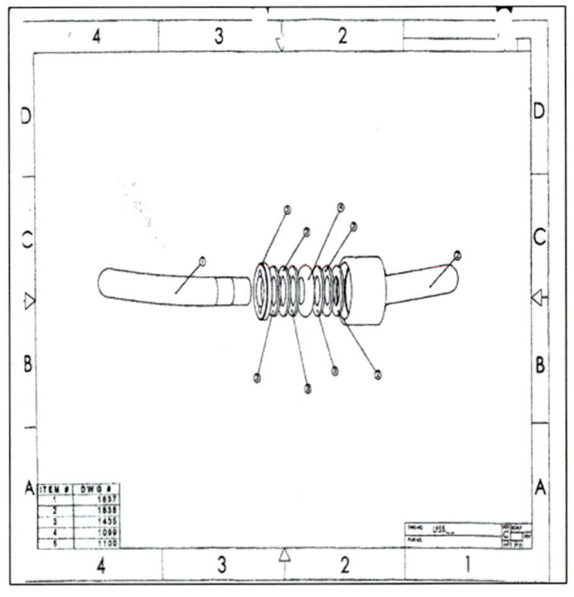

Figure 1–18   Produced from titanium alloy (Ti6Al4Va) by Scient'x USA (Scient'x USA, Maitland, FL), the Isobar TTL system consists of **(A)** a 5.5 mm diameter rod with **(B)** an integral dampener element.

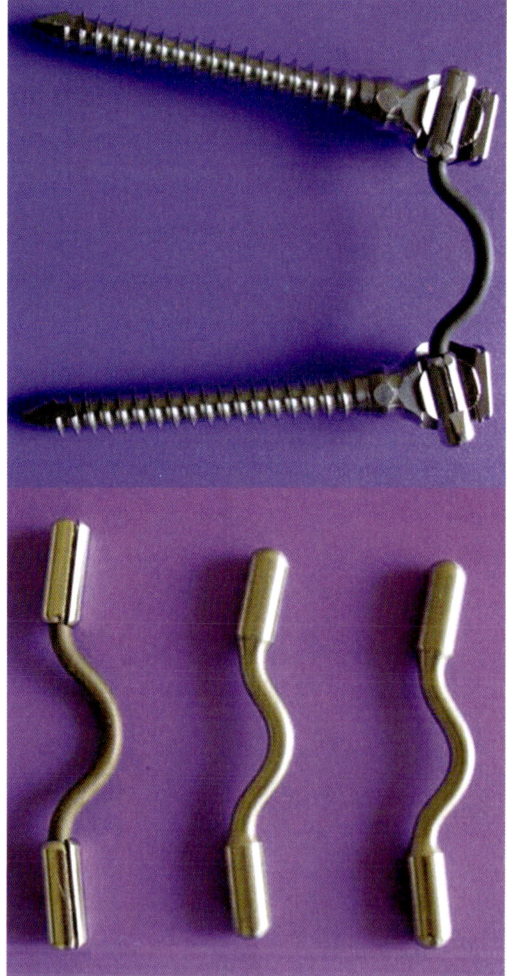

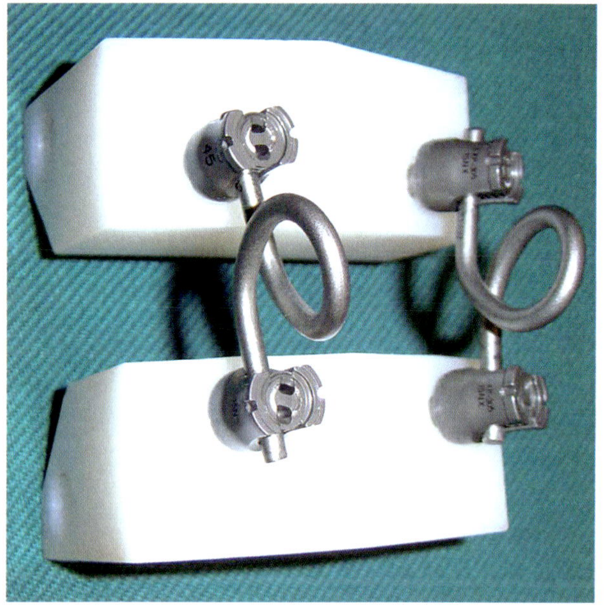

A   B

Figure 1–19   (A) The first generation Dynamic Stabilization System (DSS-I) was a C-shaped titanium spring, made of a 4 mm diameter spring grade titanium. The ends were thickened to 6 mm or fitted with a 6 mm diameter bushing for the ease of fixation to the regular pedicle screws, which can take a 6 mm rod. **(B)** The second-generation Dynamic Stabilization System (DSS-II) was an α-shaped titanium coil made of a 4 mm diameter spring-grade titanium.

References

1. Traynelis VC. Spinal arthroplasty. Neurosurg Focus 2002:13(2):E10

2. Bao QB, Yuan HA. Artificial disk technology. Neurosurg Focus 2000;(4):9

3. Le H, Thongtrangan I, Kim DH. Historical review of cervical arthroplasty. Neurosurg Focus 2004;17:E1

4. Administration USFD. Charite Artificial Disc (P040006) Approval Letter [DePuy Spine, Inc.], 2004. Available at: http://www.fda.gov/cdrh/pdf4/p040061.pdf. Accessed May 26, 2005

5. Bono CM, Garfin SR. History and evolution of disk replacement. Spine J 2004;4:145S–150S

6. Bao QB, Yuan HA. New technologies in spine: nucleus replacement. Spine 2002;27:1245–1247

7. Bao QB, McCullen GM, Higham PA, Dumbleton JH, Yuan HA. The artificial disk: theory, design and materials. Biomaterials 1996;17:1157–1167

8. Hamby WB, Glaser HT. Replacement of spinal intervertebral disks with locally polymerizing methyl methacrylate: experimental study of effects upon tissues and report of a small clinical series. J Neurosurg 1959;16:311–313

9. Nachemson A. Some mechanical properties of the lumbar intervertebral disks. Bull Hosp Joint Dis 1962;23:130–143

10. Fernström U. Arthroplasty with intercorporal endoprosthesis in herniated disk and in painful disk. Acta Chir Scand Suppl 1966;357:154–159

11. McKenzie AH. Steel ball arthroplasty of lumbar intervertebral disks: a preliminary report. J Bone Joint Surg Br 1972;54:S766

12. McKenzie AH. Fernström intervertebral disk arthroplasty: a long-term evaluation. Orthopedics International 1995;3B:313–324

13. Nachemson A. Challenge of the artificial disk. In: Weinstein J, ed. Clinical Efficacy and Outcome in the Diagnosis and Treatment of Low Back Pain. New York: Raven; 1992

14. Nachemson A. The lumbar spine: an orthopedic challenge. Spine 1976;1:59–71

15. Carl A, Ledet E, Yuan H, Sharan A. New developments in nucleus pulposus replacement technology. Spine J 2004;4:325S–329S

16. Urbaniak JR, Bright DS, Hopkins JE. Replacement of intervertebral disks in chimpanzees by silicone-Dacron implants: a preliminary report. J Biomed Mater Res 1973;7:165–186

17. Schneider PG, Oyen R. Surgical replacement of the intervertebral disk: first communication: replacement of lumbar disks with silicon-rubber: theoretical and experimental investigations [in German (author's transl)]. Z Orthop Ihre Grenzgeb 1974;112:1078–1086

18. Froning EC. Intervertebral disk prosthesis and instruments for locating same, United States Patent 3,875,595. April 8, 1975

19. Roy-Camille R, Saillant G, Lavaste F. Experimental study of lumbar disk replacement. Rev Chir Orthop Reparatrice Appar Mot 1978;64 (Suppl 2):106–107. French

20. Fassio B. French patent 2372622, 30–06. 1978

21. Fassio B, Ginestie JF. Discal prosthesis made of silicone: experimental study and first clinical cases. Nouv Press Med 1978;7(3):207

22. Horst M. Mechanical loading of the vertebral body cover plate (measurement of direct stress distribution at the interface between intervertebral disk and vertebral body). In: Junghanns H, ed. Die Wirbelsaule in Forschung und Praxis. Bd 95. Stuttgart: Hippokrates; 1982

23. Hou TS, Tu KY, Xu YK, et al. Lumbar intervertebral disk prosthesis: an experimental study. Chin Med J (Engl) 1991;104:381–386

24. Edeland HG. Suggestions for a total elasto-dynamic intervertebral disk prosthesis. Biomater Med Devices Artif Organs 1981;9:65–72

25. Kunze JD. Intervertebral disk prosthesis. United States patent 4,349,921. September 21, 1982

26. Ordway NR, Han ZH, Bao QB. Restoration of biomechanical function with the hydrogel intervertebral disk implant. Proceedings of the 21st Annual Meeting of the International Society of the Study of the Lumbar Spine. Seattle, WA, 1994:8

27. Ordway NR, Han ZH, Bao QB. Biomechanical evaluation for the intervertebral hydrogel nucleus. Proceedings of 9th Annual Meeting of the North American Spine Society. Minneapolis, MN, 1994:90–91

28. Ray CD. Prosthetic disk and method of implanting. United States patent 4,772,287. September 20, 1988

29. Ray CD. Prosthetic disk containing therapeutic material. United States patent 4.904,260. February 27, 1990

30. Ray CD, Corbin TP. Prosthetic disk containing therapeutic material. European patent 0353936, 07–02–1990. 1990

31. Ray CD, Sachs BL, Norton BK, Mikkelsen SM, Clausen N. Prosthetic disk nucleus implants: an update. In: Gunzburg R, Szpalski M, eds. Intervertebral Disc Herniation. Philadelphia: Lippincott Williams & Wilkins; 2002

32. Ray CD. The Raymedica Prosthetic Disc Nucleus (PDN®): stabilizing the degenerated lumbar vertebral segment without fusion or total disk replacement. In: Kim DH, Cammisa FP, Fessler RG, eds. Dynamic Reconstruction of the Spine. New York: Thieme; Forthcoming

33. Bertagnoli R, Schonmayr R. Surgical and clinical results with the PDN prosthetic disk-nucleus device. Eur Spine J 2002;11(Suppl 2):S143–S148

34. Klara PM, Ray CD. Artificial nucleus replacement: clinical experience. Spine 2002;27:1374–1377

35. Husson JL, Korge A, Polard JL, et al. A memory coiling spiral as nucleus pulposus prosthesis: concept, specifications, bench testing, and first clinical results. J Spinal Disord Tech 2003;16:405–411

36. Guyer RD, Ohnmeiss DD. Intervertebral disk prostheses. Spine 2003; 28:S15–S23

37. Viscogliosi AG, Viscogliosi MR, Viscogliosi JJ. Spine Arthroplasty. Spine Industry Analysis Series 2001

38. Ordway NR, Vamvani V, Zhao J, et al. Failure properties of the intervertebral disk with a hydrogel nucleus. The 44th Meeting of the Orthopaedic Research Society. New Orleans, LA, 1998:6:85

39. Ledet EH, Carl AL, Tymeson MP, Cohen B. Preliminary biomechanical evaluation of a synthetically engineered hydrogel for nucleus replacement. Proceedings of the 52nd Annual Meeting of the Congress of Neurologic Surgery. Scottsdale, AZ, 2002:314

40. Felt JC, Bourgeault CA, Baker MW. Articulating joint repair. United States patent 5888220. March 30, 1999

41. Fraser RD, Ross ER, Lowery GL, Freeman BJ, Dolan M. AcroFlex design and results. Spine J 2004;4:245S–251S

42. Steffee AD. Artificial spinal disk. European patent 0392076. October 17, 1990

43. Steffee AD. Artificial disk. United States patent 5071437. December 10, 1991

44. Steffee AD. The Steffee artificial disk. In: Weinstein JN, ed. Clinical Efficacy and Outcome in the Diagnosis and Treatment of Low Back Pain. New York: Raven; 1992

45. Enker P, Steffee A, McMillin C, et al. Artificial disk replacement: preliminary report with a 3-year minimum follow-up. Spine 1993;18:1061–1070

46. Serhan H, Kuras J, McMillin C, Persenaire M. Spinal disk prosthesis. World patent 99/20209. April 29, 1999

47. Fraser RD, Ross ER, Lowery GL, Steffe AD. Spinal disk. United States patent 6139579. October 31, 2000

48. Cunningham BW, Lowery GL, Serhan HA, et al. Total disk replacement arthroplasty using the AcroFlex lumbar disk: a non-human primate model. Eur Spine J 2002;11(Suppl 2):S115–S123

49. Büttner-Janz K, Hochschuler SH, McAfee PC. The Artificial Disc, 1st ed. Berlin: Springer-Verlag; 2003

50. Griffith SL, Shelokov AP, Buttner-Janz K, LeMaire JP, Zeegers WS. A multicenter retrospective study of the clinical results of the LINK SB Charite intervertebral prosthesis: the initial European experience. Spine 1994;19:1842–1849

51. Lemaire JP, Skalli W, Lavaste F, et al. Intervertebral disk prosthesis: results and prospects for the year 2000. Clin Orthop Relat Res 1997; 337:64–76

52. Cinotti G, David T, Postacchini F. Results of disk prosthesis after a minimum follow-up period of 2 years. Spine 1996;21:995–1000

53. Zeegers WS, Bohnen LM, Laaper M, Verhaegen MJ. Artificial disk replacement with the modular type SB Charite III: 2-year results in 50 prospectively studied patients. Eur Spine J 1999;8:210–217

54. McAfee PC, Fedder IL, Saiedy S, Shucosky EM, Cunningham BW. SB Charite disk replacement: report of 60 prospective randomized cases in a US center. J Spinal Disord Tech 2003;16:424–433

55. David T. Revision of a Charité Artificial Disk 9.5 years in vivo to a new Charité artificial disk: case report and explant analysis. Eur Spine J 2005

56. Buttner-Janz K, Schellnack K, Zippel H. Biomechanics of the SB Charité lumbar intervertebral disk endoprosthesis. Int Orthop 1989;13:173–176

57. Chedid KJ, Chedid MK. The "tract" of history in the treatment of lumbar degenerative disk disease. Neurosurg Focus 2004;16:E7

58. Marnay T. Prosthesis for Intervertebral Disks and Instruments for Implanting it. U.S. patent 5,314,477. May 24, 1994

59. Marnay T. Lumbar disk replacement: 7–10 year results with ProDisc. Eur Spine J 2002;11:S19

60. Mayer HM, Wiechert K, Korge A, Qose I. Minimally invasive total disk replacement: surgical technique and preliminary clinical results. Eur Spine J 2002;11(Suppl 2):S124–S130

61. Bertagnoli R, Kumar S. Indications for full prosthetic disk arthroplasty: a correlation of clinical outcome against a variety of indications. Eur Spine J 2002;11(Suppl 2):S131–S136

62. Zigler JE, Burd TA, Vialle EN, et al. Lumbar spine arthroplasty: early results using the ProDisc II: a prospective randomized trial of arthroplasty versus fusion. J Spinal Disord Tech 2003;16:352–361

63. LeHuec JC, Kiaer T, Friesem T, et al. Shock absorption in lumbar disk prosthesis: a preliminary mechanical study. J Spinal Disord Tech 2003;16:346–351

64. Mathews HH, Lehuec JC, Friesem T, Zdeblick T, Eisermann L. Design rationale and biomechanics of Maverick Total Disc arthroplasty with early clinical results. Spine J 2004;4:268S–275S

65. Valdevit A, Errico TJ. Design and evaluation of the FlexiCore metal-on-metal intervertebral disk prosthesis. Spine J 2004;4:276S–288S

66. Harmon PH. Anterior excision and vertebral body fusion operation for intervertebral disk syndromes of the lower lumbar spine: three- to five-year results in 244 cases. Clin Orthop Relat Res 1963;26:107–127

67. Reitz H, Joubert MJ. Intractable headache and cervico-brachialgia treated by complete replacement of cervical intervertebral disks with a metal prosthesis. S Afr Med J 1964;38:881–884

68. Cummins BH, Robertson JT, Gill SS. Surgical experience with an implanted artificial cervical joint. J Neurosurg 1998;88:943–948

69. Wigfield CC, Gill SS, Nelson RJ, Metcalf NH, Robertson JT. The new Frenchay artificial cervical joint: results from a two-year pilot study. Spine 2002;27:2446–2452

70. Porchet F, Metcalf NH. Clinical outcomes with the Prestige II cervical disk: preliminary results from a prospective randomized clinical trial. Neurosurg Focus 2004;17:E6

71. Pointillart V. Cervical disk prosthesis in humans: first failure. Spine 2001;26:E90–E92

72. Lafuente J, Casey AT, Petzold A, Brew S. The Bryan cervical disk prosthesis as an alternative to arthrodesis in the treatment of cervical spondylosis. J Bone Joint Surg Br 2005;87:508–512

73. Goffin J, Van Calenbergh F, van Loon J, et al. Intermediate follow-up after treatment of degenerative disk disease with the Bryan Cervical Disc Prosthesis: single-level and bi-level. Spine 2003;28:2673–2678

74. Goffin J, Casey A, Kehr P, et al. Preliminary clinical experience with the Bryan Cervical Disc Prosthesis. Neurosurgery 2002;51:840–845 discussion 845–847

75. Anderson PA, Sasso RC, Rouleau JP, Carlson CS, Goffin J. The Bryan Cervical Disc: wear properties and early clinical results. Spine J 2004;4:303S–309S

76. Goffin J, Komistek R, Malfouz H, Wong D, Macht D. In vivo kinematics of normal, degenerative, fused and disk-replaced cervical spines.

Annual Meeting of the American Academy of Orthopaedic Surgeons. New Orleans, PA, 2003

77. Duggal N, Pickett GE, Mitsis DK, Keller JL. Early clinical and biomechanical results following cervical arthroplasty. Neurosurg Focus 2004;17:E9

78. Anderson PA, Rouleau JP, Bryan VE, Carlson CS. Wear analysis of the Bryan Cervical Disc prosthesis. Spine 2003;28:S186–S194

79. Pimenta L, McAfee PC, Cappuccino A, Bellera FP, Link HD. Clinical experience with the new artificial cervical PCM (Cervitech) disk. Spine J 2004;4:315S–321S

80. Cunningham BW. Porous coated motion cervical disk replacement: a biomechanical, histomorphometric and biologic wear analysis in a caprine model. 18th Annual Meeting of the North American Spine Society, Total Disk Replacement Pre-Course. San Diego, CA, 2003

81. DiAngelo DJ, Foley KT, Morrow BR, et al. In vitro biomechanics of cervical disk arthroplasty with the ProDisc-C total disk implant. Neurosurg Focus 2004;17:E7

82. Bertagnoli R, Yue JJ, Pfeiffer F, et al. Early results after ProDisc-C cervical disk replacement. J Neurosurg Spine 2005;2:403–410

83. Link HD, McAfee PC, Pimenta L. Choosing a cervical disk replacement. Spine J 2004;4:294S–302S

84. Grevitt MP, Gardner AD, Spilsbury J, et al. The Graf stabilisation system: early results in 50 patients. Eur Spine J 1995;4:169–175 discussion 135

85. Freudiger S, Dubois G, Lorrain M. Dynamic neutralisation of the lumbar spine confirmed on a new lumbar spine simulator in vitro. Arch Orthop Trauma Surg 1999;119:127–132

86. Stoll TM, Dubois G, Schwarzenbach O. The dynamic neutralization system for the spine: a multi-center study of a novel non-fusion system. Eur Spine J 2002;11(Suppl 2):S170–S178

87. Senegas J. Mechanical supplementation by non-rigid fixation in degenerative intervertebral lumbar segments: the Wallis system. Eur Spine J 2002;11(Suppl 2):S164–S169

88. Senegas J. Surgery of the intervertebral ligaments, alternative to arthrodesis in the treatment of degenerative instabilities [in French]. Acta Orthop Belg 1991;57(Suppl 1):221–226

89. Senegas J, Etchevers JP, Baulny D, Grenier F. Widening of the lumbar vertebral canal as an alternative to laminectomy, in the treatment of lumbar stenosis. Fr J Orthop Surg 1988;2:93–99

90. Barbagallo G, et al. DIAM: a new soft intervertebral implant for low-back pain treatment. 12th European Congress of Neurosurgery (EANS). Lisbon, Portugal, 2003

91. Caserta S, La Maida GA, Misaggi B, et al. Elastic stabilization alone or combined with rigid fusion in spinal surgery: a biomechanical study and clinical experience based on 82 cases. Eur Spine J 2002;11 (Suppl 2):S192–S197

92. Schiavone AM, Pasquale G. The use of disk assistance prosthesis (DIAM) in degenerative lumbar pathology: indications, techniques, and results. Italian J Spinal Dis 2003;3:105–111

93. Phillips F, et al. Biomechanics of posterior dynamic stabilizing device (DIAM) after facetectomy and diskectomy. NASS 19th Annual Meeting. Chicago, IL, 2004

94. Guizzardi G, et al. The use of DIAM in the prevention of chronic low back pain in young patients operated on for large dimension lumbar disk herniation. 12th European Congress of Neurosurgery (EANS). Lisbon, Portugal, 2003

95. Sengupta DK, Mulholland RC. Fulcrum assisted soft stabilization system: a new concept in the surgical treatment of degenerative low back pain. Spine 2005;30:1019–1029 discussion 1030

96. Mulholland RC, Sengupta DK. Rationale, principles and experimental evaluation of the concept of soft stabilization. Eur Spine J 2002;11 (Suppl 2):S198–S205

97. Markwalder TM, Dubach R, Braun M. Soft system stabilization of the lumbar spine as an alternative surgical modality to lumbar arthrodesis in the facet syndrome: preliminary results. Acta Neurochir (Wien) 1995;134:1–4

98. Markwalder TM, Wenger M. Dynamic stabilization of lumbar motion segments by use of Graf's ligaments: results with an average follow-up of 7.4 years in 39 highly selected, consecutive patients. Acta Neurochir (Wien) 2003;145:209–214 discussion 214

99. Gardner A, Pande KC. Graf ligamentoplasty: a 7-year follow-up. Eur Spine J 2002;11(Suppl 2):S157–S163

100. Kanayama M, Hashimoto T, Shigenobu K, et al. Adjacent-segment morbidity after Graf ligamentoplasty compared with posterolateral lumbar fusion. J Neurosurg 2001;95:5–10

101. Brechbuhler D, Markwalder TM, Braun M. Surgical results after soft system stabilization of the lumbar spine in degenerative disk disease: long-term results. Acta Neurochir (Wien) 1998;140: 521–525

102. Hadlow SV, Fagan AB, Hillier TM, Fraser RD. The Graf ligamentoplasty procedure: comparison with posterolateral fusion in the management of low back pain. Spine 1998;23:1172–1179

103. Skinner I, Mather-Brown N, Hardcastle P. Comparative study of Graf stabilization and posterior fusion in the treatment of chronic symptomatic mechanically unstable low back syndrome. J Musculoskeletal Res 1998;2:89–100

104. Salanova C, Boulot J, Moreno P. Les resultats a moyen terme de 88 ligamemtoplasties selon Graf. Rachis 1997;9:299–303

105. Moon MS, Moon YW, Moon JL, Kim SS, Shim YS. Treatment of flexion instability of lumbar spine with Graf band. J Musculoskeletal Res 1999;3:49–63

106. Legaye J, De Cloedt P, Emery R. Supple intervertebral stabilization according to Graf: evaluation of its use and technical approach [in French]. Acta Orthop Belg 1994;60:393–401

107. Schmoelz W, Huber JF, Nydegger T, et al. Dynamic stabilization of the lumbar spine and its effects on adjacent segments: an in vitro experiment. J Spinal Disord Tech 2003;16:418–423

108. Grob D, Benini A, Junge A, Mannion AF. Clinical experience with the Dynesys semirigid fixation system for the lumbar spine: surgical and patient-oriented outcome in 50 cases after an average of 2 years. Spine 2005;30:324–331

109. Mochida J, Toh E, Suzuki K, Chiba M, Arima T. An innovative method using the Leeds-Keio artificial ligament in the unstable spine. Orthopedics 1997;20:17–23

110. Mochida J, Suzuki K, Chiba M. How to stabilize a single level lesion of degenerative lumbar spondylolisthesis. Clin Orthop Relat Res 1999;368:126–134

111. Suzuki K, Mochida J, Chiba M, Kikugawa H. Posterior stabilization of degenerative lumbar spondylolisthesis with a Leeds-Keio artificial ligament: a biomechanical analysis in a porcine vertebral model. Spine 1999;24:26–31

2

Current Concepts in Spinal Fusion versus Nonfusion

David H. Walker and Praveen V. Mummaneni

◆ **Decompression without Fusion—Cervical**

◆ **Decompression with Fusion—Cervical**

◆ **Decompression without Fusion—Lumbar**

◆ **Laminectomy versus Laminectomy with Noninstrumented Posterolateral Fusion**

◆ **Should Posterior Lumbar Fusions be Instrumented?**

◆ **Arthroplasty**
   Cervical Arthroplasty
   Lumbar Arthroplasty
   Dynamic Stabilization

◆ **Conclusion**

Cervical pathology can be treated effectively from both anterior and posterior approaches. Anterior cervical diskectomy has evolved to include interbody fusion. Plating technology, new interbody graft materials, and osteobiological materials have further advanced the anterior treatment of cervical disk disease. Posterior treatments are based upon either or both laminectomy and foraminotomy. The addition of lateral mass fusions helps prevent the complication of postlaminectomy kyphosis in patients at risk for this problem. The development of laminoplasty provides an alternative posterior technique that preserves cervical motion.

The treatment of lumbar pathology is historically based on laminectomy for decompression. Some authors propose the addition of posterolateral fusions to treat mechanical back pain and prevent progressive instability in patients with spondylolisthesis or degenerative disk disease. In the early 1990s, posterolateral fusion with pedicle screw fixation was popularized for the treatment of low back pain due to spondylosis and spondylolisthesis. Posterolateral fusion with pedicle screw fixation earned an excellent track record. Lumbar interbody fixation has emerged as another option for spinal fusion in cases of spondylosis or spondylolisthesis.

Arthroplasty and nonrigid fixation are also emerging as treatment options. Lumbar devices such as the Charité artificial lumbar disk (DePuy Spine, Raynham, MA) have already achieved U.S. Food and Drug Administration (FDA) approval while other products remain in development. Cervical devices are being actively developed and hold great promise for preserving cervical motion.

◆ Decompression without Fusion—Cervical

As recently as 1996, many authorities believed the majority of patients affected by nerve root or spinal cord compression secondary to cervical disk herniation or spondylosis were best served by anterior cervical diskectomy (ACD) alone.[1] However, problems with postoperative neck pain and instability prompted the addition of fusion to this procedure. Given current technology for anterior cervical plating and numerous alternatives for interbody spacers, ACD without fusion is rarely performed in the United States today.

Historically, laminectomy alone had been regarded as the standard posterior procedure for the treatment of multilevel cervical myelopathy in countries other than Japan. However, it fell into disfavor once sequelae such as segmental instability, kyphosis, perineural adhesions, and late neurological deterioration were recognized.[2] Studies indicated that adding fusion to laminectomy added only modest operative time and morbidity, potentially arrested spondylosis at the treated levels, and reduced the incidence of postkyphotic deformity[3] (**Fig. 2–1**). Cervical laminectomy and fusion utilizing lateral mass screws became popular, but its associated problems such as hardware failure, adjacent segment degeneration, and loss of range of motion led some to the utilization of laminoplasty.

Posterior cervical laminoplasty, first popularized in Japan due to the unusually high incidence of ossification of the posterior longitudinal ligament (OPLL), has many variations. The fundamental concept is the enlargement of the cervical canal without complete removal of the lamina while preserving cervical motion segments (**Figs. 2–2 and 2–3**).

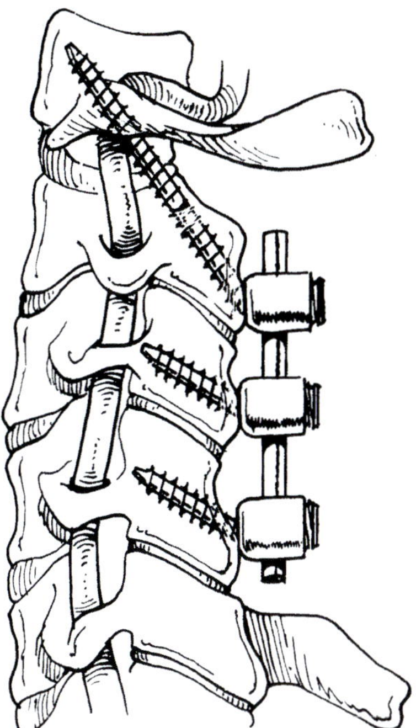

Figure 2–1 C2–C4 laminectomies with C1–C4 lateral mass fusion utilizing the Vertex Reconstruction System (Medtronic Sofamor Danek, Memphis, TN).

Proponents of laminoplasty believe the procedure preserves motion, reduces adjacent segment degeneration, and preserves the insertion points for the extensor muscles.[2] Studies comparing the results of patients with cervical spondylitic myelopathy treated with either laminectomy and fusion or laminoplasty have been performed. Heller et al[2] performed a retrospective analysis of laminectomy and fusion versus laminoplasty for the treatment of multilevel cervical

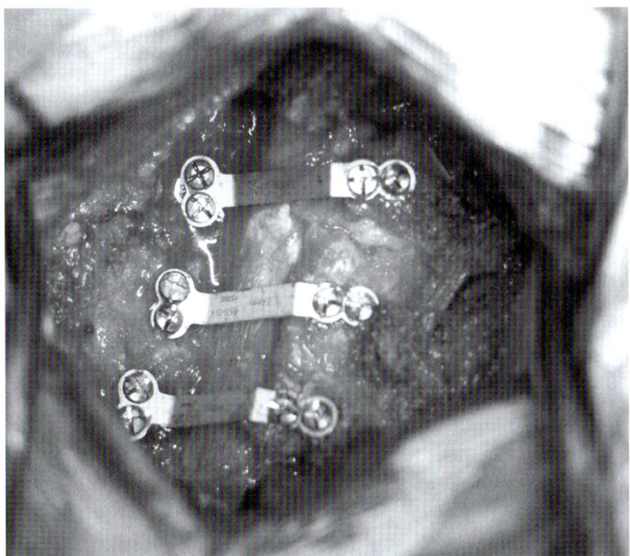

Figure 2–2 Intraoperative photograph of a laminoplasty utilizing the Centerpiece Plate Fixation System (Medtronic Sofamor Danek, Memphis, TN).

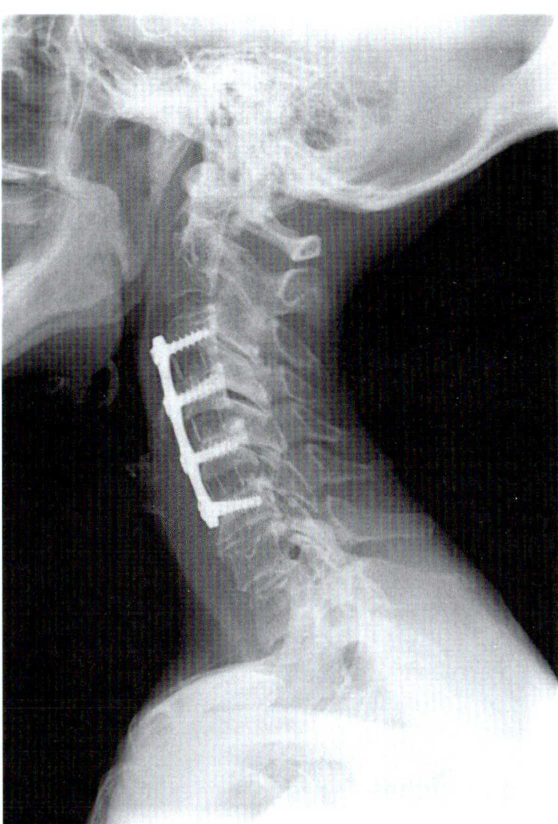

Figure 2–3 Lateral x-ray following a laminoplasty with the CenterPiece system (Medtronic Sofamor Danek, Memphis, TN).

myelopathy. Thirteen matched patients receiving either procedure were selected. Patients were matched by age, duration of symptoms, and Nurick grade. The authors concluded that patients receiving laminoplasty demonstrated greater improvements in Nurick scores with fewer operative complications.[2,4,5]

Posterior cervical foraminotomy is an option for decompression of foraminal nerve root compression. Open techniques were complicated by painful muscle-splitting incisions and prolonged recovery time secondary to muscle spasm. Minimally invasive techniques, including tube access and endoscopic technology, have opened the door to shorter recovery times and better patient tolerance. Fessler and Khoo reported on the use of microendoscopic foraminotomy (MEF) in 25 patients with cervical root compression from either foraminal stenosis or disk herniation. Twenty-six patients undergoing the standard open operation were used for a comparison. The MEF technique yielded patients with equivalent clinical results with less blood loss, shorter hospitalizations, and a much lower postoperative pain medication requirement.[6]

◆ Decompression with Fusion—Cervical

ACD with fusion (ACDF) was first described by Smith and Robinson[7] and also by Cloward[8] in the 1950s. The addition of fusion had reported benefits, including reduction of neural manipulation and neural injury, arrested spur formation or

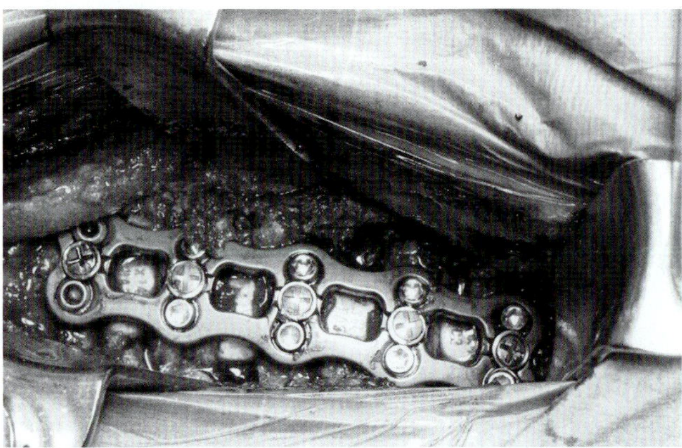

Figure 2–4   Intraoperative photograph of a multilevel anterior cervical diskectomy with fusion utilizing poly-ether-ether-ketone spacers and an ATLANTIS VISION Anterior Cervical Plate System (Medtronic Sofamor Danek, Memphis, TN).

resorption of spurs in response to fusion, reduced posterior compression as a result of unbuckling the ligamentum flavum and the posterior longitudinal ligament, and increased neuroforaminal height.[9] Initial attempts were performed without anterior plate fixation. Iliac crest autograft was usually placed as the interbody spacer. Although an excellent material to promote interbody fusion, it is associated with harvest site–related morbidity in up to 25% of patients. The potential for donor site infection and pain are limitations of its use.[10] Consequently, allograft eventually replaced iliac crest autograft as the most typical choice for an interbody spacer. When allograft is used for ACDF without

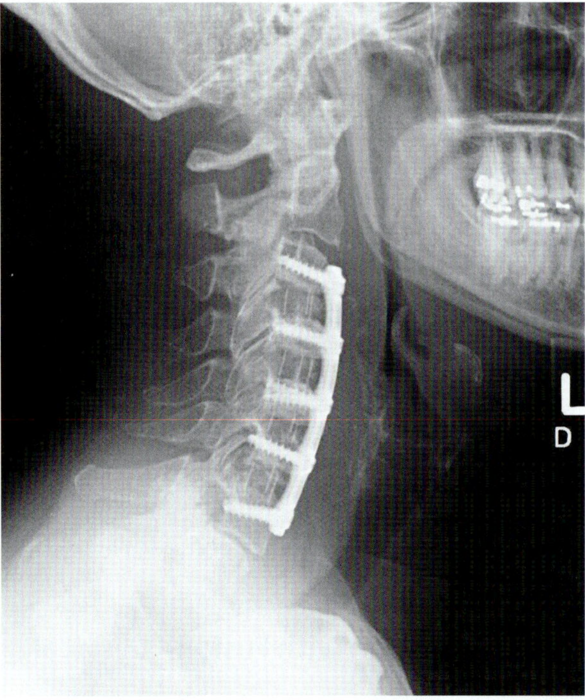

Figure 2–5   Lateral x-ray of a multilevel anterior cervical diskectomy with fusion utilizing poly-ether-ether-ketone spacers and an ATLANTIS VISION Anterior Cervical Plate System (Medtronic Sofamor Danek, Memphis, TN).

anterior plate fixation, successful fusion has been reported in 90% of single-level surgeries; however, in cases requiring two-level surgeries, the fusion rate decreases to 72% when allograft is used without supplemental plate fixation.[10] Anterior cervical plate fixation significantly improves the successful arthrodesis after single-level ACDF. A 96% fusion rate has been reported when allograft is combined with anterior cervical plate fixation. In cases requiring two-level surgery, a 91% fusion rate has been reported when allograft is used in conjunction with anterior plate fixation.[10] Drawbacks of some allograft interbody spacers include their limited supply, irregular dimensions, and the rare risk of transmitting infection (viral or bacterial). Recently, synthetic materials have been developed in an effort to overcome these limitations.

New synthetic spacers, such as poly-ether-ether-ketone (PEEK), are unlimited in supply, have regular dimensions, have similar modulus of elasticity to bone, are nonabsorbable, are radiolucent, and do not risk the transmission of infection from the donor (**Figs. 2–4** and **2–5**). When PEEK interbody spacers are combined with recombinant human bone morphogenetic protein-2 (rhBMP-2) and anterior cervical plate fixation, a 100% successful fusion rate has been reported for ACDF.[11]

◆ Decompression without Fusion—Lumbar

A study comparing surgical management (laminectomy alone) versus traditional conservative management was published by Matsunaga et al. They examined the natural history of patients with degenerative spondylolisthesis and lumbar stenosis for 10 to 18 years. Eighty-three percent of patients with neurological deficit or symptoms of neurogenic claudication refused nonsurgical treatment.[12] The issue of whether to fuse a patient during a lumbar spine procedure typically occurs in the setting of lumbar stenosis requiring multilevel laminectomy. Few would argue that a fusion procedure would not be indicated in patients undergoing single-level laminectomy/hemilaminectomy for stenosis or disk space pathology. Surgical decompression without fusion of patients with lumbar stenosis is certainly well established.

The permutations for the surgical treatment of lumbar stenosis with degenerative spondylolisthesis are many (laminectomy alone, laminectomy with posterolateral fusion, laminectomy with instrumented posterolateral fusion, transforaminal lumbar interbody fusion (TLIF), posterior lumbar interbody fusion (PLIF), anterior lumbar interbody fusion (ALIF), etc.) (**Figs. 2–6** and **2–7**). Studies examining laminectomy without fusion date back to 1976 when Cauchoix et al reported on 26 patients undergoing laminectomy with or without facetectomy.[13] Here, 25/26 - patients suffering from pain secondary to nerve root compression were immediately improved. Three of 26 patients required secondary fusion operations because of worsened listhesis. The authors stated that the only indications for accompanying fusion in the initial operation was associated low back pain in young and active patients. Lombardi et al examined three groups of patients: laminectomy with facetectomy (Group I), conservative laminectomy with preservation of the pars and facets (Group II), and laminectomy in conjunction with posterolateral fusion (Group III). Group I patients ($n = 6$) experienced good-excellent outcomes only

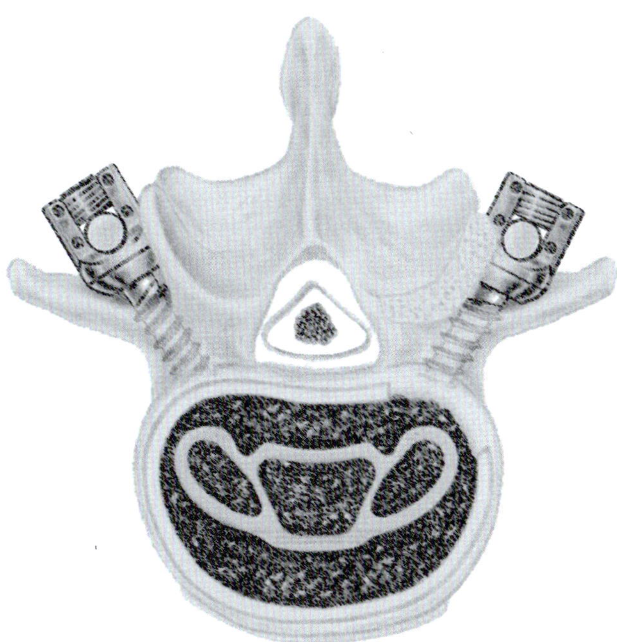

Figure 2–6 Illustration of an axial view of a transforaminal lumbar interbody fusion (TLIF) construct utilizing a poly-ether-ether-ketone boomerang cage (Medtronic Sofamor Danek, Memphis, TN).

33% of the time. Group II patients improved 80% of the time, and Group III improved 90% of the time.[14] Herron and Trippi examined 16 patients with degenerative lumbar spondylolisthesis who underwent laminectomy with partial facetectomy. The pars and facets were preserved. The average

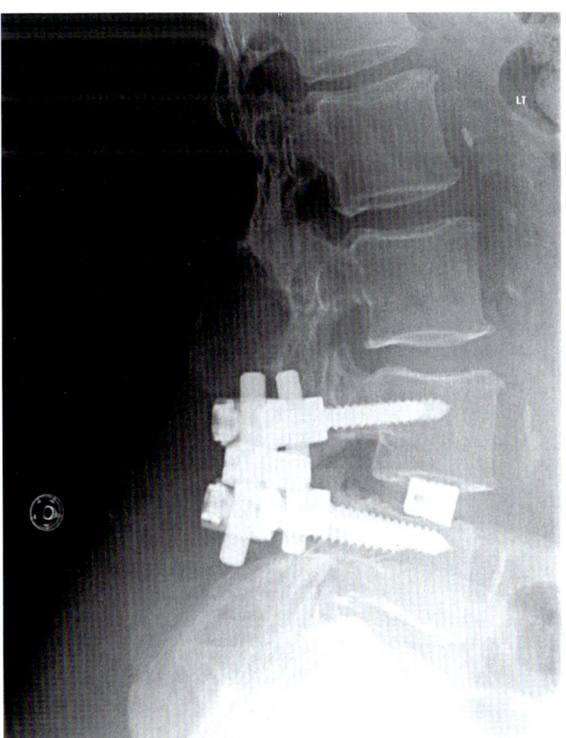

Figure 2–7 Lateral x-ray of a TLIF construct using DEVEX System titanium cage (DePuy Spine, Raynham, MA).

preoperative listhesis was 7 mm. No patient had greater than 2 mm of movement on flexion-extension views. The majority had satisfactory clinical results and none had a progression of listhesis of more than 4 mm.[15]

Poor results with laminectomy without fusion have also been documented. Dall and Rowe examined 17 patients who underwent laminectomy. Six patients underwent more aggressive facetectomies. Only nine of 17 patients experienced good results.[16] Johnson et al examined 20 patients who underwent laminectomy alone. Thirteen of 20 patients experienced progression of postoperative listhesis, and an improvement rate of only 52% was documented.[17]

◆ Laminectomy versus Laminectomy with Noninstrumented Posterolateral Fusion

As previously discussed Lombardi et al noted an 80% improvement in patients with pars/facet preserving laminectomy versus laminectomy and posterolateral fusion with a 90% good to excellent success rate. Patients were rated on a nonstandardized five-tier scale.[14] The most significant comparison of these two operative groups was published in 1991 by Herkowitz and Kurz. Fifty patients with degenerative lumbar spondylolisthesis were prospectively studied to compare the results of concomitant noninstrumented intertransverse fusion with laminectomy alone. A mean follow-up of 3 years was provided. Overall, patients who underwent arthrodesis experienced a superior clinical outcome (96% good to excellent vs 44%) based on degree of postoperative pain and degree of activity. Of note in this study, 36% of patients experienced a pseudarthrosis. All of those patients had a good to excellent outcome. The authors also noted that listhesis increased in 96% of patients without attempted fusion and 28% of patients with fusion. The age of the patient and the height of the disk space did not affect outcome. Poor clinical results were associated with progression of deformity. Increased motion in nonfused patients was associated with recurrent stenosis, back and leg pain, and mechanical instability. This study is class II evidence supporting the role of fusion in association with decompression for patients with degenerative spondylolisthesis.[18]

◆ Should Posterior Lumbar Fusions be Instrumented?

A thorough discussion of this question is certainly beyond the scope of this chapter, but several comparison studies examining the relative results of laminectomy alone, fusion without instrumentation, and instrumented fusions should be examined. One of the earliest such studies was produced by Bridwell et al. This study prospectively followed 43 patients suffering from degenerative spondylolisthesis with spinal stenosis who were placed into three treatment groups: (Group I) decompression without fusion—nine patients, (Group II) transverse process fusion with autogenous iliac crest bone graft without instrumentation—10 patients, (Group III) transverse process fusion with autogenous iliac crest bone graft with pedicle screw fixation—24 patients. They noted statistically significant progression of listhesis in Groups I and II. Higher fusion rates were reported in Group III relative to Group II. Overall, a higher proportion of patients reported clinical improvement without progressive listhesis relative to those in whom listhesis progressed.[19]

In 1997, Thomsen et al produced the Volvo Award Winner in Clinical Studies. This work examined 130 patients randomly allocated to decompression and either noninstrumented fusion or instrumented fusion. Fusion rates between the two groups, as judged by radiography, were not significantly different between the two groups. Utilizing the Dallas pain questionnaire, no significant difference in outcomes (with the exception of improved daily activities in the instrumented group) could be found between the two groups. They concluded that pedicle screw fixation increased operating room time, increased blood loss, and introduced the risk of nerve root injury without significant improvement in outcome relative to patients undergoing arthrodesis without instrumentation.[20]

Also in 1997, Katz et al produced a study comparing laminectomy alone to instrumented and noninstrumented fusion. A total of 272 patients suffering from degenerative spondylolisthesis were prospectively followed in a multicenter study involving eight surgeons. The patients were not randomized and surgeon preference, rather than objective or radiological findings, predicted the utilization of instrumentation. The placement of pedicle screw fixation was found to increase operative time, blood loss, nerve-root injury, and reoperation rate. No change in fusion rates was noted between the instrumented and noninstrumented groups. Functional outcomes improved with arthrodesis regardless of instrumentation. Relief in back pain was better in the noninstrumented group at 6 and 24 months with borderline statistical significance. Katz et al concluded that fusion was a benefit for patients suffering from stenosis with spondylolisthesis but did not believe the results justified the use of pedicle fixation techniques.[21]

In 1999, Mochida et al produced a study comparing noninstrumented laminectomy and fusion ($n = 35$), dynamic instrumented fusion (via technique of syndesmoplasty as described in their article) ($n = 33$), and rigid instrumentation ($n = 34$). Success rates between the three groups were 71%, 82%, and 91%, respectively. Fusion rates were 66%, 82%, and 91%, respectively. The role of dynamic instrumentation is unclear, though the use of rigid instrumentation does appear to significantly improve outcomes relative to noninstrumented fusions.[22]

Kimura et al proceeded to evaluate the utilization of instrumentation relative to preoperative segmental mobility in patients with single-level L4–L5 degenerative spondylolisthesis. Fifty-seven patients were retrospectively reviewed with a minimum of 2 years follow-up. Approximately half of the patients had not been instrumented (Group A) and half had undergone pedicle screw fixation (Group B) while undergoing intertransverse process fusion. Fusion rates were 82.8% versus 92.8% and satisfactory outcomes were 72.4% versus 82.1%. The authors concluded that the benefits of routine application of pedicle screw fixation were low. In patients with preoperative hypermobility (translation of > 3 mm, flexion angulation of 5 degrees, and a slip angle of ≤ 5 degrees) the slip angle tended to

increase after surgery. In these cases, the authors believed pedicle screw instrumentation may be indicated.[23]

In 2002, Christensen et al published a prospective, randomized trial that followed 129 patients with chronic low back pain for 5 years. Of those, 41 suffered from degenerative spondylolisthesis. All underwent surgery via posterior decompression with 20 of those patients receiving posterior pedicle screw instrumentation. Patients were evaluated with the Dallas pain scale questionnaire (DPQ) and the low back pain rating scale (LBPR). Patients allocated to the instrumentation group fared better statistically in the DPQ and LBPR.[24]

Upon review, the question of instrumentation has yet to be answered. With respect to fusion in general, the application of posterolateral fusions in patients with degenerative spondylolisthesis is certainly appropriate if not recommended. In the future, these discussions may become moot as technology advances and procedures providing for motion preservation begin appearing in operating rooms throughout the United States.

◆ Arthroplasty

In general, lumbar and cervical arthroplasty has widely varied applications and current points of development. Lumbar disk arthroplasty has progressed further in clinical development. Clinical trials for one device, the Charité (DePuy Spine), have progressed through the FDA's Investigational Device Exemption (IDE) to clinical availability. Clinical indications are limited. Cervical arthroplasty is not yet FDA approved but has wider applications and, perhaps, greater potential for use in the community setting. Cervical arthroplasty has, among its indications, radiculopathy. Also, surgeons performing cervical arthroplasty have significantly greater experience in the approach techniques relative to that of lumbar arthroplasty, which typically requires a vascular access surgeon. Revision surgery in the cervical spine is more familiar for the spine surgeon than anterior lumbar revision surgery.

Cervical Arthroplasty

ACDF is currently the gold standard treatment for herniated cervical disks. Arthrodesis, which was previously associated with fusion rates greater than 90% when allograft was combined with anterior cervical plate fixation, now approaches rates of 100% when the new synthetic materials such as PEEK and rhBMP-2 are used. The question arises: is cervical arthroplasty better than ACDF?

During the past decade, ACDF has been found to be associated with symptomatic adjacent-segment disease. Hilibrand et al reported that surgical intervention was necessary for 2.9% of patients annually because of symptomatic adjacent-segment disease following ACDF. Furthermore, they found that 10 years after ACDF, 25% of patients reported symptoms due to adjacent-segment disease.[25,26] In addition, Goffin et al reported that in 92% of fusion-treated patients radiographic evidence of adjacent segment degenerative disk disease was demonstrated 5 years postoperatively.[27] The cause of this adjacent-segment disease appears to be the abnormal kinematics (higher shear strains) that occur at levels adjacent to anterior cervical fusions.[10] Cervical disk arthroplasty, therefore, could be beneficial because adjacent-segment disease might be avoided by maintaining normal neck mobility.

Attempts at replacing a degenerated/herniated disk with an artificial cervical disk were made more than 10 years ago. Early designs of these implants were modeled on artificial joints (arthroplasties) implanted by orthopedists in the knees, hips, and shoulders.

Investigators in European and Australian clinical trials have demonstrated superior results when using the metal-on-metal and metal-on-polymer disks compared with ACDF; these results were based on neck disability index and arm pain intensity visual analog scale scores as well as neurological status.[10] Excessive metal debris, material fatigue with fracture, and catastrophic failure have not been shown to be problematic in the European trials, the results of which indicate that the advantages (motion maintenance and potential improved clinical outcome) of arthroplasty outweigh its disadvantages (wear debris, material fatigue, and joint failure).

In the United States, three artificial disks are undergoing prospective, randomized clinical trials in which outcomes are being compared with those demonstrated after cervical fusion. They include the Prestige CT Artificial Disc (Medtronic Sofamor Danek, Memphis, TN) (**Fig. 2–8**), Bryan Artificial Disc (Medtronic Sofamor Danek, Memphis, TN), and the ProDisc-C (Synthes, Inc., West Chester, PA). Based on the accrual of these class I data derived from comparing cervical arthroplasty with cervical interbody fusion, clinicians will be able to determine whether arthroplasty is equivalent or superior to arthrodesis.

Lumbar Arthroplasty

Current indications for lumbar disk arthroplasty are nonosteoporotic patients with one- or two-level symptomatic disk degeneration without severe facet arthropathy, segmental

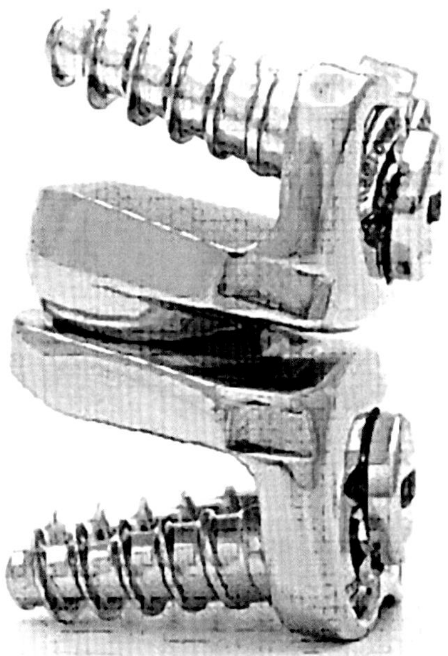

Figure 2–8 Photograph of a Prestige ST cervical arthroplasty (Medtronic Sofamor Danek, Memphis, TN).

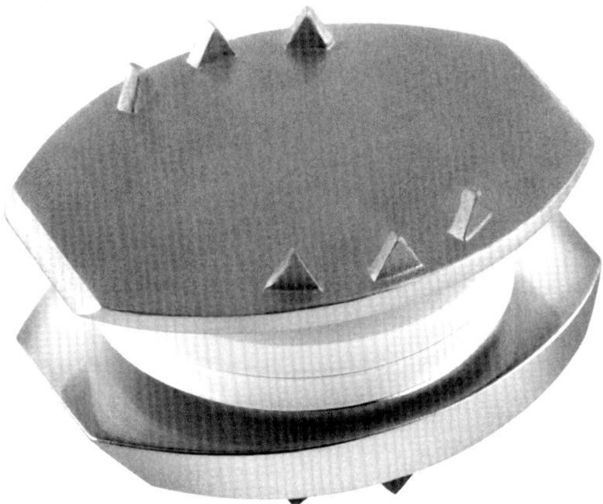

Figure 2–9 Photograph of a Charité lumbar arthroplasty (DePuy Spine, Raynham, MA).

instability, or neural element compression requiring posterior element decompression. In other words, one- or two-level diskogenic mechanical back pain primarily in the absence of radiculopathy. Devices being investigated include the Maverick (Medtronic Sofamor Danek, Memphis, TN) and ProDisc-C (Synthes, Inc., West Chester, PA). Only the Charité disk (DePuy Spine) has completed FDA trials and is currently available for implantation in the U.S. market (**Fig. 2–9**).

Dynamic Stabilization

Dynamic stabilization is a new frontier in lumbar surgery. Dynesys Dynamic Stabilization System (Zimmer Spine, Warsaw, IN) is a neutralization system for the spine consisting of a nonfusion pedicle screw stabilization system. This was developed in an attempt to overcome the inherent disadvantages of rigid instrumentation and fusion. Grob et al performed a retrospective study of 50 patients instrumented with the Dynesys system. Thirty-one patients had more than 2 years follow-up. The indications for surgery were degenerative disk disease with instability. Results indicate that both back and leg pain are, on average, still moderately high 2 years after instrumentation with the Dynesys system as determined by a visual analog pain scale. Only half of the patients declared that the operation had helped and had improved their quality of life; less than half reported improvements in functional capacity.[28] In contrast, Stoll et al conducted a prospective review of 83 consecutive patients for a variety of unstable segmental conditions. No specifics regarding length of follow-up were provided. The authors concluded that dynamic stabilization proved to be a safe and effective alternative in the treatment of unstable lumbar conditions as judged via visual analog pain scales and Oswestry disability scores.[29]

Other implants under development for the treatment of degenerative spinal disorders, without the creation of a segmental fusion, include the X-Stop device. Patients suffering from neurogenic claudication have traditionally been limited to decompressive laminectomy (with or without fusion) or a regimen of nonoperative therapies. The X STOP Interspinous Process Decompression system (St. Francis Medical Technologies, Inc., Alameda, CA), is an interspinous implant for patients whose symptoms are exacerbated in extension and relieved with flexion. This device has been available in Europe since June 2002. Zucherman et al report on a prospective randomized trial conducted at nine centers in the United States. One hundred patients received the implant and 91 underwent conservative therapy as a control. The authors concluded that X STOP offers significant improvement over nonoperative therapies at 1 year with a success rate comparable to published reports for decompressive laminectomy but with considerably lower morbidity.[30] Lee et al studied 10 elderly patients implanted with the X STOP device and examined them with postoperative magnetic resonance imaging. The cross-sectional area of the dural sack and intervertebral foramina increased by 22.3% and 36.5%, respectively. Seven of the patients were satisfied with the surgical outcome.[31] However, it should be noted that the X STOP may promote segmental lumbar kyphosis.

Prosthetic disk nucleus (PDN) replacement is yet another technology that is emerging. PDN was designed to treat patients suffering from disk herniation or degeneration. Clinical trials began in 1996 and involved implantation of two devices. Migration was the most prevalent complication in these patients. Jin et al subsequently conducted a study of 45 patients designed to test the clinical results of a single implant. Thirty patients were available for 6-month follow-up examinations. Independent analysis of patient data revealed that a "significant" proportion of patients experienced pain relief. Disk heights were improved by 19.7%. Device migration, failure, or dislocation were not noticed in any patient.[32]

◆ Conclusion

The number of treatments of cervical and lumbar spine pathologies has grown enormously over the past 20 years. Techniques of decompression have become more precise. Techniques of instrumentation have increased fusion rates. New bone graft substitutes have increased fusion rates and decreased iliac crest donor site pain. The dawning of the era of disk arthroplasty and dynamic stabilization raises new questions as to which techniques are most appropriate for the treatment of particular patients. These questions can be answered by applying outcomes-based research and evidence-based medicine.

References

1. Sonntag V. Is fusion necessary after anterior cervical diskectomy? Spine 1996;21:1111–1112

2. Heller JG, Edwards CC, Murakami H, Rodts GR. Laminoplasty versus laminectomy and fusion for multilevel cervical myelopathy. Spine 2001;26:1330–1336

3. Deutsch H, Haid RW, Rodts GE, Mummaneni PV. Postlaminectomy cervical deformity. Neurosurg Focus 2003;15:E5

4. Deutsch H, Mummaneni PV, Rodts GE, Haid RW. Posterior cervical laminoplasty using a new plating system. J Spinal Disord Tech 2004;17:317–320

5. Mummaneni P, Walker DH, Haid R, Rodts GR. Cervical myelopathy treated via stand alone instrumented laminoplasty without bone grafts: 26 prospectively followed patients. Oral presentation at the Annual Joint Section Meeting of Spine and Peripheral Nerves; March 16, 2005; Phoenix, AZ

6. Fessler RG, Khoo LT. Minimally invasive cervical microendoscopic foraminotomy: an initial clinical experience. Neurosurgery 2002; 51(Suppl 5):S37–S45

7. Smith GW, Robinson RA. The treatment of certain cervical-spine disorders by anterior removal of the intervertebral disk and interbody fusion. J Bone Joint Surg Am 1958;49:607–624

8. Cloward RB. The anterior approach for removal of ruptured cervical disks. J Neurosurg 1958;10:602–617

9. Klara P. Is fusion necessary after anterior cervical diskectomy? Spine 1996;21:1112–1113

10. Mummaneni P, Haid RW. The future in the care of the cervical spine: interbody fusion and arthroplasty. Invited submission from the Joint Section Meeting on Disorders of the Spine and Peripheral Nerves, March 2004. J Neurosurg Spine 2004;1:155–159

11. Boakye M, Mummaneni PV, Rodts GE, et al. Anterior cervical diskectomy and fusion using PEEK and BMP. Platform Presentation. Joint Section on Disorders of the Spine and Peripheral Nerves; San Diego, CA. 2004

12. Matsunaga S, Ijiri K, Hayashi K. Nonsurgically managed patients with degenerative spondylolisthesis: a 10- to 18-year follow-up study. J Neurosurg 2000;93(Suppl 2):194–198

13. Cauchoix J, Benoist M, Chassaing V. Degenerative spondylolisthesis. Clin Orthop Relat Res 1976;115:122–129

14. Lombardi JS, Wiltse LL, Reynolds J, Widell EH, Spencer C. Treatment of degenerative spondylolisthesis. Spine 1985;10:821–827

15. Herron ID, Trippi AC. L4-5 degenerative spondylolisthesis: the results of treatment by decompressive laminectomy without fusion. Spine 1989;12:534–538

16. Dall BE, Rowe DE. Degenerative spondylolisthesis: its surgical management. Spine 1985;10:668–672

17. Johnsson KE, Willner S, Johnsson K. Postoperative instability after decompression for lumbar spinal stenosis. Spine 1986;11:107–110

18. Herkowitz HN, Kurz LT. Degenerative lumbar spondylolisthesis with spinal stenosis: a prospective study comparing decompression with decompression and intertransverse process arthrodesis. J Bone Joint Surg Am 1991;73:802–808

19. Bridwell KH, Sedgewick TA, O'Brien MF, Lenke LG. The role of fusion and instrumentation in the treatment of degenerative spondylolisthesis with spinal stenosis. J Spinal Disord 1993;6:461–472

20. Thomsen K, Chrstensen F, Eiskjaer S, Hansen E. 1997 Volvo Award Winner in Clinical Studies: the effect of pedicle screw instrumentation on functional outcome and fusion rates in posterolateral lumbar spinal fusion: a prospective, randomized clinical study. Spine 1997;22: 2813–2822

21. Katz JN, Lipson SJ, Lew RA, et al. Lumbar laminectomy alone or with instrumented or noninstrumented arthrodesis in degenerative lumbar spinal stenosis: patient selection, costs, and surgical outcomes. Spine 1997;22:1123–1131

22. Mochida J, Suzuki K, Chiba M. How to stabilize a single level lesion of degenerative lumbar spondylolisthesis. Clin Orthop Relat Res 1999; 368:126–134

23. Kimura I, Shingu H, Murata M, Hashiguchi H. Lumbar posterolateral fusion alone or with transpedicular instrumentation in L4-5 degenerative spondylolisthesis. J Spinal Disord 2001;14:301–310

24. Christensen FB, Hansen ES, Laursen M, Thomsen K. Long-term functional outcome of pedicle screw instrumentation as a support for posterolateral spinal fusion. Spine 2002;27:1269–1277

25. Hilibrand AS, Carlson GD, Palumbo M, Jones PK, Bohlmann HH. Radiculopathy and myelopathy at segments adjacent to the site of a previous anterior cervical arthrodesis. J Bone Joint Surg Am 1999;81:519–528

26. Hilibrand AS, Yoo JU, Carlson GD, Bohlmann HH. The success of anterior cervical arthrodesis adjacent to a previous fusion. Spine 1997;22: 1574–1579

27. Goffin J, van Loon J, Van Calenbergh Flets. Long-term results after anterior cervical fusion and osteosynthetic stabilization for fractures and/or dislocations of the cervical spine. J Spinal Disord 1995;8: 499–508

28. Grob D, Benini A, Junge A, Mannion AF. Clinical experience with the Dynesys semirigid fixation system for the lumbar spine: surgical and patient-oriented outcome in 50 cases after an average of 2 years. Spine 2005;30:324–331

29. Stoll TM, Dubois G, Schwarzenbach O. The dynamic neutralization system for the spine: a multi-center study of a novel nonfusion system. Eur Spine J 2002;11(Suppl 2):S170–S178

30. Zucherman JF, Hsu KY, Hartjen CA, et al. A prospective randomized multi-center study for the treatment of lumbar spinal stenosis with the X STOP interspinous implant: 1-year results. Eur Spine J 2004;13: 22–31

31. Lee J, Hida K, Seki T, Iwasaki Y, Minoru A. An interspinous process distractor (X STOP) for lumbar spinal stenosis in elderly patients: preliminary experiences in 10 consecutive cases. J Spinal Disord Tech 2004;17:72–77

32. Jin D, Qu D, Zhao L, Chen J, Jiang J. Prosthetic disk nucleus (PDN) replacement for lumbar disk herniation: preliminary report with six months' follow-up. J Spinal Disord Tech 2003;16:331–337

Section II

Restoration of Cervical Motion Segment

3

Biomechanical Aspects Associated with Cervical Disk Arthroplasty

Denis J. DiAngelo and Christian M. Puttlitz

◆ **Design Rationale for Cervical Arthroplasty**

◆ **Peer-Reviewed Biomechanics Literature**

◆ **Conclusions**

Since its description in the 1950s by Cloward[1] and Robinson and Smith,[2] anterior cervical diskectomy and fusion (ACDF) has become an accepted treatment for cervical myelopathy and disk disease.[3] Clinical findings, however, have shown adverse effects of advanced degeneration at the spinal levels adjacent to fusion. The occurrence of adjacent segment degeneration with new, symptomatic radiculopathy varies between 2 and 3% of patients per year on a cumulative basis after ACDF.[4,5] An estimated 7 to 15% of patients ultimately require a secondary procedure at an adjacent level.[6,7] The increased stress placed on the adjacent segments, particularly the inferior disk, after successful ACDF may increase the rate of future symptomatic disk disease at those segments.[8–16]

More recently, spine surgeons have become interested in motion-sparing or motion-preserving spinal technologies as alternatives to fusion surgery. The goal of motion preservation is to design instrumentation or effective strategies that target the diseased intervertebral disk. These devices range from repair of local defects, such as annular tears, to complete replacement of the disk. Early clinical experience is growing; however, the biomechanics of cervical disk arthroplasty have not been fully delineated in the literature. This is mainly due to the fact that, although the literature (especially from Europe) is replete with early follow-up studies,[17–20] case reports,[21,22] survey articles,[23–26] and materials consideration with regard to disk arthroplasty designs,[27–29] there is a limited number of peer-reviewed publications on the biomechanical aspects of cervical disk replacement. This chapter provides an overview of the current research in disk arthroplasty biomechanics.

◆ Design Rationale for Cervical Arthroplasty

Cervical radiculopathy refers to pain or motor dysfunction caused by either or both mechanical deformation and inflammation of the nerve roots in the cervical spine. The etiology of radiculopathy can be diskogenic. When conservative management fails to alleviate the pain and neurological deficits caused by disk herniation, the patient is offered the option of surgical decompression of the affected nerves and spinal cord. Cervical decompression is most often accomplished via partial or complete removal of the diseased disk, providing immediate relief of pressure to the spinal cord and associated nerve roots, and treatment with an ACDF. Although ACDF has proven to be a very successful procedure,[3] fusion of a relatively mobile spinal segment is not an ideal reconstruction and can potentially lead to deleterious, long-term iatrogenic effects.

The goal of disk arthroplasty is to replace the diseased disk while preserving or restoring cervical disk motion at the operated level. The prosthesis is designed to act as an intervertebral body spacer that maintains disk space height and spinal decompression while theoretically reducing the likelihood of accelerated degeneration in adjacent disks through the preservation of normal disk kinematics at the affected disk level. It should also impart stability to the affected area that approximates what is normally seen in the native spine. Lastly, if the disk arthroplasty fails and leads to a painful pseudarthrosis, then the implantation of a disk arthroplasty device should not preclude or significantly complicate a subsequent fusion procedure.

Given that the primary aim of the cervical disk device is to maintain motion, it is important to review the ranges of "normal" or "physiological" motion that are typically present at the lower cervical (C4–C7) spinal levels. The most commonly cited source of spinal kinematic data is the classic text of White and Panjabi,[30] wherein ranges of motion for combined flexion-extension, one side lateral bending, and one side axial rotation are presented from compilations of many spine researchers. Representative values that fall in the middle of these ranges are also provided and are listed in **Table 3–1**. All three motion planes exhibit a relatively high degree of mobility at all three lower cervical levels. However, the large disparity that exists in the amount of motion afforded at each level across the general population further complicates the ability to target a specific motion for each arthroplasty design. This finding is evidenced by the large variations in ranges of sagittal, transverse, and frontal plane motions given in **Table 3–1**. Nevertheless, the goal of most disk arthroplasty designs is to approximate

Table 3–1   Native or Normal Range of Motion in the Lower Cervical Spine

Disk Level	Combined Flexion-Extension		Unilateral Lateral Bending		Unilateral Axial Rotation	
	Possible Range	Representative Value	Possible Range	Representative Value	Possible Range	Representative Value
C4–C5	13–29	20	0–16	11	1–12	7
C5–C6	13–29	20	0–16	8	2–12	7
C6–C7	6–26	17	0–17	7	2–10	6

The data indicate that the possible ranges are quite large, reflecting the significant variability across the population. (Data adapted from White and Panjabi.[30])

the normal spinal kinematics as closely as possible. The guiding rationale behind these designs is that preservation of motion offers a better clinical outcome than fusion.

Many designs have been advocated as replacements for cervical intervertebral disks that consist of either articulating or nonarticulating components constructed from various materials (**Table 3–2**). Most of these implants consist of metallic or polymeric components or both. A classification system was proposed by the Cervical Spine Study Group to better understand the similarities and differences among these design features[26] and is shown in **Fig. 3–1**. Some devices, by the nature of their geometric design, limit the amount of possible motion in certain planes or do not provide for coincident translation during rotation and are often referred to as constrained or semiconstrained. Other devices, commonly called unconstrained prostheses, rely on the perispinal soft tissue architecture and the inherent compression across the disk space to provide support and restrict the end limits of rotation and translation. The design rationale for many of these implants seeks not only to replicate the rotational kinematics of the cervical spine but also to mimic the physiological path of the center of rotation between adjacent spinal segments. Thus, based largely upon the geometry of the articulating surfaces, either a constrained design has the center of rotation fixed within the body of the implant or in the adjacent inferior or superior vertebral body, or a semiconstrained design provides a variable or changing axis of rotation but not necessarily the physiological instantaneous axis of rotation. Unfortunately, these design differences have had little impact on the overall acute kinematics, and, as discussed later, their effect on the loading mechanics of the spine remains poorly understood.

◆ Peer-Reviewed Biomechanics Literature

In response to the increasing interest in spine arthroplasty and the current concepts for disk prosthesis design, it is not surprising that the actual kinetic and biomechanical effects that cervical disk arthroplasty imparts on the spine have become more widely reported. The majority of biomechanical studies have used human cadaveric models to compare the spinal range of motion before and after implantation of the device. These studies evaluated several cervical arthroplasty disk designs that are widely available in Europe and that are undergoing investigational Food and Drug Administration (FDA) clinical trials in the United States. The following

Table 3–2   Design Parameters of Some Cervical Disk Implants

Device*	Prestige	Bryan§	ProDisc-C	CerviCore	Porous Coated Motion
Image					
Articulating materials	Metal–Metal	Metal–UHMWPE	Metal–UHMWPE	Metal–Metal	Metal–UHMWPE
Theoretical center of rotation location	Superior vertebra	Within implant	Inferior vertebra	Superior and inferior vertebra	Inferior vertebra
Initial fixation	Screws	Milled bone	Keels	Screws and spikes	Ridges

* CAUTION: Investigational devices limited by federal law (United States) to investigational use.
§ Bryan Cervical Disc System incorporates technology developed by Gary K. Michelson, MD.
UHMWPE, ultra high molecular weight polyethylene.

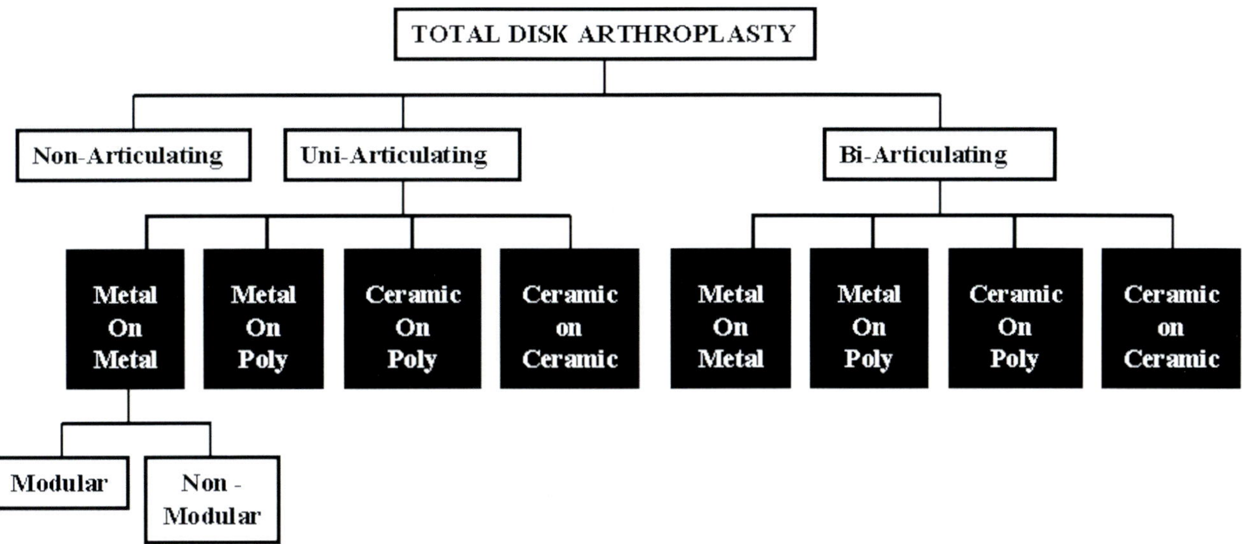

Figure 3–1   The Cervical Spine Study Group's artificial cervical nomenclature allows for classification of the different designs for cervical implants.[26]

gives a brief summary of the various studies that have been reported in peer-reviewed journals.

Two groups have reported on the biomechanical effects of implanting the ProDisc-C (Synthes Inc., West Chester, PA) device in the cervical intervertebral space. Briefly, the ProDisc-C is a semiconstrained device that uses an ultra high molecular weight polyethylene (UHMWPE) ball that articulates with a metal socket. The purported advantage of this semiconstrained device is that it will resist allowing excessive motion, thus imparting an inherent stability to the intervertebral space. Many argue that these types of devices effectively fix the center of rotation, which is commonly thought to change as one moves through the ranges of motion of the different rotational planes. DiAngelo et al investigated the motion-sparing ability of the ProDisc-C implant and compared it with the intact and single-level fused spine conditions in a human cadaveric model.[31] The spines were tested under displacement control in flexion, extension, lateral bending, and axial rotation.[32] Variations in the motion patterns were analyzed at an end limit of global (C2–T1) moment common to all spine conditions within the implanted and fused spine conditions by comparing the percent contribution of the rotation at the supe-

rior (S), operated (O), or inferior (I) motion segment units (MSUs) relative to overall rotation of those three MSUs (S + O + I). The instrumented and fused spine conditions were normalized to the harvested condition to account for intrinsic differences in tissue specimens and are shown in **Fig. 3–2** and listed in **Tables 3–3 and 3–4**. The only significant difference between the ProDisc-C and harvested (H) spines occurred in extension (57% of H), but not in combined flexion plus extension or any other individual or combined loading mode. However, fusion surgery caused a significant reduction in motion between both the harvested and the implanted spine conditions for all modes of loading.

Puttlitz et al used pure moment loading protocol, with and without a compressive follower load, to investigate how or whether the implantation of the ProDisc-C changed the kinetics of the spine.[33] They looked at both primary motions (flexion-extension, lateral bending, and axial rotation) and the coupled motion (motion in a plane that is secondary to the plane of loading) behavior of the spine. The data indicate that flexion-extension and axial rotation motion was not significantly altered after implantation of the device (**Fig. 3–3**). There was a significant difference in lateral bending motion

Table 3–3   Rotational Motion Data of Harvested, ProDisc-C, and Fused Spine Conditions

Rotational Plane	Harvested (Degrees)		ProDisc-C (Degrees)		Fusion (Degrees)	
	S + O + I	Operative	S + O + I	Operative	S + O + I	Operative
Flexion	17.79 ± 7.81	6.84 ± 4.20	21.99 ± 3.23	9.46 ± 1.99	17.85 ± 4.10	0.34 ± 0.30
Extension	14.56 ± 4.26	4.95 ± 1.30	18.92 ± 3.05	3.76 ± 1.90	11.50 ± 3.50	0.15 ± 0.13
Left lateral	13.55 ± 3.79	5.01 ± 2.30	14.16 ± 5.64	5.37 ± 3.20	10.77 ± 3.15	0.46 ± 0.42
Right lateral	9.90 ± 2.20	3.76 ± 1.48	13.99 ± 1.82	4.72 ± 2.91	9.16 ± 2.27	0.26 ± 0.27
Left axial	7.10 ± 1.93	3.88 ± 2.24	12.19 ± 6.16	5.78 ± 4.75	7.43 ± 2.70	0.95 ± 0.44
Right axial	9.22 ± 4.24	3.42 ± 1.06	14.02 ± 5.26	7.14 ± 4.48	8.95 ± 3.34	0.68 ± 0.37

S, superior; O, operated; I, inferior.

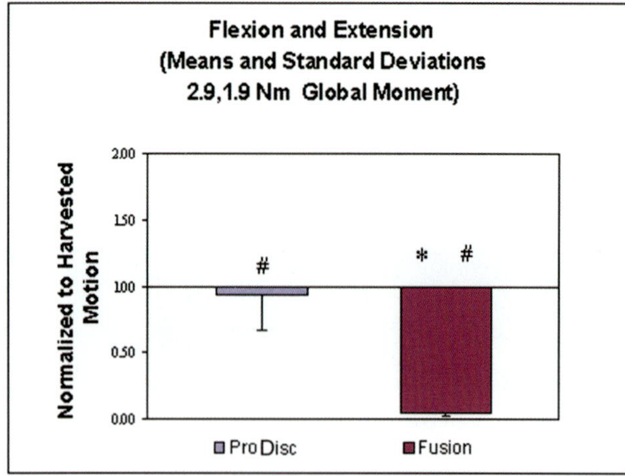

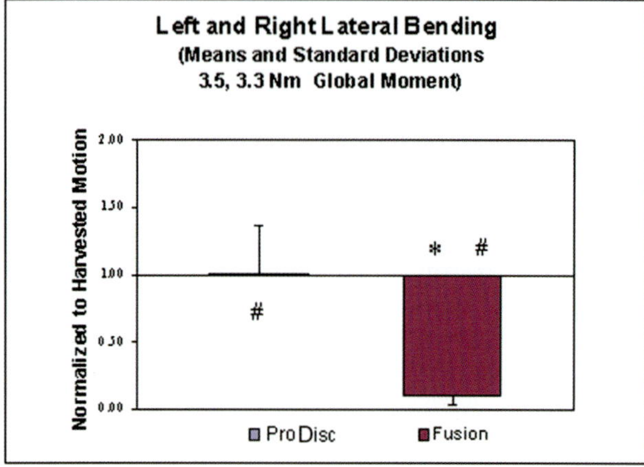

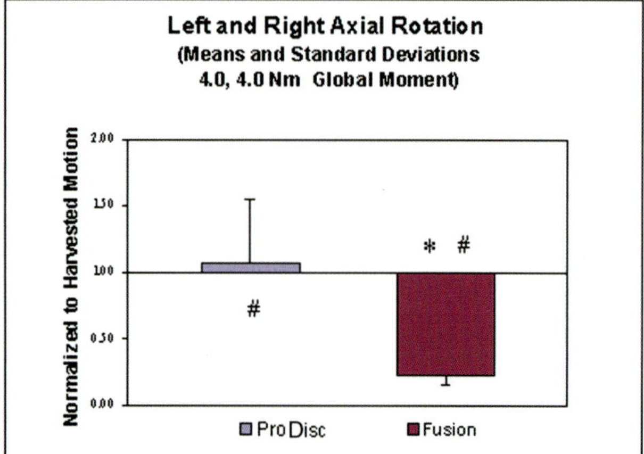

Figure 3–2 Motion segment unit rotations of the instrumented spines normalized to the harvested spine condition. *, significant difference with the harvested condition; #, significant difference between the ProDisc-C and fusion conditions.

without a compressive load; however, there was no difference in lateral bending motion before and after disk arthroplasty when a compressive load was applied. In addition, there were no significant differences in coupled motion at the affected level or at the levels above or below the level of implantation. Taken together, these two studies seem to indicate that motion obtained with the ProDisc-C device, at least in the immediate postoperative period, simulates the native motion of the spine.

Table 3–4 Rotational Motion of ProDisc-C and Fused Spines Normalized to Harvested Spine

Rotational Plane	Normalized ProDisc-C/ Harvested	Normalized Fusion/Harvested
Flexion	1.35 ± 0.51 #	0.05 ± 0.04 *#
Extension	0.57 ± 0.22 *#	0.04 ± 0.05 *#
Left lateral	1.05 ± 0.37 *#	0.13 ± 0.12 *#
Right lateral	0.92 ± 0.47 *#	0.07 ± 0.05 *#
Left axial	1.07 ± 0.88 *#	0.29 ± 0.15 *#
Right axial	1.26 ± 0.41 *#	0.24 ± 0.20 *#

*, significant difference with the harvested condition.
#, significant difference between the ProDisc-C and fusion conditions.

The Prestige Cervical Disc (Medtronic Sofamor Danek, Memphis, TN), formerly referred to as the Bristol disk, is a metal-on-metal ball and socket design with a trough in the anterior-posterior direction that allows for some translation in this direction during flexion and extension.[34] DiAngelo et al have also used a displacement protocol to investigate the kinematics of the Prestige device.[35] They reported that there were no significant differences between the intact and implanted conditions for flexion, extension, and right or left lateral bending before and after the device was installed (**Table 3–5**). In addition, the motions at the superior adjacent and subadjacent levels were not significantly different due to implantation of the device.

The Porous Coated Motion (PCM) (Cervitech Inc., Rockaway, NJ) device consists of two cobalt chrome end plates with a UHMWPE bearing surface attached to the caudal end plate. The articulating surface of the disk implant extends across the entire bearing surface providing a large radius of curvature for translational motion. The device is available in two variants: a "low profile" press-fit version for the majority of cases and a "fixed" adaptation with ventral screw fixation for cases with suboptimal carpentry or unusual loading conditions expected. The biomechanical performance of both devices after implantation were reported by McAfee et al in a cervical cadaveric study that used a pure moment loading protocol.[36] The data indicate that both the low profile and the fixed PCM were capable of restoring the acute motion profiles of the intact spine.

The previous studies are characteristic of the data that have been reported from biomechanical investigations of the cervical spine. However, other studies have started to use methodologies to discern the long-term performance of the devices. These tests were originally developed for total joint replacement (such as the hip and knee) and try to study other issues such as wear debris generation and osseointegration for long-term fixation. Anderson et al reported on a series of high cycle wear debris tests that they performed on the Bryan Cervical Disc (Medtronic Sofamor Danek, Memphis, TN).[37] The Bryan device contains two titanium end plates with a polyurethane core that allows for completely unconstrained motion. The wear testing was performed in bovine serum at 37°C and involved applying 130 N of compression coupled with repeated loadings of 4.9 degrees of flexion-extension and 3.8 degrees of axial rotation. The

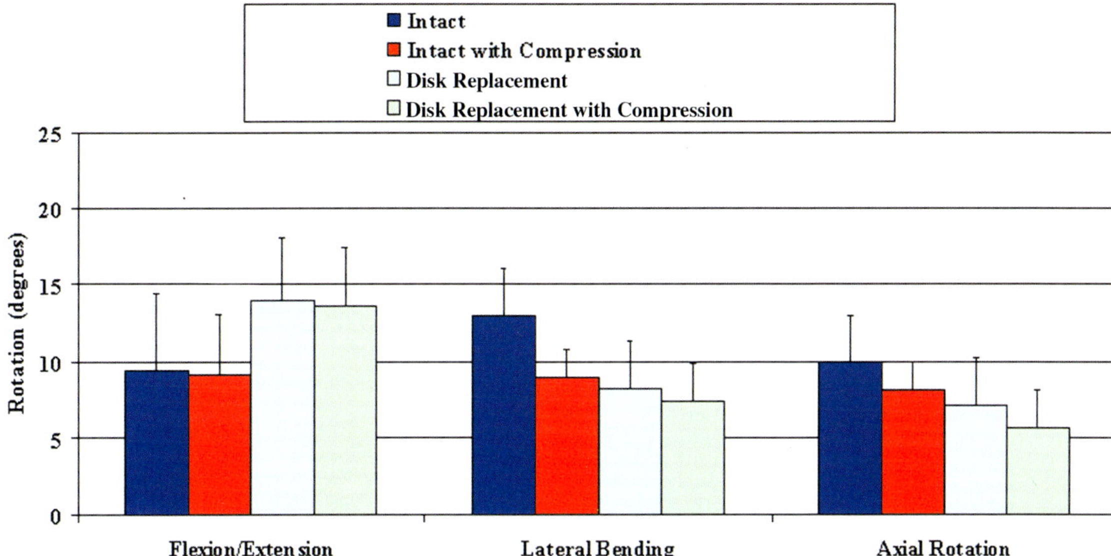

Figure 3–3 Kinetic analysis of the ProDisc-C prosthesis. The data indicate that implantation of the device replicates the intact condition, especially when a compressive follower load is applied. The only significant difference ($p < .05$.) detected in this study was between the intact condition and after disk replacement in lateral bending. This difference was not evident when the follower load was applied.

data indicate that there was a minimal height loss (0.75%) after 10 million cycles. Three test assemblies were allowed to run beyond these fatigue limits to 37.7, 39.7, and 40 million cycles. Such data provide an important insight as to the long-term survivorship of these implants.

◆ Conclusions

The advent of cervical intervertebral disk replacement represents an exciting and new frontier in the treatment of myelopathy and diskogenic pain. The ability to retain motion at the treated level while minimally affecting the motion patterns at adjacent spinal levels may represent an important step in reducing the incidence of adjacent segment disease. However, more comprehensive biome-

chanical data are needed before these arthroplasty devices are widely accepted and implanted. Although many of the disk arthroplasty implants are capable of maintaining acute motion within the three anatomical planes of movement, couple movements between these planes (i.e., axial rotation coupled with flexion-extension or lateral bending) have not been thoroughly investigated. To achieve this goal, researchers must further develop testing protocols that involve multibody, multiaxis control systems, as well as advance the current state of biomechanical testing systems to permit displacement, force, or hybrid (displacement with force feedback) control strategies.

There is also a significant vacuum of knowledge concerning how spinal loading is altered with these devices. We would caution the reader that just because the current motion data suggest that physiological kinematics/kinetics are maintained, this in no way implies that spinal loading is similarly restored. The native disk tissue is composed of a highly hydrated nucleus surrounded by a fiber-reinforced annulus. The mechanical behavior of these tissues is highly nonlinear and involves the use of fluid flow and hydrostatic support to counterbalance stresses that are seen during the activities of everyday living. The currently available arthroplasty disk designs in no way resemble the native disk from either a geometric or a material property standpoint. Intuitively, from an engineering perspective, one would expect the load transmission profile in the cervical spine to be altered after implantation of these devices. To better understand the effects of disk arthroplasty on cervical spine load mechanics, in vitro testing protocols involving force feedback control strategies for multibody spine models should be considered. Future studies using computational methods (such as the finite element technique or rigid-body dynamics analysis) to investigate and predict cervical spine load transmission will also greatly enhance the available knowledge base and facilitate the design of the next generation of disk arthroplasty designs.

Table 3–5 Kinematic Evaluation of the Prestige Cervical Prosthesis

		Recorded Moment	
Rotational Plane	Applied Global Rotation (degrees)	Intact Condition (Nm)	Bristol Prosthesis (Nm)
Flexion	22.5 ± 0.6	0.57 ± 0.25	0.47 ± 0.28
Extension	23.0 ± 0.2	1.22 ± 1.30	0.23 ± 0.22
Right lateral bending	13.5 ± 0.3	0.55 ± 0.51	0.56 ± 0.49
Left lateral bending	11.5 ± 0.2	0.74 ± 0.40	0.59 ± 0.37

Using a displacement control protocol, the investigators applied a predetermined amount of global rotation and recorded the subsequent moment needed to affect this rotation. There were no significant differences in the moment recording between the intact condition and the disk arthroplasty device.

References

1. Cloward R. The anterior approach for removal of ruptured cervical disks. J Neurol 1958;15:602–616

2. Robinson R, Smith G. Anterolateral cervical disk removal and interbody fusion for cervical disk syndrome. Bull John Hopkins Hosp 1955;96:223–224

3. Bohlman HH, Emery SE, Goodfellow DB, Jones PK. Robinson anterior cervical diskectomy and arthrodesis for cervical radiculopathy: long-term follow-up of one hundred and twenty-two patients. J Bone Joint Surg Am 1993;75:1298–1307

4. Grundy P, Nelson R. The Long-Term Outcome of Anterior Cervical Decompression and Fusion. London: British Cervical Spine Society; 1998

5. Hilibrand AS, Carlson GD, Palumbo MA, Jones PK, Bohlman HH. Radiculopathy and myelopathy at segments adjacent to the site of a previous anterior cervical arthrodesis. J Bone Joint Surg Am 1999;81:519–529

6. Baba H, Furusawa N, Imura S, Kawahara N, Tsuchiya H, Tomita K. Late radiographic findings after anterior cervical fusion for spondylotic myeloradiculopathy. Spine 1993;18:2167–2173

7. Clements DH, O'Leary PF. Anterior cervical diskectomy and fusion. Spine 1990;15:1023–1025

8. Cherubino P, Benazzo F, Borromeo U, Perle S. Degenerative arthritis of the adjacent spinal joints following anterior cervical fusion: clinicoradiologic and statistical correlation. Ital J Orthop Traumatol 1990;16:533–543

9. Cummins B, Robertson J, Gill S. Surgical experience with an implanted artificial cervical joint. J Neurosurg 1998;88:943–948

10. Eck JC, Humphreys SC, Lim TH, et al. Biomechanical study on the effect of cervical spine fusion on adjacent-level intradiskal pressure and segmental motion. Spine 2002;27:2431–2434

11. Goffin J, Geusens E, Vantomme N, et al. Long-term follow-up after interbody fusion of the cervical spine. J Spinal Disord 2004;17(2):79–85

12. Matsunaga S, Kabayama S, Yamamoto T, Yone K, Sakou T, Nakanishi K. Strain on intervertebral disks after anterior cervical decompression and fusion. Spine 1999;24:670–675

13. McAfee PC. The indications for lumbar and cervical disk replacement. Spine J 2004;4(Suppl 6):177S–181S

14. Pospiech J, Stolke D, Wilke HJ, Claes LE. Intradiskal pressure recording in the cervical spine. Neurosurgery 1999;44:379–384

15. Weinhoffer SL, Guyer RD, Herbert M, Griffith SL. Intradiskal pressure measurements above an instrumented fusion: a cadaveric study. Spine 1995;20:526–531

16. Wigfield C, Gill S, Nelson R, Langdon I, Metcalf N, Robertson J. Influence of an artificial cervical joint compared with fusion on adjacent-level motion in the treatment of degenerative cervical disease. J Neurosurg 2002;96(Suppl 1):17–21

17. Duggal N, Pickett GE, Mitsis DK, Keller JL. Early clinical and biomechanical results following cervical arthroplasty. Neurosurg Focus 2004;17:E9

18. Lafuente J, Casey AT, Petzold A, Brew S. The Bryan Cervical Disc prosthesis as an alternative to arthrodesis in the treatment of cervical spondylosis: 46 consecutive cases. J Bone Joint Surg Br 2005;87:508–512

19. Pickett GE, Mitsis DK, Sekhon LH, Sears WR, Duggal N. Effects of a cervical disk prosthesis on segmental and cervical spine alignment. Neurosurg Focus 2004;17:E5

20. Pimenta L, McAfee PC, Cappuccino A, Bellera FP, Link HD. Clinical experience with the new artificial cervical PCM (Cervitech) disk. Spine J 2004;4(Suppl 6):315S–321S

21. Sekhon LH. Two-level artificial disk placement for spondylotic cervical myelopathy. J Clin Neurosci 2004;11:412–415

22. Sekhon LH. Reversal of anterior cervical fusion with a cervical arthroplasty prosthesis. J Spinal Disord Tech 2005;18(Suppl):S125–S128

23. Albert TJ, Eichenbaum MD. Goals of cervical disk replacement. Spine J 2004;4(Suppl 6):S292–S293

24. Anderson PA, Rouleau JP. Intervertebral disk arthroplasty. Spine 2004;29:2779–2786

25. Le H, Thongtrangan I, Kim DH. Historical review of cervical arthroplasty. Neurosurg Focus 2004;17:E1

26. Mummaneni PV, Haid RW. The future in the care of the cervical spine: interbody fusion and arthroplasty. J Neurosurg Spine 2004;1:155–159

27. Oskouian RJ, Whitehill R, Samii A, Shaffrey ME, Johnson JP, Shaffrey CI. The future of spinal arthroplasty: a biomaterial perspective. Neurosurg Focus 2004;17:E2

28. Smith HE, Wimberley DW, Vaccaro AR. Cervical arthroplasty: material properties. Neurosurg Focus 2004;17:E3

29. Taksali S, Grauer JN, Vaccaro AR. Material considerations for intervertebral disk replacement implants. Spine J 2004;4(Suppl 6):231S–238S

30. White AA, Panjabi MM, eds. Clinical Biomechanics of the Spine. Philadelphia: JB Lippincott; 1990

31. DiAngelo DJ, Foley KT, Morrow BR, et al. In vitro biomechanics of cervical disk arthroplasty with the ProDisc-C total disk implant. Neurosurg Focus 2004;17:E7

32. DiAngelo DJ, Foley KT. An improved biomechanical testing protocol for evaluating spinal arthroplasty and motion preservation devices in a multilevel human cadaveric cervical model. Neurosurg Focus 2004;17:E4

33. Puttlitz CM, Rousseau MA, Xu Z, Hu S, Tay BK, Lotz JC. Intervertebral disk replacement maintains cervical spine kinetics. Spine 2004;29:2809–2814

34. Traynelis VC. The Prestige cervical disk replacement. Spine J 2004;4(Suppl 6):310S–314S

35. DiAngelo DJ, Robertson JT, Metcalf NH, McVay BJ, Davis RC. Biomechanical testing of an artificial cervical joint and an anterior cervical plate. J Spinal Disord Tech 2003;16:314–323

36. McAfee PC, Cunningham B, Dmitriev A, et al. Cervical disk replacement—porous coated motion prosthesis: a comparative biomechanical analysis showing the key role of the posterior longitudinal ligament. Spine 2003;28:S176–S185

37. Anderson PA, Sasso RC, Rouleau JP, Carlson CS, Goffin J. The Bryan Cervical Disc: wear properties and early clinical results. Spine J 2004;4(Suppl 6):303S–309S

4

Biomechanical Testing Protocol for Evaluating Cervical Disk Arthroplasty

Denis J. DiAngelo and Kevin T. Foley

◆ **Tissue-Based Biomechanical Studies**

◆ **Cervical Spine Mechanics**

◆ **Review of Biomechanical Testing Systems**

◆ **Improved Testing Protocol**
   End Mounting Configurations
   Specimen Preparation and Spine Conditions
   Nondestructive Testing Criteria

◆ **Results**
   Pinned-Pinned and Pinned-Fixed Mounting Conditions
   Modified TPF Mounting Condition

◆ **Discussion**
   Displacement versus Load Control

◆ **Conclusion**

◆ **Sources of Support**

◆ Tissue-Based Biomechanical Studies

Information used to assess the performance of spinal instrumentation or surgical techniques can come from mechanical or fatigue tests, computational studies, animal studies, in vitro studies, and clinical trials. With regard to in vitro studies, biomechanical testing on human cadaveric tissue offers a practical means for evaluating and ranking different surgical instrumentation and techniques. However, there are currently no standard tissue-based testing protocols for evaluating spinal devices. Although a variety of different testing methods have been used to study cervical spine mechanics, most testing protocols were developed to study fusion instrumentation and may not be suitable for disk arthroplasty. The most suitable method for evaluating these mobile spinal devices in vitro remains unclear.[1–4] Additionally, the different basic control strategies that have been used with the two most common methods are load control and displacement control.[2] Under load control, a pure or constant moment is typically applied to the spine in one plane of motion at a time (i.e., sagittal, frontal, or transverse). Under displacement control, the translational and rotation motions of the vertebrae are controlled.

◆ Cervical Spine Mechanics

The cervical spine consists of a series of free vertebral bodies that exhibit complex, coupled motions and loading behaviors.[5] For in vitro testing, the spinal bodies must be analyzed based on the motion/load conditions that are prescribed and applied by the testing device. The motions of interior spinal bodies not in direct contact with the testing device are measured but cannot be controlled. For the subaxial cervical spine, in vivo motion is greatest in the sagittal plane, with more rotation occurring in extension than in flexion.[5] Only small amounts of muscle activity are needed to maintain the head's orientation in an erect neutral position. Thus muscle-induced compression is small, and head weight is the typical physiological force that acts on the cervical spine. Flexion or extension of the head induces a bending-moment distribution throughout the cervical spine that increases caudally and acts in combination with the compressive (head weight) force (**Fig. 4–1**). In vitro testing methods should replicate this bending moment distribution. This chapter reviews different methods for testing the cervical spine in vitro in an attempt to identify the appropriate loading conditions that would replicate the in vivo motion response, and to help determine the most suitable method for evaluating disk arthroplasty or motion preservation devices in vitro.

◆ Review of Biomechanical Testing Systems

Simple mechanical devices continue to be used that incrementally apply pure static moments to the spine.[6] More commonly, however, programmable testing systems are used. Smith et al[7] used a material testing system (MTS) machine to study spine mechanics; the mounted specimen was highly constrained (no motion was permitted above or below the area of interest) and did not replicate physiological

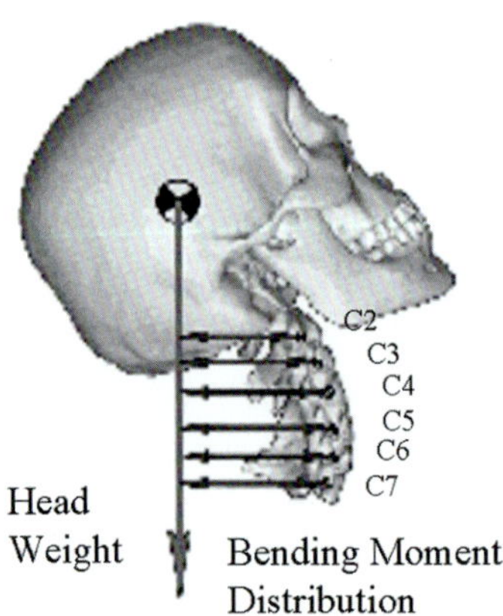

Figure 4–1 In vivo sagittal motion and mechanics of the cervical spine. This illustration depicts the caudally increasing bending moment distribution in the cervical spine (2–5 Nm), greatest at the C5–C6 level, created by continuous rotations with like polarity at each vertebral level (40 degree flexion or extension) with an axial compressive load (50 N head weight).[3,16,20,28]

motion or loading conditions. Owing to the relatively few degrees of freedom available with standard materials testing machines, custom fixtures must often be added to permit suitable movements, which often remain limited to simple scenarios (i.e., tension-compression, pure torsion, four-point bending).

Weinhoffer et al[8] added a slotted plate fixture to an MTS actuator to enable spinal rotation with nonvertical transla-tion. As the actuator moved down, the upper pot attachment was free to rotate but was constrained to follow a slotted path. The orientation of the slot imposed a specific horizon-tal versus vertical translational relationship of the upper spinal body that, in turn, was nonphysiological. Kunz et al[9] modified a 2 degree of freedom (DOF) MTS machine by adding a third rotational DOF to the base of the device. The device was used for pure moment testing with or without an axial compressive load.

James et al[10] presented a 2 DOF spine tester that regulated axial rotation with either flexion-extension or lateral bending.

Independent control of each motor prevented force feedback or force limit control features. Shea et al[11] developed a 3 DOF testing apparatus for planar analysis of spine biomechanics that provided independent control of the displacement output of each axis, but no force feedback control schemes were provided.

Wilke et al[4] developed a spine tester that applied pure moments to the superior end of a spinal construct in three orthogonal directions through the use of counterbalanced stepper motor units attached to the superior end of a spinal construct. The testing protocol was limited to pure-moment loads only. More recently, Gilbertson et al[3] employed robotics technology to study single motion segment unit (MSU) lumbar spine mechanics. Extensive modifications to the manipulator itself (at significant expense) were required and in the end the test system was limited to quasi-static analysis or pure-moment load control schemes.

◆ Improved Testing Protocol

An improved testing protocol has been developed that used a programmable single actuator biomechanical testing apparatus.[12–14] The rigid frame housed a servo driven load actuator (Industrial Device Corp., Novato, CA) commanded by a robotic controller (Adept Inc., San Jose, CA). A single-axis load cell (Transducer Technologies, Temecula, CA) was in line with the shaft of the load actuator. The other end of the load cell was coupled to end mounting fixtures that regulated the end motion and loads applied to the spinal construct. The opposing end of the construct was coupled to a six-axis force sensor (JR3 Inc., Woodland, CA), which was in turn rigidly fixed to the base of the test frame. The multiaxis load cell reported the three orthogonal forces and moments transferred through the spine in real time. With this modified approach, displacement of the spine was con-trolled and a "bending moment distribution" was induced throughout the spine via custom fixturing hardware. Other parameters were monitored to establish the upper motion limit and the total applied moments and end loads. By assigning a limit value to each parameter, the test was stopped if any limit checks were exceeded. This arrange-ment is vastly different from and superior to pure-moment methods where there is no limit check on the resultant

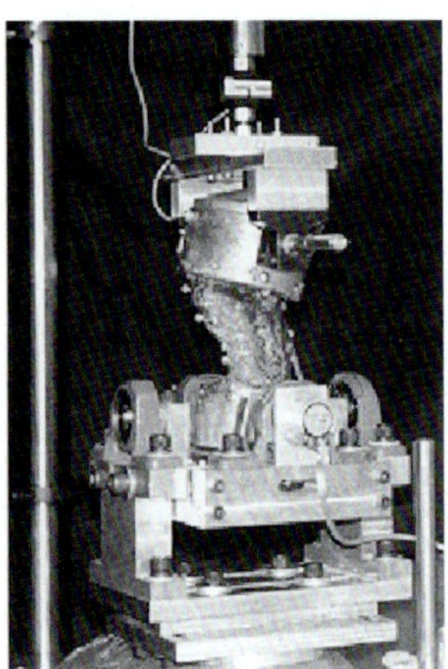

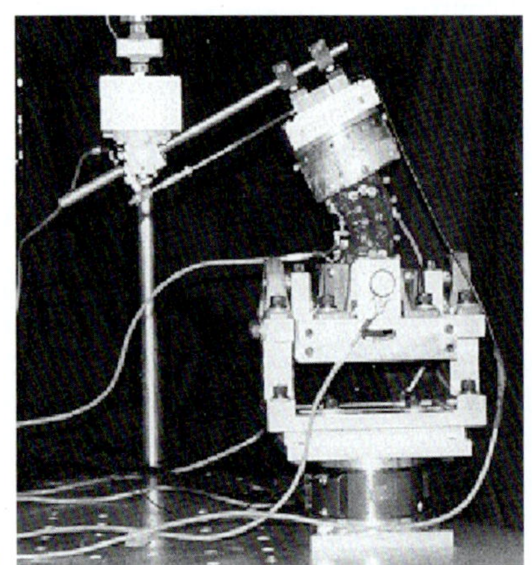

Figure 4–2 End mounting configurations. **(A)** The pinned-pinned or pinned-fixed configuration and **(B)** translational/pinned-fix configurations.

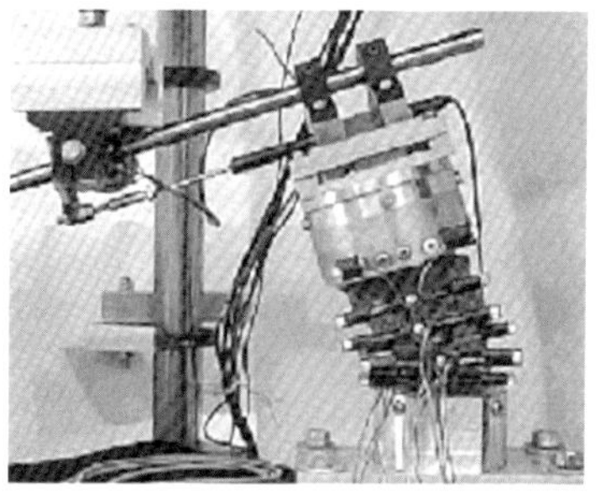

A

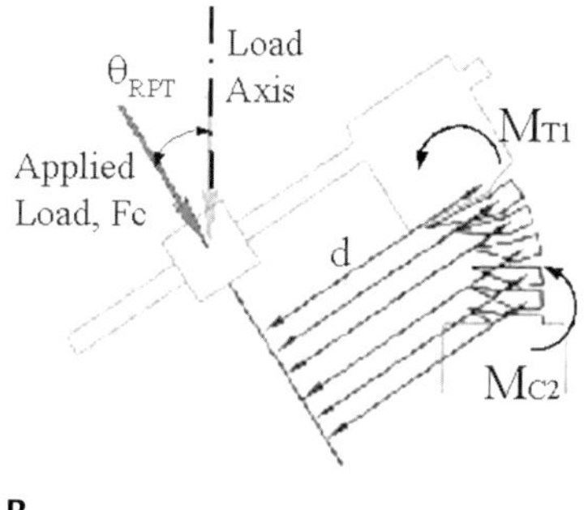

B

Figure 4–3 **(A)** Photograph of a subaxial cervical spine mounted in the testing apparatus. **(B)** Schematic of mounted specimen. With the flexion-extension axis of the spine placed eccentric to the load axis of the actuator, a compressive load (Fc) and flexion-extension bending moment ($M_{f/e}$, where $M_{f/e} = F_c {}^* d$) were induced.

global motion. Further, cervical spine studies using pure-moment protocols typically use moment values in the range of 1 to 2 Nm. However, when analyzing cervical spine instrumentation, this load level may not be sufficient to induce measurable differences in the motion response. This modified testing system was used to simulate the different end mounting configurations.

End Mounting Configurations

A sequence of tests was performed to analyze different end mounting configurations and appropriate ranges of load and motion to identify a particular set of end conditions that reproduced normal motion of the multibody spine.[13] The gold standard of motion was replication of positions considered normal by anatomists, physical therapists, and spine surgeons. Three different mounting configurations were evaluated: pinned-pinned (PP), pinned-fixed (PF), and translational/pinned-fixed (TPF) (**Fig. 4–2**). In the first test condition, the lower mounting fixtures were unclamped and free to rotate, whereas in the second condition they remained fixed. The upper mounting fixtures converted the single-controlled linear input from the load actuator to either a rotational motion or pure bending moment input alone (PP and PF condition), or to a coupled motion input (unconstrained translations and/or rotation in the sagittal plane) with a combined loading state of axial compressive force alone or with a flexion-extension bending moment (TPF configuration).

For the TPF case, the upper fixturing hardware consisted of a linear bearing and splined shaft assembly that mounted in a rotating joint attached to the actuator (**Fig. 4–3**). The linear bearing provided a virtually frictionless method for the splined shaft to move relative to the actuator, effectively eliminating the shearing forces. The flexion-extension axis of the spine was placed eccentric to the load axis of the actuator and induced a compressive load (Fc) and flexion-extension bending moment to the upper pot (M_{T1}). The specimens were mounted in an inverted neutral orientation with the T1 pot attached to the upper fixture and the C2 pot mounted to the lower base fixture, thereby inducing a greater moment at T1 than at C2 (**Fig. 4–3B**). Specimens with gross alignment deformities were not used.

A rotational displacement transducer (RDT) (Data Instruments, Acton, MA) was attached to the rotational joint connected to the actuator; this transducer measured the global rotation of the spine. A translational displacement transducer (TDT) (Data Instruments, Acton, MA) was inserted into a custom-designed plate between the upper pot and splined shaft connection; the TDT measured changes in the moment arm length. For lateral bending tests, the spine was rotated 90 degrees in the mounting fixtures, and the base remained unconstrained in axial rotation. A separate loading system was used for axial rotation. The testing arrangements for lateral bending and axial rotation are shown in **Figs. 4–4 and 4–5**.

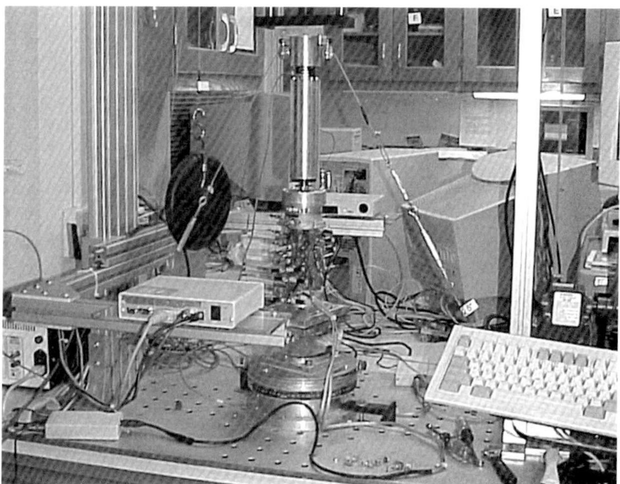

Figure 4–4   Lateral bending testing arrangement.

Figure 4–5   Axial rotation testing arrangement.

Specimen Preparation and Spine Conditions

Thirty-seven fresh human cadaveric cervical spines (C2–T1) were procured from the Medical Education Research Institute (Memphis, TN). The average age and gender of the harvested spines used was 72.6 ± 10.8 years. The spines were harvested and immediately double wrapped in plastic bags and stored at −20°C until preparation. Before preparation the spines were thawed in a refrigeration system for 12 hours. Prior to testing, the free ends of the vertebral bodies of C2 and T1 were mounted in cylindrical pots using an alignment frame that positioned the cervical spine specimen in a neutral upright orientation. The flexion-extension axis was estimated at the anterior aspect of the facet joint of each vertebra. All spines were evaluated in the six different modes of loading: flexion, extension, right and left lateral bending, and right and left axial rotation. Four specimens were used to analyze the PP and PF end mounting conditions. The remaining 33 specimens were studied using the TPF configuration.

A three-dimensional, noncontact, real-time measurement system was used to track segmental cervical motion for each testing condition.[1,15–17] For two-dimensional motion analysis, target arrays consisting of two light-emitting diodes were rigidly attached to each spinous process (**Fig. 4–3A**). The individual MSU rotations were then expressed relative to the subjacent vertebral body using principles of rigid body mechanics.

For each loading mode of the TPF condition, the relative change in the individual local MSU rotations was recorded. The individual MSU responses were expressed relative to their percent contribution to the overall global (C2–T1) rotation and compared. A one-way analysis of variance (ANOVA) with Student-Newman-Kevls (SNK) test ($p < .05$ unless otherwise stated) was used to statistically analyze the motion response for the modified testing protocol with published data for pure moment loading methods and with a set of kinematic data from Lysell.[18]

Nondestructive Testing Criteria

All tests were performed under displacement control with the subaxial (C2–T1) cervical spine positioned either in line (PP; PF) or eccentric (TPF) to the center line of the vertical linear actuator shaft. The actuator was programmed to output a triangular-shaped displacement-time waveform of 6.4 mm/sec. For each configuration, an increasing incremental displacement was applied until a target moment at T1 between 3 and 4 Nm was reached, or was stopped if any of the following limits were reached: 40 degrees of sagittal plane rotation; 5 Nm bending or torsional moment at T1, or axial compressive load of 500 N for the PP and PF configurations or 75 N for the TPF configuration. These values were based on our preliminary test findings[13] and agreed with the limits used by other researchers.[19,20] The spines were preconditioned with five cycles before formal testing. Each test trial included three loading cycles; the third cycle was analyzed.

◆ Results

Pinned-Pinned and Pinned-Fixed Mounting Conditions

For the PF configuration, minimal displacement of the actuator quickly produced a high compressive load that exceeded the allowable load limit and induced minimal amounts of vertebral motion. The PP configuration produced an unordered, bipolar motion response similar to that associated with the first mode of column buckling. Further, for both the PP and PF configurations, a nonphysiological internal moment was created in the spine. In contrast, with the TPF configuration, all vertebral bodies moved continuously with the same polarity of rotation. A distributed moment was also applied throughout the cervical spine. It was quickly established that the TPF configuration satisfied the external loading criteria necessary to replicate the in vivo motion response of the cervical spine, and all subsequent analyses and discussion of in vitro data are based on the modified TPF configuration.[5,21–24]

Modified TPF Mounting Condition

The mean relative flexion and extension MSU rotations of the harvested spine corresponding to the modified loading protocol are shown in **Fig. 4–6**. Average in vivo data from the published literature of the flexion-extension MSU rotations for

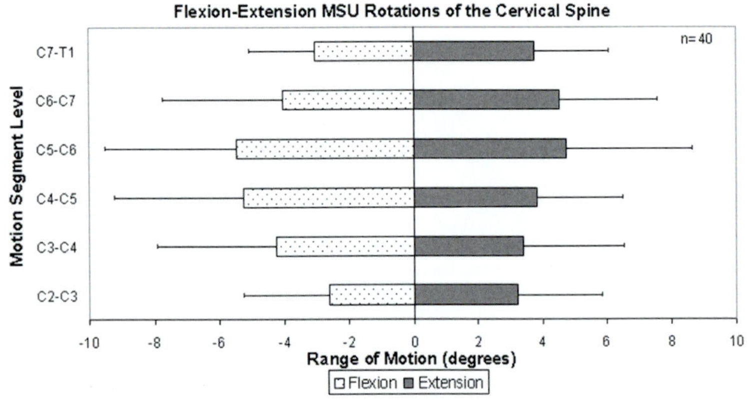

Figure 4–6 Flexion-extension motion segment unit rotations of harvested spine for modified testing protocol.

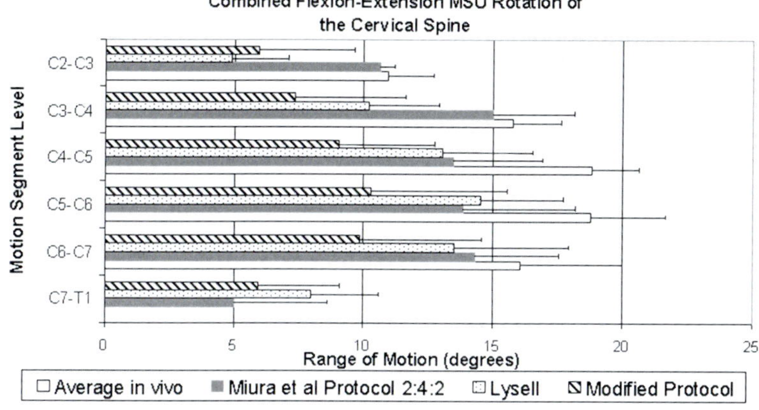

Figure 4–7 Combined flexion-extension motion segment unit (MSU) rotations for in vitro testing methods compared with published in vivo data. The greatest motion occurred at C5–C6 MSU.[21,33,34]

spinal segments C2 to C7 are plotted in **Fig. 4–7**,[5,21–23] along with the combined flexion-extension MSU rotations for the modified protocol and pure moment loading method[24] and an additional set of flexion-extension cervical motion data derived by Lysell.[18] The percent contribution of each MSU rotation expressed relative to its total global rotation for flexion and extension is shown in **Fig. 4–8**. The in vitro MSU rotational percent contribution for the modified protocol was similar to that of published in vivo data[5,21–23]; the highest range of flexion-extension motion occurred at the C5–C6 MSU, as was observed by Lysell. A significant difference occurred at C2–C3 between the modified method versus pure moment and Lysell versus pure moment. For pure moment loading, the rotational response at the lower cervical segments continued to increase slightly in magnitude moving caudally from C4 to C7. This pattern was opposite to the response for all other data.

The mean relative MSU rotations for right and left lateral bending with the modified loading protocol are shown in **Fig. 4–9**. No in vivo data were available for comparison of individual MSU rotational patterns. The combined right plus left lateral bending MSU rotations for the different in vitro methods are shown in **Fig. 4–10**. The percent contribution of each MSU rotation expressed relative to the total global rotation for lateral bending is shown in **Fig. 4–11**. The percent contributions of the individual MSU rotations

under lateral bending loads for the modified protocol were comparable to the data from Lysell. Application of a pure moment induced a significantly greater response at C3–C4 and C4–C5, which dropped off significantly across the lower segments. This pattern was not present with the modified method or with Lysell's data. Significant differences occurred at C4–C5 between modified versus pure moment and Lysell versus pure moment; and at C6–C7 and C7–T1 between modified versus pure moment, modified versus Lysell, and Lysell versus pure moment.

The mean relative axial MSU rotations of the harvested spine for the modified loading protocol are shown in **Fig. 4–12**. In vivo data from the published literature of the axial MSU rotations were available for MSU segments C2 to C7 and are plotted in **Fig. 4–13**.[5,21–24] The corresponding combined axial MSU rotations for the modified protocol and pure moment loading method[24] are also shown in **Fig. 4–13**, along with an additional set of axial cervical motion data derived by Lysell.[18] The percent contribution of each MSU rotation expressed relative to the total global rotation for axial loading is shown in **Fig. 4–14**. The in vitro MSU rotational percent contribution for the modified protocol was similar to that reported by Lysell and was comparable to published in vivo data.[5,21–23] Significant differences occurred at C6–C7 between modified versus pure moment protocols.

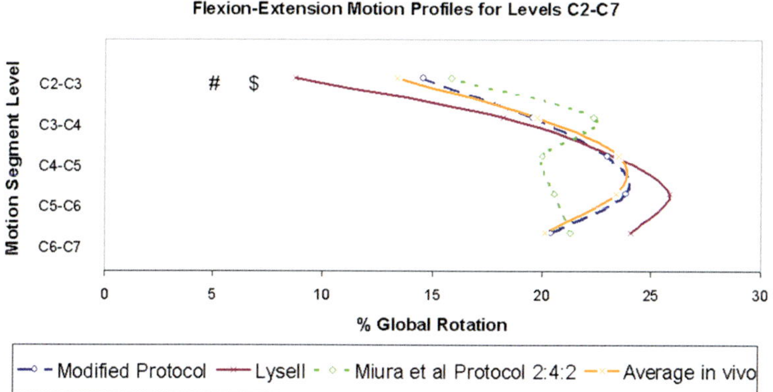

Figure 4–8 Motion segment unit contribution of global flexion-extension motion for different in vitro testing methods compared with published in vivo data. significant difference between modified and pure moment; #, significant difference between modified and Lysell; $, significant difference between pure moment and Lysell.

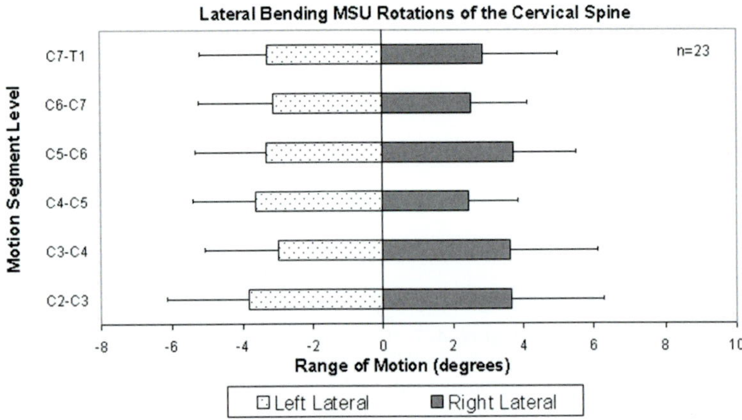

Figure 4–9   Lateral bending motion segment unit rotations of harvested spine for modified testing protocol.

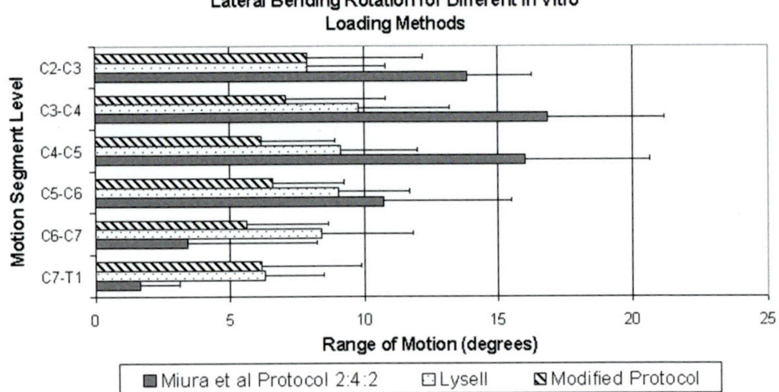

Figure 4–10   Combined lateral bending motion segment unit rotations for in vitro testing methods.

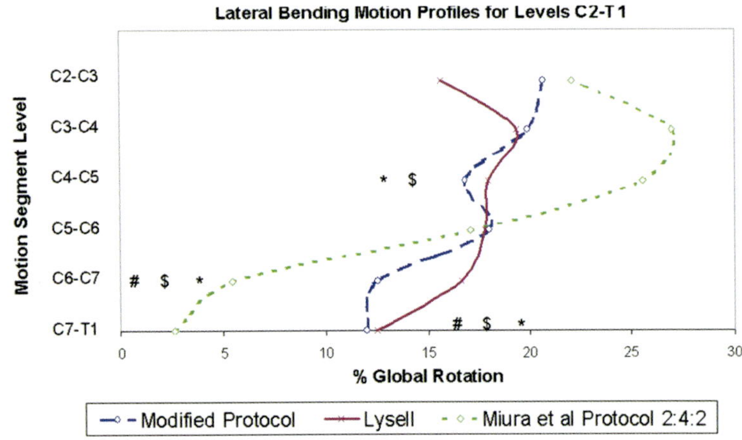

Figure 4–11   Motion segment unit contribution of global lateral bending for different in vitro testing methods. *, significant difference between modified and pure moment; #, significant difference between modified and Lysell; $, significant difference between pure moment and Lysell.

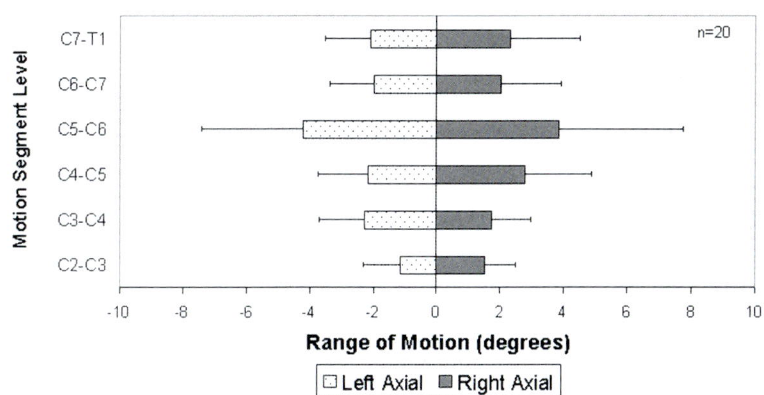

Figure 4–12 Axial motion segment unit rotations of harvested spine for modified testing protocol.

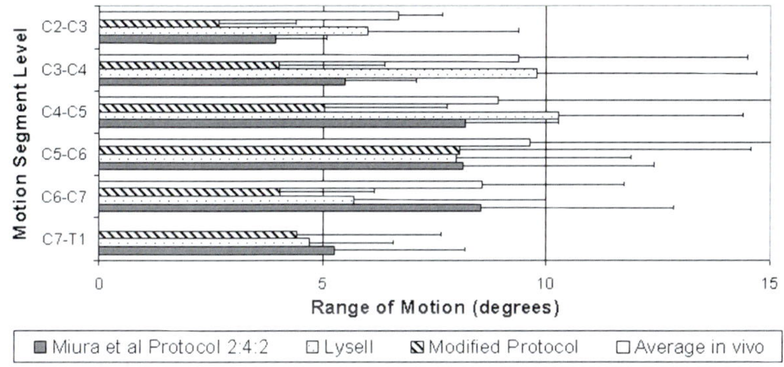

Figure 4–13 Combined axial motion segment unit rotations for in vitro testing methods compared with published in vivo data.[21,33,34]

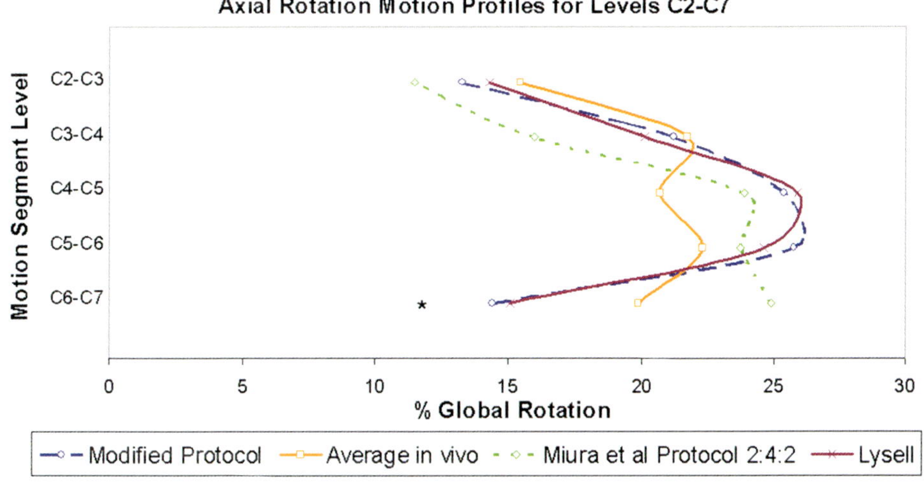

Figure 4–14 Motion segment unit contribution of global axial rotations for different in vitro testing methods compared with published in vivo data. *, significant difference between modified and pure moment ($p < .01$); #, significant difference between modified and Lysell; $, significant difference between pure moment and Lysell.

◆ Discussion

Displacement versus Load Control

A question arises as to which testing method better replicates the in vivo motion behavior of the cervical spine. Miura et al recently described a method to simulate in vivo cervical spine kinematics using a preload and pure moment protocol.[6] The technique of a follower load was used in conjunction with a pure moment. A critical detail of the follower load concept is to pass a compressive load through the instantaneous axis of rotation (IAR) of each MSU. In their study, the IAR was placed near the lateral masses and remained fixed for the flexion and extension tests. However, this IAR position was based on three cited studies,[25–27] none of which performed an error analysis on the propagation of error associated with the theoretical calculation itself, nor were the instant centers determined over small ranges of motion that typically occur between two adjacent MSUs (i.e., 2–3 degree increments). We have previously shown that the error in calculating the location of the IAR can be large (as high as $\pm$ 10 mm) for small angular changes (2–3 degrees) and that the IAR position is significantly different in flexion than in extension.[28] Further, because the axis of rotation of the cervical spine varies between flexion and extension but was constrained from moving to apply the compressive follower load, this arrangement may limit or alter the motion response.

To better understand the differences in the MSU rotation patterns for the different loading conditions, only the mean values of the percent contributions of the MSU rotations were plotted in **Figs. 4–8, 4–11, and 4–14.** For flexion-extension loading, the motion response using a pure moment protocol with a follower load was found to be representative of in vivo spine studies.[22,23,29–32] However, the combined mean flexion-extension rotational values did not always follow the in vivo pattern and in some instances went in the opposite direction or remained constant across multiple MSU levels (**Fig. 4–7**) at the region where the predominant amount of motion occurs in the cervical spine (i.e., C4–C5 and C5–C6). The trend in the data suggests that if the sample size were increased, significant differences would exist between the in vitro data and the in vivo data.

The follower load concept was developed by Patwardhan et al[33] to allow the intact spine to withstand greater compressive loads without buckling. A compressive load was applied along the bending axis of the spine to simulate the net resultant action of muscles on either side of the spine. The follower load has been successfully used to demonstrate how the intact multisegmental spine can withstand large compressive loads without buckling.[33] However, use of the follower load to study the instrumented multilevel cervical spine may artificially add more stability to the spine than occurs in vivo. When studying disk replacement or motion preservation devices, the device may or may not have a fixed axis of rotation. The location of the follower load relative to the rotational axis directly effects how the device transfers load and maintains joint stability. Further, although the follower load is traditionally applied to the flexion-extension plane, its load transferring concept also affects how the load and motion respond in the transverse and frontal planes.

More recently, a new testing method has been proposed that combines the concepts of the pure moment or flexibility method with displacement test methods, referred to as the *hybrid method*.[34] In pure moment protocols, the flexibility of different spinal constructs was compared at the same end limit of moment. With the hybrid method, the spinal constructs are still tested under load control with pure moments, but the end limit conditions are compared at a common end limit of rotational displacement achieved by the intact/harvested spine condition. It is hypothesized that the changes due to a nonfusion or fusion device will over time lead to the complementary changes in motion at the remaining adjacent spinal levels. It was further suggested that during daily living activities of the spine patient, the individual will attempt to move the treated spinal region in a similar manner as before the surgery, thereby applying additional stress to the free spinal segments and causing the compensatory changes to occur. However, two significant limitations exist with this approach. Even though the patient may attempt to achieve the same movement limits after surgery as before, the compensation may not concentrate at only the adjacent segments in the treated region but may occur at other regions of the entire spine. Another concern with this testing rationale is that it is subject to the same limitations and drawbacks as with the pure moment/flexibility testing method. Further, when the altered (injured, instrumented) spine condition is pushed to the same end limit of rotation as the intact/harvested spine condition, the compensatory changes in the motion and loads at the adjacent disks and facet joints have been shown to be nonphysiological (**Fig. 4–14**). As such, the output motion and load response for this hybrid protocol have minimal clinical relevance and can be considered only as a standardized approach to compare spinal constructs in a nonphysiological manner.

◆ Conclusion

When evaluating the performance of disk arthroplasty or motion preservation devices, not only should the instrumented level be analyzed but changes at the adjacent and remaining segments should be included in the analysis. As such, the preferred testing protocol is one that most closely follows the in vivo pattern for all spinal segments of the cervical spine. An improved biomechanical testing protocol was developed that better replicated the physiological motion response of the cervical spine. In contrast, application of the pure moment/flexibility method or the hybrid testing method does not replicate the physiological response and is less suited for evaluating disk arthroplasty and nonfusion hardware.

◆ Sources of Support

Tissue procurement was coordinated through Medical Education and Research Institute (MERI, Memphis, TN). Henry Bonin and Brian Kelly for assistance with data processing and manuscript preparation and Eve Blair, Thomas Jansen, Jaclyn Kuspiel, Brian Morrow, John Schwab, Amanda Thomas, and Keith Vossel for technical assistance with the experimental tests.

References

1. DiAngelo DJ, Foley KT, Vossel KA, Rampersaud YR, Jansen TH. Anterior cervical plating reverses load transfer through multilevel strut-grafts. Spine 2000;25:783–795

2. Goel VK, Wilder DG, Pope MH, Edwards WT. Biomechanical testing of the spine: load-controlled versus displacement-controlled analysis. Spine 1995;20:2354–2357.

3. Gilbertson LG, Doehring TC, Livesay GA, Rudy TW, Kang JD, Woo SL. Improvement of accuracy in a high-capacity, six degree-of-freedom load cell: application to robotic testing of musculoskeletal joints. Ann Biomed Eng 1999;27:839–843

4. Wilke HJ, Wolf S, Claes LE, Arand M, Wiesend A. Influence of varying muscle forces on lumbar intradiskal pressure: an in vitro study. J Biomech 1996;29:549–555

5. White AA III, Panjabi MM. Clinical Biomechanics of the Spine. 2nd ed. Philadelphia: Lippincott Williams & Wilkins; 1990

6. Miura T, Panjabi MM, Cripton PA. A method to simulate in vivo cervical spine kinematics using a compressive preload. Spine 2002;27:43–48

7. Smith SA, Lindsey RW, Doherty BJ, Alexander J, Dickson JH. An in vitro biomechanical comparison of the orosco and ao locking plates for anterior cervical spine fixation. J Spinal Disord 1995; 8:220–223

8. Weinhoffer SL, Guyer RD, Herbert M, Griffith SL. Intradiskal pressure measurements above an instrumented fusion: a cadaveric study. Spine 1995;20:526–531

9. Kunz DN, McCabe RP, Zdeblick TA, Vanderby R Jr. A multi-degree of freedom system for biomechanical testing. J Biomech Eng 1994;116:371–373

10. James KS, Wenger KH, Schlegel JD, Dunn HK. Biomechanical evaluation of the stability of thoracolumbar burst fractures. Spine 1994; 19:1731–1740

11. Shea M, Edwards WT, White AA, Hayes WC. Variations of stiffness and strength along the human cervical spine. J Biomech 1991;24:95–107

12. Chen J. Development of a flexible biomechanical testing apparatus. MS Thesis, University of Tennessee-Memphis, 1996

13. DiAngelo DJ, Faber HB, Dull ST, Jansen TH. Development of an in vitro experimental protocol to study the extensional mechanics of the cervical spine. In: Simon B, ed. Advances in Bioengineering. New York: American Society of Mechanical Engineers; 1997;BED36:211–212

14. DiAngelo DJ, Jansen TH, Eckstein EC, Foley KT, Dull ST. Measurements for the in vitro failure of multi-level instrumented cervical spine. In: Simon B, ed. Advances in Bioengineering. New York: American Society of Mechanical Engineers; 1997;BED36:223–224

15. DiAngelo DJ, Robertson JT, Metcalf NH, McVay BJ, Davis RC. Biomechanical testing of an artificial cervical joint and an anterior cervical plate. J Spinal Disord Tech 2003;16:314–323

16. DiAngelo DJ, Vossel KA, Jansen TH. A multi-body optical measurement system for the study of human joint motion. In: Yogannathan AP, ed. Advances in Bioengineering. New York: American Society of Mechanical Engineers; 1998;BED39:195–196

17. Foley KT, DiAngelo DJ, Rampersaud YR, Vossel KA, Jansen TH. The in vitro effects of instrumentation on multilevel cervical strut-graft mechanics. Spine 1999;24:2366–2376

18. Lysell E. Motion in the cervical spine: an experimental study on autopsy specimens. Acta Orthop Scand 1969;(Suppl 123):1–61

19. Parsons JR, Zimmerman MC, Lee CK, Langrana NA. Examination of the failure mode of several cervical spine fixation devices. In: Langrana NA, Friedman MH, Grood ED, eds. Bioengineering Conference. New York: American Society of Mechanical Engineers; 1993;24:175–178

20. Pelker RR, Duranceau JS, Panjabi MM. Cervical spine stabilization: a three-dimensional, biomechanical evaluation of rotational stability, strength, and failure mechanisms. Spine 1991;16:117–122

21. Amevo B, Macintosh JE, Worth D, Bogduk N. Instantaneous axes of rotation of the typical cervical motion segment, I: An empirical study of technical errors. Clin Biomech (Bristol, Avon) 1991; 6:31–37

22. Dvorak J, Froehlich D, Penning L, Baumgartner H, Panjabi MM. Functional radiographic diagnosis of the cervical spine: flexion/extension. Spine 1988;13:748–755

23. Lind B, Sihlbom H, Nordwall A, Malchau H. Normal range of motion of the cervical spine. Arch Phys Med Rehabil 1989;70:692–695

24. Miura T, Panjabi MM, Cripton PA. Stability of three strut-graft constructs for multi-level cervical corpectomy [abstract]. In: Proceedings of the 2001 Cervical Spine Research Society. Rosemont, IL: Cervical Spine Research Society; 2001:55–56

25. Amevo B, Worth D, Bogduk N. Instantaneous axis of rotation of the typical cervical motion segments: a study in normal volunteers. Clin Biomech (Bristol, Avon) 1991;6:111–117

26. Dvorak J, Panjabi MM, Novotny JE, Antinnes JA. In vivo flexion/extension of the normal cervical spine. J Orthop Res 1991;9:828–834

27. van Mameren H, Sanches H, Beursgens J, Drukker J. Cervical spine motion in the sagittal plane, II: Position of segmental averaged instantaneous centers of rotation: a cineradiographic study. Spine 1992;17:467–474

28. DiAngelo DJ, Vossel KA, Foley KT. The instant axis of rotation of the cervical spine in flexion and extension [abstract.] In: Proceedings of the 2000 Cervical Spine Research Society. Rosemont, IL: Cervical Spine Research Society; 2000:203–204

29. Dvorak J, Panjabi MM, Grob D, Novotny JE, Antinnes JA. Clinical validation of functional flexion/extension radiographs of the cervical spine. Spine 1993;18:120–127

30. Holmes A, Wang C, Han ZH, Dang GT. The range and nature of flexion-extension motion in the cervical spine. Spine 1994;19: 2505–2510

31. Penning L. Normal movements of the cervical spine. AJR Am J Roentgenol 1978;130:317–326

32. Ordway NR, Seymour RJ, Donelson RG, Hojnowski LS, Edwards WT. Cervical flexion, extension, protrusion, and retraction: a radiographic segmental analysis. Spine 1999;24:240–247

33. Patwardhan AG, Havey RM, Ghanayem AJ, et al. Load carrying capacity of the human cervical spine in compression is increased under a follower load. Spine 2000;25:1548–1554

34. Goel VK, Panajabi MM. Adjacent level effects: design of a new testing protocol and finite element model simulations of disk replacement. In: Goel VK, Panajabi MM, eds. Roundtables in Spine Surgery. Vol 1. St. Louis: Quarter Medical; 2005:45–55

5

Cervical Disk Arthroplasty: Rationale, Indications, and Clinical Experience

Moe R. Lim, Joon Y. Lee, and Alexander R. Vaccaro

◆ **Rationale for Cervical Total Disk Replacement**

　Possible Prevention of Adjacent Segment Degeneration and Disease

　Avoidance of Pseudarthrosis

　Avoidance of Iliac Crest Bone Graft Donor Site Morbidity

　Potential Avoidance of Postoperative Dysphagia

◆ **Potential Disadvantages of Cervical Total Disk Replacements**

◆ **Indications for Cervical Total Disk Replacement**

　Cervical Total Disk Replacement in the Treatment of Adjacent Segment Disease

◆ **Current Designs of Cervical Total Disk Replacements**

　Prestige Cervical Disk Replacement (Medtronic Sofamor Danek, Memphis, TN)

　Bryan Cervical Disc (Medtronic Sofamor Danek, Memphis, TN)

　Porous Coated Motion (Cervitech, Rockaway, NJ)

　ProDisc-C (Synthes, Inc., West Chester, PA)

　CerviCore (Stryker Spine, Allendale, NJ)

◆ **Pros and Cons of the Various C-TDR Designs**

◆ **Conclusion**

Anterior cervical diskectomy and fusion (ACDF) is one of the most reliable procedures in spine surgery for relief of symptoms due to a herniated disk and produces satisfactory results in 90 to 95% of patients with cervical radiculopathy or myelopathy.[1] Despite the excellent results of this existing treatment, there has been much recent interest in cervical total disk replacement (C-TDR) as an alternative to ACDF. A portion of the drive to accept C-TDR can be attributed to the interests of the spine implant industry. Unlike fusion in the peripheral joints, short or single-level fusions and subsequent loss of mobility in the subaxial cervical spine result in no functional limitations. However, there exist multiple legitimate problems associated with ACDF that C-TDRs have the potential to address: adjacent segment degeneration and disease, iliac crest bone graft donor site morbidity, pseudarthrosis, and postoperative dysphagia.

◆ Rationale for Cervical Total Disk Replacement

Possible Prevention of Adjacent Segment Degeneration and Disease

Retrospective radiographic studies have demonstrated that many patients develop degenerative changes at levels adjacent to segments treated by ACDF.[2–5] In a series of 180 patients treated with ACDF with greater than 5-year follow-up, 92% of the patients were found to have new degeneration or progression of degeneration at levels adjacent to the fusion.[4] In a recent study of 44 patients who had anterior cervical corpectomy and fusion, magnetic resonance imaging was performed after mean 18 months of follow-up. New degenerative changes adjacent to the fused segment were seen in 75% of the patients. The majority of these patients with radiographic changes (referred to as adjacent segment degeneration), however, remained asymptomatic.[5]

In contrast, *adjacent segment disease* refers to the subset of patients who develop new radiculopathy or myelopathy due to degeneration of a motion segment adjacent to the site of a previous anterior cervical fusion. Hilibrand et al reviewed 374 patients with 409 noninstrumented anterior cervical fusions who were followed for up to 21 years. They found that adjacent segment disease, symptomatic enough to warrant further surgical treatment, occurred at a relatively constant rate of 2.9% per year. C5–C6 and C6–C7 were the levels most likely to develop adjacent segment disease. Survivorship analysis predicted that adjacent segment disease may affect more than one fourth of all patients within 10 years after an anterior cervical fusion.[6]

Whether these degenerative changes are the result of increased mechanical forces on the levels adjacent to a fusion or whether these changes merely represent the natural progression of the degenerative disease process is yet to be determined. Likely, both factors have a role in the etiology of adjacent segment disease. A long-term 5- to 9-year follow-up after ACDF with plating for trauma detected a 60% incidence of asymptomatic adjacent segment degeneration. The high incidence of adjacent degeneration in a patient population without preexisting spondylosis points to the significance of the effect of the fusion on the adjacent levels.[7] However, it must be noted that adjacent level degeneration may also be related to the use of instrumentation in these patients. Park and Riew have described the entity of adjacent level ossification secondary to encroachment of the adjacent disk space by cervical plates.[8]

Multiple studies suggest that the immobility of the fused segment has detrimental biomechanical effects on the adjacent levels. These detrimental effects have been quantified as compensatory increases in adjacent segmental motion and elevation in adjacent intradiskal pressures during cervical motion. In two cadaveric studies, intradiskal pressures at adjacent levels were measured before and after ACDF at C5–C6. Both studies found that intradiskal pressures were increased during flexion and extension at both the caudal and cephalad adjacent levels. Dmitriev et al found that C4–C5 experienced a 48% increase in intradiskal pressure and the C6–C7 experienced a 125% increase in intradiskal pressure. Eck et al found that the pressure increased by 73% at C4–C5 and by 45% at C6–C7.[9,10]

Other cadaveric studies have also shown that segmental motion is increased at levels adjacent to a fusion.[10–14] Eck et al found that during flexion, motion increased at both adjacent levels, with greater increases at the cephalad level. However, during extension, greater increases in motion occurred at the caudal level.[10] Summers et al found that increases in adjacent motion were greater after a two-level fusion compared with a single-level fusion.[12] Using slightly different testing methods, Fuller et al similarly demonstrated increased motion in nonfused levels and that increased bending moments were required to achieve the same amount of global sagittal motion. However, they found that motion was not increased disproportionately at the motion segments immediately adjacent to the fusion.[11]

Additional cadaveric studies have suggested that the adverse biomechanical effects of fusion on adjacent levels can be prevented by C-TDR. Dmitriev et al found that the intradiskal pressures adjacent to a C-TDR when using a Porous Coated Motion (PCM) prosthesis (Cervitech, Rockaway, NJ) were significantly less than the pressures adjacent to a fusion. No differences in intradiskal pressure were recorded between the native spine and the spines implanted with a C-TDR under any loading conditions.[9] Two additional cadaveric studies using two different C-TDR implants (Prestige I; Medtronic Sofamor Danek, Memphis, TN, and ProDisc-C; Synthes, Inc., West Chester, PA) found that C-TDRs maintained the normal kinematics of the cervical spine. Simulation of fusion significantly reduced motion at the fusion level, which was compensated for by increased motion at the adjacent segments. In contrast, the use of a C-TDR did not alter the motion patterns at either the C-TDR level or adjacent segments.[13,14]

The findings of these biomechanical cadaveric studies have been verified by the results of clinical studies. Wigfield et al performed a prospective randomized study and compared the motion at levels adjacent to a single-level C-TDR (12 patients, Prestige I) to that of a fusion (13 patients).[15] In the fusion group, adjacent-level motion increased from preoperative levels by 5% at 6 months to 15% at 12 months. The increase in motion mainly occurred in disks that were preoperatively normal. At 1 year after surgery, the levels next to a fusion had significantly greater motion than the levels next to a C-TDR. However, a slight reduction in adjacent-level motion was observed in the C-TDR group when compared with preoperative range of motion (ROM). The significance of the decrease in adjacent motion with C-TDR is unknown. In contrast, Duggal et al found that patients with single-level C6–C7 C-TDRs (Bryan Cervical Disc; Medtronic Sofamor Danek, Memphis, TN) had restoration of normal physiological cervical spine kinematics. Motion at both the C-TDR level and adjacent levels was unchanged from the preoperative measurements.[16,17]

Current clinical evidence to support the contention that C-TDR can prevent adjacent segment degeneration/disease consists of a recent study comparing the rate of adjacent segment degeneration in two prospective single-level cervical diskectomy cohorts. One cohort of 187 patients were treated by fusion with a cage, whereas the other cohort of 80 patients were treated with a C-TDR (Bryan). The two cohorts were followed using similar methodologies. At 2-year follow-up, 27% of the fusion patients had developed new radiographic changes of disk degeneration, compared with 14% in C-TDR patients. Adverse events of neck, shoulder, or arm pain developed in 32% of the fusion patients compared with 1% of the C-TDR patients. The rates of reoperation for adjacent segment disease were similar (3.2% in fusion vs 2.5% in C-TDR).[18] Unfortunately, because of the nonrandomized nature of the study, only limited conclusions could be made. The authors also did not examine whether the quantity of preserved motion in the C-TDR group correlated with the incidence of adjacent segment degeneration.[18] Only long-term follow-up of ongoing prospective randomized studies comparing C-TDR to ACDF will determine whether C-TDR can prevent or decrease the incidence of adjacent segment disease.

Avoidance of Pseudarthrosis

The rate of pseudarthrosis following ACDF depends on multiple patient and nonpatient factors such as smoking status, use of anti-inflammatory medications, and host immunocompetency, and surgical factors such as number of levels fused, use of autograft versus allograft bone, and use of instrumentation. In a series of studies by Wang et al, for a one-level ACDF using autograft, the nonunion rate was 4% if plated and 8% if not plated.[19] For a two-level ACDF, the nonunion rate was 0% if plated and 25% if not plated.[20] For a three-level ACDF the pseudarthrosis rate was 18% if plated and 37% if not plated.[21] Fortunately, ~50% of the patients with nonunion will remain asymptomatic at 2 years and 33% will remain asymptomatic at 5 years.[22] However, ~50% of the patients will require revision surgery.[23]

With C-TDR, the risk of pseudarthrosis is virtually eliminated. However, for the C-TDR to be stable long term, bony ingrowth into the prosthesis end plates is required. The porous coating of the Bryan C-TDR has demonstrated bony ingrowth ranging from 10 to 50% in chimpanzee models and 20 to 50% in human explant retrieval studies.[24] The porous surface of the PCM C-TDR has been shown to have 48% surface ingrowth in a baboon model.[25] This amount of ingrowth compares favorably to that seen in stable total hip arthroplasties and is likely sufficient for long-term C-TDR implant stability.

Avoidance of Iliac Crest Bone Graft Donor Site Morbidity

A current advantage of C-TDR over ACDF is that C-TDR does not require autologous iliac crest bone grafting and thus bone graft harvesting morbidities can be avoided.[26] In a retrospective, questionnaire-based investigation of 134 patients who underwent single-level ACDF, acute morbidities related to the iliac crest bone graft were reported at the following rates: ambulation difficulty, 51%; extended antibiotic usage, 8%; persistent drainage, 4%; wound dehiscence, 2%; and need for incision and drainage, 1.5%. At an average of 4 years after surgery, pain at the donor site was reported by 26% of patients with a mean Visual Analogue Scale (VAS) score of 3.8. Chronic use of pain medication for iliac crest pain was required by 11.2% of patients. Abnormal sensation at the donor site was reported by 16%, but only 5.2% reported discomfort with clothing. A functional assessment revealed iliac crest-related impairments at the following rates: ambulation, 13%; recreational activities, 12%; work activities, 10%; activities of daily living, 8%; sexual activity, 8%; and household chores, 7%.

The current gold-standard graft source for anterior cervical fusion is the use of autologous iliac crest bone graft. However, the recent introduction of fusion-enhancing biologics may decrease the need for autograft once this technology is adapted for use in the cervical spine.[27,28] In addition, increasing evidence shows that the use of allograft and plate fixation provides a safe and effective alternative to autograft.[29-32]

Potential Avoidance of Postoperative Dysphagia

One month after anterior cervical surgery, ~50% of patients still experience dysphagia.[33] This subjective symptom has been validated by abnormal postoperative videofluoroscopic swallow evaluations.[34] Although the prevalence of dysphagia gradually decreases to ~18% at 6 months, 12% of patients are still symptomatic at 1 year. Age, female gender, and multiple operated levels have been identified as risk factors for persistent postoperative dysphagia.

A possible cause of postoperative dysphagia is the retraction pressure placed on the esophagus during the anterior cervical procedure. A recent study revealed that implantation of C-TDRs may place less pressure against the esophagus than ACDF plating. ACDFs or C-TDR (PCM, with no fixation screws) implantations were performed in cadavers through a 4 cm transverse incision while esophageal pressures were monitored. Cervical plating resulted in significantly greater intraesophageal pressures than C-TDR. It was postulated that cervical plating required more traction to insert the convergent contralateral drill, tap, and screws. Because disk arthroplasty does not require more contralateral retraction, less pressure is theoretically placed against the esophagus.[35]

One possible additional risk factor for postoperative dysphagia relates to the bulkiness of anterior surface internal fixation. In a recent prospective study, the prevalence of dysphagia was compared in patients who underwent ACDF with use of a thin, narrow plate versus a wide, thicker plate.[36] The two plates had very similar rates of dysphagia at 1 month postop (~50%). However, at 2 years, the prevalence of dysphagia was significantly higher for the bulkier plate (14% vs 0%). Because bulky anterior hardware may have a causative role in postoperative persistent dysphagia, the use of C-TDRs with no anterior profile (Prestige STLP, Bryan, ProDisc-C, and PCM) may lower the incidence of this complication.

◆ Potential Disadvantages of Cervical Total Disk Replacements

Several potential disadvantages of cervical disk arthroplasty exist. It is important to realize that symptomatic radiculopathy and myelopathy are caused by combined static and dynamic neural compression.[37-40] Because motion at the diseased level is retained with C-TDRs, there may be greater potential for failure to relieve symptoms due to dynamic factors or for recurrent symptoms at the same level ("same level disease"). With ACDF, the static component can be decompressed and the dynamic component can be eliminated by fusion. With C-TDR, dynamic neural compression will remain unless a more aggressive decompression is performed. More aggressive decompression may mean greater blood loss and higher risks of neural or vascular injury. In addition, there exist no objective criteria for what represents an adequate decompression. Even if individual surgeons have developed their own set of criteria, these criteria are based on the amount of decompression necessary to achieve good clinical results with fusion. Current criteria for adequate decompression may become obsolete in the setting of a C-TDR.

Contrary to these contentions, short-term results of randomized trials suggest equivalent clinical outcomes of ACDF and C-TDR. However, these trials are being conducted by surgeons with vast experience in performing an anterior cervical decompression. With wider release of these implants to the general population, good results may become less predictable. With ACDF, the room for error in performing a decompression is high. In fact, it has been shown that equally good outcomes can be achieved regardless of whether direct uncovertebral joint decompression is performed.[41] With C-TDR, performing a decompression may be more critical in achieving successful short-term outcomes. Reports of C-TDR revisions for inadequate decompression have already begun to surface.[42-44]

In the long term, successful ACDF also eliminates motion and thus halts progression of spondylotic spurs. In fact, fusion often leads to spur resorption. With motion preserved in C-TDR, however, spondylotic spurs may recur, leading to late symptom recurrence at the same level.[45] Further follow-up may reveal that we have traded a relatively low incidence of adjacent segment disease for a higher incidence of same-level disease.

Other potential disadvantages of C-TDRs include increased cost, neurological injury due to posterior implant dislodgement, implant failure, and need for revision. Fortunately, the approach and potential need for corpectomy in revision C-TDR are known to most spine surgeons.

◆ Indications for Cervical Total Disk Replacement

The current indications for cervical disk replacement are identical to those for ACDF (i.e., radiculopathy or myelopathy caused by one or more levels of anterior compression). These are patients who present with a neural compressive lesion causing upper extremity weakness, paresthesias, and pain, with or without lower extremity hyperreflexia. The varied diagnosis may include soft tissue disk herniation with radiculopathy, spondylotic radiculopathy, disk herniation with myelopathy, and spondylotic myelopathy.

As more experience with these devices accrues, however, the indications may expand or contract. For example, C-TDRs may encounter problems with same-level disease and symptom recurrence in older patients with spondylotic spurs and degenerated facet joints. Indications may then become narrowed to younger patients with soft disk herniations. These patients are typically younger with normal facet joints and may have more predictable results with motion preservation.

On the other hand, indications could also expand to include patients with diskogenic axial neck pain. Interestingly, the indication for lumbar total disk replacement is primarily diskogenic axial low back pain. In contrast to the indications for C-TDR, neural compressive lesions such as spinal canal stenosis or herniated nucleus pulposus are considered to be contraindications to lumbar TDR.[46] There are limited data to indicate that patients with refractory axial neck pain and degenerative disk disease limited to one or two levels can benefit from ACDF. These same patients may benefit from C-TDR.[47,48]

Contraindications for C-TDR include (1) conditions unlikely to be improved by C-TDR (axial neck pain related to facet arthropathy, cervical myelopathy caused primarily by posterior compression); (2) deformity (cervical scoliosis, postlaminectomy kyphosis); (3) potential for C-TDR instability (posterior element insufficiency, cervical segmental instability); (4) potential for inadequate end plate integrity (osteoporosis, metabolic bone diseases); and (5) potential for poor results (prior infection, ossification of the posterior longitudinal ligament, ankylosing spondylitis, rheumatoid arthritis).

Cervical Total Disk Replacement in the Treatment of Adjacent Segment Disease

C-TDR may have a specific role in treating adjacent segment disease next to an established fusion. Revision fusion for adjacent disease is challenging due to high rates of pseudarthrosis and postoperative dysphagia.[49–51] The difficulty in obtaining fusion adjacent to a prior fusion may be due to an unfavorable biological milieu and a large differential in stiffness between the fusion and the adjacent open disk space.[45] With C-TDR, the need for fusion is eliminated, although bony ingrowth is still necessary. C-TDR may also decrease the potential for progression of disease to the next adjacent level. A cadaveric biomechanical study has shown that there is increased motion at a level adjacent to a two-level fusion versus a one-level fusion and second-level C-TDR.[12]

With revision fusion for adjacent disease, the index plate is removed to provide space for a new plate to be extended to the additional level. The multilevel dissection required to remove the index plate likely contributes to a higher incidence of postoperative dysphagia and respiratory compromise.[33,52,53] If a C-TDR (without screw fixation) is used, there is no need to remove the index plate, and the multilevel dissection can be avoided. Of note, the novel concept of an add-on extension plate to treat adjacent disease may also accomplish the same goal.[54]

◆ Current Designs of Cervical Total Disk Replacements

At the time of this writing, three C-TDR devices are undergoing Investigational Device Exemption (IDE) studies in the United States: the Prestige ST, the Bryan, and the ProDisc-Cervical (ProDisc-C). The Prestige ST and Bryan have completed enrollment for comparison to ACDF with allograft and plate. The inclusion criteria are for single-level disk herniations with radiculopathy or myelopathy or both with minimal spondylosis and no substantial adjacent-level degeneration. Two other prostheses are in pre-IDE development: the PCM and the CerviCore Cervical Intervertebral Disc Replacement (Stryker Spine, Allendale, NJ). All prostheses allow motion in flexion-extension, lateral bending, and axial rotation.

Prestige Cervical Disk Replacement (Medtronic Sofamor Danek, Memphis, TN)

The Prestige ST (**Fig. 5–1**) is the fourth generation of a two-piece, uniarticulating, metal-on-metal, minimally constrained

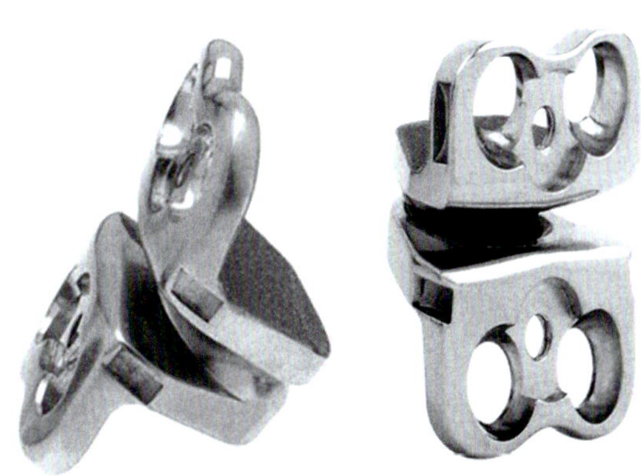

Figure 5–1   The Prestige ST is the fourth generation of a two-piece, uniarticulating, metal-on-metal, minimally constrained cervical total disk replacement (C-TDR) with anterior screw fixation.

C-TDR with anterior screw fixation. This implant has undergone the longest period of clinical evaluation of all the C-TDRs. It was originally invented by B.H. Cummins at the Frenchay Hospital in Bristol, U.K., in 1989.[55] The articulation was an upside-down ball and socket design with the concavity on the caudal end plate and the convexity on the cephalad end plate. The device was implanted in a series of 20 patients with cervical myelopathy, radiculopathy, or severe pain. Nineteen of the 20 patients had a prior congenital or surgical fusion. The inventor found that motion of the prosthesis was preserved in 89% of the patients at up to 5 years postop. Sixteen of the 20 patients noted clinical improvement. Wear debris and heterotopic ossification were not observed. There was, however, a high complication rate with seven cases of screw pullout or breakage, one transient hemiparesis due to drill injury, one reoperation to remove a loose device, one joint subluxation associated with persistent dysphagia, and three cases of mild persistent dysphagia. The high complication rates were attributed to the use of a uniform-sized device without the ability to accommodate the size to the individual patient's anatomy.

The Cummins Bristol prosthesis was redesigned to the Prestige I in 1998 by Medtronic Sofamor Danek. The major design change was the conversion of the ball and socket articulation to a ball and trough articulation. The ball and trough allowed independent anterior-posterior translation with flexion-extension and a mobile instantaneous flexion-extension center of rotation. Prestige I (also known as the Frenchay device) was evaluated prospectively in 17 patients requiring revision surgery to treat adjacent segment disease. The mean operative time was 143 minutes. The mean blood loss was 316 mL. There were no wound or prosthesis infections. Two patients had transient voice hoarseness, which resolved at 3 and 6 months. At 4 years postsurgery, clinical outcome measures including the Neck Disability Index (NDI) and SF-36 showed good improvement, especially in light of the end-stage nature of this challenging patient population. However, due to the small number of patients, statistical significance was not achieved. In regard to prosthesis function, all devices were mobile at 2 years, with an average ROM of 6.5 degrees. At 4 years, the average ROM was 5.7 degrees.

There were notable complications of Prestige I in nine patients. Two patients had persistent arm pain due to incomplete decompression. One resolved at 12 months. The other needed revision surgery for a foraminotomy at an adjacent level. Four patients had persistent neck pain with neck extension; the first patient's symptoms developed at 6 months, the second developed pain after a motor vehicle accident, the third was found to have two broken caudal screws at 6 months and developed neck pain at 2 years, and the fourth patient had a loose prosthesis that was removed and fused at 12 months. A second well-functioning implant was removed at 3.5 years to place a plate over the diseased adjacent level. Two further patients had progression of myelopathy. One underwent a laminectomy at two levels below the prosthesis and developed kyphosis at the intervening level, requiring an anterior posterior fusion. The second patient, who suffered progression of myelopathy and subluxation at C6–C7 below a

C4–C5 implant, required a posterior fusion from C5–C7 and demonstrated no motion of the implant after 12 months due to the fusion.[42,56,57]

In 1999, the Prestige I end plates were redesigned to be more anatomical and a roughened surface was added to promote bony ingrowth (Prestige II). The Prestige II has been compared with an uninstrumented autograft ACDF for single-level disease in a randomized prospective trial with 55 patients enrolled. At 12 months, the C-TDR demonstrated angular motion with a mean value of 5.9 degrees. At 2-year follow-up, the C-TDR patients had greater improvement in NDI and VAS, and SF-36 mental and physical scores compared with ACDF. Motion was retained in all C-TDRs.[58]

The current version, Prestige ST, was introduced in 2002 and is currently being implanted in the U.S. FDA IDE study. The Prestige ST is a two-piece implant constructed of stainless steel with a metal-on-metal ball and trough articulation. Constrained locking screws inserted through the anterior flanges achieve initial fixation of the two articulating components to the vertebral bodies. The major design change between the Prestige II and Prestige ST is a 2 mm reduction in the height of the anterior flanges. The 2.5 mm thickness of the anterior flanges is comparable to many cervical plates. The end plates are grit-blasted to allow bony ingrowth for long-term fixation.

Wear testing of 10 million cycles in flexion-extension and 5 million cycles of coupled axial rotation and lateral bending has been performed on the Prestige ST. The mean volumetric wear was 0.57 mm^3/million cycles. Assuming 400,000 cycles per year,[59] at 10 years the volumetric wear of the Prestige is calculated to be more than 10-fold lower than metal-on-metal total hip arthroplasty and more than 100-fold lower than metal-on-polyethylene total hip arthroplasty.[56,60] On explant retrieval analysis, wear was considerably less than predicted in simulators. There were no failures of the device due to a reaction to wear debris, fracture, polymer oxidation, or metal corrosion. The inflammatory response seen in the periprosthetic tissues was minimal.[61]

The most recent version of the Prestige is the Prestige STLP, which is constructed of a unique combination of titanium alloy and ceramic titanium carbide (**Fig. 5–2**). Instead of screws through anterior flanges, initial fixation of the Prestige STLP is achieved by two small keels on the end

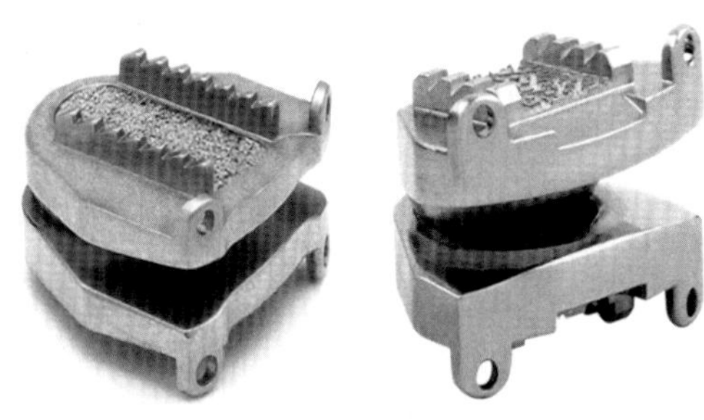

Figure 5–2   The Prestige STLP is the most recent version of the Prestige. It is constructed of a unique combination of titanium alloy and ceramic titanium carbide.

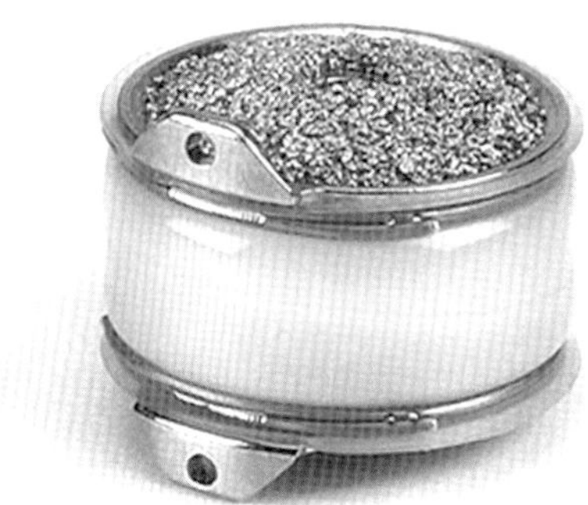

Figure 5–3   The Bryan prosthesis has been the subject of the largest clinical experience of the cervical total disk replacements (C-TDRs). Since January 2000, more than 5500 of these devices have been implanted.

plates. This eliminates the anterior profile of the implant, simplifies implantation, and allows unrestricted multilevel implantation. However, it has the potential to destroy more bone stock if removal is required. The Prestige STLP is currently in the enrollment phase of a U.S. IDE trial and is available outside the United States.

Bryan Cervical Disc (Medtronic Sofamor Danek, Memphis, TN)

The Bryan prosthesis (**Fig. 5–3**) has been the subject of the largest clinical experience of the C-TDRs. Since January 2000, more than 5500 of these devices have been implanted. It is a one-piece, biarticulating, unconstrained device. The porous coated titanium alloy end plates articulate with the polyurethane core, which allows for motion and shock absorption. A unique polyurethane flexible membrane surrounds the entire articulation and forms a sealed space containing a saline lubricant to reduce friction and prevent migration of wear debris. The instantaneous center of rotation is variable and is in the center of the disk space. Initial stability of the implant is achieved by precise milling of the vertebral end plates. Concavities are milled into the end plates to create a surface for bony ingrowth and to provide a press-fit for initial stability.

Wear and immune response to the Bryan C-TDR have been studied in simulators, animals, and human retrievals. In wear testing, failure (defined as end plate metal-to-metal contact) occurred at ~40 million cycles. A mean volumetric wear of 0.48 mm^3/million cycles was noted. Assuming 400,000 cycles per year, at 10 years, the volumetric wear of the Bryan is calculated to be more than 10-fold lower than metal-on-metal total hip arthroplasty and more than 100-fold lower than metal-on-polyethylene total hip arthroplasty. On retrieval analysis, wear on the specimens was considerably less than predicted in simulators. There was no failure of the device, fracture, polymer oxidation, or metal corrosion.[61] In a caprine model, periprosthetic tissue revealed birefringent ellipitical particles. There was minimal to no inflammatory response to particles observed in local tissues, spinal canal tissues, liver, spleen, and draining lymph nodes. This lack of a rigorous inflammatory response was also seen in human retrieval periprosthetic tissue.[62,63]

Two prospective observational European clinical studies on the Bryan have been initiated. In 2000, a single-level study was initiated and 103 patients were enrolled. In 2001, the two-level study was initiated and 43 patients have been implanted. In the one-level study, 73 patients have had at least 2-year follow-up and 71% of the patients demonstrated good or excellent results based on modified Odom's criteria. In the two-level study, 30 patients have had at least 1-year follow-up and 80% of the patients were rated as good or excellent. The SF-36 physical and mental outcomes measures were improved postoperatively and maintained at 2-year follow-up. The outcomes were similar to that of historical data on ACDF, primarily related to adequate decompression and patient selection.

Radiographic analysis of the Bryan in the European studies showed no evidence of subsidence. Motion of at least 2 degrees was observed in 93% of the one-level patients at 2 years and in 86% of the two-level patients at 2 years. The average ROM was 7.4 degrees. Restricted ROM was thought to be related to intraoperative malpositioning with misaligned shells. The complications included three revision decompressions, two cases of temporary migration of the implants (< 3 mm, one anterior and one posterior, thought to be related to incomplete milling of the end plates), one cerebrospinal fluid leak, one esophageal injury, and four hematoma evacuations.[44,63,64] Other international experience with the Bryan includes clinical series from Australia and Canada. Sekhon reported on 11 cases of cervical myelopathy treated with 15 Bryan prostheses from New South Wales, Australia. At an average 18-month follow-up, there were improvements in Nurick grade by 0.91 grades and Oswestry Neck Disability Index score by 42 points. Using Odom's criteria, 91% of the patients had good/excellent outcomes.[65] Two patients had adverse outcomes. One patient with persistent neck and arm pain developed heterotopic ossification posterior to the prosthesis, leading to an inadvertent interbody fusion at 17 months postop. The second patient was readmitted 10 days after surgery for acute worsening myelopathy. Imaging revealed kyphotic angulation at her two prostheses but no persistent cord compression. Her symptoms resolved with steroid therapy.[43]

In a report from Ontario, Canada, Duggal et al described 26 patients who underwent single- or two-level implantation of the Bryan C-TDR for either or both radiculopathy and myelopathy. At mean follow-up of 12 months, a statistically significant improvement in the mean NDI scores was seen and there was a trend toward improvement in the SF-36 physical component. Mean ROM was 7.8 degrees and motion preservation was noted at up to 24 months postsurgery.[66]

Porous Coated Motion (Cervitech, Rockaway, NJ)

The PCM prosthesis (**Fig. 5–4**) was originally designed by Paul C. McAfee but has been modified by the developers of the lumbar Charité total disk replacement (DePuy Spine, Raynham, MA). It is a two-piece, uniarticulating,

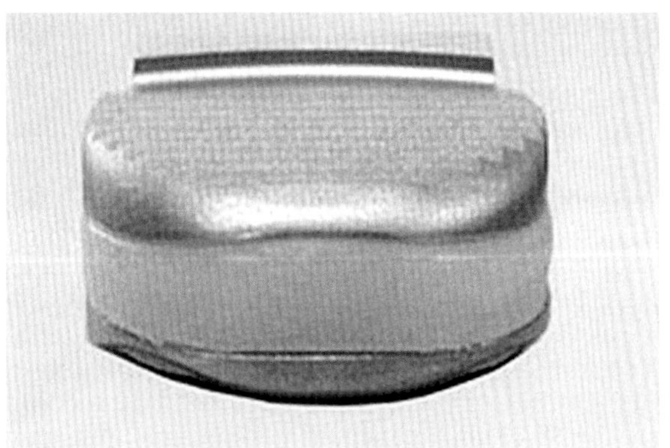

Figure 5–4   The Porous Coated Motion (PCM) prosthesis was originally designed by Paul C. McAfee but has been modified by the developers of the lumbar Charité total disk replacement.

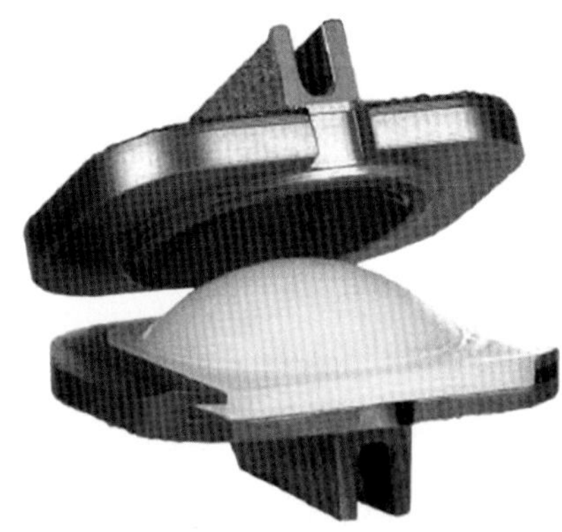

Figure 5–5   The ProDisc-C is a three-piece, uniarticulating ultra high molecular weight polyethylene on cobalt-chromium (UHMWPE on CoCr) device. It is the cervical version of the lumbar ProDisc.

metal-on-polyethylene unconstrained device. The cobalt-chromium (CoCr) end plates have been shaped to maximize loading in the more dense lateral vertebral body surfaces.[67] The serrations on the end plates allow initial fixation with a press-fit in the vertebral bodies. The end plate–vertebral body interface is composed of two ultrathin layers of titanium with electrochemically coated calcium phosphate in a 1:1 ratio (TiCaP). This surface has been shown to have excellent surface ingrowth in a baboon model.[25] The PCM articulation is the time-tested ultra high molecular weight polyethylene on cobalt-chromium (UHMWPE on CoCr) combination. The articulating surface of this prosthesis extends across the entire end plate surface, creating a large radius of articulation. The large radius of curvature allows near physiological unconstrained anterior-posterior translation with flexion-extension motion. It is the only C-TDR prosthesis without inherent ROM limitations. Instead, the limits of ROM are guided by the soft tissue sleeve.[67] The standard press-fit PCM has no anterior profile. However, if bony preparation is suboptimal or the anatomy is aberrant, then the Augmented PCM can be used. The Augmented PCM allows screw fixation to the vertebral bodies through anterior flanges.

Between December 2002 and October 2003, 81 PCM C-TDRs were implanted in 53 patients at the Mattos Pimenta Clinic in São Paulo, Brazil. Forty-three patients had primary degenerative disk disease and 10 patients had adjacent segment disease. Implantations were performed at one to three levels. The average operative time was 50 minutes per level and the average estimated blood loss was 50 mL. Average hospitalization was 1 day. No cervical collars were used postoperatively. One patient was noted to have 4 mm anterior displacement of the prosthesis at 3 months postop, which was asymptomatic. There was one case of heterotopic ossification. Clinical evaluation with VAS and NDI revealed continuing improvements in all categories at the latest 1-year follow-up. Using Odom's criteria, 97% of the patients were rated as good/excellent. Eighty-seven percent of the patients were able to return to their baseline level of employment at 3 weeks.[68] Following this pilot study and the initiation of a European multicenter observational trial led by Prof. Alan

Crockard of London, a submission to begin U.S. clinical trials of the PCM is currently under review by the FDA.

ProDisc-C (Synthes, Inc., West Chester, PA)

The ProDisc-C (**Fig. 5–5**) is a three-piece, uniarticulating UHMWPE-on-CoCr device. It is the cervical version of the lumbar ProDisc. The end plates are composed of a cobalt-chrome alloy covered with a plasma-sprayed porous titanium alloy on the bone–end plate interface. An upright keel enhances initial fixation of the porous end plates. The polyethylene spacer inserts into the caudal end plate and articulates with the superior end plate. It is a pure ball and socket joint with a fixed axis of rotation that is near the center of the disk space. The axis of rotation is fixed in the vertebral bone below the disk space.

Early results of the FDA IDE randomized, controlled, multicenter trial to assess the safety and efficacy of the ProDisc-C have become available. In one center, 34 patients with cervical radiculopathy and single-level disease were randomized to ACDF (17 patients) with allograft/plating or to the ProDisc-C (17 patients). Patient outcomes were assessed using neurological function, VAS, NDI, and SF-36 scores. At 6-month follow-up, neurological improvement was seen in 84% of the ACDF and 82% of the ProDisc-C patients. All patients showed significant improvement in pain and disability. There was no significant difference between the treatment groups. At the ProDisc-C level, the average motion was 6.2 degrees in flexion and 7.4 degrees in extension. No complications were noted in the fusion group. One ProDisc-C patient developed heterotopic ossification at 6 months leading to autofusion with a good clinical result.[69] In another center of the same multicenter study, 27 patients were randomized to ACDF or ProDisc-C. Operative time averaged 79 minutes for ProDisc-C and 75 minutes for ACDF. Estimated blood loss was 63 mL for ProDisc-C compared with 126 mL for ACDF. There were no intraoperative, neurological, vascular, or wound complications in either group. Adverse events of dysphagia, dysphonia, and interscapular pain were similar in the two treatment groups. All patients showed improvements in pain and disability.[70]

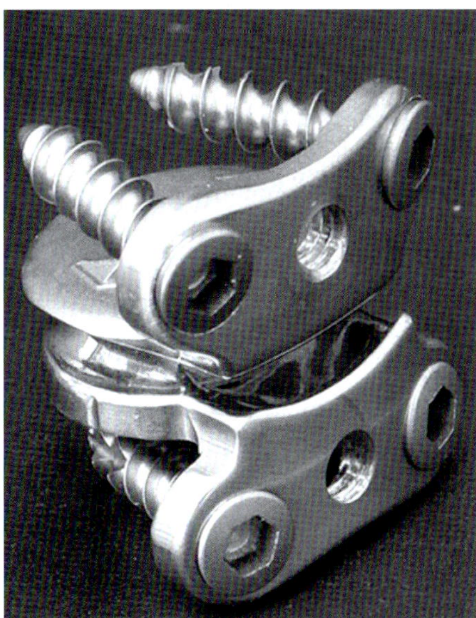

Figure 5–6   The CerviCore is a two-piece, uniarticulating, metal-on-metal device. The saddle-shaped articulation purportedly allows a flexion-extension moving center of rotation in the vertebral body below the prosthesis yet allows the center of rotation for lateral bending to be in the vertebral body above the prosthesis.

CerviCore (Stryker Spine, Allendale, NJ)

The CerviCore (**Fig. 5–6**) is a two-piece, uniarticulating, metal-on-metal device. The saddle-shaped articulation purportedly allows a flexion-extension moving center of rotation in the vertebral body below the prosthesis yet allows the center of rotation for lateral bending to be in the vertebral body above the prosthesis. Fixation is via screw through anterior flanges. At this time, no results are publicly available of simulator, animal, cadaveric, or clinical studies on the CerviCore C-TDR.

◆ Pros and Cons of the Various C-TDR Designs

Multiple similarities and differences exist between the various current C-TDR designs. All models allow flexion-extension, lateral bending, and axial rotation motions. However, the articulation materials are different. The time-tested joint arthroplasty articulation material combination is metal-on-polyethylene (ProDisc-C and PCM). Although this articulation has been associated with osteolysis related to particulate wear debris in synovial joints, no similar problems have been seen in the synovium-free cervical disk space. Metal-on-metal articulations are found in the Prestige and CerviCore designs. Metal-on-metal peripheral joint arthroplasties have shown none to minimal osteolysis at midterm follow-up. However, this articulation raises two potential concerns. In peripheral joints, synovial fluid is necessary to lubricate the metal-on-metal articulation. The long-term function of a similar articulation in a synovial fluid-free environment of the cervical disk space is unknown. Also, elevated blood levels of metal ions and hypersensitivity lymphocytic immunological responses of unknown significance have been recently reported in metal-on-metal peripheral joint replacements.[71] The Bryan C-TDR is unique in its shock-absorbing titanium-on-polyurethane articulation. The long-term durability of this articulation has not been clinically studied. The flexible sheath surrounding the Bryan C-TDR is able to retain the lubricating saline but also retains wear debris with potential for third-body wear and has potential to rupture.

The current C-TDRs all have porous ingrowth surfaces at the end plate–vertebral body interface for long-term fixation. Their methods of initial fixation, however, differ. The screw fixation of the Prestige ST, CerviCore, and Augmented PCM have an elevated anterior profile with the potential to cause persistent dysphagia and does not allow adjacent multilevel implantation. There has also been a high rate of screw-related complications in the earlier versions of the Prestige. However, screws may be more appropriate if a significant portion of the vertebral body surface is resected during the decompression or in the setting of suboptimal carpentry and end plate preparation. Also, this fixation method is simple and similar to ACDF and anterior plating. In contrast, the vertebral body milling required to achieve a stable press-fit of the Bryan requires multiple interdependent steps. The milling process has also been anecdotally linked to heterotopic ossification and autofusion of the C-TDR level. However, heterotopic ossification has been reported with most of the other designs as well. The ProDisc-C, the Prestige STLP, and the standard PCM can be implanted with ease without the need for screw fixation or milling. The ProDisc-C's keel is unique and provides additional initial fixation. However, concerns have been raised over the need to remove excessive bone stock around the keel if the well-fixed prosthesis requires removal.

The current C-TDR designs have varying levels of constraint. Nonconstrained devices are more likely to allow reproduction of normal or near normal physiological joint kinematics. They also have the potential to significantly reduce stress at the bone–implant interface. However, nonconstrained devices are more likely to dislocate and surpass normal physiological motion. In the cervical spine, dislocation of a C-TDR could have catastrophic consequences. In contrast, constrained devices are less likely to dislocate. The kinematics are controlled more by the prosthesis itself and less by the soft tissue sleeve. This allows controlled motion. However, the motion may be less physiological. Constrained devices may also allow less ROM and increase stress at the end plate–bone interface. Lack of motion at the end plate–bone interface is crucial for long-term stability of the implant. Proceeding from most to least constrained are the ProDisc-C, Prestige ST/CerviCore, Bryan, and PCM. The PCM is unique in that there are no internal limits to ROM of the prosthesis. The large radius of curvature of the articulation allows increased anterior-posterior translation. For the Bryan, the nucleus articulation between the two end plates may produce similar constraint as the Charité lumbar disk replacement. The ball in trough and ball in saddle articulations of the Prestige ST and CerviCore allow anterior-posterior sliding independent of flexion-extension. The ball and socket articulation of the ProDisc-C is the most constrained of the current C-TDRs. Anterior-posterior translation is not possible independent of flexion-extension. Because of its inherent stability, the ProDisc-C may have a unique indication to restore stability to the cervical spine, such as in mild spondylolisthesis or in cases of iatrogenic instability due to surgical decompression.

◆ Conclusion

Cervical total disk replacement represents an exciting new frontier in spine surgery. The role of these new devices in the future of the field, however, is yet to be determined. The ultimate evaluation of the success of C-TDRs will depend on minimum 5-year follow-up results of currently ongoing multicenter, prospective, randomized, controlled trials. Surgeon preference between the various C-TDR designs will ultimately be based on clinical outcomes, unique indications, ease of implantation, maintenance of motion, and incidence of complications.

References

1. Bohlman HH, Emery SE, Goodfellow DB, Jones PK. Robinson anterior cervical diskectomy and arthrodesis for cervical radiculopathy: long-term follow-up of one hundred and twenty-two patients. J Bone Joint Surg Am 1993;75:1298–1307

2. Baba H, Furusawa N, Imura S, Kawahara N, Tsuchiya H, Tomita K. Late radiographic findings after anterior cervical fusion for spondylotic myeloradiculopathy. Spine 1993;18:2167–2173

3. Hunter LY, Braunstein EM, Bailey RW. Radiographic changes following anterior cervical fusion. Spine 1980;5:399–401

4. Goffin J, Geusens E, Vantomme N, et al. Long-term follow-up after interbody fusion of the cervical spine. J Spinal Disord Tech 2004;17:79–85

5. Kulkarni V, Rajshekhar V, Raghuram L. Accelerated spondylotic changes adjacent to the fused segment following central cervical corpectomy: magnetic resonance imaging study evidence. J Neurosurg 2004;100(Suppl 1 Spine):2–6

6. Hilibrand AS, Carlson GD, Palumbo MA, Jones PK, Bohlman HH. Radiculopathy and myelopathy at segments adjacent to the site of a previous anterior cervical arthrodesis. J Bone Joint Surg Am 1999;81:519–528

7. Goffin J, van Loon J, Van Calenbergh F, Plets C. Long-term results after anterior cervical fusion and osteosynthetic stabilization for fractures and/or dislocations of the cervical spine. J Spinal Disord 1995;8:500–508 discussion 499

8. Park JB, Riew KD. Timing of adjacent level ossification development (ALOD) secondary to anterior cervical plates. Paper presented at: Meeting of the Cervical Spine Research Society, 2004; Boston, MA

9. Dmitriev A, Cunningham B, Hu N, Sell G, Vigna F, McAfee PC. Adjacent level intradiskal pressures following a cervical total disk arthroplasty: an in-vitro human cadaveric model. Paper presented at: Meeting of the Cervical Spine Research Society, 2004; Boston, MA

10. Eck JC, Humphreys SC, Lim TH, et al. Biomechanical study on the effect of cervical spine fusion on adjacent-level intradiskal pressure and segmental motion. Spine 2002;27:2431–2434

11. Fuller DA, Kirkpatrick JS, Emery SE, Wilber RG, Davy DT. A kinematic study of the cervical spine before and after segmental arthrodesis. Spine 1998;23:1649–1656

12. Summers HD, Gullickson MA, Ghanayem AJ, et al. Effect of cervical arthroplasty vs. fusion on adjacent segment kinematics. Paper presented at: Meeting of the Cervical Spine Research Society, 2004; Boston, MA

13. DiAngelo DJ, Foley KT, Morrow BR, et al. In vitro biomechanics of cervical disk arthroplasty with the ProDisc-C total disk implant. Neurosurg Focus 2004;17:E7

14. DiAngelo DJ, Roberston JT, Metcalf NH, McVay BJ, Davis RC. Biomechanical testing of an artificial cervical joint and an anterior cervical plate. J Spinal Disord Tech 2003;16:314–323

15. Wigfield C, Gill S, Nelson R, Langdon I, Metcalf N, Robertson J. Influence of an artificial cervical joint compared with fusion on adjacent-level motion in the treatment of degenerative cervical disk disease. J Neurosurg 2002;96(Suppl 1):17–21

16. Duggal N, Pickett GE, Rouleau JP. Kinematic analysis of the Bryan cervical disk prosthesis. Paper presented at: Meeting of the Cervical Spine Research Society, 2004; Boston, MA

17. Goffin J, Komistek R, Malfouz H, Wong DA, Macht D. Poster 236: In vivo kinematics of normal, degenerative, fused and disk-replaced cervical spines. Paper presented at: Annual Meeting of the American Academy of Orthopaedic Surgeons, 2003; New Orleans, LA

18. Robertson J, Papadopoulos SM, Traynelis VC. Assessment of adjacent segment disease in patients treated with cervical fusion or cervical arthroplasty: a prospective 2-year study. Paper presented at: Meeting of the Cervical Spine Research Society, 2004; Boston, MA

19. Wang JC, McDonough PW, Endow K, Kanim LE, Delamarter RB. The effect of cervical plating on single-level anterior cervical diskectomy and fusion. J Spinal Disord 1999;12:467–471

20. Wang JC, McDonough PW, Endow KK, Delamarter RB. Increased fusion rates with cervical plating for two-level anterior cervical diskectomy and fusion. Spine 2000;25:41–45

21. Wang JC, McDonough PW, Kanim LE, Endow KK, Delamarter RB. Increased fusion rates with cervical plating for three-level anterior cervical diskectomy and fusion. Spine 2001;26:643–646 discussion 646–647

22. Phillips FM, Carlson G, Emery SE, Bohlman HH. Anterior cervical pseudarthrosis: natural history and treatment. Spine 1997;22:1585–1589

23. Newman M. The outcome of pseudarthrosis after cervical anterior fusion. Spine 1993;18:2380–2382

24. Anderson PA, Jensen WK, Rouleau JP. Bone ingrowth in retrieved Bryan cervical disk prosthesis. Paper presented at: Meeting of the Cervical Spine Research Society, 2004; Boston, MA

25. McAfee PC, Cunningham BW, Orbegoso CM, Sefter JC, Dmitriev AE, Fedder IL. Analysis of porous ingrowth in intervertebral disk prostheses: a nonhuman primate model. Spine 2003;28:332–340

26. Silber JS, Anderson DG, Daffner SD, et al. Donor site morbidity after anterior iliac crest bone harvest for single-level anterior cervical diskectomy and fusion. Spine 2003;28:134–139

27. Lanman TH, Hopkins TJ. Early findings in a pilot study of anterior cervical interbody fusion in which recombinant human bone morphogenetic protein-2 was used with poly(L-lactide-co-D,L-lactide) bioabsorbable implants. Neurosurg Focus 2004;16:E6

28. Baskin DS, Ryan P, Sonntag V, Westmark R, Widmayer MA. A prospective, randomized, controlled cervical fusion study using recombinant human bone morphogenetic protein-2 with the CORNERSTONE-SR allograft ring and the ATLANTIS anterior cervical plate. Spine 2003;28:1219–1225 discussion 1225

29. Young WF, Rosenwasser RH. An early comparative analysis of the use of fibular allograft versus autologous iliac crest graft for interbody fusion after anterior cervical diskectomy. Spine 1993;18:1123–1124

30. Samartzis D, Shen FH, Matthews DK, Yoon ST, Goldberg EJ, An HS. Comparison of allograft to autograft in multilevel anterior cervical diskectomy and fusion with rigid plate fixation. Spine J 2003;3:451–459

31. Kaiser MG, Haid RW Jr, Subach BR, Barnes B, Rodts GE Jr. Anterior cervical plating enhances arthrodesis after diskectomy and fusion with cortical allograft. Neurosurgery 2002;50:229–236 discussion 236–228

32. Balabhadra RS, Kim DH, Zhang HY. Anterior cervical fusion using dense cancellous allografts and dynamic plating. Neurosurgery 2004;54:1405–1411 discussion 1411–1402

33. Bazaz R, Lee MJ, Yoo JU. Incidence of dysphagia after anterior cervical spine surgery: a prospective study. Spine 2002;27:2453–2458

34. Smith-Hammond CA, New KC, Pietrobon R, Curtis DJ, Scharver CH, Turner DA. Prospective analysis of incidence and risk factors of dysphagia in spine surgery patients: comparison of anterior cervical, posterior cervical, and lumbar procedures. Spine 2004;29:1441–1446

35. Tortolani PJ, Cunningham B, Vigna F, Hu N, Zorn CM, McAfee PC. Intraesophageal retraction pressure during anterior cervical plating versus cervical disk replacement: a cadaveric study. Cervical Spine Research Society Annual Meeting Poster, 2004; Baltimore, MD

36. Lee MJ, Bazaz R, Furey CG, Yoo JU. The incidence of dysphagia in anterior cervical surgery as a function of plate design: a prospective study. Paper presented at: Meeting of the Cervical Spine Research Society, 2004; Boston, MA

37. Kitagawa T, Fujiwara A, Kobayashi N, Saiki K, Tamai K, Saotome K. Morphologic changes in the cervical neural foramen due to flexion and extension: in vivo imaging study. Spine 2004;29:2821–2825

38. Holmes A, Han ZH, Dang GT, Chen ZQ, Wang ZG, Fang J. Changes in cervical canal spinal volume during in vitro flexion-extension. Spine 1996;21:1313–1319

39. Yoo JU, Zou D, Edwards WT, Bayley J, Yuan HA. Effect of cervical spine motion on the neuroforaminal dimensions of human cervical spine. Spine 1992;17:1131–1136

40. Nuckley DJ, Konodi MA, Raynak GC, Ching RP, Mirza SK. Neural space integrity of the lower cervical spine: effect of normal range of motion. Spine 2002;27:587–595

41. Shen FH, Samartzis D, Khanna N, Goldberg EJ, An HS. Comparison of clinical and radiographic outcome in instrumented anterior cervical diskectomy and fusion with or without direct uncovertebral joint decompression. Spine J 2004;4:629–635

42. Wigfield CC, Gill SS, Nelson RJ, Metcalf NH, Robertson JT. The new Frenchay artificial cervical joint: results from a two-year pilot study. Spine 2002;27:2446–2452

43. Sekhon LH. Cervical arthroplasty in the management of spondylotic myelopathy: 18-month results. Neurosurg Focus 2004;17(3):E8

44. Goffin J, Van Calenbergh F, van Loon J, et al. Intermediate follow-up after treatment of degenerative disk disease with the Bryan Cervical Disc Prosthesis: single-level and bi-level. Spine 2003;28:2673–2678

45. Albert TJ, Eichenbaum MD. Goals of cervical disk replacement. Spine J 2004;4(Suppl 6):292S–293S

46. Huang RC, Lim MR, Girardi FP, Cammisa FP Jr. The prevalence of contraindications to total disk replacement in a cohort of lumbar surgical patients. Spine 2004;29:2538–2541

47. Palit M, Schofferman J, Goldthwaite N, et al. Anterior diskectomy and fusion for the management of neck pain. Spine 1999;24:2224–2228

48. Garvey TA, Transfeldt EE, Malcolm JR, Kos P. Outcome of anterior cervical diskectomy and fusion as perceived by patients treated for dominant axial-mechanical cervical spine pain. Spine 2002;27:1887–1895 discussion 1895

49. Lowery GL, Swank ML, McDonough RF. Surgical revision for failed anterior cervical fusions: articular pillar plating or anterior revision? Spine 1995;20:2436–2441

50. Hilibrand AS, Yoo JU, Carlson GD, Bohlman HH. The success of anterior cervical arthrodesis adjacent to a previous fusion. Spine 1997;22:1574–1579

51. Zdeblick TA, Hughes SS, Riew KD, Bohlman HH. Failed anterior cervical diskectomy and arthrodesis: analysis and treatment of thirty-five patients. J Bone Joint Surg Am 1997;79:523–532

52. Frempong-Boadu A, Houten JK, Osborn B, et al. Swallowing and speech dysfunction in patients undergoing anterior cervical diskectomy and fusion: a prospective, objective preoperative and postoperative assessment. J Spinal Disord Tech 2002;15:362–368

53. Sagi HC, Beutler W, Carroll E, Connolly PJ. Airway complications associated with surgery on the anterior cervical spine. Spine 2002;27:949–953

54. Fassett DR, Apfelbaum RI, Clark R, Bachus KN, Brodke DS. Biomechanical analysis of a new concept: an add-on extension plate for adjacent-level anterior cervical fusion. Paper presented at: Meeting of the Cervical Spine Research Society, 2004; Boston, MA

55. Cummins BH, Robertson JT, Gill SS. Surgical experience with an implanted artificial cervical joint. J Neurosurg 1998;88:943–948

56. Traynelis VC. The Prestige cervical disk replacement. Spine J 2004;4(Suppl 6):310S–314S

57. Robertson JT, Metcalf NH. Long-term outcome after implantation of the Prestige I disk in an end-stage indication: 4-year results from a pilot study. Neurosurg Focus 2004;17:E10

58. Robertson J, Porchet F, Brotchi J, et al. A multicenter trial of an artificial cervical joint for primary disk surgery. Paper presented at: Spine Arthroplasty Society, 2002; Montpelier, France

59. Kostuik JP. Intervertebral disk replacement: experimental study. Clin Orthop Relat Res 1997;337:27–41

60. Haid RW, Buchholz PA, Rouleau JP. Performance of metal-on-metal and polyurethane-on-metal artificial cervical disks in spinal stimulators. Paper presented at: Meeting of the Cervical Spine Research Society, 2004; Boston, MA

61. Anderson PA, Rouleau JP, Toth JM, Riew KD. A comparison of simulator-tested and -retrieved cervical disk prostheses: invited submission from the Joint Section Meeting on Disorders of the Spine and Peripheral Nerves, March 2004. J Neurosurg Spine 2004;1:202–210

62. Anderson PA, Rouleau JP, Bryan VE, Carlson CS. Wear analysis of the Bryan Cervical Disc prosthesis. Spine 2003;28:S186–S194

63. Anderson PA, Sasso RC, Rouleau JP, Carlson CS, Goffin J. The Bryan Cervical Disc: wear properties and early clinical results. Spine J 2004;4(Suppl 6):303S–309S

64. Goffin J, Casey A, Kehr P, et al. Preliminary clinical experience with the Bryan Cervical Disc Prosthesis. Neurosurgery 2002;51:840–845 discussion 845–847

65. Sekhon LH. Cervical arthroplasty in the management of spondylotic myelopathy. J Spinal Disord Tech 2003;16:307–313

66. Duggal N, Pickett GE, Mitsis DK, Keller JL. Early clinical and biomechanical results following cervical arthroplasty. Neurosurg Focus 2004;17(3):E9

67. Link HD, McAfee PC, Pimenta L. Choosing a cervical disk replacement. Spine J 2004;4(Suppl 6):294S–302S

68. Pimenta L, McAfee PC, Cappuccino A, Bellera FP, Link HD. Clinical experience with the new artificial cervical PCM (Cervitech) disk. Spine J 2004;4(Suppl 6):315S–321S

69. Murrey DB, Darden BV, Laxer EB, et al. Early results of a randomized controlled clinical trial comparing ProDisc-C and ACDF for cervical radiculopathy. Cervical Spine Research Society Annual Meeting Poster, 2004; Charlotte, NC

70. Patel AI, Talbert SD, Lam C, Janssen ME. Comparison of single-level ACDF versus ProDisc-C: preliminary results of a randomized prospective study. Paper presented at: Meeting of the Cervical Spine Research Society, 2004; Boston, MA

71. Willert HG, Buchhorn GH, Fayyazi A, et al. Metal-on-metal bearings and hypersensitivity in patients with artificial hip joints. a clinical and histomorphological study. J Bone Joint Surg Am 2005;87:28–36

6

Spinal Kinetics Cervical Disc

Daniel H. Kim, Michael L. Reo, Janine Robinson, and Steve Moscaret

◆ **Clinical Use of Artificial Disks**

◆ **Design of the Spinal Kinetics Cervical Disc**

   Polymer Nucleus

   Fiber Annulus

   Sheath

   End Plates

   Keels

   Trial

   Chisel

   Implant Introducer

   Tamp

◆ **Surgical Technique**

◆ **In Vitro Testing**

   Fatigue and Wear Testing

   Static and Dynamic Characterization

   Migration and Expulsion Test

   Biomechanics Cadaver Study

◆ **Preclinical Studies**

◆ **Clinical Feasibility**

◆ **Conclusion**

The spine can succumb to degenerative changes due to skeletal aging or a genetic predisposition. In time, the direct vascular supply to the vertebrae and disks decreases, and both undergo the accumulated effects of axial loading. The rate at which skeletal degenerative changes occur differs on an individual basis, depending in part upon the forces absorbed by the spine throughout an individual's life. The resulting decreases in water and oxygen content, and metabolic efficiency lead to a disk that is more compressed, less elastic, and more prone to tear and rupture. The polysaccharide gel in the nucleus may deteriorate and lead to redistribution of pressure loads. This redistribution may stress the annulus, leading to disk material protrusion or herniation. As the degeneration progresses, the collagen in the disk is altered and the stress-bearing ability of the disk is reduced along with the disk space height.[1] As a result, the biomechanical burden is shifted to the adjacent vertebral structures. At each vertebral level, there are three distinct motion segments—two at the facet joint complex and one at the disk space. Changes in any part of this motion segment are ultimately compensated by the adjoining parts of the functional spine unit.

Ironically, degenerative changes in biological tissues are usually the body's attempt to heal. If damage exceeds the local healing process, a hypermobile spinal segment could lead to further instability. The body's response to instability would be to further immobilize the motion segments of the vertebral elements. This results in osteophyte or spur formation along the ligaments, joint capsule, and peridiskal area. This cascade of degenerative changes was first described by Kirkaldy-Willis and Yong-Hing and can be subdivided into three stages: dysfunction, instability, and restabilization.[2] The stage of dysfunction may involve one or more of the following changes: outer annular tears and separation of the end plate, synovial reaction, and cartilage destruction. The clinical and radiographic findings are minimal or absent. The instability stage involves disk resorption and loss of disk space height. Further, capsular laxity in the facets may develop, leading to subluxation. Clinical and radiographic findings are more apparent. In the restabilization stage, the severe degenerative changes lead to osteophyte formation and stenosis.

As a result of the body's reactive changes, areas around the degenerated motion segment of the vertebral column enlarge with new reactive tissue and bony formation. Unfortunately, these reactive changes, such as formation of osteophytes, and ligamentous and facet hypertrophy, can sometimes lead to neural compression requiring surgical intervention. Furthermore, multiple levels of disk degeneration may lead to the reversal of normal cervical curvature. All of these changes can result in symptoms of pain and weakness, and, ultimately, debilitation.

Degenerative disk disease thus describes a normal process of aging, and thus the term *disease* is perhaps a misnomer. Typically, it represents a natural aging process, rather than a true disease state, which nevertheless can be a painful and debilitating process. Pain arising from this process may be divided into neurocompressive or mechanical on the basis of the anatomical pain generators. The important step in the initial evaluation of patients with neck pain is determining the pain generator and the presence of radiculopathy, myelopathy, or both.

◆ Clinical Use of Artificial Disks

Total lumbar disk replacements have been used in Europe since the 1980s, with reported clinical success similar to interbody fusions despite the lack of long-term prospective randomized clinical trials.[3,4] The SB Charité (DePuy Spine, Raynham, MA, a Johnson & Johnson Company) is currently the most widely implanted total disk replacement. In 2005, the SB Charité was approved for commercialization by the U.S. Food and Drug Administration (FDA). In addition, there are other prospective randomized studies ongoing in the United States for lumbar artificial disks.

Enthusiasm for cervical arthroplasty came about in the late 1990s. The first human trial involving a cervical prosthesis was reported in 1998.[5] The Prestige (Medtronic Sofamor Danek, Memphis, TN), formerly known as the Bristol disk, is a two-piece stainless steel metal-on-metal design. A British trial comparing the Bristol disk versus autologous graft fusion demonstrated increase in adjacent-level movement in the fusion group as compared with the Bristol disk group at 1-year follow-up.[6] Medtronic's Bryan Cervical Disc, another investigational device, consists of a polyurethane nucleus that is situated between two end plates. As with the lumbar artificial disks, there are multiple, prospective, randomized cervical disk trials ongoing in the United States.

◆ Design of the Spinal Kinetics Cervical Disc

The Spinal Kinetics Cervical Disc (Spinal Kinetics, Inc., Redwood City, CA) is a novel artificial disk that is intuitively designed to replicate the natural disk (**Fig. 6–1**). It will maintain the appropriate motion and resistance of a functional spinal unit when the natural disk has become diseased and needs to be removed. Essential to replicating the natural motion and resistance is the assembly of the core construct, which is made of an elastomeric material that is surrounded by a redundant polymer fiber construct. The compressible core is designed to simulate the function of a nucleus and the

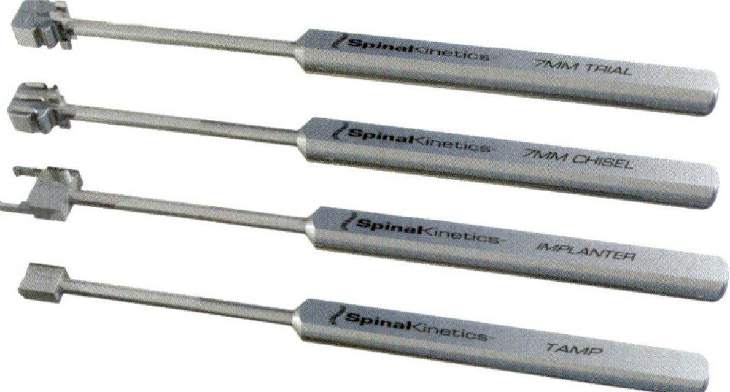

Figure 6–2   Spinal Kinetics Instruments consist of the Trial, Chisel, Implant Introducer, and Tamp.

fibers are designed to simulate the annulus. These are attached to titanium alloy end plates in a unique manner that allows the physiological range of motion in flexion, extension, lateral bending, and axial rotation, as well as compression. The core and fibers work in concert to produce this physiological motion and stiffness. The disk also has a polymer sheath encasing the core and fiber construct to inhibit any tissue ingrowth, as well as capture potential wear debris. The superior and inferior end plates are attached to the vertebral body via three small keels on each end plate. The end plates and keels are coated with titanium plasma spray to promote osseointegration. The Spinal Kinetics Cervical Disc system consists of six components (Polymer Nucleus, Fiber Annulus, Sheath, End Plates, Keels) that are intended to be used with the Spinal Kinetics Instruments (Trial, Chisel, Implant Introducer, Tamp) (**Fig. 6–2**).

Polymer Nucleus

The Polymer Nucleus replicates a natural nucleus in stiffness and, in part, modes of motion. It is constructed from polyurethane that has optimized properties to match the natural disk's stiffness.

Fiber Annulus

The Fiber Annulus simulates a human annulus by providing "semiconstrained" or "physiologically constrained" modes of motion. It is assembled from high tensile strength polymeric fibers wound in four redundant layers around the Polymer Nucleus.

Sheath

The Sheath is a tissue barrier for the Fiber Annulus and Polymer Nucleus. It also inhibits the migration of potential wear debris from the assembly of the Polymer Nucleus and Fiber Annulus. It is a polyurethane component similar to the Polymer Nucleus.

End Plates

The End Plates are the bone interface and rigid support for the entire assembly. On the superior and inferior surfaces of the end plate, commercially pure titanium is coated via a plasma

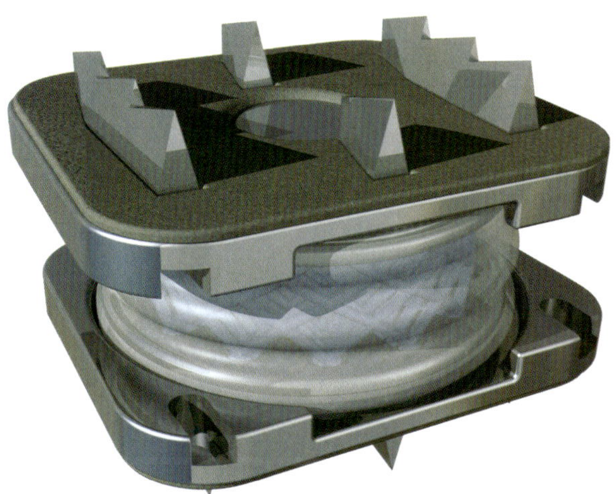

Figure 6–1   The Spinal Kinetics Cervical Disc is a novel, artificial disk that is intuitively designed to replicate the natural disk.

spray for the purpose of osseointegration. The end plates are symmetrical relative to the caudal and cephalad directions.

Keels

The Keels are three anterior-posterior-oriented features on the end plates. The Keels provide acute fixation while healing proceeds.

Trial

The Trial is designed to assist the surgeon in confirming the appropriate Spinal Kinetics Cervical Disc size and location.

Chisel

The Chisel is designed to create grooves into the superior and inferior vertebral body end plates for insertion of the Spinal Kinetics Cervical Disc keels.

Implant Introducer

The Implant Introducer, to which the Spinal Kinetics Cervical Disc is attached, is designed to aid the surgeon in deploying the disk into the intervertebral disk space.

Tamp

The Tamp facilitates final positioning of the implant within the intervertebral space.

◆ Surgical Technique

The patient is positioned supine. After general endotracheal anesthesia, the head is placed in a foam headrest. A rolled sheet is placed behind the shoulders to extend the neck and support the lordotic cervical curve. The left-sided approach is preferred to minimize recurrent laryngeal nerve injury. For C5–C6 and C6–C7 levels, the incision is placed at the level of the cricoid cartilage. A prominent bony tubercle on the C6 transverse process can be palpated to help guide incision placement. A transverse skin incision is made from the midline to the lateral edge of the sternocleidomastoid muscle (SCM). The platysma muscle is divided transversely. The medial border of the SCM and carotid sheath are retracted laterally, in this case to the patient's left side. The omohyoid and sternothyroid muscles are then retracted medially along with the trachea and esophagus. An 18 gauge needle is inserted into the C5–C6 intervertebral disk space and fluoroscopy is used to localize the desired level. A self-retaining retractor system is positioned as shown in Fig. 6–3. Blade teeth are inserted underneath the longus colli muscles. A second retractor with longer, smooth-tipped blades is positioned perpendicularly to the placed retractors to complete the exposure. Caspar distraction pins are placed into the midportions of the vertebral bodies above and below the operative disk space in a cephalad angle. The disk space is distracted via the use of distractor pins. A rectangular opening is created by incising the anterior longitudinal ligament and annulus at the desired level. The anterior and marginal osteophytes should be removed to facilitate implant insertion

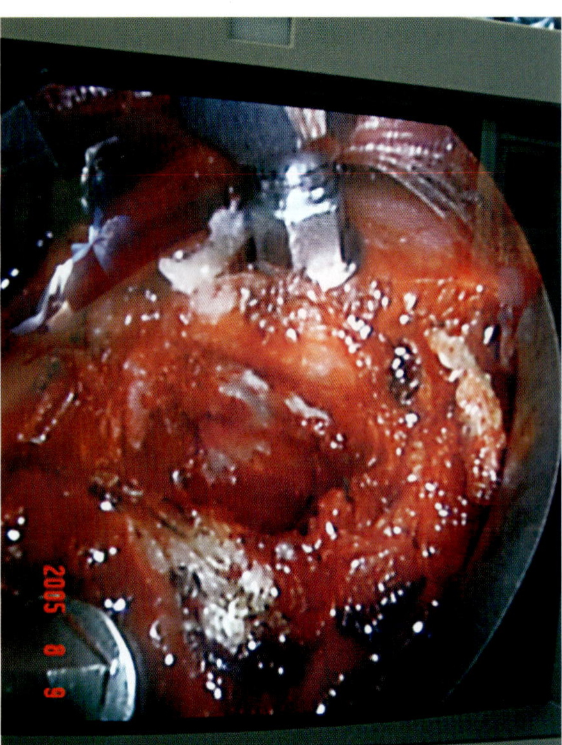

Figure 6–3   A diskectomy has been performed.

and positioning. A complete and effective posterior/lateral decompression is critical for the long-term effectiveness of any artificial disk. Care should be taken to minimize excessive end plate preparation because this could weaken the subchondral bone resulting in possible disk implant subsidence. Once the diskectomy is completed (**Fig. 6–3**) the Trial is inserted to determine the appropriate size and position of the implant (**Fig. 6–4**). After implant sizing is determined the

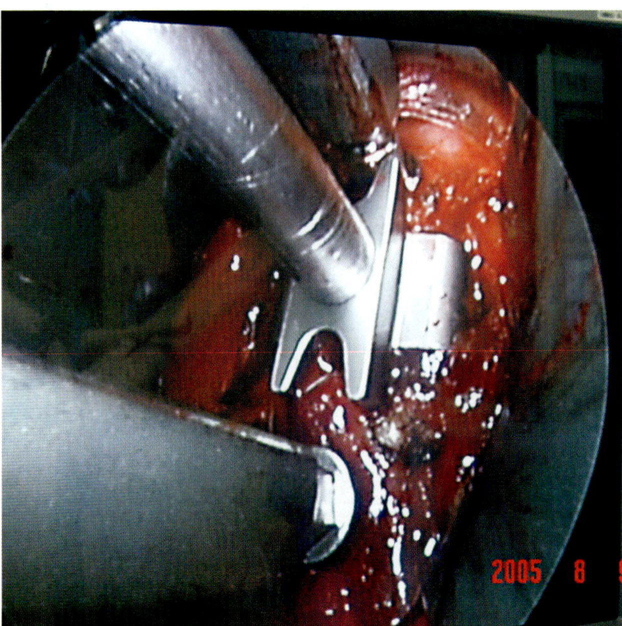

Figure 6–4   The Spinal Kinetics Cervical Disk Trial is inserted to determine the appropriate size and position of the implant.

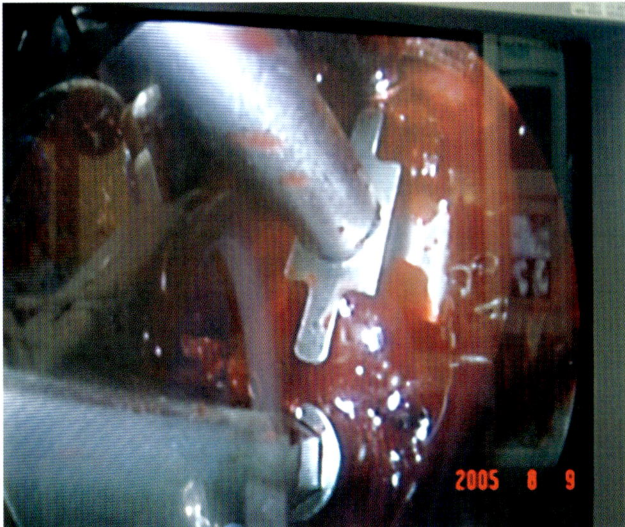

Figure 6–5   Under radiographic guidance the Chisel is tapped into the superior and inferior vertebral end plates creating the channels for the acute fixation keels on the implant.

Trial is removed and the Chisel is introduced (**Fig. 6–5**). Under radiographic guidance the Chisel is tapped into the superior and inferior vertebral end plates, creating the channels for the acute fixation keels on the implant. The Chisel is removed after proper posterior positioning has been achieved via radiographic assessment. The Spinal Kinetics Cervical Disc is a one-piece implant that is loaded into the Implant Introducer (**Figs. 6–6, 6–7**). The keels on the implant

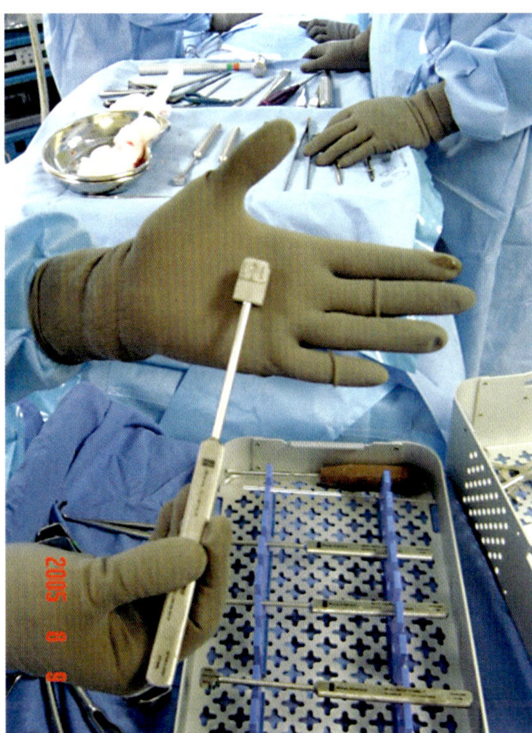

Figure 6–6   The Implant Introducer, to which the Spinal Kinetics Cervical Disc is attached, is designed to aid the surgeon in deploying the disk into the intervertebral disk space.

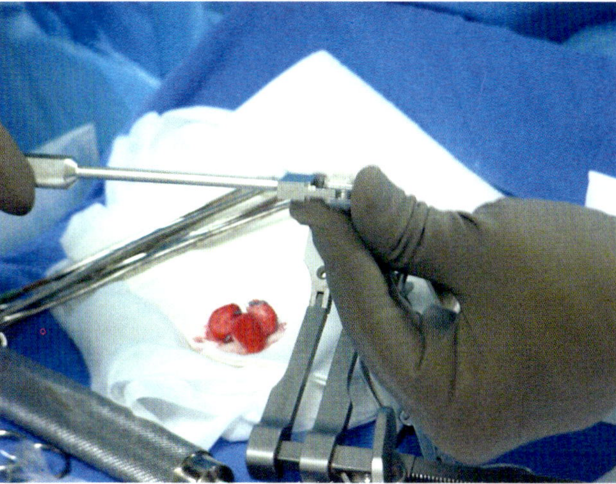

Figure 6–7   Preparing to insert the disk into the intervertebral disk space.

are aligned with the grooves that were cut by the Chisel. Under radiographic guidance the implant is tapped into the vertebral segment. Final positioning of the implant is assessed from a lateral and anteroposterior (AP) radiographic view. The Tamp may be used to facilitate any additional implant positioning as needed within the intervertebral space. Distraction pins and retractors are removed and hemostasis is carefully performed. The platysmal layer is closed separately with fine, absorbable sutures. Fine interrupted subcuticular stitches are used next to cosmetically reapproximate the skin.

◆ In Vitro Testing

The Spinal Kinetics Cervical Disc underwent a comprehensive set of studies to evaluate the performance and safety of the device.

Fatigue and Wear Testing

The Spinal Kinetics Cervical Disc underwent challenging fatigue- and wear-testing verification in flexion-extension and lateral bending and torsion to ascertain the functional and wear debris characteristics of the device. The device was tested at an appropriate cycling frequency through a minimum 10 million cycles in a physiological solution under a preload. Periodically, the testing solution was removed with the wear debris and evaluated for size, shape, quantity, and material composition of the debris.

Static and Dynamic Characterization

The Spinal Kinetics Cervical Disc underwent testing to generate fatigue-life characterization curve of load versus number of cycles in compression, compression-shear, and torsional modes of motion (**Fig. 6–8**). The dynamic testing ran through 10 million cycles at its high cycle limit, and it was conducted in a physiological solution at appropriate loads and torques. Static testing was conducted to characterize maximum functional or mechanical failure limits.

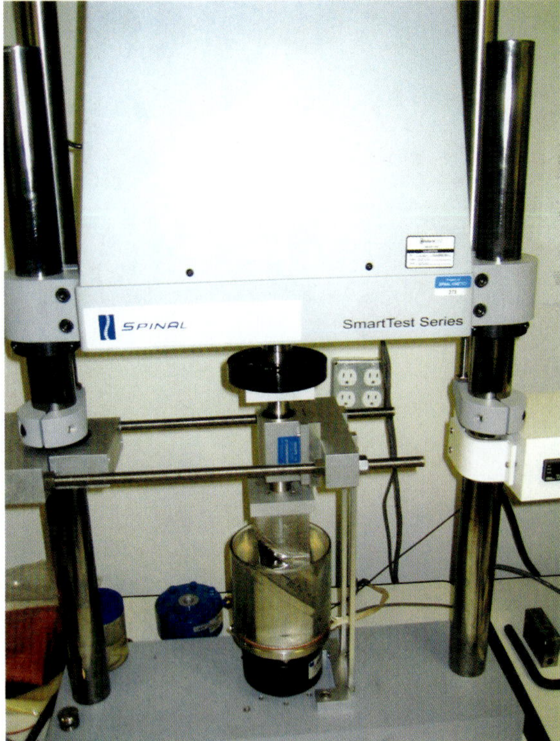

Figure 6–8 The Spinal Kinetics Cervical Disc underwent testing to generate fatigue-life characterization curve of load versus number of cycles in compression, compression-shear, and torsional modes of motion. The dynamic testing ran through 10 million cycles at its high cycle limit, and it was conducted in a physiological solution at appropriate loads and torques. Static testing was conducted to characterize maximum functional or mechanical failure limits.

Migration and Expulsion Test

The Spinal Kinetics Cervical Disc is designed with Acute Fixation Technology (AFT) to ensure adequate purchase with the bone post implantation. However, it is beneficial to demonstrate that fixation up to the point of bone formation. The migration and expulsion testing was designed to study the movement of the disk replacement in cadaver bone through a natural range of motion under normal and excessive loads.

Biomechanics Cadaver Study

Range of motion, stiffness, torque, and instantaneous axis of rotation (IAR) are some of the key aspects of a total artificial disk's (TAD's) biomechanical performance. The Spinal Kinetics Cervical Disc has undergone this testing to show its performance relative to the natural disk and competitive technologies.

Results from all in vitro tests demonstrated that the Spinal Kinetics Cervical Disc is physiological, safe, and robust in its design and function.

◆ Preclinical Studies

The Spinal Kinetics Cervical Disc was studied in a caprine animal model for the purposes of evaluating the biological response in the spine region of an animal model. Disk

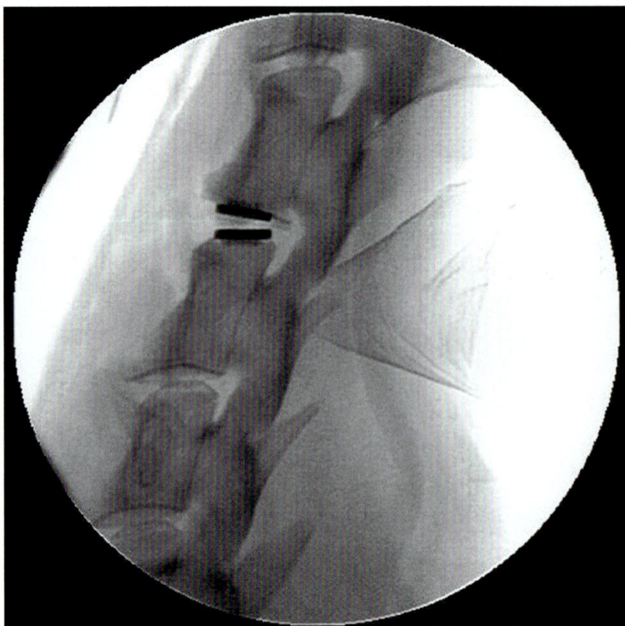

Figure 6–9 The Spinal Kinetics Cervical Disc was studied in a caprine animal model for the purpose of evaluating the biological response in the spine region of an animal model. Disk implantation consisted of single- and double-level procedures. Pictured here is the single-level procedure.

implantation consisted of single- and double-level procedures (**Fig. 6–9**). Tissue analysis was conducted for the functional spine units, including the spinal cord, perivertebral tissues, regional draining lymph nodes, liver lobe, and spleen, all of which were prepared for histological analysis. There were neither significant microscopic lesions nor any particulate material for any of the tissue samples. The amount of osseointegration and attachment was determined to be commensurate with the duration of implantation (**Fig. 6–10**).

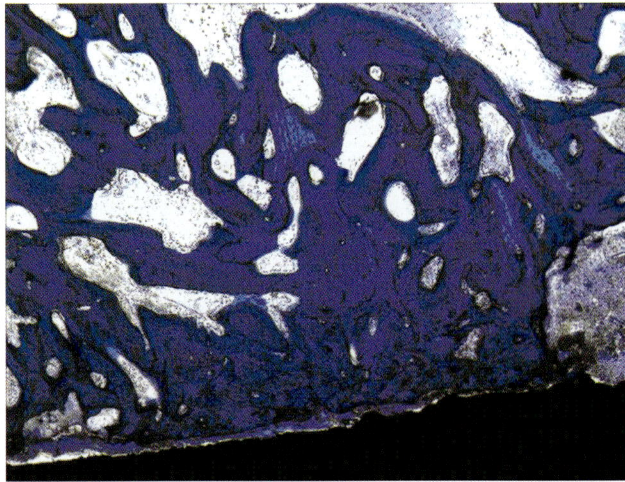

Figure 6–10 Tissue analysis was conducted for the functional spine units, including the spinal cord, perivertebral tissues, regional draining lymph nodes, liver lobe, and spleen, all of which were prepared for histological analysis. There were neither significant microscopic lesions nor any particulate material for any of the tissue samples. The amount of osseointegration and attachment was determined to be commensurate with the duration of implantation.

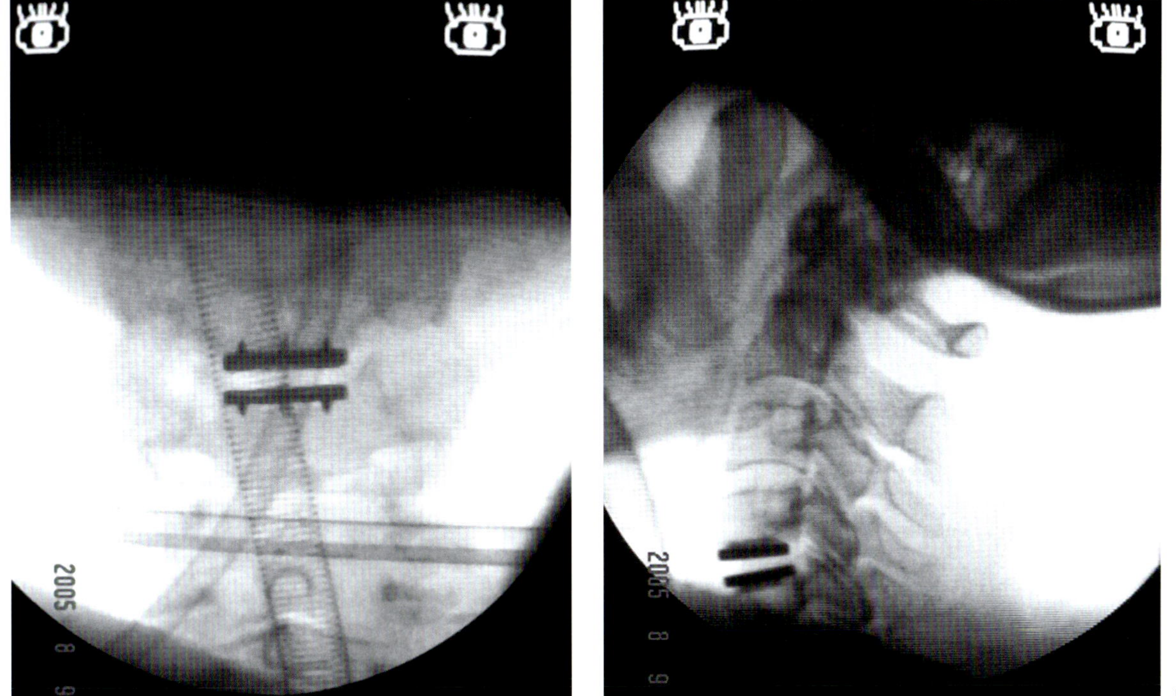

Figure 6–11   **(A)** Anteroposterior intraoperative image. **(B)** Lateral intraoperative image.

◆ Clinical Feasibility

Spinal Kinetics initiated a nonrandomized clinical feasibility trial outside the United States with a follow-up at 6 weeks and 3 months postprocedure. The primary objective of this study was to determine the preliminary safety and feasibility of the Spinal Kinetics Cervical Disc for use with patients undergoing single-level (**Fig. 6–11A,B**) or two-level cervical spinal procedures, as measured by overall patient success. Pain assessment and quality of life questionnaires were administered during the follow-up period to determine patient satisfaction and qualitative pain relief. Neurological exams, neck disability index, and SF-36 scoring were administered to determine overall procedural success and patient satisfaction. Radiographic follow-up was also completed for each patient at 6 weeks and 3 months postprocedure. Implanted disk levels as well as adjacent levels were assessed in flexion-extension and lateral bending (**Fig. 6–12A,B**). At the time of this writing,

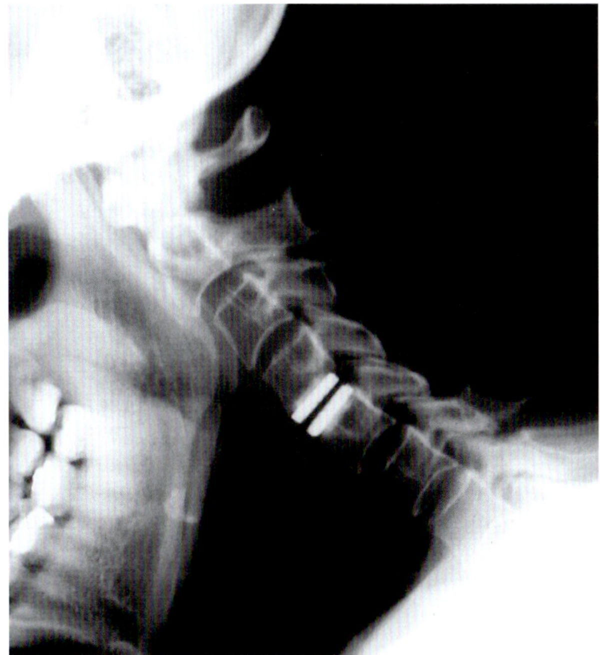

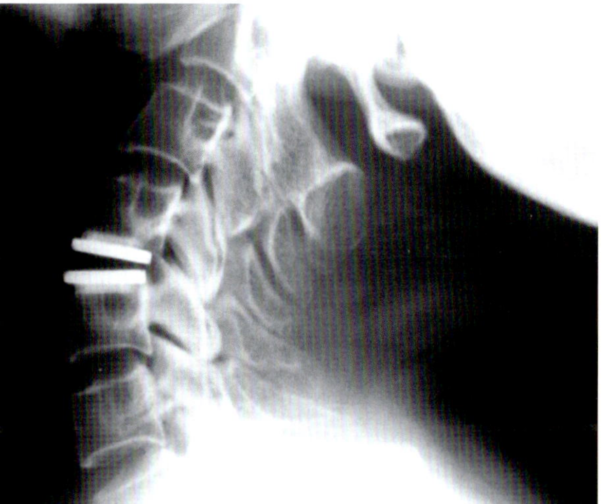

Figure 6–12   **(A)** Six-week flexion radiograph. **(B)** Six-week extension radiograph.

preliminary results were being gathered for the 6-week and 3-month follow-up on these initial patients.

Also at the time of this writing, a prospective, randomized, clinical trial protocol for the Spinal Kinetics Cervical Disc was under review by the U.S. FDA.

◆ Conclusion

The Spinal Kinetics Cervical Disc is a true next-generation total disk replacement. It addresses the biomechanics of a natural disk by incorporating an artificial fiber annulus and compressible nucleus. Currently, the Spinal Kinetics Cervical Disc is embarking on extensive international clinical work and will commence a U.S. clinical trial. The results of the initial clinical work show the Spinal Kinetics Cervical Disc to be a safe device that has demonstrated beneficial outcomes for the patient. To date, there have been no device-related complications, and a future planned prospective, randomized, clinical trial these authors believe will demonstrate the continued safety and effectiveness of the Spinal Kinetics Cervical Disc.

References

1. Naylor A. Intervertebral disk prolapse and degeneration: the biochemical and biophysical approach. Spine 1976;1:108–114
2. Kirkaldy-Willis WH, Yong-Hing K. The pathophysiology of degenerative disease of the lumbar spine. Orthop Clin North Am 1983;14:491–504
3. Griffith SL, Shelokov AP, Buttner-Janz K, LeMaire JP, Zeegers WS. A multicenter retrospective study of the clinical results of the LINK SB Charité intervertebral prosthesis: the initial European experience. Spine 1994;19:1842–1849
4. Lemaire JP, Skalli W, Lavaste F, et al. Intervertebral disk prosthesis: results and prospects for the year 2000. Clin Orthop Relat Res 1997;337:64–76
5. Cummins BH, Robertson JT, Gill SS. Surgical experience with an implanted artificial cervical joint [see comment]. J Neurosurg 1998;88:943–948
6. Wigfield CC, Nelson RJ. Nonautologous interbody fusion materials in cervical spine surgery: how strong is the evidence to justify their use? Spine 2001;26:687–694

7

Bryan Cervical Disc Device

Robert Hacker

◆ **Bryan Cervical Disc Features**

◆ **The Bryan Arthroplasty Procedure**
  Preoperative Planning
  Operative Setup
  Site Preparation
  Neural Element Decompression
  Device Placement

◆ **Clinical Experience**
  Methods
  Outcome Assessment
  Results

◆ **Summary**

The treatment of degenerative cervical disk disorders is one of the most satisfying aspects of a neurosurgeon's or an orthopedic spine surgeon's practice. In general, those patients with pathology requiring surgical treatment present with classic findings, complaints, and imaging studies that make the diagnosis of myelopathy and radiculopathy due to disk disease straightforward. The surgical options commonly employed have been extensively studied and their efficacy and safety are well documented. Most importantly, patient outcomes are uniformly satisfying with acceptable morbidity and a mortality rate well below 1%.[1,2] In light of the endorsement of the current surgical treatment of degenerative cervical disk disorders, one could reasonably wonder why an entirely new approach such as cervical disk arthroplasty need be considered.

The impetus to pursue arthroplasty in the cervical spine is not due to outright failure of current surgical options. Rather, it arises from a desire to avoid the shortcomings and inherent morbidities that accompany those approaches.

In the treatment of radiculopathy and myelopathy, ventral removal of compressive disk space lesions is easily achieved with an anterior microdiskectomy. However, subsequent fusion eliminates the motion segment, changing spinal biomechanics in the process. Adjacent segment hypermobility and progressive adjacent segment degeneration have been documented in several reports. Hilibrand et al looked at adjacent segment disease following cervical arthrodesis.[3,4] They noted symptomatic disease defined as new onset radiculopathy or myelopathy appropriate for surgical treatment occurring annually in nearly 3% of their patients.[3] Radiographic evidence of adjacent segment degeneration can be much higher. Goffin et al found more than 90% of patients treated with fusion had evidence of adjacent segment degenerative disk disease 5 years after surgery.[5] Whether or not adjacent segment degenerative disk disease is accelerated by

fusion or simply an expression of multilevel degenerative disease has not been conclusively answered in the medical literature. Perhaps tilting the scales in favor of fusion as a significant contributing factor is further consideration of Goffin et al's paper.[5] They compared rates of subsequent adjacent segment disease in patients fused for degenerative disk disease to those undergoing fusion for trauma and found no significant difference. Thus fusion appears to be an independent variable in regard to the breakdown of the adjacent segment because the trauma patients were not undergoing an operation for a degenerative condition.

Sagittal plane balance is frequently altered with anterior cervical procedures. Subsidence of the interbody fusion graft and kyphosis of the fused segment are known iatrogenic deformities associated with the fusion procedure.[6,7] This loss of lordosis may hasten adjacent segment degeneration because changes to both local and distant intervertebral alignment will alter biomechanics of the spine.

Even when fusion does not accompany anterior cervical diskectomy, loss or impairment of mobility of the treated segment is predictable. In one study, ~90% of patients treated with anterior microdiskectomy without arthrodesis went on to spontaneous fusion, with most experiencing kyphotic change.[8] Anterolateral foraminotomy has been advocated by a few authors as a method of preserving the disk while providing decompression.[9,10] The procedure removes the ipsilateral uncovertebral joint or portions of it to expose and remove the offending pathology. Excellent results have been reported by one surgeon retrospectively reviewing his own results.[9] However, the procedure has not enjoyed uniform success. Another report showed that reoperation was required in 30% of the patients treated with that procedure. In addition, the same authors found only 52% of their patients experienced good or excellent outcomes.[11]

A posterior approach such as laminoforaminotomy may be considered as an option for neural element decompression that does not compromise the motion segment. Although this approach can provide satisfying results for foraminal disk herniations, many surgeons are uncomfortable applying this technique to large or medially positioned lesions, especially if osteophytic change is recognized.

Other morbidity associated with anterior cervical fusion depends on the choices the surgeon makes in regard to technique. Iliac crest graft harvest is associated with chronic hip pain in nearly 30% of patients.[12] Plate fixation, currently in vogue, has been shown to contribute to dysphagia, especially when thick or rough-surfaced plates are used.[13] Finally, pseudarthrosis is a well-known complication of anterior cervical fusion. Depending on graft material, number of levels fused, and smoking history, a pseudarthrosis rate as high as 50% has been reported.[14] The treatment of pseudarthrosis often necessitates a second operation. Another drawback of fusion is the months of activity restriction that most surgeons impose postoperatively on their patients. This has little to do with the recovery from radiculopathy or myelopathy. Rather, this convalescent period is imposed to achieve a solid fusion.

Avoiding fusion may be motivation enough to entertain a surgical alternative without even considering the issue of motion preservation. Absent degenerative deformity or instability, fusion is performed primarily to mitigate the iatrogenic damage created during decompression for treatment of radiculopathy and myelopathy.

◆ Bryan Cervical Disc Features

Cervical disk arthroplasty devices are classified according to their makeup. Composed of polymer (polyurethane core) and metal (titanium end plates), the Bryan Cervical Disc prosthesis (Medtronic Sofamor Danek, Memphis, TN) is categorized as a metal-on-poly device (**Fig. 7–1**). Currently, all other metal-on-poly cervical arthroplasty devices have ultra high molecular weight polyethylene (UHMWPE) cores. UHMWPE has a higher modulus of elasticity than polyurethane, making it less compressible.[15] The compressibility of the Bryan core allows it to accommodate sudden axial loads, similar to a shock absorber on an automobile. The dome-shaped, polished titanium end plates are merged with a polyurethane sheath. The sheath prevents fibrous tissue ingrowth and contains particulate debris generated by the moving surfaces. Located inside this shell is the donut-shaped polyurethane nucleus. At the top and bottom of the device are filling ports that allow sterile saline instillation prior to insertion. The saline functions as a lubricant. The device is axially symmetric and also symmetric in a caudad to cephalad direction.

Stability of insertion describes the resistance the device has to extrusion before biological incorporation occurs. For the Bryan disk, this is dependent on fixed interspace distraction and a drilling tool that "mills" concavities in the adjacent vertebral body end plates that conform to the device's dome-shaped titanium end plates. Ligamentous tension from distraction of the interspace combined with the milled vertebral body end plates results in an interference or a "hand in glove" fit providing initial stability. No screw fixation is utilized with the Bryan device. Ultimately, fixation depends on bony ingrowth into the porous end plates. Ingrowth is a feature found solely with the Bryan device. Currently, other cervical arthroplasty devices that rely on biological fixation use a titanium plasma spray that is an ongrowth surface.

The Bryan disk is axially symmetric and unconstrained in the normal range of cervical spine motion. It also has a mobile center of rotation like a normal cervical disk. Device flexion and extension of 11 degrees can occur on an infinite number of radii. The device allows for coupled motions of angulation and rotation. These parameters, combined with translation of up to 2 mm, allow the Bryan disk to mimic normal disk function. As mentioned earlier, the Bryan device is also able to absorb sudden axial loads. This is unique among cervical arthroplasty devices.

Like all implanted devices, particularly those that incorporate motion, some degree of device deterioration and component debris is expected with cervical disk arthroplasty. With repetitive motion a certain amount of the device's mass will be shed into the surrounding tissues, with the potential for distant transport as well. Particulate matter is of concern in synovial joint arthroplasty and has been linked to osteolysis and subsequent implant failure. The disk space is classified as an amphiarthrodial joint. It does not have a synovium. Instead, it is connected to bony surfaces by fibrous and cartilaginous tissue only.

Because the joint lacks synovium, concerns for a focal reaction to wear debris are not as acute. Although particle toxicity or an immune response to debris is a potential concern, the materials in the Bryan device have a long history of orthopedic and cardiac surgery usage without undue concern about toxicity.[16] Debris created from the articulation between the nucleus and the metallic end plates is theoretically contained by the sheath, preventing a biological reaction.

Detailed wear analysis within a motion simulator showed that after 10 million cycles the Bryan device lost 0.75% of its mass. Animal studies found debris in the tissues in one of two chimpanzees and four of nine goats. All goats were implanted

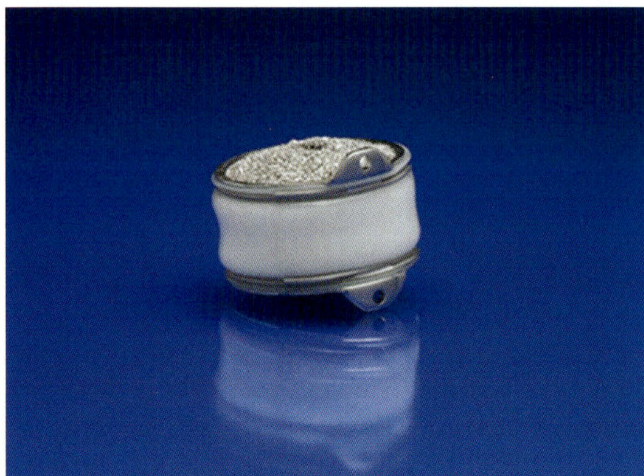

Figure 7–1 The Bryan disk device has porous titanium end plates that promote bony ingrowth. Device diameters range from 14 to 18 mm with one height. The metal tabs on the right side of the figure attach to the insertion instrument and also eliminate the risk of device migration into the central canal.

with the spine in a flexed orientation, creating a worst-case environment for sheath abrasion against posterior bone unique to the goat model. Particle generation and release were achieved, allowing the development team to evaluate particle morphology and biological response. Particles averaging 3.9 m were noted in the loose connective tissue of the epidural space without an inflammatory response. This is in contrast to control group animals with cervical plates that had more debris and inflammatory responses identified.[16]

Of the several thousand Bryan devices implanted, thus far only one report describing device explantation has appeared in the literature.[17] In that report, 11 devices were removed from patients either for ongoing pain not relieved by the index procedure or for treatment of an infection. On average, devices had been implanted for 1 year. Laboratory evaluation of those devices showed no evidence of oxidative degradation or instability of the core.

◆ The Bryan Arthroplasty Procedure

Common to all arthroplasty procedures is the need for exacting placement technique. Suboptimal position will impair full range of motion of any arthroplasty device. Poor positioning may alter wear characteristics and increase the risk of device extrusion. Because initial insertion stability of the device is related to close approximation of the domed device end plates to the concavities that are milled in the opposing vertebral body end plates, site preparation is a critical portion of the operation. There are five separate phases to the Bryan cervical disk arthroplasty procedure: preoperative planning, operative setup, arthroplasty site preparation, neural element decompression, and device placement.

Preoperative Planning

Besides the usual selection criteria for cervical spine surgery, the surgeon should determine that the candidate has preserved motion at the anticipated treatment level prior to considering arthroplasty as a treatment option. A device is unlikely to return motion to a partially or completely autoarthrodesed segment. Loss of sagittal plane balance on preoperative cervical spine radiographs should be carefully considered because the arthroplasty Bryan device is not able to restore a loss of lordosis. If kyphosis is thought to contribute to the patient's symptoms the device may not be as good a surgical choice as fusion. Although a stiffer arthroplasty device could conceivably improve sagittal balance, the trade-off would be less mobility and increased concerns about spontaneous fusion.

Sizing the device is easily done with preoperative computed tomographic (CT) or magnetic resonance imaging (MRI) scan. Given that the vertebral bodies are distracted and shaped to a predetermined height, only the diameter is measured. This step establishes presumptive sizing only because the implant size is determined intraoperatively.

Operative Setup

This includes those steps that occur in the operating room prior to making an incision. The surgeon must use lateral fluoroscopy to ensure that the patient's position on the table is consistent with the neutral cervical spine posture. When a surgeon performs an anterior cervical fusion, the patient's neck is typically extended. That inclination must be avoided with arthroplasty. If the patient's neck is extended prior to arthroplasty, the device will be flexed when the patient assumes a neutral posture. Because the device allows for 11 degrees of flexion, a portion of the device's overall flexion capacity would already be used prior to the patient attempting to bend the neck forward. Thus the patient would not have full flexion. Similarly, if the patient's neck is flexed at the time of device insertion, neutral posture will cause the device to be extended and the amount of further extension will be limited.

Of equal importance is the ability to see the entire operative area on lateral fluoroscopy. Taping of the shoulders is nearly always required for any large patient or when insertion is planned at the C6–C7 level. To aid in positioning the device accurately from right to left, an anteroposterior view is obtained to avoid rotation or tilt of the neck. Once lateral fluoroscopy is established, a scout lateral fluoroscopic view with a goniometer (essentially a plumb line attached to a ruler) fixed to the image intensifier is obtained. This view aids in determining the "angle" of the intervertebral disk. Rarely is the patient positioned such that the disk space is perpendicular to the floor. In most cases, the disk space inclines such that ventral to dorsal movement deeper into the disk interspace also results in caudad to cephalad movement. To ensure that the device properly contacts the vertebral end plates, the surgeon must position the device parallel to the interspace. Most often an angle of 15 to 20

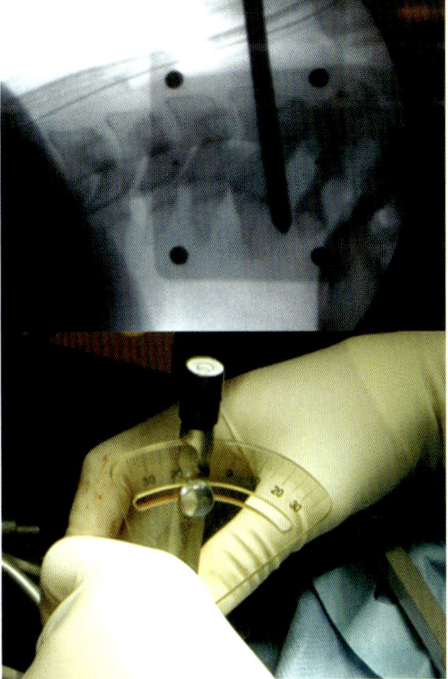

Figure 7–2 Prior to making an incision, a goniometer is used to measure the angle of the interspace relative to a true perpendicular approach (above). Intraoperatively, a bubble level is used with the angle measurement tool to ensure a parallel approach to the interspace (below).

degrees is encountered (**Fig. 7–2**). The fluoroscope is also helpful in placing the skin incision.

Site Preparation

A standard skin incision is fashioned on the surgeon's preferred working side with sharp dissection to the proposed interspace. The author most often follows the plane of dissection along the medial border of the omohyoid muscle. Identifying the superior laryngeal nerve for procedures at the C3–C4 level and dividing the superior thyroid artery for procedures at C6–C7 are helpful. Handheld retractors are used during initial exposure and mobilization of the soft tissues. The precervical fascia is opened to the disk level above and below the proposed treatment level. The longus colli muscles are reflected so that the bases of the transverse processes at the proposed arthroplasty level are visualized, ensuring adequate dissection for self-retaining retractor placement. The anterior annulus is widely incised. Disk material is debrided, including the cartilaginous end plates. Osteophyte formation at the anterior margin of the superior end plate of the disk space is often removed with a Kerrison rongeur or bur so that interspace distraction later in the procedure doesn't cause asymmetric opening of the interspace. Caution should be exercised during this step because aggressive bone removal will reduce distraction and may result in a loss of lordosis during subsequent steps.

The distraction process commences with sequential placement of instruments that gently stretch the ligamentous attachments of the disk annulus and facet capsules. They are removed and a centering tool accurately defines the midline. Next, a distraction wedge is tamped into the disk space. With the wedge simultaneously distracting the vertebral bodies and acting as an anchor, a frame to direct and hold the power instruments used in subsequent steps is slid over the top of the wedge and secured with posts that screw into the vertebral bodies. This milling guide is positioned parallel to the

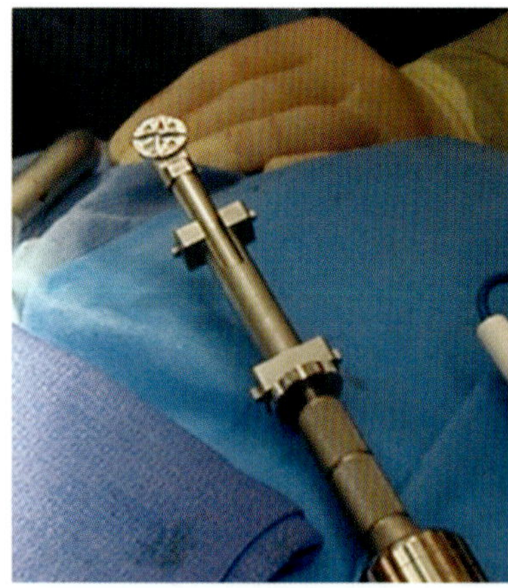

Figure 7–4 The milling disk is attached to the electric drill in preparation for milling of the vertebral body end plates.

disk space. Additional stability for the milling guide is obtained with a table-mounted support arm.

With the milling guide attached, the surgeon uses fluoroscopy to measure the anterior and posterior margins of the disk space (**Fig. 7–3**). This is a critical step to ensure that an appropriate-sized device is selected. Stability and function depend on the device covering as much of the vertebral body diameter as possible and engaging the ring apophysis for support. A small device may be more prone to extrusion and also may not have full motion. The milling guide helps direct a power-driven bur that smoothes the end plates into parallel surfaces. This makes the end plates suitable for the shaping of concavities cephalad and caudad to seat the Bryan disk, which is the next step.

After determining the appropriate size Bryan disk to insert, the device is delivered to the sterile field along with a milling disk (**Fig. 7–4**). The milling disk diameter corresponds to the device diameter. It is essential for preparing the concavities in the vertebral end plates so that the device will be engaged not only by ligamentous compression but by

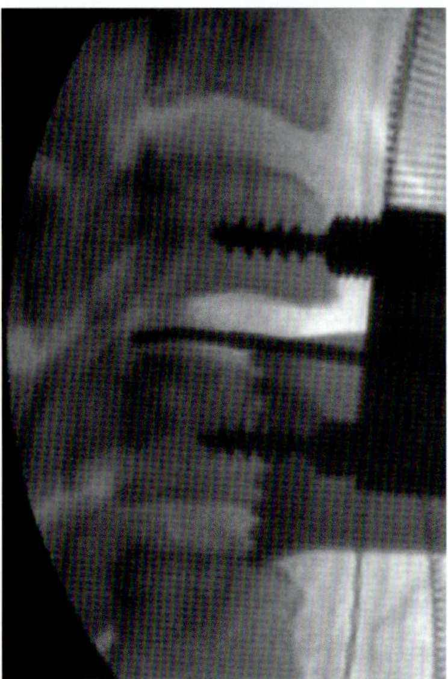

Figure 7–3 Measurement of the posterior margin of the disk space is obtained using fluoroscopy. The milling guide has been secured using threaded anchoring pins.

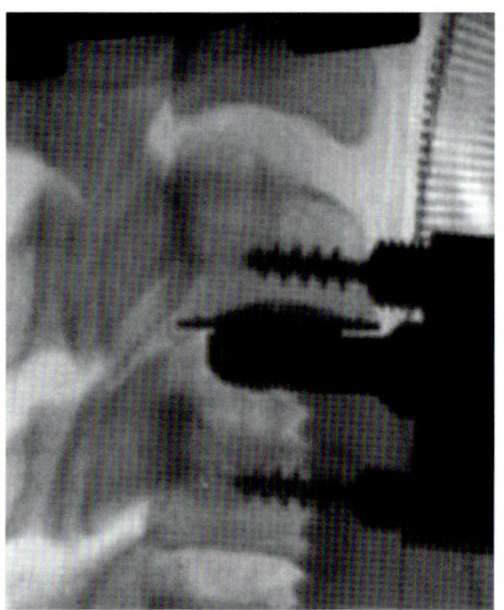

Figure 7–5 In this patient the milling disk is being used to shape the inferior aspect of the C3 vertebral body. The concavity milled corresponds to the domed end plate of the Bryan disk.

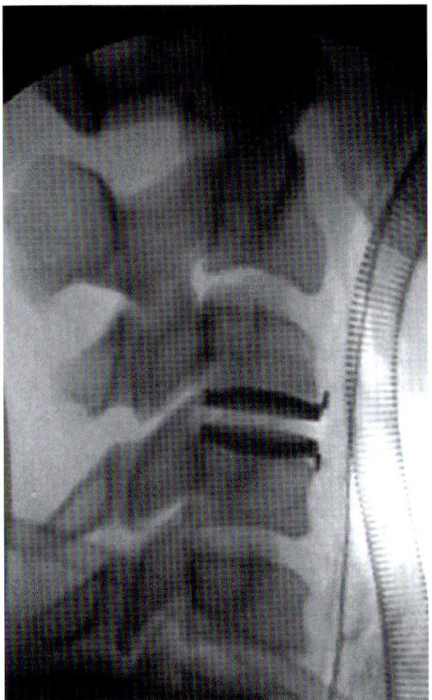

Figure 7–6 The device is seen intraoperatively. Correct sizing ensures that the entire span of the end plate is in contact with the device.

a hand-in-glove approximation of the device surfaces and the end plates. The convex milling tool has positive stops in the milling guide that prevent overpenetration of the end plates. After completing the short milling step, no further site preparation is necessary for device insertion (**Fig. 7–5**).

Neural Element Decompression

This step is essentially the same as for any other anterior diskectomy. An interspace distractor can be slipped over the anchoring posts that previously held the milling guide for additional exposure. The operating microscope is routinely utilized during this part of the procedure. It is the author's preference to take down the posterior longitudinal ligament and annulus and visualize the thecal sac as well as the origin of both nerve roots, resecting the posterior aspect of the uncovertebral joint unilaterally or bilaterally as necessary. Extensive resection of osteophytes at the posterior margin of the disk space and resection of several millimeters of the vertebral body margin may also be performed without compromising the insertion stability of the Bryan device. Hemostasis is achieved with bipolar forceps and powdered hemostatic agents soaked in thrombin. The concavities within the end plates are routinely allowed to have persistent oozing of blood so as not to blunt the biological incorporation of the device.

Device Placement

Device insertion now proceeds with instillation of saline into the Bryan device followed by seal plug placement and fixation of the disk onto the insertion tool. The device is then pressed into the milled concavities in the end plates and released from the insertion tool. Direct inspection and fluoroscopic confirmation of placement take place prior to closure (**Fig. 7–6**).

◆ Clinical Experience

An Investigational Device Exemption (IDE) was granted by the U.S. Food and Drug Administration (FDA) allowing a clinical study of the safety and effectiveness of the Bryan disk device in the United States. The author's experience with the Bryan device is based on participation in that IDE study.

Methods

This was a controlled randomized prospective study with the control group receiving cervical fusion with allograft and plate fixation. The study was limited to patients requiring surgical treatment at one level for either or both radiculopathy and myelopathy, with or without neck pain. Imaging studies were required to confirm disk hernia or spondylotic compression. Treatment was limited to C3–C4 through C6–C7. A minimum of 6 weeks of conservative therapy was required except when myelopathy was identified. Patients with previous cervical spine procedures were excluded. Radiographic evidence of significant degeneration at the proposed treatment level such as a marked loss of height, subluxation, or loss of motion resulted in patient exclusion.

Outcome Assessment

Multiple follow-up evaluations over a 2-year period with radiographs and clinical data looking at the safety and effectiveness of the device compared with a control group formed the basis for assessing outcomes. Achieving success depended on meeting all of the following:

1. Improved pain and function
2. Maintained or improved neurological status
3. Radiographic documentation of device motion
4. Avoidance of adverse events

Outcome measurements included the neck disability index (NDI), patient global assessment (Odom's criteria), (SF-36), and the neurological examination case Report Form. Independent assessment of SF-36 radiographs was performed to evaluate motion.

Results

The author enrolled a total of 55 patients in the clinical study. Of these patients, 27 had Bryan disk devices inserted and 28 underwent anterior fusion. Follow-up is currently ongoing with data collected at 3, 6, 12, and 24 months. Several patients have already reached the 2-year follow-up mark.

The control and investigational groups were quite similar in regard to age, male:female ratio, and preoperative working status. There was a statistically significant difference in regard to smoking, with more smokers in the fusion group. Hospital stay, blood loss, and treated level did not vary significantly between the two groups. Operative time differed between the two groups averaging 52 minutes for the anterior fusion group and 82 minutes for the arthroplasty patients. (**Table 7–1**). The author found that familiarity with

Table 7–1   Treatment Parameters for Control and Experimental Groups

	Surgery and Discharge Information				
	Operative Time (h)	Blood Loss (mL)	Hospital Stay (day)	Treatment Levels (n)	External Orthosis (n)
Investigational	1.4 ± 0.3	46.1 ± 28.6	0.8 ± 0.4	1 C3–C4 2 C4–C5 14 C5–C6 9 C6–C7	27 None, 0 Soft collar
Control	0.9 ± 0.2	56.0 ± 42.6	0.8 ± 0.6	2 C4–C5 16 C5–C6 10 C6–C7	1 None, 27 Soft collar

the procedure resulted in shorter operative times for arthroplasty patients treated later in the study.

Both groups found marked improvement in arm pain compared with their preoperative status (**Fig. 7–7**). SF-36 data, both physical and mental component scores, showed a similar improvement over time for both groups, with the Bryan group showing numerically better values at each data point. Evaluation of neck symptoms using the neck pain and NDI scores showed an interesting outcome. Although both the experimental and the investigational groups showed statistically significant improvement compared with their preoperative status on early postoperative evaluations, only the Bryan disk patients maintained a statistically significant improvement at the 2-year follow-up point (**Fig. 7–8A,B**). No patient in the study suffered a major neurological or systemic complication. Complications recorded included failed fusion which was noted in one control group patient. One arthroplasty patient developed a wound hematoma requiring return to the operating room the same day for evacuation. Another arthroplasty patient ultimately underwent operation for adjacent level radiculopathy and was treated with cervical fusion as dictated by study guidelines. Two patients, one from each group, had transient postoperative dysphonia that completely resolved. One patient who was initially planned for Bryan disk insertion was switched intraoperatively to fusion because thyroid goiter markedly impaired exposure.

Postopertive radiographs confirmed motion in every Bryan disk case (**Fig. 7–9A,B**). No peridiskal calcifications were noted in any case. All patients received ant-inflammatory drugs for 2 weeks postoperatively, which appears to eliminate heterotopic calcifications. Some authors have reported improved motion postoperatively with the Bryan disk. They opine that relief of preoperative neck and arm pain allows for a return of motion.[18] A comparison of preoperative and postoperative films in the author's series showed essentially identical motion on 1-year follow-up x-rays. Films taken earlier occasionally showed increased motion that returned to preoperative levels by 1 year.

Other authors have reported their experience with the Bryan device as well. Goffin et al have published their results with the Bryan disk device. They found 93% of the patients in their single-level study showed motion ≥ 2 degrees. The effectiveness of the device was evaluated considering each patient's pain, neurological examination, and range of motion on x-rays. Eighty-five percent of their series was regarded as having a successful outcome.[19] Similar results were reported by Lafuente et al with 91% of their Bryan disk patients maintaining motion on x-rays at 1-year follow-up. They also noted "highly significant improvement" in visual analog scores, SF-36, and NDI postoperatively.[20]

Goffin et al provided extended follow-up data on 82 of their original study patients seen 2 years after surgical treat-

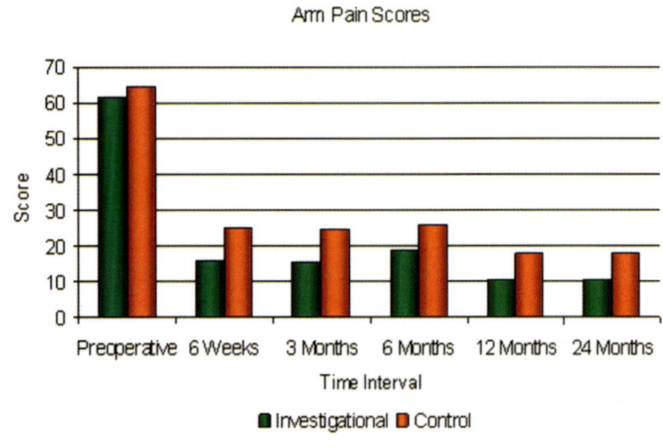

Figure 7–7 Results of arm pain for the control and device groups in the author's study.

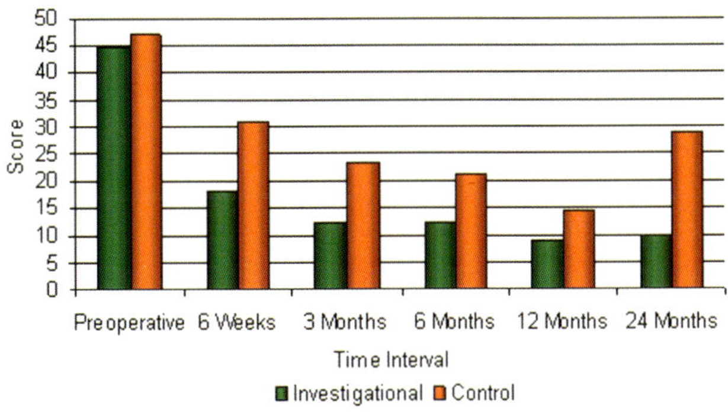

A

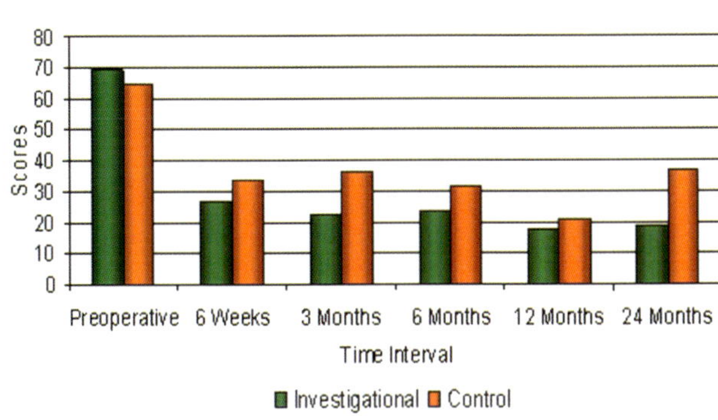

B

Figure 7–8 Results of **(A)** neck pain and **(B)** neck disability index. Significantly better results are noted in the Bryan patients for both parameters at 2 years.

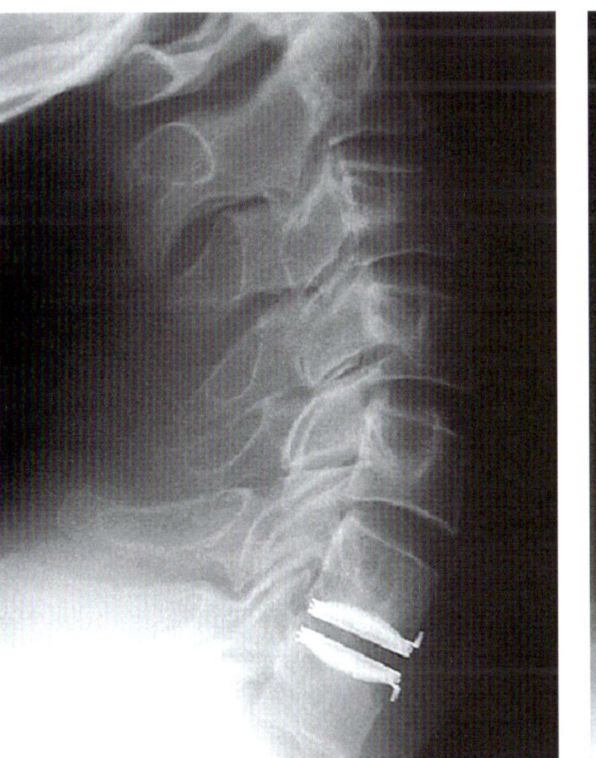

A

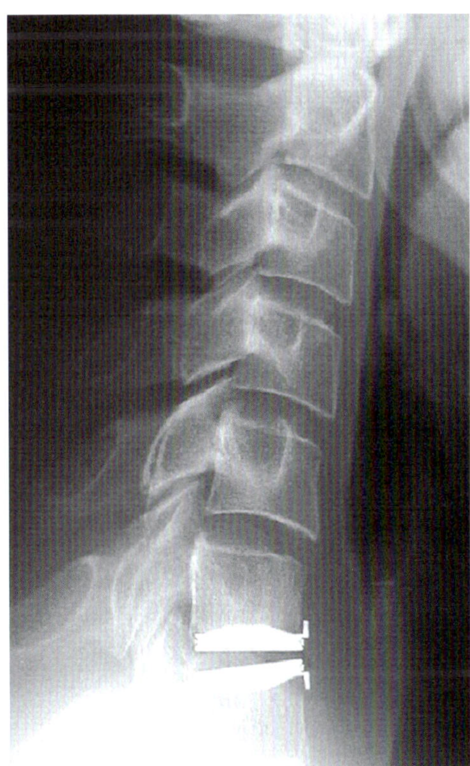

B

Figure 7–9 **(A)** Flexion and **(B)** extension lateral views after placement of a Bryan disk at C6–C7. At 1 year, range of motion was identical to preoperative motion films.

ment. They found preserved motion in 86% with continued satisfying results.[21] Four-year follow-up data available on 27 of these patients suggest improvement is enduring. Of the 26 with motion present preoperatively, 23 patients showed preserved mobility at the 4-year mark.[22]

◆ Summary

Worldwide, the Bryan disk device has been implanted in a 10-fold greater number of patients than all other cervical arthroplasty devices combined. The author's personal experience and that of others suggests the device is safe and effective for degenerative cervical disk disorders associated with myelopathy and radiculopathy. Whether the device will play a role in the treatment of neck pain as an isolated entity remains to be studied. Although the results of a com-prehensive controlled study with extended follow-up are currently pending, it is the author's opinion that the device will supplant fusion as the treatment of choice for certain carefully selected patients. The potential benefits of preserving motion at the disk interspace are intriguing. This combined with the avoidance of a fusion eliminates some of the obvious drawbacks of the status quo. Of greater interest is whether preserving motion at the treated disk level lessens the occurrence of symptomatic adjacent segment disease. One report has offered early evidence that Bryan arthroplasty does appear to prevent or delay the development of symptoms from adjacent levels.[23]

Although arthroplasty has compared well to fusion, extended follow-up is necessary to determine the scope of its application. Experience says that we must carefully evaluate a new procedure's safety, effectiveness, and utility before embracing it as a standard of care.

References

1. Hacker RJ. A randomized prospective study of an anterior cervical interbody fusion device with a minimum of 2 years of follow-up results. J Neurosurg 2000;93(Suppl 2):222–226
2. Cloward RB. The anterior approach for removal of ruptured cervical disks. J Neurosurg 1958;15:602–616
3. Hilibrand AS, Yoo JU, Carlson GD, Palumbo MA, Jones PK, Bohlman HH. Radiculopathy and myelopathy at segments adjacent to the site of a previous anterior cervical arthrodesis. J Bone Joint Surg Am 1999;81:519–528
4. Robbins MM, Hilibrand AS. Post-arthrodesis adjacent segment degeneration. In: Vaccaro A, Anderson DG, Crawford A, Benzel E, Ragan J, eds. Complications of Pediatric and Adult Spinal Surgery. New York: Dekker;2004:125–146
5. Goffin J, Geusens E, Vantomme N, et al. Long-term follow-up after interbody fusion of the cervical spine. J Spinal Disord Tech 2004; 17:79–85
6. Hacker RJ, Cauthen JC, Gilbert TJ, Griffith SL. A prospective randomized multicenter clinical evaluation of an anterior cervical fusion cage. Spine 2000;25:2646–2655
7. Geer C, Selden NRW, Papadopoulos SM. Anterior cervical plate fixation in the treatment of single-level cervical disk disease. J Neurosurg 1999;90:410A
8. Savolainen S, Rinne J, Hernesniemi J. A prospective randomized study of anterior single-level cervical disk operations with long-term follow-up: surgical fusion is unnecessary. Neurosurgery 1998;43:51–55
9. Jho HD. Microsurgical anterior cervical foraminotomy for radiculopathy: a new approach to cervical disk herniation. J Neurosurg 1996; 84:155–160
10. Johnson JP, Filler AG, McBride DQ, Batzdorf U. Anterior cervical foraminotomy for unilateral radicular disease. Spine 2000;25:905–909
11. Hacker RJ, Miller CG. Failed anterior cervical foraminotomy. J Neurosurg 2003;98(Suppl 2):126–130
12. Sawin PD, Traynelis VC, Menezes AH. A comparative analysis of fusion rates and donor-site morbidity for autogeneic rib and iliac crest bone grafts in posterior cervical fusions. J Neurosurg 1998;88:255–265
13. Lee MJ, Bazaz J, Furey CG, Yoo JU. The incidence of dysphagia in anterior cervical surgery as a function of plate design: a prospective study. Paper presented at: Annual Meeting of the Cervical Spine Research Society; December 9, 2004; Boston, MA
14. Martin GJ, Haid RW, MacMillan M. Anterior cervical diskectomy with freeze-dried fibula allograft: overview of 317 cases and literature review. Spine 1999;24:852–859
15. Anderson PA, Rouleau JP. Intervertebral disk arthroplasty. Spine 2004;29:2779–2786
16. Anderson PA, Rouleau JP, Bryan VE, Carlson CS. Wear analysis of the Bryan Cervical Disc prosthesis. Spine 2003;28(20S):S186–S194
17. Anderson PA, Rouleau JP, Toth JM, Riew KD. A comparison of simulator-tested and- retrieved cervical disk prostheses. J Neurosurg Spine 2004;1:202–210
18. Duggal N, Pickett GE, Rouleau JP. Kinematic analysis of the Bryan Cervical Disc prosthesis. Paper presented at: Annual Meeting of the Cervical Spine Research Society; December 9, 2004; Boston, MA
19. Goffin J, Van Calenbergh F, van Loon J, et al. Intermediate follow-up after treatment of degenerative disk disease with the Bryan Cervical Disc prosthesis: single-level and bi-level. Spine 2003;28: 2673–2678
20. Lafuente J, Casey AT, Petzold A, Brew S. The Bryan Cervical Disc prosthesis as an alternative to arthrodesis in the treatment of cervical spondylosis: 46 consecutive cases. J Bone Joint Surg Br 2005;87: 508–512
21. Goffin J, Casey A, Kehr P, et al. Two-year results from a European study of the Bryan Cervical Disc system. Paper presented at: Annual Meeting of the American Association of Neurological Surgeons; April 18, 2005 New Orleans, LA
22. Goffin J. Personal communication, April, 2005
23. Robertson JT, Papadopoulos SM, Traynelis VC. Assessment of adjacent segment disease in patients treated with cervical fusion or cervical arthroplasty: a prospective 2-year study. Paper presented at: Annual Meeting of the Cervical Spine Research Society; December 9, 2004; Boston, MA

8

Prestige Cervical Artificial Disk

James T. Robertson

◆ **The Prestige I**

◆ **The Prestige II Disk**

◆ **The Prestige ST**

◆ **The Prestige STLP Disk**

◆ **The Prestige LP**

◆ **Prestige LP Surgical Technique**

◆ **Conclusion**

The Prestige family of disks traces its lineage back to the Cummins (Bristol) Artificial Cervical Joint (**Fig. 8–1**). The late Brian Cummins, senior consultant in neurosurgery at Frenchay Hospital in Bristol, U.K., became concerned about the need for repeated surgical therapy in patients with degenerative spinal disk disease undergoing anterior cervical fusion, particularly after two or more previous surgically or congenitally acquired fusions. Prof. Cummins recognized the potential clinical benefit of an artificial cervical joint and in 1989 began consultation with Colin Walker, head of the Department of Medical Engineering at Frenchay Hospital (DMEFH).

Several concepts were considered; however, they ultimately elected to place a prosthetic joint in the intervertebral space after a standard anterior diskectomy. Several prototypes were manufactured in the DMEFH and in early 1991 the initial design was produced for clinical trial. The prosthetic joints were individually produced in the medical engineering shop and were made of Type 316 stainless steel (composition D: BS7262: part 1: 1990 and ISO5832-1: 1987). The prosthesis was basically a ball and socket joint that allowed flexion-extension, axial rotation, lateral bending, and, by making the ball slightly smaller than the saucer, slight translation. Fixation was initially achieved with a single anterior bone screw through each anterior flange. After the joint was placed in the first five patients, an additional screw site was added to the anterior flange of the joint and the screw sites were adjusted to ensure a more stable interface. The first five joints had simple stainless steel fracture screws. Subsequently, A-O locking screws were used to affix the joint anteriorly to the vertebral body. However, these screws were made of titanium, which added a variant metal to the process.

Between February 1991 and August 1996, 22 joints were placed in 20 patients. All patients provided detailed informed consent before undergoing this innovative surgical procedure. Nineteen of the 20 cases were associated with previous surgical or congenital fusions at single and multiple levels of the cervical spine. Patients were operated because of symptomatic adjacent segment cervical stenosis, spondylosis, or herniated disk with associated myelopathy, radicu-

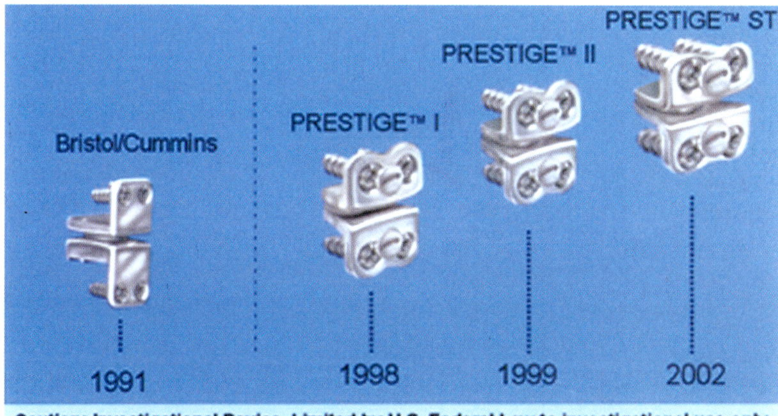

Figure 8–1   Metal/metal cervical disk clinical history.

lopathy, or, in one case, intractable pain. The joint appeared to be stable, it preserved motion, and it was both biomechanically and biochemically compatible. Subsidence was not observed despite several incidences of fixation screw fracture. After review in July 1996 of the medical records, examination of the patients, and obtaining delayed cervical spine motion x-rays, the results revealed this prosthesis to be suitable for cervical disk replacement.[1]

Most of the patients reported improvement after joint placement. However, complications occurred in a significant number of these cases. The complications were due in part to poor screw placement, the use of a single uniform-sized joint regardless of the patient's anatomy, and, in one case, improper manufacturing of the joint, which ultimately led to surgical removal. At the time of removal, the joint was firmly embedded in bone and had a smooth, synovial-like scar tissue lining anteriorly. On review, this joint was shown to have an improper ball and socket size differentiation preventing symmetrical fitting.

◆ The Prestige I

Subsequent to Cummins's retirement in 1996, Steven Gill, an associate in the department of neurosurgery, suggested that the female component of the joint be modified to an oval shape, which would allow translation with flexion and extension. Simultaneously, Sofamor Danek purchased the intellectual property and entered into a collaborative agreement with Gill and the department of neurosurgery at Frenchay Hospital. Gill and the biomedical engineers at Sofamor Danek entered into a team relationship, which led to the development of the Prestige I disk (Medtronic Sofamor Danek, Memphis, TN). The major improvements over the original disk included a reduced anterior profile and a fixed-angle screw geometry. A bone screw locking mechanism based on anterior cervical plate technology was incorporated, similar to the Orion Anterior Cervical Plate (Medtronic Sofamor Danek, Memphis, TN). The socket (female component) was changed to an oval "trough" so that the ball component could slide, allowing for physiological anterior-posterior translation with flexion and extension of the cervical spine. The size of the device was reduced to 8 mm in height and 14 mm in depth.

The Prestige I disk clinical experience began in 1998 in an ethics committee-approved clinical study at Frenchay Hospital.[2] The prospective clinical trial was limited to 17 patients with end-stage disease, represented by adjacent symptomatic disk disease developing after congenitally or surgically acquired adjacent cervical fusions. The patients were followed according to strict protocol for 4 years postoperatively. Clinical and radiographic parameters were evaluated at each follow-up interval along with patient-completed outcome questionnaires.

Clinical improvement was demonstrated in all outcome measures evaluated. A 27% improvement in the Neck Disability Index was seen at 48 months postoperative. The mean flexion-extension angulation at 48 months was within 2 degrees of mean preoperative angulation. Complications were similar to those seen with anterior cervical diskectomy and fusion procedures. Postoperative pain was minimal and early discharge without cervical collars was routine. One patient required device removal approximately 3 years and 3 months postoperatively due to a preexisting adjacent segment symptomatic degenerative disk, which required anterior cervical fusion. The device was maintaining motion prior to removal and, at surgery, no wear debris was observed. A histological examination of periexplant tissues revealed no host response.

In summary, the Prestige I disk demonstrated clinical longevity, lack of subsidence, and motion maintenance in a small cohort of end-stage patients.

◆ The Prestige II Disk

The Prestige II disk (**Fig. 8–2**) incorporated several design improvements and led to additional clinical studies. The modifications from the Prestige I disk involved a slightly reduced anterior profile and roughened end plates for enhanced interbody fixation. It was sized in 8 mm heights, and 12 mm and 14 mm depths. In 1998, a prospective, randomized clinical trial was initiated in four centers in Europe and Australia. Patients with primary single-level cervical disk disease producing either or both radiculopathy and myelopathy were randomized prospectively to receive anterior cervical diskectomy with either fusion or artificial cervical disk placement. Ethics committee approval of the study, as well as patient informed consent, was obtained at all centers prior to randomization. The patients were evaluated pre- and postoperatively with serial flexion-extension x-rays at 6 weeks and at 3, 6, 12, and 24 months. At the same intervals, the patients had pre- and postoperative neck disability indexes, visual analog pain scales, SF-36 general health scores, and neurological examinations assessing the reflex, motor, and sensory function. Fifty-four patients were enrolled in the trial. Clinical and radiographic results revealed similar improvement in both treatment groups. Most outcome measures tended to favor the Prestige II disk; however, the differences between the groups were not statistically significant. Radiographic results demonstrated that the Prestige disk maintains cervical motion at the treated level without adjacent segment compromise. Complications were similar in the two groups. This was the first study to compare cervical fusion to cervical arthroplasty in a prospective randomized fashion.

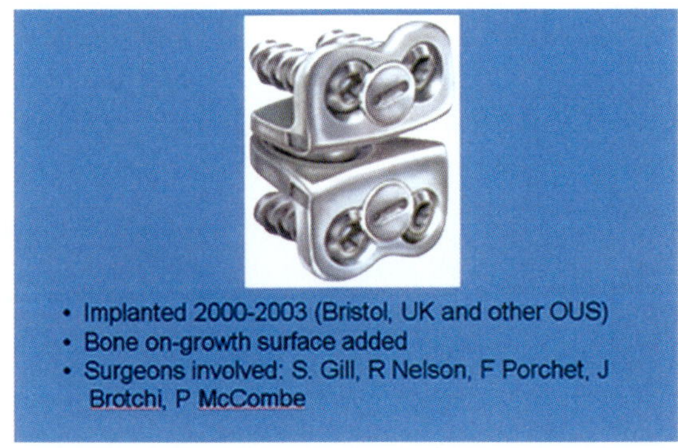

Figure 8–2   Prestige II.

◆ The Prestige ST

After this favorable surgical experience, and with surgical and engineering collaboration, the artificial disk was again modified by further reducing the anterior profile of the Prestige II and creating several additional sizes (6, 7, 8, and 9 mm heights, and 12 and 14 mm depths) to better accommodate patient anatomical variation. This modification, the Prestige ST, has—after appropriate institutional review board (IRB) approval and patient concurrence—undergone an Investigational Device Exemption (IDE) study involving 550 patients randomized either to the Prestige ST disk or anterior fusion after anterior cervical discectomy. Twenty-five centers participated and the protocol has been completed with 2-year postoperative follow-up now under way. Early results appear to be positive for the Prestige ST disk.

◆ The Prestige STLP Disk

The Prestige STLP device was the next step in the Prestige program. This stainless steel device does not achieve fixation via anterior bone screws, but rather through a porous end plate contact and dual stabilization rails. The device was evaluated in several centers in Europe and Australia. To date, the results are excellent, and surgeons appreciate the ease of insertion and ability to treat adjacent levels.

◆ The Prestige LP

The latest device in the Prestige program is the Prestige LP (**Fig. 8–3**). The design and sizes are similar to the Prestige STLP, but the device is made of a titanium ceramic composite. It has excellent longevity on biomechanical testing and minimal wear debris. This device allows for magnetic resonance imaging with minimal metallic artifact. Because there are no anterior bone screws, the device achieves stabilization

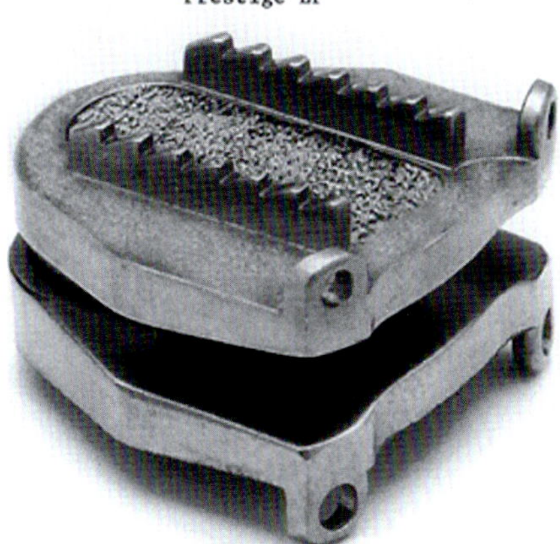

Figure 8–3   Prestige LP.

through a porous end plate contact with the vertebral bodies and dual stabilization rails. The device has been implanted in Europe, Australia, and the United States through an IDE trial.

◆ Prestige LP Surgical Technique

The cervical spine is placed in a neutral position with excess extension avoided. After a standard anterior discectomy and careful osteophyte removal, the end plates are shaped flat and parallel, sparing as much cortical bone as possible (**Fig. 8–4**). Appropriately sized rasps are included in the surgical set to help achieve appropriate shaping of the disk space. Sizing trials are inserted in the interspace to ensure alignment and to determine device dimensions (**Fig. 8–5**). Channels are created in the end plates to accommodate the rails of the device to reduce impaction of the cervical spine. To accomplish this, four holes are drilled using a trial with a captured drill guide, then a channel cutter is gently impacted. The Prestige LP is

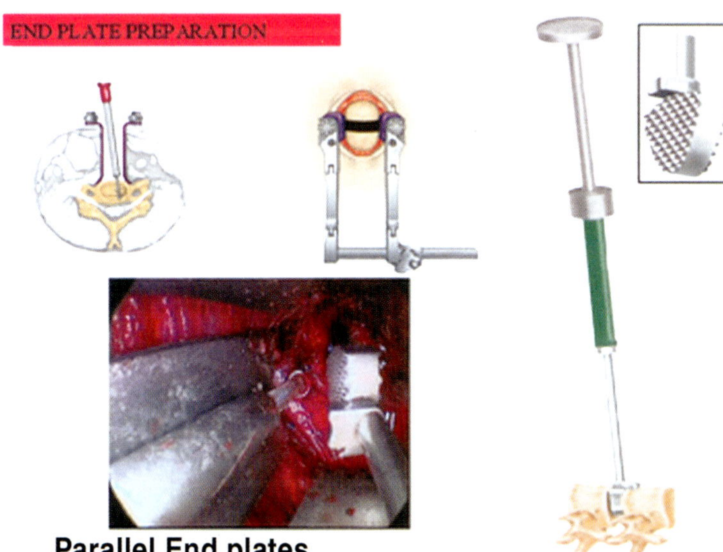

Figure 8–4   End plate preparation: parallel end plates.

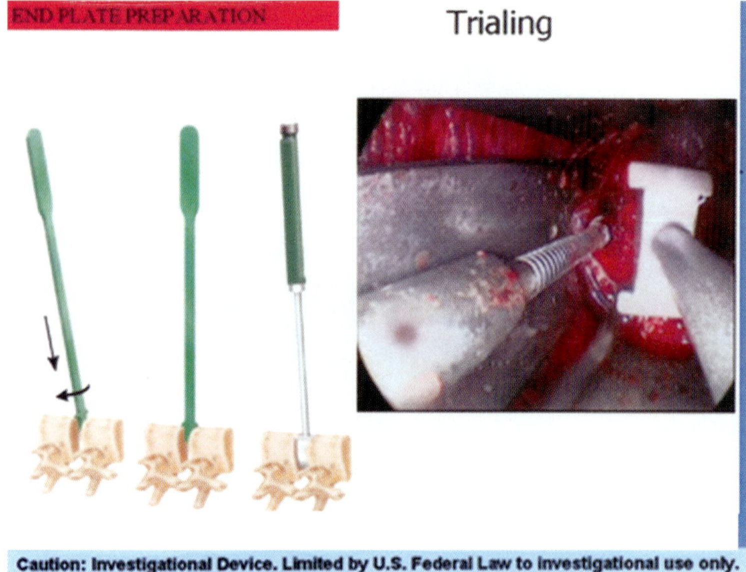

Figure 8–5   End plate preparation: trialing.

inserted with minimal interspace distraction (**Figs. 8–6, 8–7**). Positioning of the trials and rasps can be assessed under lateral fluoroscopy. Routine closure of the wound follows. The time required for the procedure is comparable to an anterior diskectomy and fusion. Bracing is not necessary, and early discharge within 24 hours is common. Typically, the patient is allowed to resume light activities and encouraged to move the neck as desired. Postoperative films reveal excellent motion comparative to preoperative evaluation (**Fig. 8–8**).

◆ Conclusion

It is anticipated that the Prestige ST and subsequently the Prestige LP will become available in the United States for surgical use potentially as early as 2007. It is also anticipated that the Prestige ST device will be the first to market in the United States. The clinical history, simplicity, reliability, and ease of placement of the Prestige ST and Prestige LP should make the devices favorably received by spine surgeons.

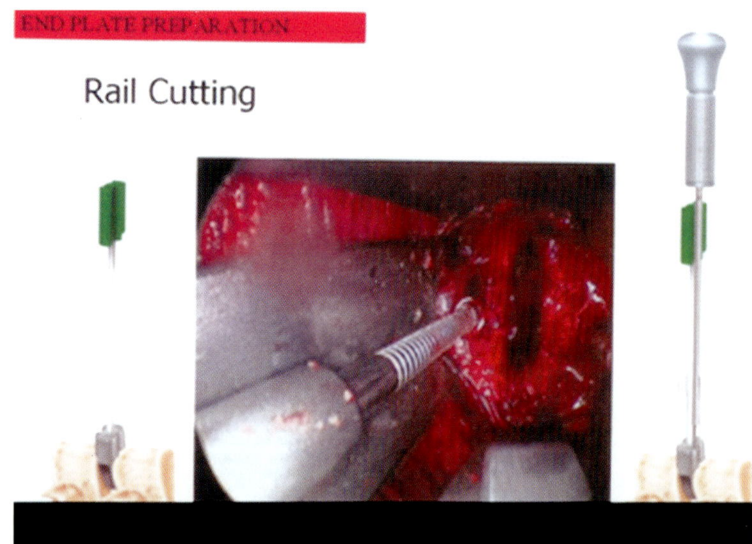

Figure 8–6   End plate preparation: rail cutting.

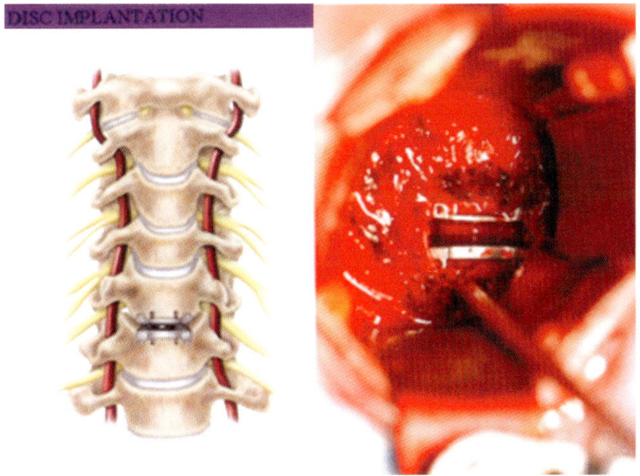

Figure 8–7   Disk implantation.

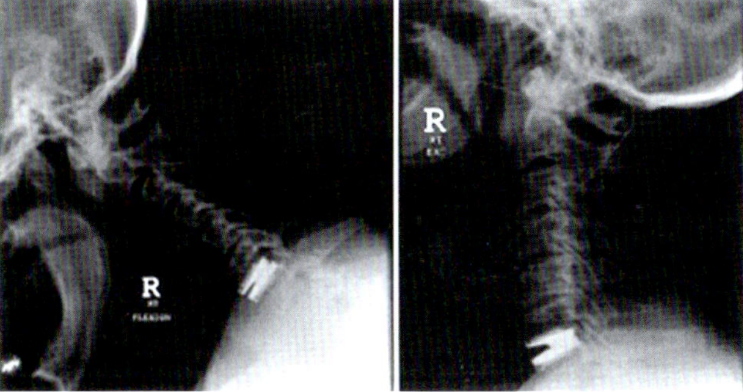

Figure 8–8   Postop films.

References

1. Cummins B, Robertson J, Gill S. Surgical experience with an implanted artificial cervical joint. J Neurosurg 1998;88:943–948

2. Wigfield C, Gill S, Nelson RJ, Metcalf NH, Robertson JT. The new Frenchay artificial cervical joint: results from a two-year pilot study. Spine 2002;22:2446–2452

9

ProDisc-C Cervical Artificial Disk

Gerard K. Jeong, Frank P. Cammisa, and Federico P. Girardi

◆ **ProDisc-C Cervical Disk Prosthesis**

◆ **Surgical Technique**

◆ **Clinical Results**

◆ **Complications**

◆ **Summary**

Since its original description in the 1950s by Cloward and Robinson and Smith, anterior cervical diskectomy and fusion (ACDF) has become the standard for operative treatment of radiculopathy and myelopathy due to one- to two-level cervical degenerative disk disease.[1,2] However, the detrimental effects of arthrodesis on adjacent motion segments at longer follow-up have been demonstrated. Hilibrand et al observed the occurrence of symptomatic adjacent segment disease at a relatively constant incidence rate of 2.9% per year on a cumulative basis during the 10-year postoperative follow-up.[3] Using survival analysis methods, the authors predicted that 25.6% of the patients who had an anterior cervical arthrodesis would have new disease at an adjacent level within 10 years after the operation. Other investigators have reported that an estimated 7 to 15% of patients ultimately require a secondary procedure at an adjacent level.[4,5] Whether the rate of adjacent symptomatic disk disease is accelerated due to the increased stress placed on the adjacent motion segments, particularly the subjacent motion segment, following successful fusion remains controversial.[6] Due to the long-term effects of fusion on adjacent motion segments, motion preservation and nonfusion technologies have met renewed interest.

The early clinical experience with a variety of cervical disk prostheses is growing. The premise behind artificial vertebral disk implantation is that abnormal motion will be corrected, the intervertebral space height will be restored, the physiological curvature and instantaneous axis of rotation will be normalized, the corrected normal intervertebral motion will be maintained over time, and the patients will experience pain relief and return of function.

The ProDisc-C cervical disk prosthesis is a relatively new device with limited clinical experience compared with its counterparts such as the Bryan (Medtronic Sofamor Danek, Memphis, TN), Cummins (or Bristol, Frenchay), or Prestige (Medtronic) disk prostheses.[7-17] At present, the ProDisc-C is under the U.S. Food and Drug Administration Investigational Device Exemption (IDE) study. This chapter reviews the specific features, theoretical advantages/disadvantages, and biomechanical considerations of the ProDisc-C implant (Synthes, Inc., West Chester, PA). The chapter also discusses the early clinical results from case series and from the ongoing multicenter, prospective, randomized, controlled

clinical trial comparing the safety and effectiveness of the ProDisc-C cervical implant to ACDF in the treatment of symptomatic cervical disk disease. Some of the early device-related complications reported in a few European case series are described here as well.

◆ ProDisc-C Cervical Disk Prosthesis

The ProDisc-C cervical disk is a metal-on-polymer implant (**Fig. 9–1**). It consists of two forged cobalt-chromium-molybdenum (CoCrMo) alloy end plates and an ultra high molecular weight polyethylene (UHMWPE) inlay element, which is fixed to the inferior prosthetic end plate. The

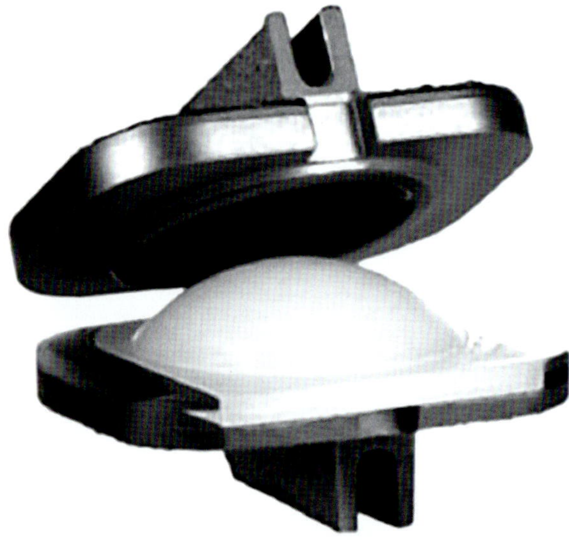

Figure 9–1 ProDisc-C cervical prosthesis is a semiconstrained, ball and socket design with fixed axis of rotation. It consists of two forged cobalt-chromium-molybdenum alloy end plates and an ultra high molecular weight polyethylene inlay element, which is fixed to the inferior prosthetic end plate. The metal end plates have two vertical fins for immediate fixation in the end plates and are plasma sprayed with titanium for long-term fixation through osseointegration.

UHMWPE wear rate was 40- to 50-fold less than typical wear rate shown for hip and knee prosthesis in multiaxis simulator testing. The metal end plates are plasma sprayed with titanium and have two vertical fins for fixation in the end plates. A keel cutting chisel with a safety block mechanism is used to prepare the host bone for the keeled end plates. The keels, a design unique to the ProDisc-C cervical prosthesis and the ProDisc lumbar prosthesis, provide immediate fixation of the prosthetic end plate in each adjacent vertebral end plate, whereas the surface roughness of the plasma-sprayed titanium end plate surface provides not only a high coefficient of friction to augment immediate implant fixation but also long-term stability through bony ongrowth.

The ProDisc-C is a semiconstrained, ball and socket design with fixed axis of rotation. Whether the semiconstrained nature of the ProDisc-C may provide a more optimal balance between motion preservation, ease and consistency of implantation, and neurological fitness than a noncon-strained disk prostheses is unknown.

The theoretical advantages of the ProDisc-C device are (1) the absence of anterior plate-like fixation/hardware common to many other disk prostheses, (2) immediate stability provided by the end plates' keel fixation, and (3) the possibility of multilevel application.

The theoretical concerns of the ProDisc-C may be divided into concerns inherent with any motion-preserving disk prosthesis and concerns specific to the ProDisc-C device. General concerns include revision capabilities, ectopic bone formation, autofusion, and persistent or recurrent neural compression, which is inherent with any motion-preserving procedure because posterior osteophytes may not resorb as they do in arthrodesis. Device-specific concerns include the possibility of a more difficult revision procedure and signifi-cant host bone loss because extraction of the keeled device may sacrifice a substantial portion of host bone, especially when performed at multiple levels. Sagittal-splitting verte-bral body fracture following preparation or implantation of the keeled prosthesis is also a concern, especially in multilevel applications. Theoretical concerns regarding UHMWPE wear and osteolysis are also specific to the ProDisc-C because many of the available cervical disk prostheses employ a metal-on-metal design.

Lastly, the theoretical concern of the dynamics and kine-matics of the ProDisc-C has been raised. The instantaneous axis of rotation (IAR) in the normal cervical spine is not fixed and dependent upon the specific motion performed. In the normal cervical spine, the location of the IAR varies depending on the type of motion. In flexion-extension, the IAR lies along the anterior border of the vertebral body; in axial rotation, it lies in the center of the vertebral body; whereas in lateral bending, the IAR translates in the superior-inferior direction. Whether the ProDisc-C, a semiconstrained device with a fixed axis of rotation, can adequately replicate or reproduce the motion of the normal motion segment remains a topic of investigation.

A recent biomechanical study has demonstrated that the kinematics of the ProDisc-C are similar to those in the normal cervical motion segment. Despite having a fixed center of rotation, the ProDisc-C prosthesis was found to reasonably preserve the physiological distribution of the IAR, which in turn may decrease loosening forces and facet joint strain.[18]

Interestingly, the investigators found that, despite the level of constraint in the prosthesis, there appeared to be some translational motion in the IAR depending on the specific motion, which suggests the influence of other anatomical stabilizing structures as well as the ability of the disk to accommodate such motion.

Recent studies have also demonstrated that the dynamics of the ProDisc-C closely replicate those in the normal motion segment. In a multilevel human cadaveric model, DiAngelo et al demonstrated that the ProDisc-C implant did not alter the motion patterns of flexion, lateral bending, and axial rotation at either the instrumented level or adjacent seg-ments compared with the harvested condition.[19] The only significant difference between the ProDisc-C and harvested spine conditions occurred in extension, in which only 57% of motion of the harvested spine was obtained with the cervical prosthesis.

The authors also demonstrated that a simulation of a one-level fusion significantly reduced motion at the surgical site, for which it was compensated by increased motion at adjacent segments. This increased adjacent segment motion may accelerate degeneration of adjacent disk segments. As a result, they argued that use of a prosthetic total disk replace-ment device to treat symptomatic degenerative cervical disk disease may minimize or alleviate adjacent segment disease associated with fusion surgery.

Sliva et al also demonstrated that the kinematics and range of motion (ROM) of the operated and adjacent motion segments were fairly well preserved following one-level disk replacement with the ProDisc-C prosthesis compared with the harvested, native condition.[20] A significant increase in flexion-extension ROM, axial rotation, disk height, and lor-dosis of the affected segment was found after insertion of the ProDisc-C prosthesis in cadaveric testing ($p < .05$). Adjacent segment disk pressures and ROM did not show a significant difference following prosthetic insertion, except in extension where there was a significant increase ($p < .05$).

◆ Surgical Technique

The patient is positioned in the supine or in slight reverse Trendelenburg's position on the operating table. The head may be stabilized with Gardner-Wells tongs on a horseshoe frame. A standard anteromedial approach is performed. A transverse skin incision over the corresponding level is made and preferably over a skin crease if possible for cosmesis. The platysma may be split longitudinally or transversely. Blunt dissection allows the sternocleidomas-toid and carotid sheath to be mobilized laterally and the strap muscles, trachea, and esophagus medially. The disk and vertebral bodies can now be palpated. The longus colli are elevated. It is important at this point to mark the midline for subsequent central positioning of the prosthesis. We perform a relatively wide exposure of the vertebral elements to allow better visualization for an adequate decompression.

After the initial annulotomy, we attempt to remove only the cartilaginous portion of the end plate using a combination of rongeurs, curettes, and a bur. We recommend minimal end plate disruption if possible to preserve the subchondral bone for seating of the prosthesis and to avoid subsidence of the implant. When indicated, the posterior osteophytes, posterior annulus, and uncinate processes are removed as part of the anterior decompression. We release the posterior longitudinal ligament to remove any extruded disk fragments as needed. A thorough central and lateral decompression is of paramount importance in the setting of motion preservation because the resorption of vertebral osteophytes, which occurs following arthrodesis, does not occur in arthroplasty cases. A blunt nerve hook is used to inspect centrally and the foramen to confirm the adequacy of the central and lateral decompression, respectively.

Following wide decompression, the reconstruction begins with placing trial implants in an increasingly stepwise fashion to confirm the appropriate width and height of the final prosthesis. The central or midline position is then rechecked and may be confirmed fluoroscopically or radiographically prior to making the cuts for the end plate keels. Once the midline has been confirmed, the keel-cutting chisel is guided over the prosthesis trial to produce the grooves for the prosthetic end plate keels. The chisel and trial are then removed. The appropriately sized final prosthetic end plates are then seated into the upper and lower bodies. The end plates are then distracted to allow the inlay UHMWE polyethylene element to be inserted into the inferior prosthetic end plate. Distraction is then released, and appropriate positioning of the prosthesis is confirmed with anteroposterior and lateral fluoroscopy (**Figs. 9–2 and 9–3**).

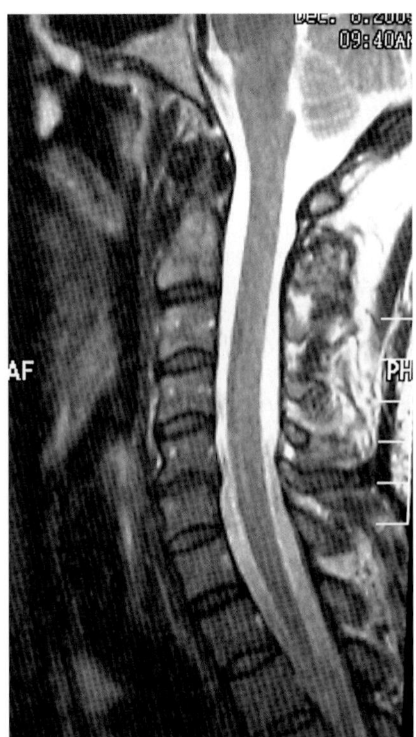

Figure 9–2   Magnetic resonance imaging sagittal view of a 45-year-old female demonstrating isolated cervical degenerative disk disease at C5–C6. Her clinical symptoms of neck pain and radicular pain along the C6 dermatome correlated with her preoperative imaging findings.

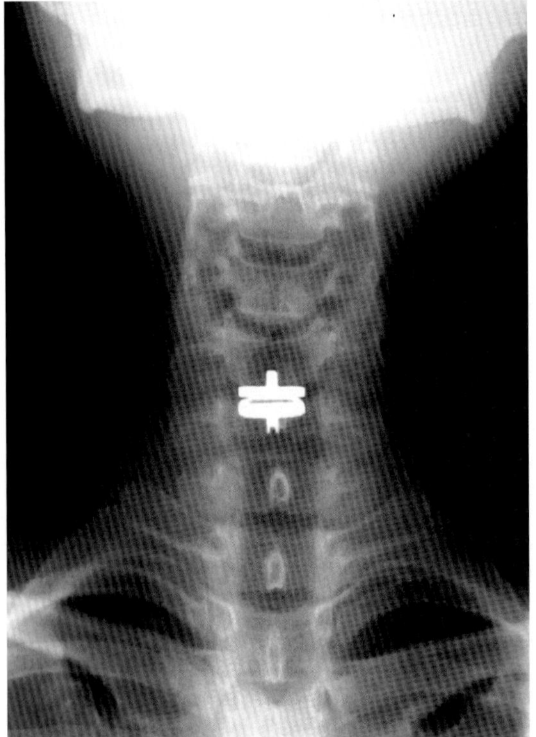

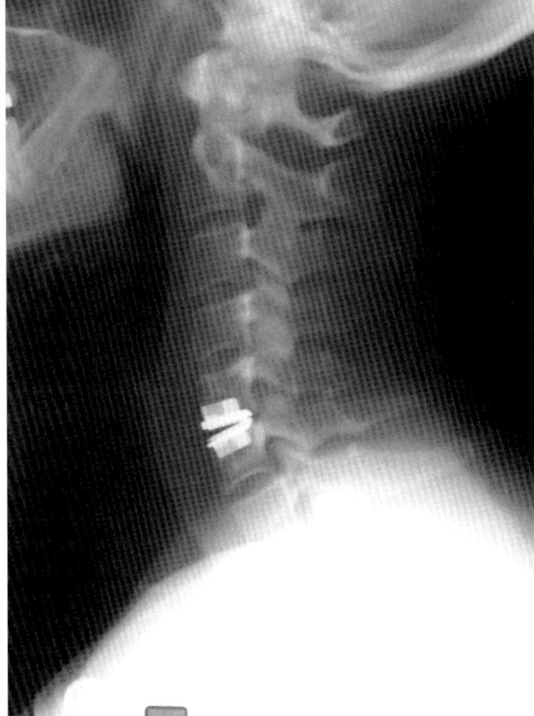

Figure 9–3   **(A)** Anteroposterior and **(B)** lateral radiograph of the same 45-year-old female following C5–C6 arthroplasty with the ProDisc-C prosthesis at 11-month follow-up. The keels of the end plate are appropriately positioned in the midline between the uncinate processes and along the spinous processes.

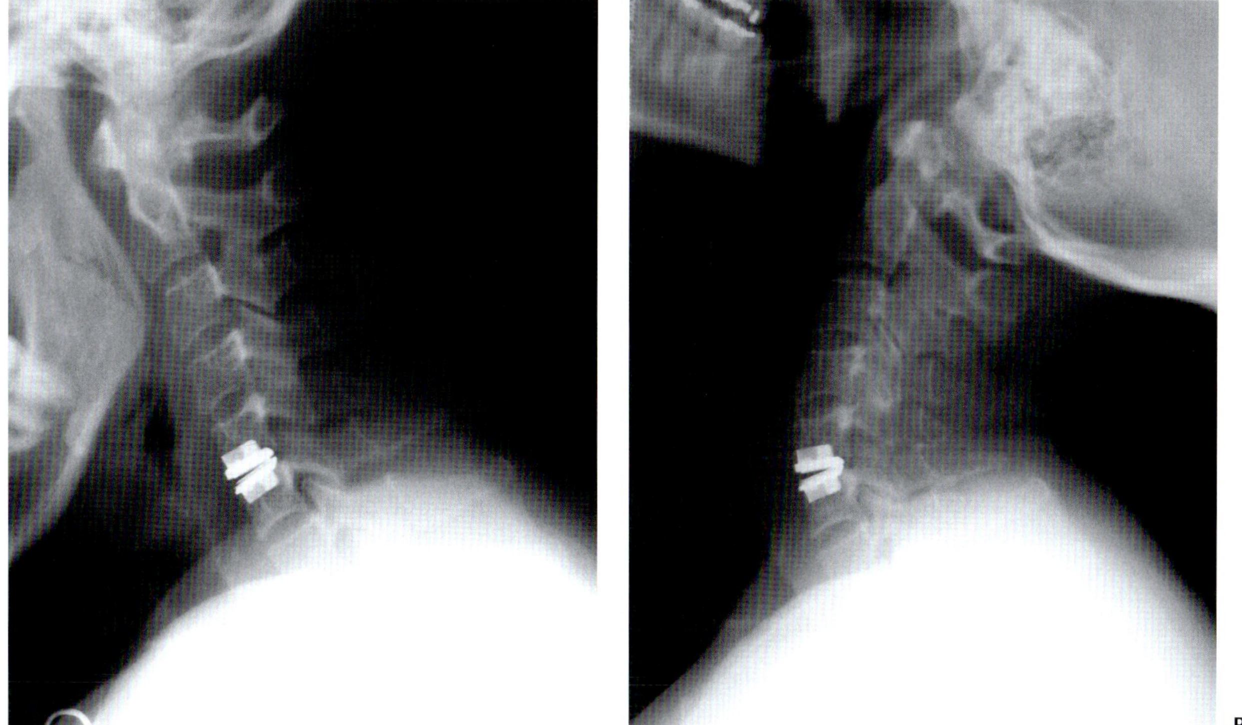

Figure 9–4 **(A)** Dynamic flexion lateral and **(B)** extension lateral radiographs at most recent follow-up demonstrating preservation of the C5–C6 motion segment. Clinically, the patient has experienced complete resolution of her neck pain and radicular symptoms.

Postoperatively, the patient is placed in a soft collar and usually discharged by the second postoperative day. The collar is then discontinued at 2 weeks, although patients are allowed to move in the collar as tolerated (**Fig. 9–4A,B**).

◆ Clinical Results

Clinical experience in cervical disk arthroplasty has been much greater in Europe and Australia. Although clinical trials in the United States are ongoing, the experience with the ProDisc-C cervical prosthesis is limited compared with the Bryan, Cummins, and Prestige disk prostheses, which have been implanted worldwide for more than 10 years. At the time of this writing, there is only one published study reporting the clinical results of cervical disk arthroplasty with the ProDisc-C prosthesis.[21]

Bertagnoli et al reported their initial safety and efficacy data using the ProDisc-C for the treatment of symptomatic cervical spondylosis.[21] The preliminary results were promising. Twenty ProDisc-C prostheses were implanted in 16 patients for symptomatic cervical disk disease with and without radiculopathy/myelopathy; four patients had two-level procedures performed. They reported significant improvements in neck pain, arm pain, and disability scores by 3 months. These improvements were sustained up through 1 year postoperatively. No additional fusion surgeries were performed at the affected or adjacent levels. There were no surgical or device-related complications (subsidence, loosening, dislocation, metallic or UHMWPE component failure, or allergic reaction) found in their series. They not only demonstrated a significant restoration of affected disk height from 3 mm preoperatively to 8 mm postoperatively ($p < .001$) but also found significantly increased motion of the treated segment from 4 degrees preoperatively to 12 degrees postoperatively ($p < .004$).

The remaining studies have not yet been published but have been presented. Bertagnoli reported more recent results of a larger prospective, nonrandomized series of 101 patients with 140 ProDisc-C implants.[22] He reported a substantial decrease in pain intensity scores, neck pain frequency scores, and arm pain frequency scores at 1 year postoperatively. He also reported a high rate of patient satisfaction with 91% of the patients satisfied or completely satisfied with the outcome of the procedure.

The preliminary data from the current FDA multicenter, prospective, randomized clinical trial comparing ProDisc-C to ACDF have now been reported by various investigators.[23–27] The results from the various centers have been similar in demonstrating the initial safety and efficacy of the ProDisc-C prosthesis. Both ACDF and ProDisc-C groups have reported significant improvement in pain and function tests following surgical intervention. No differences in pain scores or functional outcome scores have been found between the two treatment groups; however, in contrast to the ACDF group, motion at the operated segment has been found to be maintained in the ProDisc-C group. There have been no device-related complications reported in any of the U.S. centers conducting the trial.

Murrey et al presented their early results from the prospective, randomized, controlled clinical trial comparing ProDisc-C and ACDF for cervical radiculopathy.[27] Forty-four patients were enrolled with 22 patients in each treatment arm. They found no significant difference between the two groups in motor and neurological function, visual analog scale (VAS) arm pain scores, VAS neck pain scores, neck disability index (NDI), and short form (SF)-36 pain scores. Although both treatment groups demonstrated significant improvements in pain and function compared with preoperatively, the ProDisc-C group was found to have significantly improved flexion-extension ROM at the treated level compared with preoperatively and to the ACDF group ($p < .05$). The investigators concluded that at early clinical follow-up the ProDisc-C disk replacement was found to be equally safe and efficacious as ACDF for the treatment of cervical radiculopathy and to allow restoration of early ROM postoperatively.

Delamarter et al also reported the early-term results from the prospective, randomized FDA clinical trial of ProDisc-C versus ACDF.[26] They found significant improvements in clinical outcome scores (VAS scores, ODI) in both the anterior cervical discectomy fusion (ACDF) and ProDisc-C groups at 6-, 12-, and up to 24-month follow-up. They also found that, unlike in the fusion group, flexion-and-extension motion and lateral bending were well preserved compared with preoperatively in the ProDisc group. Flexion-extension improved from 11 degrees preoperatively to 12.5 degrees postoperatively. Lateral bending was well preserved from 5.9 degrees preoperatively to 5 degrees postoperatively. The authors concluded that ProDisc cervical disk arthroplasty preserved motion at the affected segments without compromising clinical outcomes at early-term follow-up. Mehren et al also demonstrated restoration and improvement in global ROM and sagittal contour/alignment following monosegmental and multisegmental disk arthroplasty with the ProDisc-C.[28] Following one-level disk replacement, global ROM improved from a mean of 7.5 degrees preoperatively to 12 degrees postoperatively. Mean cervical lordosis as performed using the Rechtman-Borden method improved from 6 to 9 mm following single-level disk replacement and improved from 5 to 8.5 mm following multiple-level disk replacement.

The preliminary results for the FDA clinical trial of ProDisc-C versus ACDF for the treatment of symptomatic cervical degenerative disk disease are promising and have demonstrated the initial safety and efficacy of the ProDisc-C device. Longer-term safety and efficacy studies are in progress; the results will determine the ultimate role of ProDisc-C and other cervical disk prostheses in the treatment of cervical disk disease and in the prevention of adjacent segment disease.

◆ Complications

Although the clinical results appeared at least comparable with fusion techniques, there have been device-related complications reported in European centers investigating the ProDisc-C. Grochulla et al reported two cases in 40 patients in which prosthetic insertion was aborted and salvaged using a standard fusion because of intraoperative implant-related complications.[29] They attributed these complications to the technique of implantation and its potential risk for neurological injury. They also reported one case in which ossification at the prosthetic motion segment occurred and two cases of subsidence of the implant into the adjacent vertebra.

Suchomel et al reported two cases in 40 patients in which a sagittal split of the vertebral body occurred during chiseling of the grooves in the body for preparation of the keeled end plates.[30] In both cases, the fracture occurred at the intermediate vertebral body of a two-level disk replacement and in women with small vertebral bodies. As a result, the investigators cautioned its use in multilevel cases in patients with small vertebral body dimensions.

◆ Summary

The ProDisc-C cervical disk prosthesis is a relatively new device with limited clinical experience compared with its counterparts such as the Bryan, Cummins (or Bristol, Frenchay), or Prestige disk prostheses. Its specific features include a semiconstrained, ball and socket design, metal-on-polyethylene interface, end plate keels for immediate fixation, and titanium coating for long-term fixation. The kinematics and dynamics of the cervical motion segment implanted with the ProDisc-C prosthesis have been shown to closely approximate that of the normal motion segment in biomechanical studies. At present, the ProDisc-C is under the U.S. FDA IDE study. The preliminary clinical results from case series and from the ongoing prospective, randomized clinical trials have demonstrated the ProDisc-C to be safe and as efficacious as ACDF in the treatment of symptomatic cervical disk disease. Early device-related complications have been reported in a few European case series; however, no device-related complications, autofusion, or ectopic bone formation have yet been reported in any of the clinical trials in the United States. Intermediate- and long-term studies will determine the safety and efficacy of the ProDisc-C in the treatment of cervical disk disease and in the prevention of adjacent segment disease.

References

1. Cloward RB. The anterior approach for removal of ruptured cervical disks. J Neurosurg 1958;15:602–617
2. Robinson RA, Smith GW. Anterolateral cervical disc removal and interbody fusion for cervical disc syndrome. Bull Johns Hopkins Hosp 1955;96:223–224
3. Hilibrand AS, Carlson GD, Palumbo MA, Jones PK, Bohlman HH. Radiculopathy and myelopathy at segments adjacent to the site of a previous anterior cervical arthrodesis. J Bone Joint Surg Am 1999;81:519–528
4. Baba H, Furusawa N, Imura S. Late radiographic findings after anterior cervical fusion for spondylotic myeloradiculopathy. Spine 1993;18:2167–2173
5. Cherubino P, Benazzo F, Borromeo U, Perle S. Degenerative arthritis of the adjacent spinal joints following anterior cervical spinal fusion: clinicoradiologic and statistical correlations. Ital J Orthop Traumatol 1990;16:533–543
6. Hilibrand AS, Robbins M. Adjacent segment degeneration and adjacent segment disease: the consequences of spinal fusion? Spine J 2004;4(Suppl 6):190S–194S
7. Bryan VE Jr. Cervical motion segment replacement. Eur Spine J 2002;11(Suppl 2):S92–S97
8. Pickett GE, Duggal N. Artificial disc insertion following anterior cervical discectomy. Can J Neurol Sci 2003;30:278–283

9. Duggal N, Pickett GE, Mitsis DK, Keller JL. Early clinical and biomechanical results following cervical arthroplasty. Neurosurg Focus 2004;17:E9

10. Goffin J, Casey A, Kehr P, et al. Preliminary clinical experience with the Bryan Cervical Disc prosthesis. Neurosurgery 2002;51:840–845 discussion 845–847

11. Goffin J, Van Calenbergh F, van Loon J, et al. Intermediate follow-up after treatment of degenerative disc disease with the Bryan Cervical Disc prosthesis: single-level and bi-level. Spine 2003;28: 2673–2678

12. Sekhon LH. Cervical arthroplasty in the management of spondylotic myelopathy: 18-month results. Neurosurg Focus 2004;17:E8

13. Sekhon LH. Two-level artificial disc placement for spondylotic cervical myelopathy. J Clin Neurosci 2004;11:412–415

14. Cummins BH, Robertson JT, Gill SS. Surgical experience with an implanted artificial cervical joint. J Neurosurg 1998;88:943–948

15. Porchet F, Metcalf NH. Clinical outcomes with the Prestige II cervical disc: preliminary results from a prospective randomized clinical trial. Neurosurg Focus 2004;17:E6

16. Robertson JT, Metcalf NH. Long-term outcome after implantation of the Prestige I disc in an end-stage indication: 4-year results from a pilot study. Neurosurg Focus 2004;17:E10

17. Wigfield CC, Gill SS, Nelson RJ, Metcalf NH, Robertson JT. The new Frenchay artificial cervical joint: results from a two-year pilot study. Spine 2002;27:2446–2452

18. Demetropoulous C, et al. Biomechanical evaluation of the cadaver cervical spine instant axis of rotation following single-level disc replacement with a fixed axis of rotation. Scientific presentation at the Annual Meeting of the Spine Arthroplasty Society 2005, May 4–7, New York, NY

19. DiAngelo DJ, Foley KT, Morrow BR, et al. In vitro biomechanics of cervical disc arthroplasty with the ProDisc-C total disc implant. Neurosurg Focus 2004;17:E7

20. Sliva C, et al. Biomechanical evaluation of the cadaver cervical spine kinematics following single-level disc replacement with the ProDisc-C prosthesis. Poster presentation at the Annual Meeting of the Spine Arthroplasty Society 2005, May 4–7, New York, NY

21. Bertagnoli R, Yue JJ, Pfeiffer F, et al. Early results after ProDisc-C cervical disc replacement. J Neurosurg Spine 2005;2:403–410

22. Bertagnoli R. ProDisc-C. Clinical results. Scientific presentation at the Annual Meeting of the Spine Arthroplasty Society 2005, May 4–7, New York, NY

23. Janssen M, et al. Cervical disc arthroplasty: preliminary results of a randomized prospective study of single-level ACDF versus ProDisc-C for the management of cervical spondylosis. Poster presentation at the Annual Meeting of the Spine Arthroplasty Society 2005, May 4–7, New York, NY

24. Petrizzo AM, et al. Preliminary results of the ProDisc-C clinical IDE trial. Poster presentation at the Annual Meeting of the Spine Arthroplasty Society 2005, May 4–7, New York, NY

25. Darden BV, et al. Early results of a randomized controlled clinical trial comparing ProDisc-C and ACDF for cervical radiculopathy. Poster presentation at the Annual Meeting of the Spine Arthroplasty Society 2005, May 4–7, New York, NY

26. Delamarter RB, et al. Cervical disc replacement: intermediate-term follow-up (1–2 years) of range of motion and clinical outcomes with the ProDisc-C prosthesis. Scientific presentation at the Annual Meeting of the Spine Arthroplasty Society 2005, May 4–7, New York, NY

27. Murrey D, et al. Early results of a randomized controlled clinical trial comparing ProDisc-C and ACDF for cervical radiculopathy. Scientific presentation at the Annual Meeting of the Spine Arthroplasty Society 2005, May 4–7, New York, NY

28. Mehren C, et al. Curvature and range of motion before and after cervical disc replacement with ProDisc-C. Scientific presentation at the Annual Meeting of the Spine Arthroplasty Society 2005, May 4–7, New York, NY

29. Grochulla F, et al. Cervical total disc replacement with ProDisc-C: first experiences and clinical results. Poster presentation at the Annual Meeting of the Spine Arthroplasty Society 2005, May 4–7, New York, NY

30. Suchomel P, et al. ProDisc-C cervical disc prosthesis in the first 40 patients. Half-year evaluation of results. Poster presentation at the Annual Meeting of the Spine Arthroplasty Society 2005, May 4–7, New York, NY

10

PCM (Porous Coated Motion) Artificial Cervical Disc

Luiz Pimenta, Roberto C. Díaz, Paul C. McAfee, and Andy Cappuccino

◆ **Indications for Cervical Arthroplasty**

◆ **The Design of the PCM (Porous Coated Motion) Artificial Cervical Disc**

◆ **Clinical Study**
  Single and Multiple Levels with the PCM

◆ **Complications**

◆ **Evaluation of the Bone Ingrowth Characteristics in the Implant–Bone Interface Gaps**

◆ **Conclusion**

Cervical disk arthroplasty is a recently introduced option for patients otherwise undergoing anterior cervical diskectomy and fusion (ACDF) for nontraumatic indications. To the greatest extent possible in spine surgery, ACDF as a treatment for radicular and myelopathic symptoms represents a gold standard with long-term clinical experience, established indications, and reproducible clinical and surgical results.[1] However, shortcomings of ACDF remain, including loss of segmental motion, possible adverse impacts upon adjacent segments,[2] perioperative immobilization, bone graft site morbidity, pseudarthrosis with reoperation, and hardware failures. Because the incidences of the aforementioned are very low, any potential replacement treatment must meet a high standard.

Cervical disk arthroplasty is a promising alternative, having been introduced as a means to allow motion preservation and potential avoidance or minimization of adjacent level degeneration while providing the requisite postdecompression height, stability, and alignment maintenance. Ideally, restoration of the normal kinematics of the lower cervical spine as outlined by White and Panjabi[3] is the desired goal of cervical arthroplasty. To this end, total disk replacement arthroplasty has been reported to restore motion in the cervical spine.[4]

◆ Indications for Cervical Arthroplasty

In general, the indications for anterior cervical disk arthroplasty are similar to the traditional indications for anterior cervical decompression (i.e., radiculopathy or myelopathy caused by either one or two levels of anterior cervical compression).[5–9] Symptoms of arm weakness, paresthesia, and unremitting radicular pain with or without lower extremity hyperactive reflexes with documentation of a neural

compressive lesion are generally accepted as requiring anterior cervical decompression. Following decompression, the surgical goals are the restoration of the intervertebral and neuroforaminal height to prevent recurrence of neurological compression. Cervical disk arthroplasty aims to achieve this restoration while maintaining the prevalence of motion in an ideally natural fashion. In some instances, for example, in patients with a congenitally narrow spinal canal and myelopathy, the maintenance of motion may be undesirable. This distinction has prompted the formation of specific cervical disk arthroplasty indications according to Pimenta et al and McAfee[10,11] (**Table 10–1**). Inevitably, with experience, critical review of clinical outcomes, and the advancement of the technology and techniques, further clarification and stratification of indications for arthroplasty as opposed to fusion will be defined.

◆ The Design of the PCM (Porous Coated Motion) Artificial Cervical Disc

Several criteria are to be considered in the design of devices for cervical disk arthroplasty.[12] All device designs, like the PCM (Porous Coated Motion) Artificial Cervical Disc (Cervitech, Inc., Rockaway, NJ), pursue the following implant design and material–related objectives:

◆ Maintenance of implant longevity and having predictable and physiologically tolerable wear properties

◆ Motion creating surfaces designed to permit motion in a physiologically desirable fashion

◆ The ability to maintain position in the intervertebral space under the variety of anticipated loading situations

◆ Augmentation of the stability of the spinal segment

Table 10–1 Indications for Cervical Disk Arthroplasty

Clinical inclusion criteria	Patients 20 to 70 years old Degenerative disk disease with radicular or spinal cord compression
Clinical exclusion criteria	Metabolic and bone disease Patients in terminal phase of chronic disease Patients with pyogenic infection or active granulomatosis Patients with neoplastic or traumatic disease of the cervical spine
Indications for the press-fit (no screws) model	Radicular compression Herniation of the nucleus pulposus of C3–C4 to C7–T1 Anterior medullary compression Cervical spondylosis Nuclear magnetic resonance imaging evidence of mechanical compression of neural elements Nontraumatic segmental instability Neurological compression of one, two, three or four levels from C3–C4 to C7–T1 Primary degenerative disk disease Degenerative adjacent segment disease
Indications for the flanged version (with screw fixation), in addition to the above	Suboptimal carpentry, understood as an irregular cut in the preparation of the vertebral end plate Anterior vertebral subluxation $\geq$ 3.5 mm Anatomical variation or previous surgery predisposing the segment to higher loads
Contraindications to PCM disk arthroplasty	Ossification of the posterior longitudinal ligament Ankylosing spondylitis Spondylolisthesis with posterior element lesion Narrow cervical canal, anterior-posterior diameter < 10 mm Severe arthritis of the facet joints Overt instability or posterior column inadequacy

The PCM implant is designed much like a joint surface replacement in that it provides an articulating surface between two end plates that bond to the adjacent vertebrae. Given the critical design parameters and the novel nature of cervical disk replacement, selection of familiar materials and design attributes were favored over those less proven or with less clinical experience. The biomaterials chosen, ultra high molecular weight polyethylene (UHMWPE) and cast cobalt-chromium-molybdenum (CoCrMo) alloy to form the articulating bearing surface, represent gold standard materials from the field of joint replacement. Compression-molded sheet polyethylene was preferred for its more favorable and predictable deformation properties versus the durable but brittle, highly cross-linked polyethylene. The end plate surfaces are coated with a titanium-calcium-phosphate (TiCaP) coating providing both a surface featuring 75 to 300μ pores and a biochemically favorable interface for bone ingrowth. Pioneered in the field of dental implants, this coating has been utilized by the lumbar SB Charité Artificial Disc (DePuy Spine, Raynham, MA) prostheses implanted outside of the United States since 1998, and very favorable bone ingrowth characteristics have been documented in animal studies.[13] The resulting electrochemical contoured surface is also stronger than prostheses using plasma spray hydroxyapatite (HA) coating.

The cervical vertebral end plates are substantially rectangular in shape, with the highest bone density in the lateral and dorsal regions.[14] Similarly the PCM implant end plate is greater in width than in depth, reflecting the desirability of a large surface area for maximum support and subsidence resistance.

Longitudinal rows of unidirectional ridges provide pullout resistance along the implant's vertebral interface (**Fig. 10–1**), but with consideration given to the eventuality of implant revision, embedded fins or sharp projections were avoided, reducing the likelihood of either partial corpectomy or extensive bone grafting in a revision situation. Only the extent of bone resection typically employed for ACDF is needed for preparation of the PCM prosthesis, and excessive reaming or table-mounted fixation jigs are not utilized. Given reports of heterotopic ossification and "spontaneous" postoperative fusion across the vertebral levels, possibly enhanced by excess bone resection or reaming,[15] end plate preservation is encouraged and incorporated in the implant design criteria. In the event that supplemental fixation to the "press-fit" is desired, a version of the prosthesis that is fixed with screws to the anterior surface of the vertebral body is available. These design variations are similar to those described for other cervical disk prostheses.[16,17]

Selection of the shape and curvature of the articulating surface is a critical design element in cervical disk replacement implant design. Based on anatomical reviews of the normal translational component present in cervical segmental motion and the location of the naturally occurring center of rotation, a large radius of curvature mimicking the normal cervical motion arc was selected (**Fig. 10–2**).

A comparison of ranges of motion of cadaveric spinal segments with intact, destabilized, fused, and both varieties of PCM cervical disk replacements confirmed the ability of the cervical disk replacement implants to maintain the motion properties of the intact spinal segment, versus the destabilized and fused segments[8] (**Fig. 10–3**). The study further delineated the role of the posterior longitudinal ligament (PLL) as a stabilizing entity and determined the durability and stability of the implant in a caprine model. Additionally, the ability to image and assess the cervical spinal canal in the area of the prosthesis was evaluated. Representative computed tomographic (CT) scan axial images through the maximum mass of the prosthesis showed the preserved ability to rule out further compressive spinal cord lesions. At 6-month follow-up in the caprine model, there was an absence of cellular reaction and no granulation tissue response to any particulate wear debris. Dmitriev et al[18] performed an in vivo biomechanical study to compare the differences between the effects of a spinal arthrodesis versus PCM cervical arthroplasty on the adjacent cervical disk pressures above and below. The results correlated quite well with the premise of an adverse influence of fusion on adjacent segment degenerative changes. Similar intradiskal pressures were recorded between the intact condition and the total disk replacement reconstruction at both adjacent levels

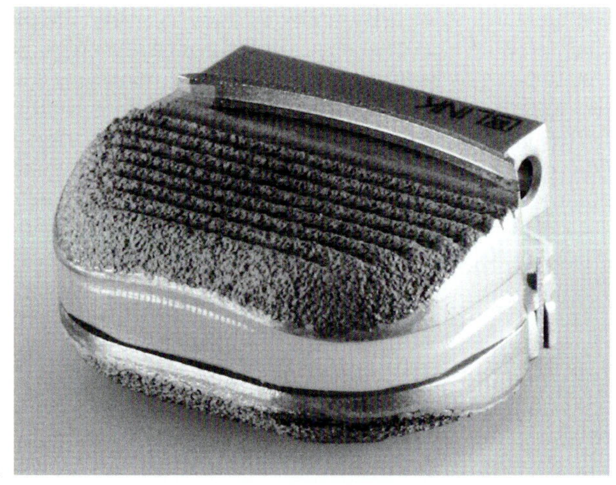

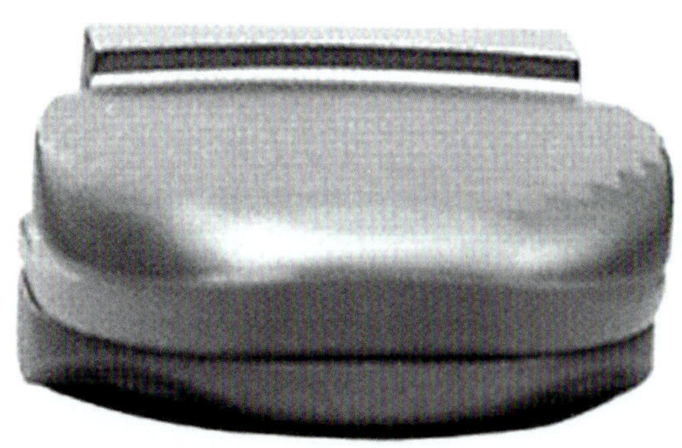

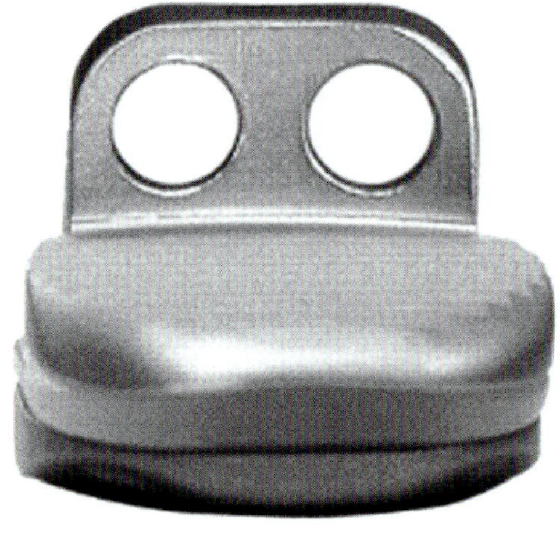

Figure 10–1   PCM (Porous Coated Motion) Artificial Cervical Disc. **(A)** PCM. **(B)** Press-fit version. **(C)** Flanged version. The PCM cervical disk implant features wide, porous coated surfaces with ridges to interface with the adjacent vertebrae.

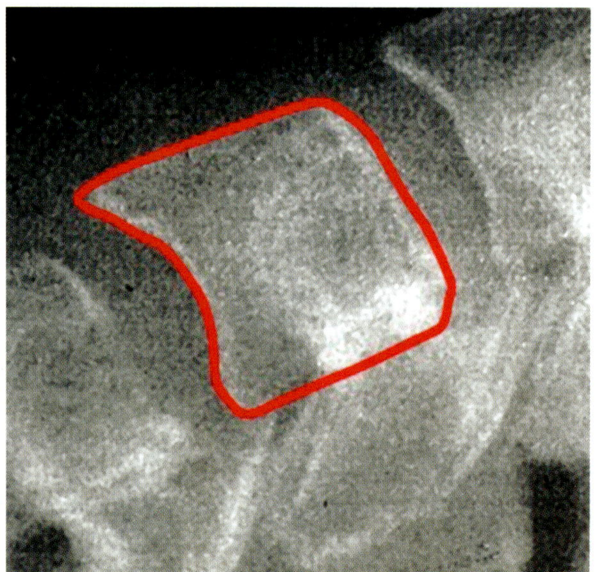

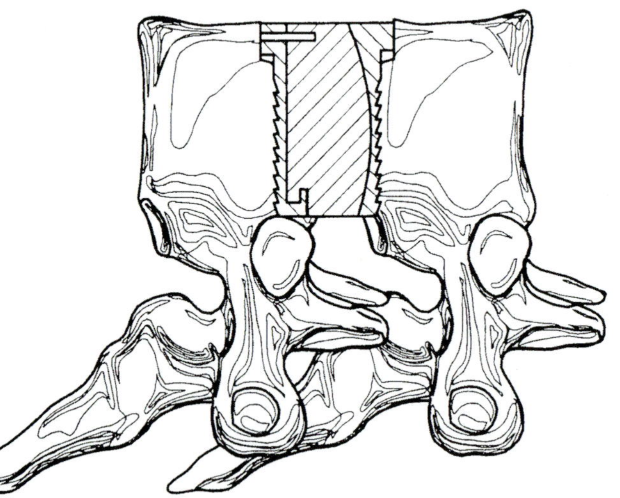

Figure 10–2   **(A)** X-ray lateral view of the vertebral body. **(B)** A large radius of curvature to the articulating surface is designed to mimic the translational component of the cervical intersegmental motion.

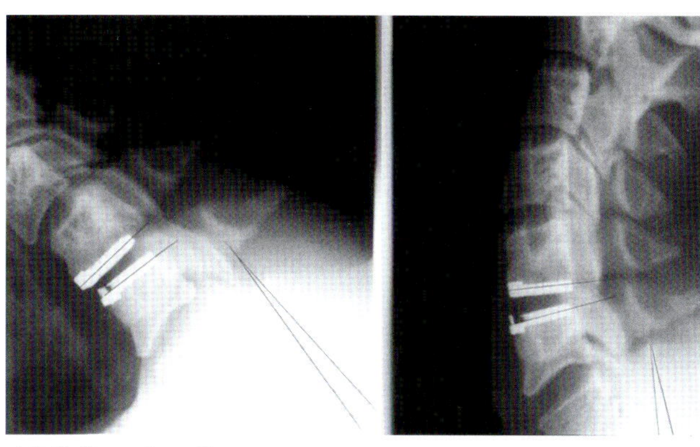

15 Months Post-op
7 Degrees Flexion + 9 Degrees Extension
= 16 Degrees Flexion-Extension Arc

Figure 10–3   Low-profile PCM (Porous Coated Motion) device C5–C6. Postoperative flexion and extension cervical spine radiographs demonstrate 16 degrees of motion and slight physiological translation at extremes of motion. The mean average range of motion value at the final of the follow-up was 8.3 degrees (±4.2 degrees).

under all loading modes. However, in axial rotation testing the intradiskal pressure values produced under flexion-extension and, at the caudal level, for both arthrodesis treatments were significantly higher than the means obtained for intact and arthroplasty groups ($p < .05$).

◆ Clinical Study

We recently reported our clinical experience utilizing the PCM implant.[20] Since December 2002 to December 2004, information on clinical and radiographic outcomes following cervical total disk replacement has been collected prospectively using standardized outcome assessment scores. Patients received implants at one level in 51% of the cases, two levels in 38% of cases, three levels in 7% of cases, and four levels in 4% of cases. Clinical indications for treatment were radiculopathy and cervical myelopathy. Approach and neural decompression were performed in a standard left-sided Smith-Robinson fashion, with complete decompression and PLL removal followed by implantation of the PCM artificial cervical disk. The mean age of the patients was 45 years (range: 28–63). Eighteen cases were performed as complex revision procedures, including treatment of one patient with a previous replacement using the Bryan Cervical Disc System (Medtronic Sofamor Danek, Memphis, TN), one patient with previous cage–plate fusion, three patients with failed lordotic fusion cages, and 12 patients presenting with adjacent segment disease following previous anterior cervical disk fusion. The study includes 115 patients to date. For each, eligible patient demographic information, employment status, and return-to-work status were prospectively recorded. Operative details including the type of procedure (single-, two-, three-, or four-level), duration of the surgery, blood loss, complications, and the size and version of the device used were recorded. All patients enrolled underwent a complete neurological examination prior to surgery and at

each follow-up visit postoperatively. The neck disability index (NDI), visual analog scale (VAS), Treatment Intensitive Grade Test (TIGT) questionnaires, and Odom criteria were used to assess pain and functional outcomes preoperatively and on intervals of 1,3,6,9,12,15, 18,21, and 24 months postsurgery. Static and dynamic cervical radiographs were obtained at 1 week, and 1,3,6,9,12,15,18, 21, and 24 months postoperatively. All adverse outcomes and complications related to the procedure were noted.

At 24-month follow-up, patients enrolled included 67 women and 48 men. The levels of disk implantation included C3–C4 (19 procedures), C4–C5 (33 procedures), C5–C6 (85 procedures), C6–C7 (54 procedures), and C7–T1 (two procedures). The mean length of surgery was 80.7 minutes. Blood loss ranged from 50 to 850 mL, with a mean of 113 mL. Almost all patients (92%) were discharged within 24 hours of surgery. Patients did not receive a cervical collar postoperatively. Procedures were performed at one-level procedure in 51% of patients, at two levels in 38%, at three levels in 7%, and at four levels in 4%. In six patients receiving two-level procedures, the implanted levels were not adjacent.

The mean clinical values are favorable after 2 years. Whereas the mean preoperative VAS score was 7.3, it was 4.07 at 1 week follow-up, 2.8 at 1 month, and maintained at 3.4 after 2 years. The mean preoperative NDI value was 45, becoming 28.4 at 1-week follow-up, 21.85 at 1 month, and 24.1 (the final score) at 2-year follow-up. The same occurs with the TIGT, where the mean preoperative value was 10.64, becoming 6.41 at 1-week follow-up, 5.3 at 1-month follow-up, and 4.94 at 2-year follow-up.

Single and Multiple Levels with the PCM

It is accepted that multilevel arthrodesis has less favorable clinical outcomes than single-level arthrodesis.[20] We prospectively evaluated the short- and long-term clinical results for single and multiple total cervical artificial disk replacement.

In patients implanted for single-level disease, the mean NDI was 45.7 initially and 28 at 2-year follow-up. In addition, the VAS showed scores of 73.3 before the surgery and 35 at the 2-year follow-up. Patients with two-level disease showed a mean average of 45.8 in the NDI score and 77 for the VAS score before surgery, changing to 16 and 30 at 2-year follow-up, respectively. Patients with multilevel implantation (receiving three or four disk prostheses) obtained an NDI and a VAS of 42.6 and 75, respectively, before their surgery and two and 10 at the 2-year follow-up. In the single-level group the NDI and the VAS score diminished 38.7% and 38.6%, respectively. For the two levels, the NDI diminished 65% and the VAS diminished 61.4%, along with the multilevel 95.3% and 86.6%, respectively. Of 41 patients implanted for single-level disease, the Odom outcomes at 2-year follow-up were clinically defined as excellent in 12.8%, good in 73.5%, and fair in 13.7%. In the two-level group, 16.3% were determined to be excellent, 74.3% good, and 9.4% fair at 2-year follow-up. Finally, for the multilevel group, 20.8% were rated as excellent and 79.2% as good.

Disk arthroplasty represents a safe surgical procedure for those patients with multiple levels affected

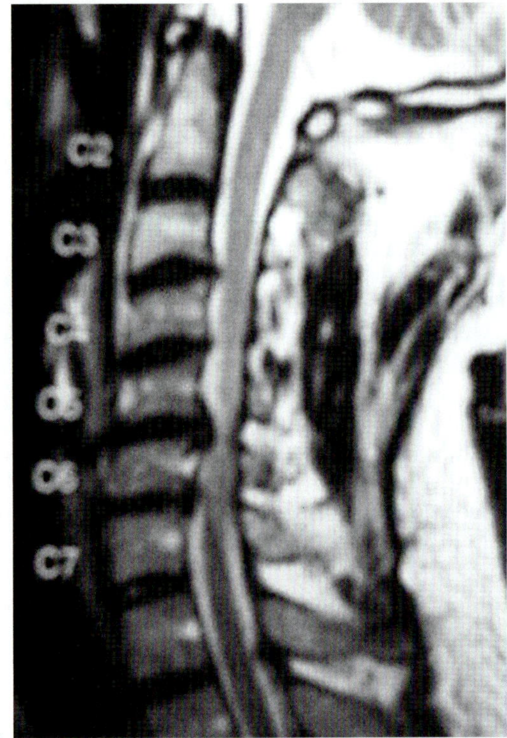
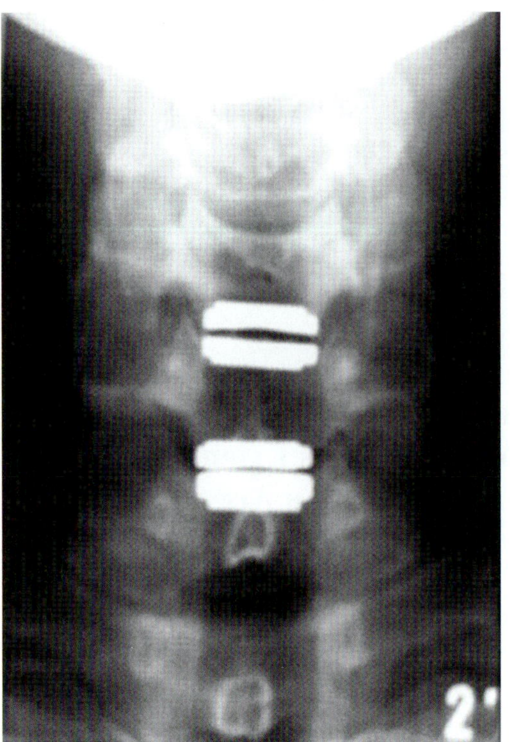
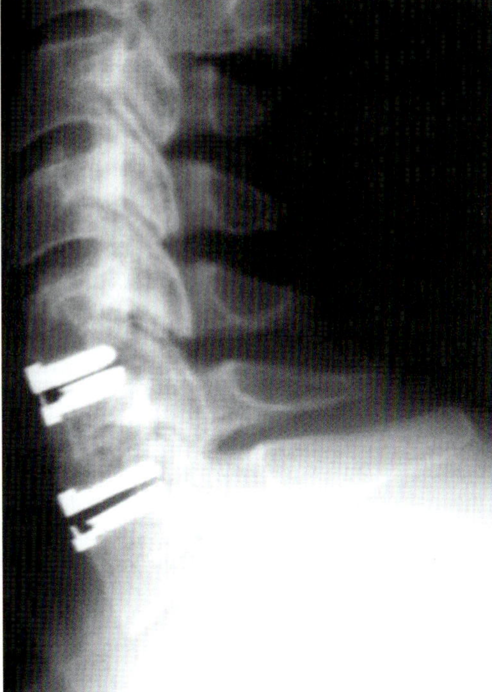

Figure 10–4   A two-level PCM (Porous Coated Motion) arthroplasty. **(A)** This 48-year-old woman presented with myelopathy with bilateral arm weakness and hyperactive lower extremity reflexes. The preoperative magnetic resonance imaging (MRI) indicates two-level anterior spinal cord compression from herniated disks at C5–C6 and C6–C7. **(B,C)** After undergoing two-level anterior spinal decompression, the patient had PCM double-level implantations at C5–C6 and C6–C7.

(**Figs. 10–4 and 10–5**). Furthermore, the clinical results appear to be even superior to those in single-level patients. Such favorable results may be reflective of the ability to maintain or even restore the global motion and alignment of the cervical spine. It seems that what occurs with multilevel arthroplasty is the opposite of the arthrodesis outcomes.[21,22]

◆ Complications

The failure rate for cervical disk arthroplasty is unknown, and although numerous studies show improvement in pain and function, details about the failures,[23,24] including approach and decompression complications, technical intraoperative

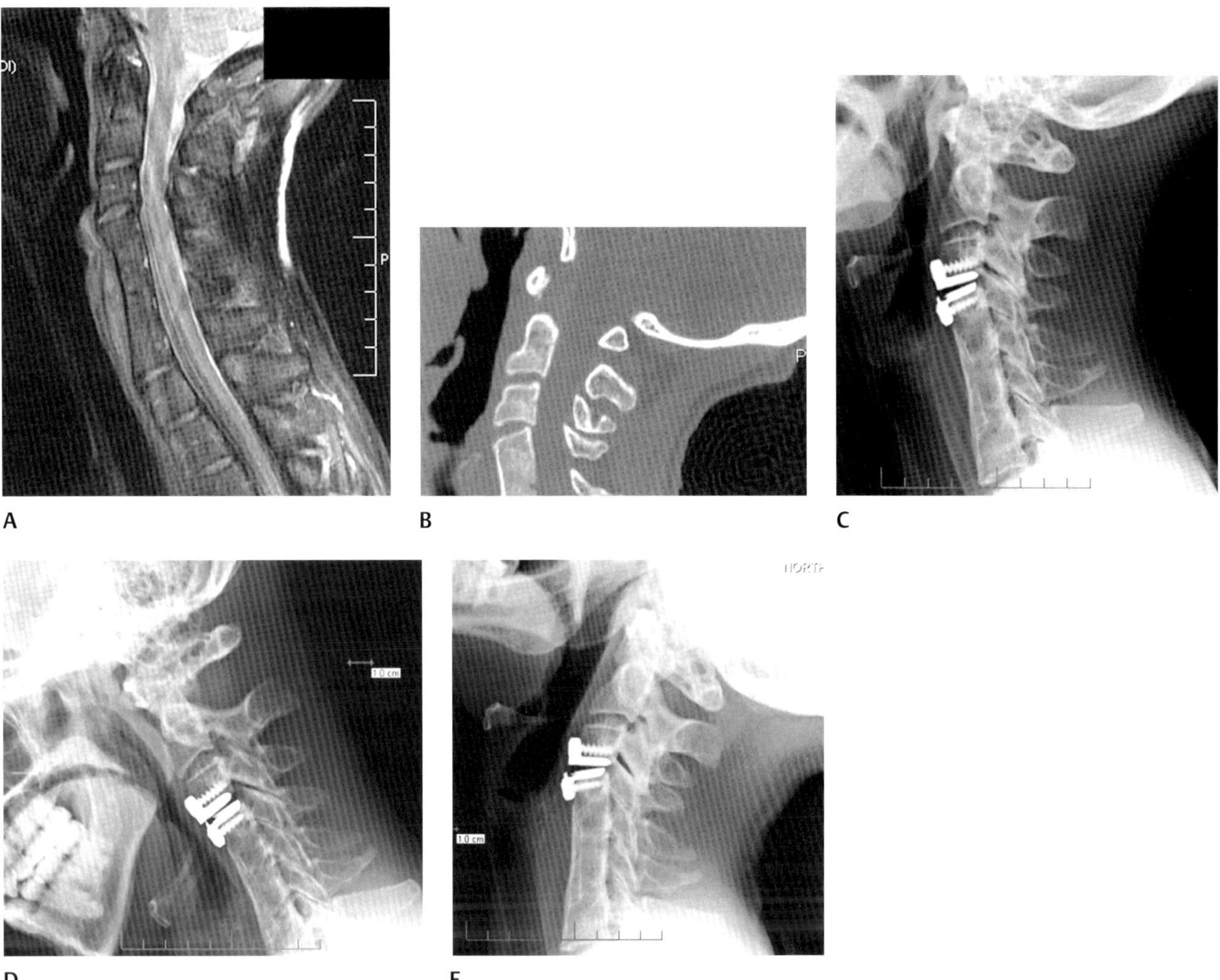

Figure 10–5 Fixed PCM (Porous Coated Motion) prosthesis. A 45-year-old woman presented with a previous arthrodesis C4–C5, C5–C6, and C6–C7 secondary to traumatic subluxation 5 years earlier. **(A)** The preoperative magnetic resonance imaging (MRI) and **(B)** computed tomography (CT) showed adjacent-level disease C3–C4. This woman presented with myelopathy with bilateral arm weakness and hyperactive upper extremity reflexes. **(C)** After undergoing single-level anterior decompression, the patient had PCM flange–fixed implantation at C3–C4. **(D)** Postoperative 6-month flexion. **(E)** Extension cervical spine radiographs demonstrate a good range of motion.

complications, postoperative malposition, device displacement, arthrodesis, and infection, are not presented. Also, different complications will likely require different revision strategies and solutions.

One of the most beneficial aspects of ACDF is the exceptionally low rate of intraoperative and short-term postoperative complications. Decades of refinement in surgical and grafting techniques combined with modern internal fixation technology have rendered the procedure virtually free of complications. Cervical disk arthroplasty procedures, although undoubtedly benefiting similarly from these refinements represented in cervical spine surgery, will have to match the high standards set by the ACDF operation.

Complications in cervical disk arthroplasty procedures may be considered as in the following categories: procedure related, implant related, fixation related, alignment related, stability related, and movement related (dynamic). Several of these complications, especially those in the first category, are familiar from traditional ACDF procedures. However, the introduction of disk arthroplasty in the cervical spine does introduce new variations or entirely new complications, particularly in the latter category[25] (**Table 10–2**).

In our series, no approach-related complications with the standard Smith-Robinson technique occurred. There were no permanent esophageal or tracheal injuries. No incorrect levels were operated. Two cases of cerebrospinal fluid leakage occurred intraoperatively during the end plate preparation. This was resolved with compress intraoperatively and without need for additional surgery. No postoperative hematomas occurred.

No complications were presented during preparation of the end plates and device implantation procedures. Although implants were occasionally removed and reinserted intraoperatively following trial flexion-extension motion, no short-term surgical reexploration to replace or remove the prosthesis was necessary.

Secondary to an excessive intraoperative lordotic position, two patients developed postoperatively vertebral

Table 10–2 Categories of Cervical Disk Arthroplasty Complications

Complication	Anterior Cervical Diskectomy and Fusion	Cervical Disk Arthroplasty
I. Procedure related	Esophageal injury Laryngeal nerve injury Vascular injury Inadequate decompression Cerebrospinal fluid leakage	Esophageal injury Laryngeal nerve injury Vascular injury Inadequate decompression Cerebrospinal fluid leakage
II. Implant related	Graft subsidence Graft failure Plate/screw breakage	Implant subsidence Implant fracture Implant wear Translatory misalignment
III. Fixation related	Plate/screw loosening Graft migration Pseudarthrosis	Implant loosening Implant migration Screw loosening
IV. Alignment related	Loss of lordosis Loss of disk height	Loss of lordosis Loss of disk height
VI. Stability related	Adjacent segment stress	Hypermobility Traumatic instability
VII. Movement related	None, if successful	Heterotopic ossification Dynamic neural compression

"pseudosubluxation." This abnormal translation alignment found in x-rays without clinical correlation never needed revision and preserved normal range of motion during further follow-ups.

No implant or screw loosening was seen. Four disk prostheses (2.05% of implanted disks) showed anterior device migration and received revision. All patients were revised with motion-preserving procedures with either PCM augmented with screw fixation or a motion-preserving vertebral replacement device. Any new motor or sensory symptoms and signs were associated with these complications, and all cases were observed during periodic follow-up.

No loss of disk height, hypermobility, or traumatic instability was encountered. In two patients with preoperative kyphosis, the overall cervical alignment remained kyphotic postoperatively. All the other kyphotic patients' sagittal balance was corrected following arthroplasty. No new kyphotic alignments were demonstrated.

No dynamic neural compression was presented. One patient showed a heterotopic bone ossification grade 3, without clinical correlation.

◆ Evaluation of the Bone Ingrowth Characteristics in the Implant–Bone Interface Gaps

One of the major objectives of artificial disk implantation is to achieve bone ingrowth for secure long-term fixation of the prosthesis. The PCM Artificial Cervical Disc is provided with a TiCaP porous coating intended to facilitate bone attachment. We reviewed prospectively the anterior and medial periprosthetic gaps left during implantation at 3,6, 12, and 24 months to evaluate the occurrence of bone ingrowth.[27]

The bone approximation on the sagittal x-ray films was reviewed across a 2 cm long interface between the bone and the artificial disk in both the medial and the anterior aspects.

The results were reported as a percentage of the total length covered by extracortical bone. Absence of bone of a thickness greater than 1 mm was considered a periprosthetic gap. Gaps remained evident in seven patients at 6-month follow-up and averaged 30% of the interface. Among patients reaching 12- and 24-month follow-up, gaps averaged 20% and 19.6% of the interface, respectively. For all patients reaching 2-year follow-up, with and without identified gaps, the average percentage of the bone–prosthesis interface that was not covered by bone formation was 11% in the anterior aspect and was 7.3% in the medial aspect. The incidence of periprosthetic gaps identified in postoperative imaging was 13.8% at 3-month follow-up, and 8% at the 6-month follow-up. The size of the gaps appeared to reduce during the postoperative period. The successful mid- and long-term fixation of the PCM disk device may be dependent upon reduction of periprosthetic gaps and achievement of bone ingrowth over a large percentage of the implant–bone interface.

◆ Conclusion

Cervical arthroplasty with the PCM artificial disk provides favorable clinical and radiographic outcomes. The PCM device restores normal neuroforaminal height and can preserve cervical motion. Following single-level cervical arthroplasty with the PCM disk, radiographic and clinical outcome measures were encouraging when compared with historical data of ACDF and preliminary reports of other cervical disk replacements. Contrary to ACDF, the outcomes in patients treated at multiple levels do not decline relative to single-level counterparts. Periodic radiographic evaluation during the 2-year follow-up period following cervical disk arthroplasty is critical because implant-related complications have occurred without immediate clinical consequences. However, PCM complications, results, and a small surgical revision rate appear to indicate that cervical disk arthroplasty is a safe and effective procedure.

References

1. Bohlman HH, Emery SE, Goodfellow DB, Jones PK. Anterior cervical diskectomy and arthrodesis for cervical radiculopathy: long-term follow-up of one hundred and twenty-two patients. J Bone Joint Surg Am 1993;75:1298–1307

2. Hilibrand AS, Carlson GD, Palumbo MA, Jones PK, Bohlman HH. Radiculopathy and myelopathy at segments adjacent to the site of a previous anterior cervical arthrodesis. J Bone Joint Surg Am 1999; 81-A:519–528

3. White AA, Panjabi MM. Kinematics of the spine. In: White AA, Panjabi MM, eds. Clinical Biomechanics of the Spine. Philadelphia: JB Lippincott; 1990:86–125

4. Pimenta L, McAfee PC, Cappuccino A, Bellera FP, Link HD. Clinical experience with new artificial cervical PCM (Cervitech) disc. Spine J 2004;4:315S–321S

5. Bryan VE. Cervical motion segment replacement. Eur Spine J 2002;11:S92–S97

6. Cummins BH, Robertson JT, Gill SS. Surgical experience with an implanted artificial cervical joint. J Neurosurg 1998;88:943–948

7. Goffin J, Calenbergh F, van Loon J, et al. Intermediate follow up after treatment of degenerative disc disease with the Bryan Cervical Disc prosthesis: single-level and bi-level. Spine 2003;28:2673–2678

8. McAfee PC, Cunningham BW, Dmitriev A, et al. Cervical disc replacement—porous coated motion prosthesis: a comparative biomechanical analysis showing the key role of the posterior longitudinal ligament. Spine 2003;28:S167–S185

9. Pointillart V. Cervical disk prosthesis in humans: first failure. Spine 2001;26:E90–E92

10. Pimenta L, McAfee PC, Cappuccino A, Bellera F, Link HD. Clinical experience with the new artificial cervical PCM (Cervitech) disc. Spine J 2004;4(Suppl 6):315S–321S

11. McAfee PC. The indications for lumbar and cervical disc replacement. Spine J 2004;4(Suppl 6):177S–181S

12. Link HD. Choosing a cervical disc replacement. Spine J 2004;4(Suppl 6):294S–302S

13. McAfee PC, Cunningham BW, Orbegoso CM, Sefter JC, Dmitriev AE, Fedder IL. Analysis of porous ingrowth in intervertebral disc prostheses: a nonhuman primate model. Spine 2003;28:332–340

14. Link HD. Choosing a cervical disc replacement. Spine J 2004;4(Suppl 6):294S–302S

15. McAfee PC, Cunningham BW, Devine J, Williams E, Yu-Yahiro J. Classification of Heterotopic Ossification (HO) in Artificial Disk Replacement. J Spinal Disord Tech 2003;16(4):384–389

16. Bryan VE. Cervical motion segment replacement. Eur Spine J 2002;11:S92–S97

17. Cummins BH, Robertson JT, Gill SS. Surgical experience with an implanted artificial cervical joint. J Neurosurg 1998;88:943–948

18. Dmitriev AE, Cunningham BW, Hu N, Sell S, Vigna F, McAfee PC. Adjacent level intradiscal pressure and segmental kinematics following a cervical total disc arthroplasty. Spine 2005;30:1165–1172

19. McAfee PC, Pimenta L, Crockard A, et al. Porous Coated Motion prosthesis (PCM): cervical disc replacement: a report of 189 discs in 112 patients. Presented at AANS/CNS Joint Spine Section, Phoenix AZ, March 9–12, 2005

20. Lowery GL, McDonough RF. The significance of hardware failure in anterior cervical plate fixation: patients with 2- to 7-year follow-up. Spine 1998;23:181–187

21. Geisler FH, Caspar W, Pitzen T, Johnson TA. Reoperation in patients after anterior cervical plate stabilization in degenerative disease. Spine 1998;23:911–920

22. Lowery GL, McDonough RF. The significance of hardware failure in anterior cervical plate fixation. patients with 2- to 7-year follow-up. Spine 1998;23:181–187

23. Kostuik J. Complications and surgical revision for failed disc arthroplasty. Spine J 2004;4:289S–291S

24. Duggal N, Pickett GE, Mitsis DK, Keller JL. Early clinical and biomechanical results following cervical arthroplasty. Neurosurg Focus 2004;17:E9

25. Pimenta L, Diaz R, McAfee P, Cappuccino A, Cunningham B. Complications in total cervical disk replacement. Presented at the 5th Annual Meeting of the Spine Arthroplasty Society, New York, May 4–8, 2005·

26. Pimenta L, McAfee P, Crockard A, et al. Evaluation of bone gap filling after PCM artificial cervical disc implantation in a 2-year radiographic follow-up study. Presented at the 73rd Annual Meeting of the American Association of Neurological Surgeons. New Orleans, LA, April 16–21, 2005

11

Cervidisc Concept: Six-Year Follow-Up and Introducing Cervidisc II: DISCOCERV

Aymen S. Ramadan, Véronique Maindron-Perly, and Peggy Schmitt

- ◆ **Material**
  Cervidisc Design Features (Fig. 11–1)
- ◆ **Method**
- ◆ **Complications**
- ◆ **Subsidence**

- ◆ **Technical Surgical Points**
  Uncus Drilling
  Posterior Longitudinal Ligament Opening
  Blood Loss, Operative Time
- ◆ **Clinical Evaluation**
- ◆ **Conclusion**

The time has come to evaluate the results, at 6 years, of 52 implanted Cervidiscs (Scient'x USA, Maitland, FL). Cervidisc is a mobile cervical prosthesis, first implanted June 11, 1999, in Geneva. It is made of a ceramic mobile interface surrounded by a coating of titanium, zirconium, and hydroxyapatite (**Fig. 11–1**).

We are happy to present the encouraging results obtained with this first-generation Cervidisc. Substantial lessons have been learned and have led to Cervidisc II, a second generation, called the Discocerv (Scient'x), which is ready for a multicenter study.

At this 6-year evaluation, it may be too early to know the effect of a prosthesis on the adjacent segment(s). However, adjacent segment disease remains the challenge and the real justification of a prosthesis implantation.

◆ Material

Cervidisc Design Features

The features and goals of the Cervidisc are:

Increased patient comfort Avoidance of fusion, reduction of risk of herniation at adjacent levels, reduction of adjacent segment disease (i.e., transition syndrome)

Preserved long-lasting mobility for segment Increased anterior range of motion (ROM) by a maximum of 20 degrees, increased posterior ROM by a maximum of 10 degrees, increased left-right ROM by a maximum of 5 degrees each

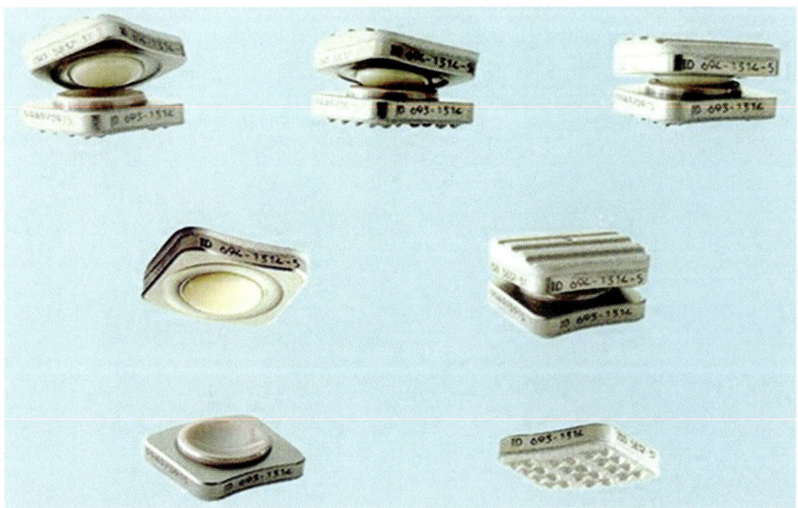

Figure 11–1 Cervidisc.

Table 11–1   Population Sex, Age, Period, and Number of Procedures

	Mobile Cervical Prosthesis Cervidisc
Period	June 11, 1999 to December 15, 2003
Number of procedures	46
Gender	31F/15M
Age at surgery	49 (SD 8.78, range 25–70)

Table 11–2   Summary of the Groups[a]

Group	Description	n
A	One single level	23
B	Two levels (one Cervidisc, one cage underneath)	18
C	Already fused between C5–C7	5

[a]Implanted Cervidisc n = 46.

Modular implant design Spherical motion through well-known and proven "head-cup coupling," zirconium/ Al_2O_3 ceramics coupling gives excellent tribology, predefined lordotic angle of 4 degrees, two different shapes for cranial component: straight, various heights (7,8,9 mm), plate size (14 × 13 mm), end plates with teeth giving good bony anchorage, hydroxyapatite coating accelerating osseointegration

Easy surgical technique Well-known and proven surgical technique from cervical fusions, one-stage insertion of the entire prosthesis, only one ancillary tool for insertion

◆ Method

Between June 11, 1999 and December 15, 2003, the Cervidisc was implanted in 52 patients by the same neurosurgeon. Six cases were removed from the study (see Complications). The remaining forty-six patients were reviewed for long-term follow-up. There were 31 females and 15 males, aged 25 to 70 years, with a mean age of 49, as shown in **Table 11–1**.

The 46 patients were divided into three groups (**Table 11–2**):

◆ Group A: One-level Cervidisc (*n* = 23), C5–C6 level (*n* = 16), C6–C7 level (*n* = 7)

◆ Group B: Two-level procedures (18), interbody fusion cage at one level and Cervidisc at the other level

◆ Group C: Cases previously fused at C5–C6–C7 levels (*n* = 5)

Seven Cervidiscs were implanted at C4–C5, 31 at C5–C6, and eight at C6–C7. Three sizes were implanted: H3-7 mm (*n* = 15), H4-8 mm (*n* = 24), H5-9 mm (*n* = 7).

All patients had suffered from neck and radicular pain. Radicular pain was due to a herniated disk in the majority of cases, except for three bony compressions at the Cervidisc instrumented level.

All patients were questioned for neck and arm pain at the last control during May 2005. Visual analog scale (VAS) evaluation is shown in **Fig. 11–2**.

All patients were reviewed with dynamic x-rays screening six incidences (**Fig. 11–3**). X-rays were all assessed for mobility, device placement, and subsidence.

	Cervical pain	Arm pain
no pain	35	38
light pain (VAS 0-2)	2	5
medium pain (VAS 3-5)	9	3
heavy pain (VAS 6+)	0	0

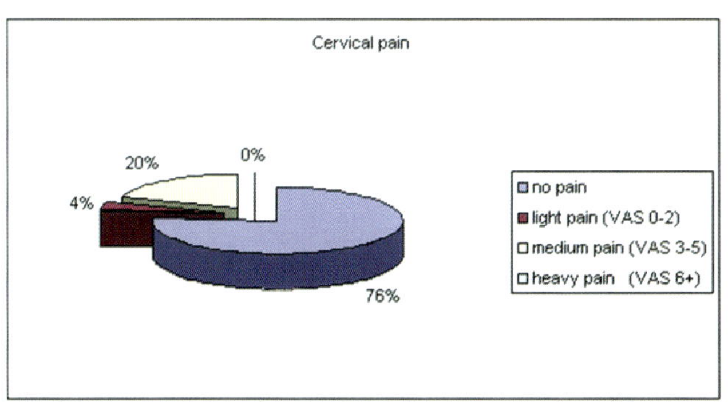

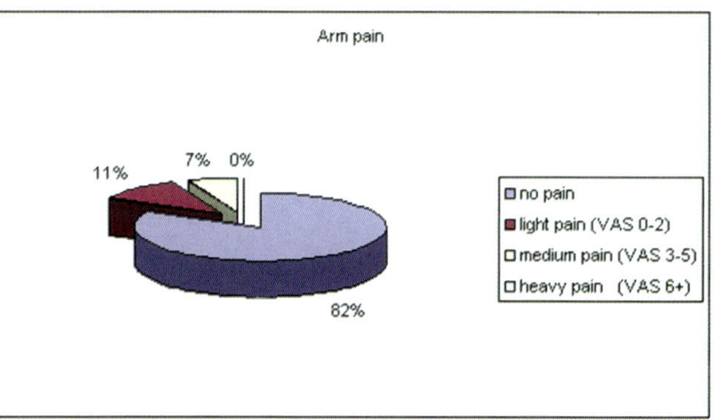

Figure 11–2   Pain evaluation. Pain before surgery was set at 10. Postoperative pain was evaluated with VAS, separating neck and arm pain.

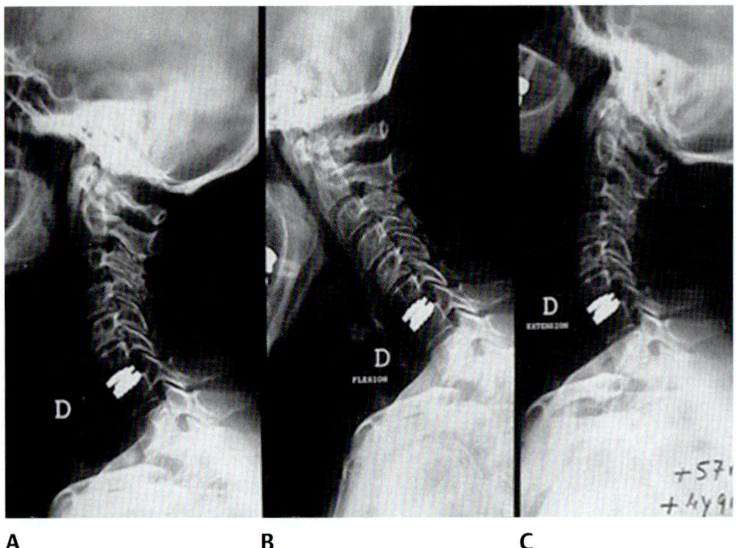

Figure 11–3 Patient from group A at 57 months. **(A)** Profile x-ray showing the implantation of the Cervidisc at C6–C7. **(B)** Flexion. **(C)** Extension.

◆ Complications

The six retrieved cases are represented in **Table 11–3.** Four devices had to be removed because of severe neck pain, with cervical kyphosis (group A, C5–C6) in one case. The second one was caused by pseudarthrosis (group B, C5–C6). The third was the only one operated at three levels (61-year-old female) with a mobile Cervidisc implanted between two interbody fusion cages. Unfortunately the whole system collapsed at 4 months. The fourth (group C) was a misplaced device to the left side that had to be replaced by a fusion. One patient had diskitis after diskography at adjacent level with abscess. The last patient had a calcified traumatic neck hematoma with a fusion at 6 years.

◆ Subsidence

Twenty patients of 46 had subsidence of the device (43%). Subsidence was always an impaction in the lower vertebra. However, despite the high incidence of subsidence, 96% of the artificial disks still had mobility 18 to 68 months later (**Figs. 11–4 and 11–5**).

The new Cervidisc II, Discocerv, has been modified to possess much smoother edges and a slightly larger shape to fit the empty disk space (**Fig. 11–6**).

Table 11–3 Complications (Retrieved Disks)

Complications	n	Percentage of the Group
Total patients	6	12
Group A	1	4
Group B	3	14
Group C	2	29

◆ Technical Surgical Points

Uncus Drilling

The controversy about drilling the lateral unci to preserve long-term mobility remains open. It is obvious that the problem of subsidence arises, increasing the risk of fusion when the uncinate processes are in contact. We had no secondary fusion after drilling. Quite the opposite, we believe that it is more important to drill the uncus on both sides, and avoid the drilling of the "plateaux," with the risk of further subsidence. The device is then inserted under gentle and adequate distraction after opening the posterior longitudinal ligament (PLL).

Nevertheless, it must be emphasized that the lateral drilling bears a risk to the vertebral artery and veins with resultant bleeding. This is the case with older patients with degenerative bony compression. In six instances, this bleeding, which generally stopped when distraction was released, did not permit the insertion of a Cervidisc and a cage-fusion was achieved.

Posterior Longitudinal Ligament Opening

We all agree that the PLL has to be opened, especially in the presence of a herniated disk and to avoid leaving a sequestrated disk fragment behind. As mentioned, the mobile device has to be inserted in a position of distraction: this positioning will secure the device between the vertebral bodies without hindering the intersegmental motion at the level of the device. To achieve this goal, three craniocaudal heights of the upper part of the Cervidisc are provided (7,8,9 mm).

Blood Loss, Operative Time

Blood loss was negligible, with no complications. Operative time is within the same range as for a decompression-fixation procedure (**Table 11–4**).

Subsidence	n	Total population percentage
Total population	20	43%
Group A	11	23%
Group B	9	20%

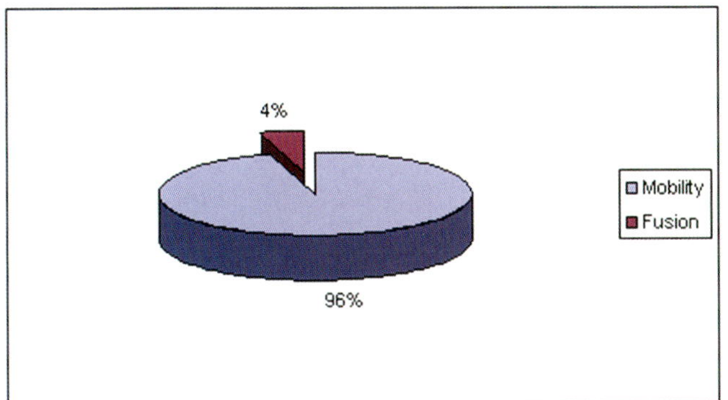

Figure 11–4 Subsidence and mobility percentages.

◆ Clinical Evaluation

Postoperative pain was evaluated with VAS, separating neck and arm pain. Pain before surgery was set at 10.

- Cervical pain: 76% completely relieved, 4% light pain (VAS 0–2), medium pain 20% (VAS 3–5)
- Arm pain: 82% no pain, 11% light pain, 7% medium pain

All patients answered Yes! when asked if they would "do it again."

In **Fig. 11–6** of the second-generation Cervidisc, the Discocerv, notice that the cupula remains underneath, which differs from the semiconstraint polyethylene of other devices (PCM, Cervitech, Inc., Rockaway, NJ; ProDisc-C, Synthes, Inc., West Chester, PA) or the metal-metal device (Prestige, Medtronic Sofamor Danek, Memphis, TN) or the nonconstraint Bryan Cervical Disc System (Medtronic Sofamor Danek, Memphis, TN). We don't believe it affects ROM and nor any incidence on the whole cervical spine. Biomechanical studies compared ROM on cadaver spines and showed practically no difference (**Fig. 11–7**).

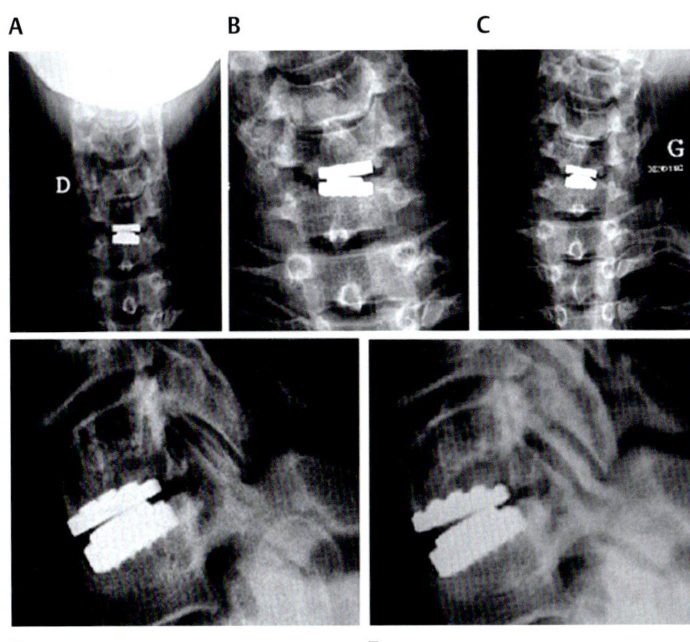

Figure 11–5 Patient from group A, at 49 months, showing disk mobility despite the subsidence. **(A)** Anteroposterior x-ray. **(B,C)** Lateral bending. **(D,E)** Flexion-extension.

Table 11–4 Operative Time

	Operative Time	No. of Patients
Group A	75 min (SD 28, range 43–150)	23
Group B	131 min (SD 35, range 61–200)	18
Group C	65 min (SD 23, range 48–105)	5
Total	96 min (SD 41, range 43–200)	46

◆ Conclusion

It has become obvious that we are now on our way to replacing the human cervical disk by a mobile cervical prosthesis. The success of the first-generation Cervidisc has opened the door to a bright future and success for the second-generation Cervidisc, the Discocerv.

The main drawback of the first-generation Cervidisc was subsidence. It is crucial to minimize drilling of the plateau to retain some of the end-plate structure. This is essential to ensure

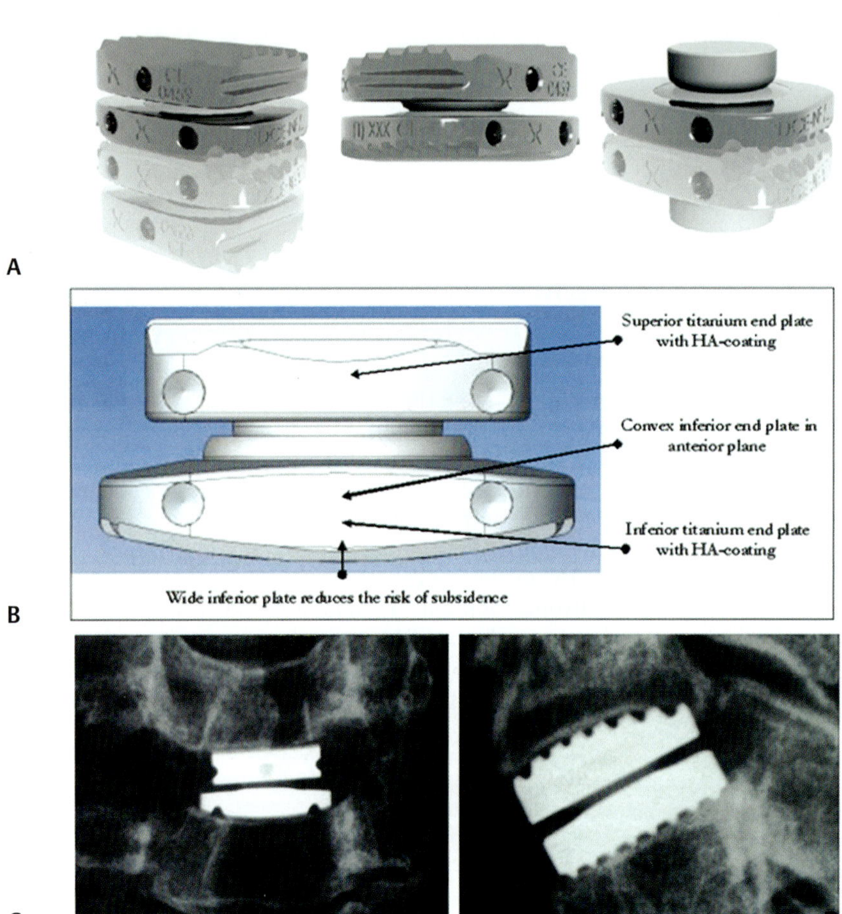

Figure 11–6 **(A)** Cervidisc II-Discocerv device. **(B)** Design features of Cervidisc II, second generation, the Discocerv. **(C)** Postoperative x-rays, anteroposterior and **(D)** lateral views.

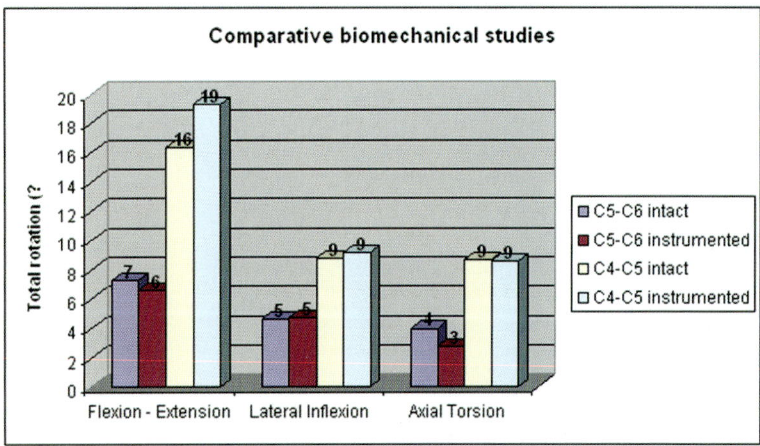

Figure 11–7 Comparison of mobility properties between the cadaver intact disk and the Cervidisc II-Discocerv instrumented levels.

good osseointegration of the floor of the device because the majority of subsidence was seen within the lower vertebral body. For this reason, the new generation has a larger lower device platform, allowing greater stability and harmony with the bone.

The clinical evaluation clearly shows that we can obtain results comparable to those with fusion, and this is equally true for the assessment of neck pain (80% relief) and radicular pain (93% relief).

Despite the high incidence of subsidence (43%), the end results show 96% mobility of the Cervidisc and only 4% with fusion. The two cases considered to be fused are part of group B, which means we have a Cervidisc on top of a fusion.

A study is under way to determine the relation between uncus drilling and the preservation of ROM. There is much less need of any drilling in cases of compression by a herniated disk with a preserved height of the disk itself. The drilling becomes more hazardous in cases of bony compression and disk degeneration. These cases might need overdrilling, with the risk of awakening the plateau and thus causing subsidence.

Another study is needed on the relation between the degree of mobility and subsidence. In all our cases, subsidence did not affect the ROM obtained, within the ROM and security of the device itself.

12

CerviCore Cervical Intervertebral Disk Replacement

Steven S. Lee, Kenneth J. H. Lee, Jean-Jacques Abitbol, and Jeffrey C. Wang

◆ **Design Philosophy**

◆ **Materials Testing**

◆ **Preclinical Testing**

◆ **Current Clinical Trials**

◆ **Conclusion**

A surgical option besides fusion for cervical disk disease has been elusive until recently. With advances in biomechanics and design philosophy, disk replacement surgery has emerged to provide a viable alternative to fusion surgery. The force advancing this "motion preservation" philosophy is the theoretical prevention of adjacent segment disease that is purported to occur after fusion of a motion segment.

Several theories have implied that fusion is directly related to the development of adjacent disease. Cadaver studies have shown that disk pressure above and below a simulated fusion segment during flexion increase 73% and 45%, respectively.[1] Motion at a segment adjacent to a fusion also increases up to 40%.[2]

It is believed that the use of a total disk replacement system can preserve physiological motion at adjacent levels. This has been postulated to prevent disk disease at a normal adjacent level and reduce the morbidity and poorer outcomes of revision surgical procedures.

Other benefits of disk replacement surgery include maintenance of a physiological range of motion, decreased morbidity related to fusion procedures, and an earlier return to function and activity.

◆ Design Philosophy

The CerviCore Cervical Intervertebral Disk Replacement prosthesis (Stryker Spine, Allendale, NJ) was developed with an innovative saddle-shaped articulation (**Fig. 12–1**). It is a cobalt chromium metal-on-metal articulation that more closely matches physiological motion than constrained ball and socket or single center of rotation designs. From C3–C4 to C6–C7 in the cervical spine, maximum range of motion in flexion-extension is 10 degrees. In lateral bending and axial rotation, it is 11 degrees and 7 degrees, respectively.[3] The center of rotation is in the superior vertebral body during lateral bending and in the inferior body during flexion-extension (**Figs. 12–2 and 12–3**).

The motion provided by the opposing saddle-shaped bearing surfaces is 7.5 degrees in both flexion-extension and lateral bending (**Fig. 12–4**). More importantly, the center of rotation is maintained below the device in flexion-extension and above it in lateral bending, simulating natural physiological motion.

A unique feature of the saddle articulation is preservation of the distraction seen across the intervertebral space during the coupled motion required for axial rotation.

Within the first 3 degrees of axial rotation, there is no axial distraction. Once rotation goes beyond 3 degrees, the radii of curvature of the two articulating surfaces are slightly different to allow the distraction motion seen during normal cervical motion segment mobility (**Fig. 12–5**).

Implantation of the device is intuitive and simple for the surgeon. The operative technique is similar to anterior cervical diskectomy and plating for fusion. The upper baseplate has a domed vertebral contact surface. The lower baseplate has a flat vertebral contact surface.

To augment fixation, there are three teeth that anchor into the subchondral bone. A titanium plasma spray is present for later help with bony ingrowth in long-term fixation.

◆ Materials Testing

High-frequency fatigue testing was performed with six implants in preclinical trials.[4] The implants were subjected to 10 million cycles of cyclic compressive loading with an average load of 70 N. All of the devices survived axial fatigue testing with no observable or mechanical compromise of the implant.

Wear debris retrieval of the bearing surfaces was found to be negligible. The total volume of cobalt debris was calculated to be 0.000002 cm^3 per million cycles, whereas chromium debris was 0.000216 cm^3 per million cycles. No evidence of cavitation or pitting was seen in photomicrographs.

Although wear markings were seen on the articulating surfaces of the prosthesis, no component failed to perform

"

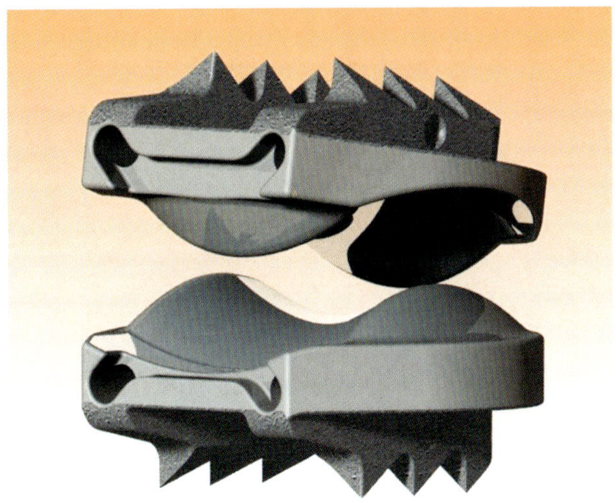

A

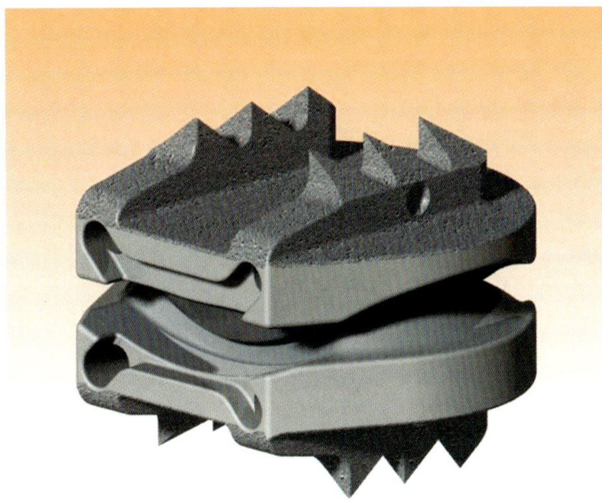

B

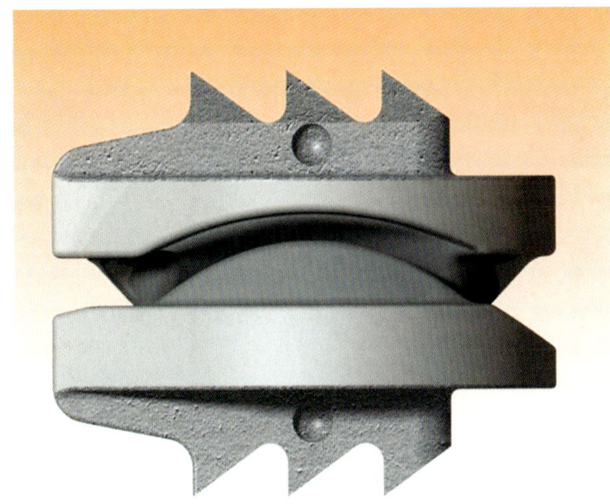

C

Figure 12–1 The CerviCore Cervical Intervertebral Disk Replacement device. **(A)** Detailed view of the unique saddle articulation. **(B)** Oblique view outlining the anchoring teeth and plasma titanium spray to augment fixation. **(C)** Profile view of the device.

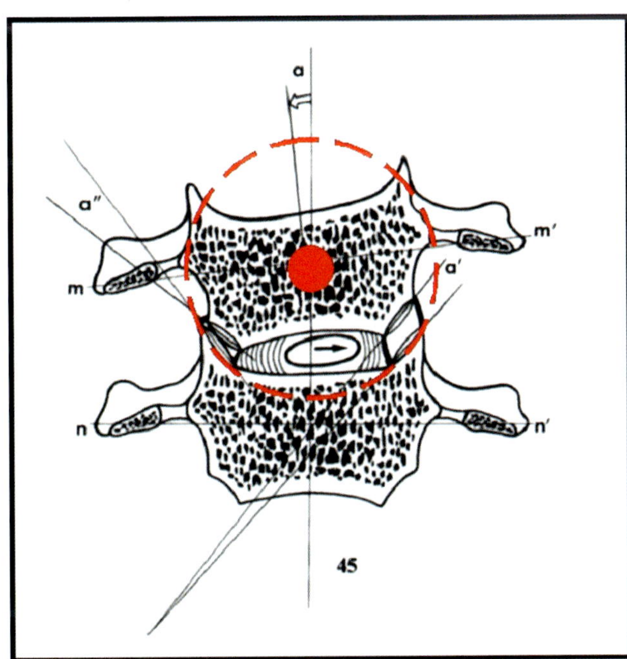

Figure 12–2 Range of motion in lateral bending. Note that the center of rotation lies in the superior vertebral body.

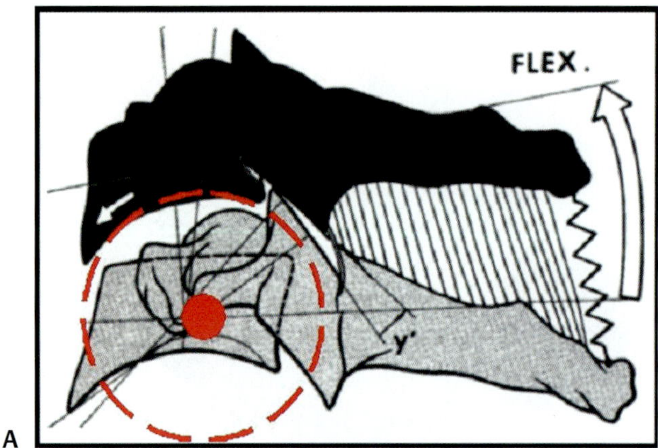

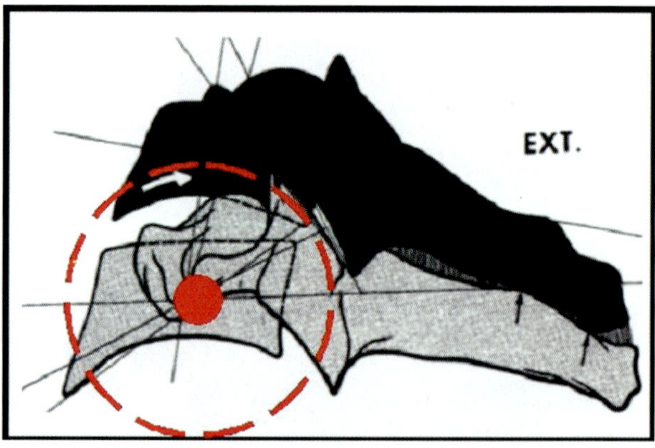

Figure 12–3   Range of motion in **(A)** flexion and **(B)** extension. Note that the center of rotation is in the inferior vertebral body.

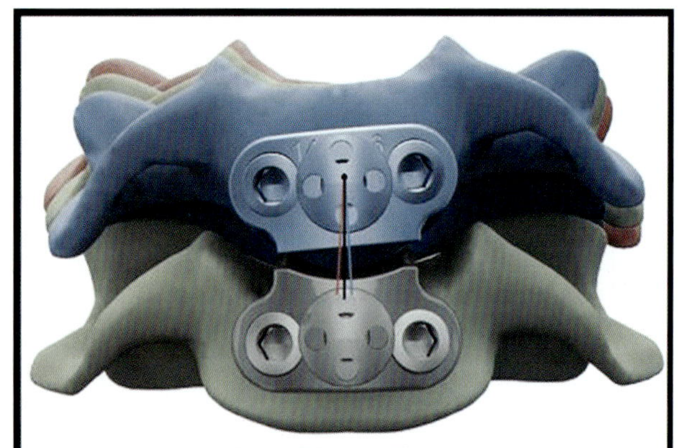

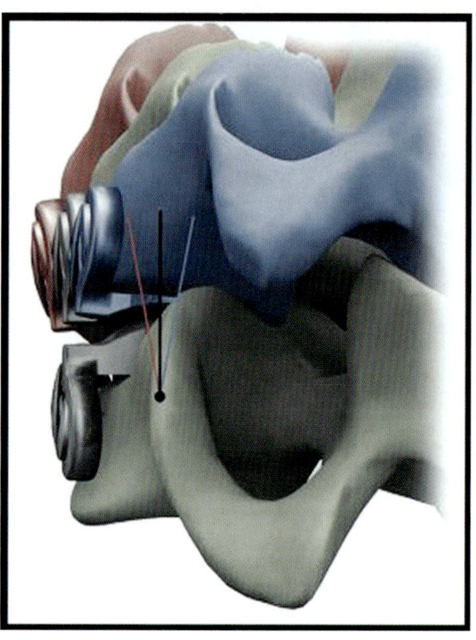

Figure 12–4   The range of motion provided by the CerviCore Cervical Intervertebral Disk Replacement device. The centers of rotation in lateral bending and flexion-extension have been positioned in their respective vertebral bodies. **(A)** A range of ±7.5 degrees with a center of rotation (COR) below the device for flexion-extension. **(B)** A range of ±7.5 degrees with a COR above the device for lateral bending.

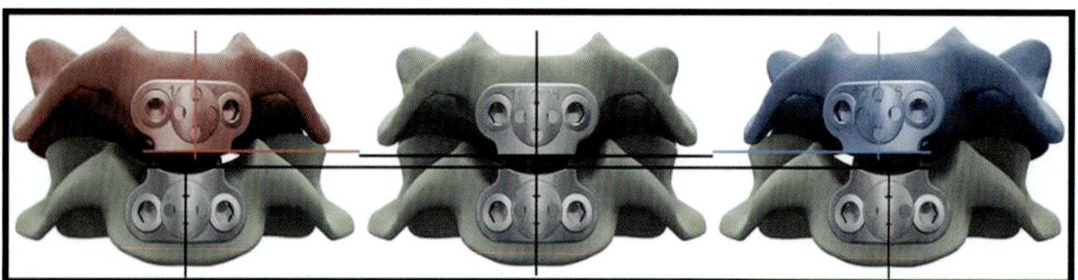

Figure 12–5   Axial rotation of the device is coupled with a distraction motion because of the unique saddle-shaped design of the articulating surfaces.

within the designed range of motion. This saddle design appears to be feasible in cases where large loads are rare and geometric constraints make a traditional ball and socket design difficult. The cervical spine provides just such a situation.

◆ Preclinical Testing

Preclinical trials in rabbits were performed to determine the biocompatibility of this device in vivo (unpublished data). Devices were implanted at C4–C5 in animals. Standard tissue analysis was performed for the surrounding lymph tissue, liver, lungs, kidneys, spleen, and surrounding spinal column and tissues.

Histological review at 90 days postimplantation in the surgical animals showed no abnormal pathology in all tissues in all animals. Furthermore, there were no signs of dark-staining material that would represent cobalt-chromium (CoCr) metallic debris, and no inflammation was present.

◆ Current Clinical Trials

At the time of this writing, there are no reported clinical results in peer-reviewed journals of the CerviCore device. It remains under investigational status and approval is pending prospective clinical trials. Therefore, this device is limited by U.S. law to investigational use.

◆ Conclusion

The CerviCore disk appears to have promising features to make it a successful option for cervical disk disease. The design philosophy attempts to re-create the natural biomechanical movements of the cervical disk in vivo.

Mechanical testing of the disk appears to re-create many of the natural motions of a healthy cervical disk. Current trials are in place to determine the clinical outcomes of the CerviCore disk replacement. If successful, this will be a viable alternative, or maybe even preferable, to disk fusion surgery.

References

1. Eck JC, Humphreys SC, Lim TH, et al. Biomechanical study on the effect of cervical spine fusion on adjacent-level intradiscal pressure and segmental motion. Spine 2002;27:2431–2434
2. Fuller DA, Kirkpatrick JS, Emery SE, Wilber RG, Davy DT. A kinematic study of the cervical spine before and after segmental arthrodesis. Spine 1998;23:1649–1656
3. Dvorak J, Antinnes JA, Panjabi M, Loustalot D, Bonomo M. Age and gender related normal motion of the cervical spine. Spine 1992; 17(Suppl 10):S393–S398
4. Valdevit A, Kambic H, Errico JP, Zubok R, Salveston B. Characteristics of a saddle joint: an alternative geometry for bearing surfaces. Transactions of the Orthopaedic Research Society, 51st Annual Meeting, Feb. 20–23, 2005.

Section III

Restoration of Lumbar Motion Segment
A. Lumbar Nucleus Replacement

13

Prosthetic Disk Nucleus Partial Disk Replacement: Pathobiological and Biomechanical Rationale for Design and Function

Charles Dean Ray, Joseph E. Hale, and Britt K. Norton

◆ **The Pathophysiology of the Degenerating Disk**

◆ **Biomechanical Considerations for Partial Disk Replacements**

Geometry

Strength and Stiffness

Device Testing

Range of Motion

Center of Rotation

Fixation

Function of the Annulus

Function of the Facet Joints

Failure Mode

Surgical Procedure

◆ **Summary**

The normally hydrated nucleus provides annular fiber stretch, which then stabilizes the intervertebral segment. The normal pressure inside the nucleus, resulting from body weight and muscular contraction, is several times that of arterial pressure so the nucleus and internal annulus have no intrinsic circulation. The limited metabolism of these tissues is therefore essentially anaerobic. The limited nerve supply of the annulus is found only in its outer layers where the lower pressure permits neurovascular structures to exist. Studies have shown that significant changes in fluid transmission through the end plate are the likely initiator of the degenerative cascade. This progressive deterioration and dehydration of the nucleus with associated buckling of the circular laminated annulus and narrowing of the disk often lead to mechanical disruption of the annulus structure with both mechanical and chemical irritation of its outermost belt of free nerve endings. These effects often result in both diskogenic pain and segmental instability. At present, the term *partial disk replacement (PDR)* is used in reference to prosthetic nucleus devices, although in the future, prosthetic annuli or end plates might utilize a similar nomenclature. Prosthetic nuclei function by obliterating the degenerated toxigenic nucleus while replicating its lifting force, restoring annular tension. This uplifting force generally reduces torsional instability with its traction on the free nerve endings, restabilizes the motion segment, and expectantly halts further degenerative changes. This chapter reviews the rationale of the prosthetic disk nucleus PDR device design based on pathophysiological and mechanical parameters. Specific details of the Raymedica PDN prosthetic disk nucleus are given in Chapter 14 and elsewhere.[1,2]

◆ The Pathophysiology of the Degenerating Disk

The intradiskal nucleus tissue, well hydrated from birth until middle adult age, is principally composed of a powerful hygroscopic material, quite unlike any other body tissues. It is a complex of saccharides (polysaccharide sugars) and amino acids. This glycosaminoglycan has a core of hyaluronic acid, the most powerful hygroscopic tissue in nature, plus a small content of short collagen fibers. These tissues are synthesized in situ under optimal conditions. From fetal life onward the nucleus is normally completely surrounded and isolated from other body fluids by a multilayered, complex laminated type I collagen belt, the annulus (**Fig. 13–1**). In that the internal pressure within the nucleus is far higher than arterial, the nucleus tissue is essentially anaerobic and markedly hypoxic (**Fig. 13–2**). Vertical loading, osmotic diffusion, and normal motions of the disk aid in transferring metabolites in and out of a small microvascular bed outside the end plates adjacent to, but independent of, the quasi-venous circulation of the vertebral spongiosa. This exchange of fluids across the end

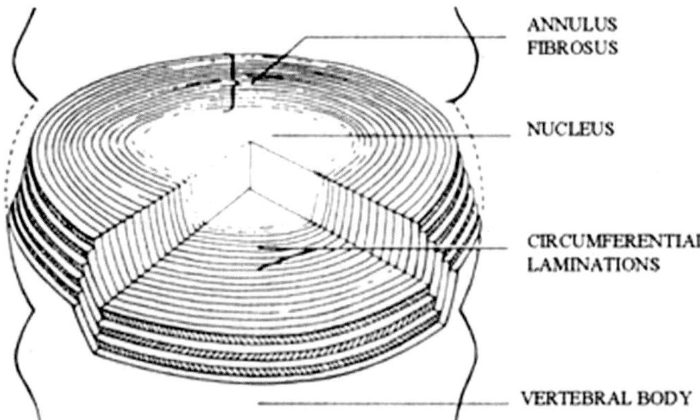

Figure 13–1 A cross-sectional diagram of the human disk space illustrating the circumferential laminations of the annulus fibrosus (as many as 24 at the lumbosacral level) and the contained hydrogel nucleus tissue (glycosaminoglycan). This hygroscopic tissue absorbs water and swells, exerting substantial upward and centrifugal pressure to maintain annulus height and stabilize the segment. The nucleus is normally at very high pressure (up to 6 atmospheres, ~5000 mm Hg), prohibiting any direct circulation or nerve supply. The internal tissues are therefore anaerobic and accumulate potentially toxic substances that are normally diluted through the end plates to pass into extrinsic circulation. Annular tears may release these substances to reach the outer annulus innervation producing severe diskogenic pain.

plates is slow (having a 4- to 8-hour cycle) and produces an approximate 15 to 20% daily change in both gel hydration and associated volume, or a rise and fall of ~1 to 2 mm in disk height per lumbar segment, depending on spine loading. The transmission of nutrients effectively filters out large circulating fractions from the blood, resulting in an isolation of the nucleus tissue. The incoming filtered nutrients are partially catabolized into by-products that are anaerobic, neurotoxic, and potentially pain producing. But, when these products pass out through the end plates they become diluted as they enter the microcirculation mentioned earlier. The nucleus can thus be thought of as the engine of the disk where the end plate microcirculation provides its fuel. Alterations in the end plate transmission of nutrients and catabolic by-products are thus the most likely cause of nucleus starvation, loss of water-binding ability with associated degenerative dehydration, hyperaccumulation of the toxins, and collapse of the

disk. As acid metabolites accumulate and the pH falls the synthesis and regeneration of nucleus and inner annular tissues ceases, further accelerating diskal degeneration.

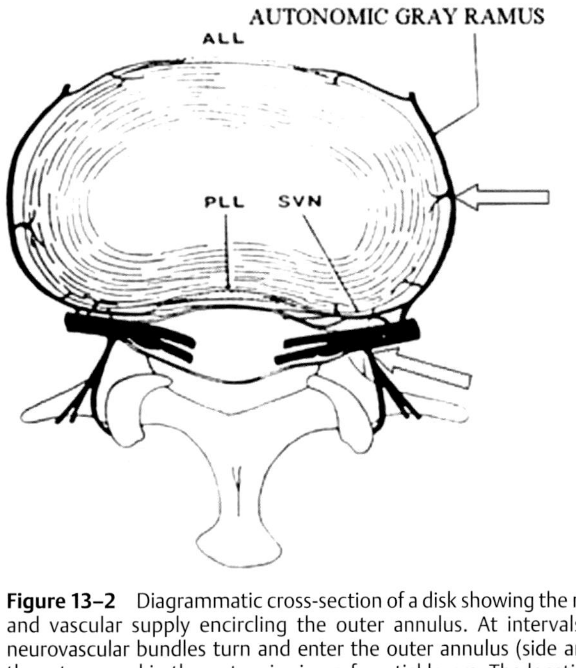

With failure of transference, the by-products of normal intradiskal anaerobic metabolism can markedly increase. These include lactic acid, phospholipase A_2, stromalysins, metalloproteinases, and other potentially neurotoxic substances. Should these escape via annular tears or defects and reach the free nerve endings of the outer layers of the annulus, or reach nearby nerve ganglia, severe, recurrent back and leg pain and potential spinal nerve damage can result.[2] Further, degenerative delamination of layers in axial rotation can produce traction on the free nerve endings that cross the layers resulting in stretch-induced pain. As already indicated, diskogenic pain can therefore result from chemical or physical (torsional) stimulation of the polymodal pain-transmitting, free nerve endings in the outer annular belt. Nonetheless, the vast majority of degenerated disks, for a variety of interesting and in part unknown reasons, are essentially painless.

The annular collapse causes a tearing of its fibers from the vertebral outer ring, resulting in torsional instability and "traction" spur formation along with the delamination of annular belts. The classical degenerative cascade of disk dehydration, collapse, loss of flexibility, and delaminated buckling as discussed earlier, as far as is now known, cannot be repaired or reversed[3] (**Figs. 13–3 and 13–4**). Medication,

Figure 13–2 Diagrammatic cross-section of a disk showing the nerve and vascular supply encircling the outer annulus. At intervals the neurovascular bundles turn and enter the outer annulus (side arrow) there to spread in the outer six circumferential layers. The location of the sensory ganglia with ventral and dorsal branches is indicated by the lower arrow. ALL, anterior longitudinal ligament; PLL, posterior longitudinal ligament; SVN, sino-vertebral nerve.

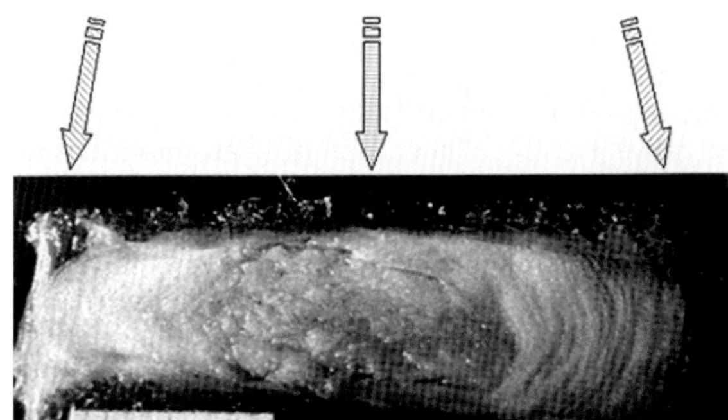

Figure 13–3 Photograph of cross-section of normal human intervertebral disk illustrating the distribution of normal, downward forces (arrows) evenly across the disk space, end plate, and epiphyseal ring margins. Nucleus hydrogel glycosaminoglycan expansion lifts the space, tightens annular fibers, and maintains flexible stability.

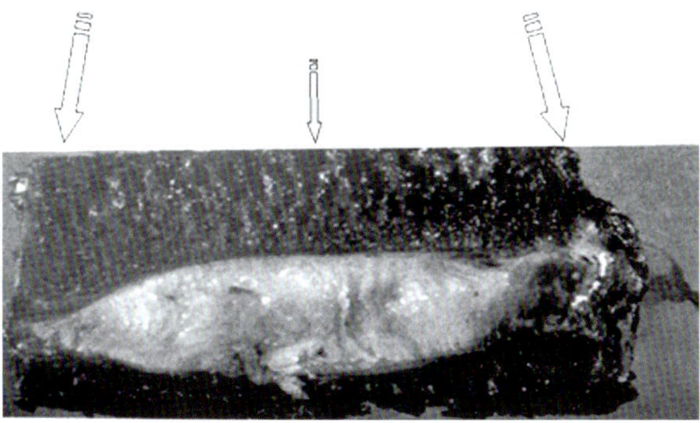

Figure 13–4   Photograph of cross-section of degenerated human intervertebral disk illustrating the loss of supporting counterforce across the end plate due to loss of water-binding nucleus substance. Early degeneration loosens the annulus and promotes instability, but with continuing marked degeneration the space ultimately becomes stable and often rigid.[3]

exercise, spinal column traction, and all other conservative, nonsurgical means that may be generally beneficial during early degeneration do not appear to be capable of halting or reversing the progressively advancing degenerative cascade. Current standard surgical treatments of this disorder are focused on obliteration of the abnormal, frequently painful disk structures by fusion or total diskal replacement. Prosthetic disk nucleus devices, with only one of the few existing designs now in broad commercial use and others in various stages of development, were conceived as a more physiological and anatomical solution to disk degeneration.

◆ Biomechanical Considerations for Partial Disk Replacements

The pathomechanics of diskogenic pain provide the rationale for replacing the degenerated disk nucleus with a prosthetic device. The effective goals of a prosthetic disk nucleus should be twofold: to alleviate diskogenic pain by removing the diseased nucleus and to maintain or restore the biomechanics of the affected motion segment. The result should inhibit torsional stimulation of the free nerve endings in the outer annulus as well as halt the progression of the degenerative cascade. In contrast to total disk replacement (TDR) devices, a PDR works in concert with the existing annulus and longitudinal ligaments to restore segmental stability and motion. Clinical applications of the PDR (currently, only the Raymedica PDN device) show that it is indicated for patients with earlier degenerative disk disease; that is, having moderate degenerative changes in the nucleus and annulus, with minimal degeneration of the facet joints and adjacent ligamentous tissues. Certainly, complete restoration of diskal biomechanics to that of a healthy, intact disk, although highly desirable, is not a realistic goal given the nature and extent of the degeneration present. Nonetheless, because the patient's activity level is often severely compromised by diskogenic pain, even a moderate increase in mobility from pain reduction is usually perceived as beneficial and certainly preferable to fusion with its complete loss of segment mobility. Preservation or improvement in diskal biomechanics is also likely to impede potential degeneration of adjacent

vertebral segments. Several studies regarding disk biomechanics and the effects of aging and degeneration have been published, such as by White and Panjabi[4] and Pope.[5] The biomechanical indications and requirements specific to prosthetic nucleus devices are a unique subset of those of the disk and have been explored by pioneers in this field. Notwithstanding, many of the biomechanical considerations for nucleus replacement are similar to those defined for artificial intervertebral (total) disk replacement as documented by Eijkelkamp et al.[6] Clearly, additional unique aspects arise, in part due to the remaining tissues adjacent to the nucleus.

Geometry

Prosthetic nucleus devices attempt to produce a minimal disruption of the annulus during implantation while removing sufficient nucleus tissue to provide room for the implant. The nucleus cavity is the geometric boundary for implanted PDR devices. Individual variation in the shape of the end plates can be substantial, particularly regarding the extent of intradiskal biconcavity. This latter variability derives from initial anatomy plus the degree of disk degeneration and change in lifting force by the nucleus.[7] Prosthetic nucleus devices must either be individually customized or sufficiently conformable to adapt to the variety of end plate shapes seen clinically. Definition of the boundary between the nucleus and annulus can blur with both age and degeneration, where nuclear material becomes striated and annular material thickens. Therefore, despite the use of preoperative imaging studies, the final cavity dimensions may not be known until device implantation. Further, the implants need to be adjustable in either or both width and length to accommodate individual dimensions of the enucleated cavity or be sufficiently narrow and short to accommodate the smallest cavity. Of equal importance is the distribution of the lifting force across as much of the prepared end plate surfaces as possible. Myers et al reported both nucleus and outer disk dimensions among healthy and degenerated lumbar disks as measured from preoperative patient magnetic resonance imaging (MRI) films.[8]

Variations in disk height that are observed in healthy tissues show poor statistical correlations to factors such as subject height, gender, and age.[7,9] Decreases in disk height with degeneration introduce additional variability, making it difficult to establish the optimal height for a nucleus replacement device. Moreover, with degeneration there is often a decrease in extensibility of the annular fibers as well as of surrounding tissues, limiting possible height restoration. PDR devices require either infinite height adjustability to accommodate for such variations, such as attainable with an in situ solidifying injectable material, or that they be available in a range of device heights. The use of an intraoperative sizing method such as an inflatable balloon, trial device, or sizing instrument may be used to determine the desired height of an implant. One of us (CDR) conducted a clinical study (unpublished) attempting the use of an intradiskal balloon to measure height and volume of the empty nucleus cavity, but on sufficient inflation the balloon always ejected.

Strength and Stiffness

The load borne by a PDR depends on two major elements: the morphology and condition of the supportive elements of the motion segment and the stiffness of the prosthesis. Adams and Hutton reported that the facets carry 15% of the total axial compression load when the segment is in a neutral position and up to 40% of the load when the segment is in extension and axial rotation.[10] Yang and King reported facet load mean values of 25.1% and 11.0% for two- and three-segment tests of cadaveric lumbar spines, respectively.[11] The remainder of the load is carried primarily by the vertebral column, being transferred between vertebrae through the annulus and nucleus. The disk nucleus hydrostatic lifting force or pressure and the intact annulus bear the load in compression. Stress profilometry indicates that in the normal disk the pressure in the annulus is roughly the same as that in the nucleus, indicating disk load distribution is a ratio between nucleus/end plate area and the total disk area. Using Myers et al's data[8] and approximating the shape of the disk as an ellipse, the nucleus is estimated to be 39 to 43% of the total disk area. Broberg reported estimates of 45 to 50%.[12] These values indicate that a PDR should generally bear 30 to 40% of the load on the spine to preserve normal load sharing. At the highest loads ever expected in the spine, 7500 to 8000 N reported for vertebral bone failure, the PDR could be subjected to compressive loads as high as 3200 N.[13-15]

As noted, the annulus becomes thicker (bulging) as degeneration progresses. Thus the load distribution is altered, with the annulus bearing an increasing share. This shift further degrades the mechanical integrity of annulus tissue until, as Kirkaldy-Willis et al pointed out, the degeneration finally restabilizes itself by an effective collapse of the disk.[3] Nucleus replacement attempts to reestablish balance of load distribution between the annulus and nucleus, as well as between the anterior and posterior elements of the spine.

Softer device designs, such as those based on polyvinyl alcohol, are unable to bear a significant compressive load due to their low compressive modulus (near that of the natural nucleus). These devices appear to be effective only if they function like the natural nucleus in the presence of a hydrostatically sealed or fully healed annulus. Stiffer device designs will have the ability to share in at least part of the load on the spine without the need for a fully sealed annulus, resulting in a shift of part of the load from the annulus back to the nucleus. Should the device be too stiff, however, there may be excessive end plate accommodation or subsidence and the load progressively borne again by the annulus. The stiffness of the intact disk is nonlinear; as the magnitude of the applied load increases the resulting deformation or compressibility of the tissue decreases (**Fig. 13–5**).[16] This nonlinear overall effect is important in preserving and improving diskal biomechanics. Firm elastomeric PDR device designs, including those utilizing hydrogels, seem best suited to provide a proper nonlinear compressive response across the entire range of physiological loads.[14]

Device Testing

PDR devices require extensive biological and mechanical testing to determine the nature and extent of any tissue

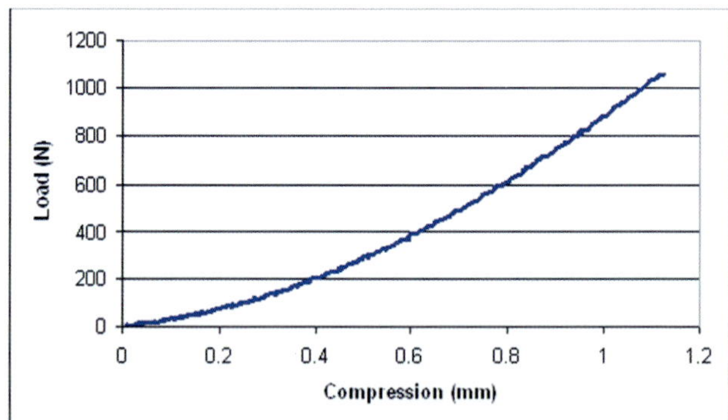

Figure 13–5 Graph showing typical nonlinear compressive behavior of an intact cadaveric lumbar motion segment.[22]

reactivity toward the polymers employed and to mechanically characterize the device. Present bioreactivity testing includes the search for toxic free monomers, potential polymer breakdown products, and other toxic agents through extraction testing and the extensive use of both in vitro and in vivo tests. Unfortunately, there is no suitable animal model for mechanical acceptance and endurance testing, although some experts arguably feel that baboon implant studies should be performed. Mechanical testing is largely performed using standard biomechanical protocols employing programmable force/endurance machinery with or without fixed human cadaveric specimens. Current U.S. Food and Drug Administration (FDA) guidelines for evaluation of spinal implants are based on traditional approaches developed for major joint arthroplasty and more appropriately applied to total disk replacement. Because disk nucleus replacement preserves much of the surrounding tissue structures, additional challenges arise with biomechanical (preclinical) device evaluation.

The FDA has an extensive menu of tests that must be performed, many at great expense, to predict safety and to a limited extent, potential efficacy of spinal implants.

Range of Motion

Current PDR designs minimize disruption of not only the annulus but the longitudinal ligaments and facets as well. It is the condition of all these structures that will determine the degree of motion restoration. A patient may experience an increased range of motion (ROM) almost immediately following device implantation as a result of pain relief, but the degree of motion preservation or restoration is limited by permanent changes in all the peridiskal structures related to aging and degeneration. Persistent loss of disk height, just as with immobilized joints, is generally associated with permanent shortening of the collagen fibers. These changes in such fibers have been well documented.[17-19] Although a PDR device may work to restore tension to the annulus, it may not be able to fully restore disk height due to these permanent morphological changes in annulus fibers.

Center of Rotation

By preserving nearly all the connective and supportive tissues of the motion segment, the PDR device is especially well suited to preserving the center of rotation of the motion segment. In general, devices that can result in load distribution similar to that of the healthy disk will likely have a superior ability to preserve the center of rotation. This preservation is also facilitated by some freedom of device movement within the nucleus cavity, as discussed next.

Fixation

None of the current PDR designs are intended to be anchored in place. This freedom mimics the natural nucleus. One reason for this freedom is the lack of suitable tissue to which to attach the device because one is usually dealing with an annulus weakened by the degeneration process, and violation of the end plate using studs or screws may initiate a fusion process. Although PDR clinical experience is as yet relatively limited (the PDN by Raymedica, Inc, Minneapolis, MN, having by far the largest and earliest experimental and clinical experience to date), device movement inside the nucleus cavity has been observed, similar to that seen in studies of the natural nucleus.[10,20] Unfortunately, movement of the device past the outer perimeter of the annulus was also noted in the earlier versions of this device causing sciatica in the same manner as a disk herniation.[21] Fortunately, design changes in the PDN device and surgical method have yielded marked improvements in undesirable displacements, suggesting that the problem may be resolved through proper device design and site preparation rather than by fixation.

Function of the Annulus

As noted in the earlier discussion of disk pathophysiology, the annulus plays a vital role in stability of the healthy disk through maintenance of tension of the annulus fibers. Degeneration/dehydration of the nucleus leads to collapse and loss of disk height and fiber tension. Studies regarding collagen repair and regeneration have demonstrated the importance of restoring fiber tension.[17–19] Thus, in reestablishing disk height, nucleus replacement seeks to extend annulus fibers and restore tension.

Function of the Facet Joints

Patients selected for PDR device implantation should have minimal degenerative changes in facets (i.e., minimal changes in facet geometry and no more than moderate patient discomfort). By taking a significant share of the load on the spinal column and restoring diskal biomechanics, the PDR device is thus likely to aid in preserving long-term function of the facets.

Failure Mode

Clinical experience with PDR devices to date indicates two primary failure modes: either device displacement or device subsidence into the vertebral end plates. Device extrusion presents in a manner similar to disk herniation, and the surgical response and options are the same. With no primary fixation and likely little encapsulation in the avascular disk space, PDR devices can be repositioned, replaced, or removed with relative ease. Minimal tissue disruption at both implantation and removal preserves the option for subsequent treatment with a total disk replacement or arthrodesis.

Surgical Procedure

Although PDR designs vary widely, the common feature is a reduced profile upon insertion and expanded shape once in the disk space. This feature provides the ability for many designs to be implanted through a variety of open approaches: unilateral posterior, transforaminal, lateral (through the psoas muscle), and anterior retroperitoneal.[20] The choice of approach may depend on the presence of a sequestered nucleus fragment, the maneuvering space allowed by the geometry of the posterior elements, individual anatomical considerations, or the availability of specific instrumentation. PDR designs that offer increased compressibility may also be implantable through endoscopic instrumentation.[20,22]

The surgical procedure for insertion of a PDR typically entails creating an opening in the annulus to remove the degenerated nucleus and insert the device; this opening necessarily compromises the integrity and stability of the annulus. Adequate removal of the degenerated nucleus can be difficult depending on the surgical approach, with the posterior approach offering the greatest challenge in the removal of material contralateral to the annular access. Sealing the opening to isolate the contents of the disk space (i.e., preventing fluid flow in/out of the disk space or device extrusion) also presents a considerable challenge. The potential for repair or healing of the injured annulus is severely limited by the tissue's sparse vascular supply.

◆ Summary

The biomechanical considerations discussed in this chapter are not intended to be an exhaustive list, but rather provide a starting point for understanding the pathobiological and biomechanical rationale for design and function of a PDR device. Critical considerations for different devices may vary and are influenced strongly by the design of the device, the choice of material(s), and the interaction of both with the surrounding tissues.

References

1. Ray CD. Lumbar interbody threaded prostheses. In: Brock M, Mayer HM, Weigel K, eds. The Artificial Disc. Berlin; New York: Springer-Verlag; 1991:53–67

2. Ray CD. The artificial disc: introduction, history, and socioeconomics. In: Weinstein, JN, ed. Clinical Efficacy and Outcome in the Diagnosis and Treatment of Low Back Pain. New York: Raven; 1992: 205–225

3. Kirkaldy-Willis WH, Wedge JH, Yong-Hing K, Reilly J. Pathology and pathogenesis of lumbar spondylosis and stenosis. Spine 1978;3:319–328

4. White AA, Panjabi MM. Clinical Biomechanics of the Spine. Philadelphia: Lippincott Williams & Wilkins; 1990

5. Pope MH. Disc biomechanics and herniation. In: Gunzburg R, Szapalski M, eds. Lumbar Disc Herniation. Philadelphia: Lippincott Williams & Wilkins; 2002:3–21

6. Eijkelkamp MF, van Donkelaar CC, Veldhuizen AG, van Horn JP, Huyghe JM, Verkerke GJ. Requirements for an artificial intervertebral disc. Int J Artif Organs 2001;24:311–321

7. Miller JAA, Schmatz C, Schultz AB. Lumbar disc degeneration: correlation with age, sex and spine level in 600 autopsy specimens. Spine 1988;13:173–178

8. Myers M, Shazly K, Sherman T, Steere K. Normal and degenerated nucleus pulposus dimensions: an MRI analysis. Paper presented at: Annual Meeting of the International Society for Study of the Lumbar Spine (ISSLS); May 2000; Adelaide, Australia

9. Berry JL, Moran JM, Berg WS, Steffe AD. A morphometric study of human lumbar and selected thoracic vertebrae. Spine 1987;12:362–367

10. Adams MA, Hutton WC. The mechanical function of the lumbar apophyseal joints. Spine 1983;8:327–330

11. Yang KH, King AI. Mechanism of facet load transmission as a hypothesis of low-back pain. Spine 1984;9:557–565

12. Broberg KB. On the mechanical behaviour of intervertebral discs. Spine 1983;8:151–160

13. McNally DS, Shackleford IM, Goodship AE, Mulholland RC. In vivo stress measurement can predict pain on discography. Spine 1996;21:2580–2587

14. Jager M, Luttmann A. The load on the lumbar spine during asymmetrical bi-manual materials handling. Ergonomics 1992;35:783–805

15. Adams MA, McNally DS, Chinn H, Dolan P. Posture and the compressive strength of the lumbar spine. Clin Biomech (Bristol, Avon) 1994;9:5–14.

16. Bain A, Sherman T, Norton B, Hutton W. A comparison of the viscoelastic properties of a prosthetic disc nucleus and the human intervertebral disc. Paper presented at: Annual Meeting of the International Intradiscal Therapy Society (IITS); June 2000; Williamsburg, VA

17. Frank CB. Ligament healing: current knowledge and clinical applications. J Am Acad Orthop Surg 1996;4:74–83

18. Hayashi K. Biomechanical studies of the remodeling of knee joint tendons and ligaments. J Biomech 1996;29:707–716

19. Skutek M, van Griensven M, Zeichen J, Brauer N, Bosch U. Cyclic mechanical stretching of human patellar tendon fibroblasts: activation of JNK and modulation of apoptosis. Knee Surg Sports Traumatol Arthrosc 2003;11:122–129

20. Ray CD. The PDN prosthetic disc-nucleus device. Eur Spine J 2002;11(Suppl 2):S137–S142

21. Wilder DG, Pope MH, Frymoyer JW. The biomechanics of disc herniation and the effect of overload and instability. J Spinal Disord 1988;1:16–32

22. Ray CD, Schönmyer R, Kavanaugh SA, Assell R. Prosthetic disc nucleus implants. Revista di Neurorad 1999;12(Suppl 1):157–162

14

The Raymedica Prosthetic Disk Nucleus (PDN): Stabilizing the Degenerated Lumbar Vertebral Segment without Fusion or Total Disk Replacement

Charles Dean Ray

◆ **Materials and Methods**

◆ **Patient Selection**

◆ **Posterior Approach**

◆ **Anterior, Lateral, and Posterolateral Approaches**

◆ **Postoperative Care**

◆ **Results**

◆ **Comments**

◆ **Conclusion**

◆ **Acknowledgments**

The Raymedica prosthetic disk nucleus (PDN; Raymedica, Inc., Minneapolis, MN) has undergone substantial polymeric, mechanical, biocompatibility, toxicological, and clinical implantability research and development (R&D) for several years. These and subsequent product modifications have required nearly 16 years of R&D to define and determine the validity of the author's vision regarding this specific device and its applicability for reasonably and painlessly restoring and reproducing the natural functions lost in painful degeneration of lumbar intervertebral disks.[1] In achieving these goals the need for more complicated obliterative fusion or total disk replacement procedures in selected patients is eliminated. An estimated 4000 patients have been implanted internationally to date using the PDN device, either in its earlier paired design or in the more recent singular PDN-SOLO device.[2,3] International commercial use of any medical device results in difficult and sometimes impossible collection of clinical data, or the data often arrive slowly and not always completely. Therefore, definitive information with follow-up examinations has been obtained in only several (~12 of 20) of the earliest cases going back as far as over 9 years and ~300 of the more recent cases. These data generally were obtained following standard protocols with some local variation. But a more recent, controlled cohort is under way using standardized clinical outcomes assessment methods (listed later in this chapter) approved by the U.S. Food and Drug Administration (FDA). The PDN implant is neither a strictly mechanical device nor a free intradiskal polymer or metallic construct or total disk replacement. It is a true nuclear prosthesis that performs much as the original, natural central intradiskal nucleus tissue. Thus this long-term implantable device is unique.[4,5] A few more recent nucleus replacement devices have been reported at clinical congresses, but no substantial clinical data have yet been published.

In general, for restoring normal or nearly normal conditions of body structures it is preferable to replicate the natural structure and function and not simply to obliterate them. Through contemporary biological and materials sciences, solutions to regeneration or replacement of tissues and structures or organs arise from technologies outside of, but parallel to, medicine and surgery. Technical details of the PDN implants are reviewed following here. Utilizing a protocol with well-recognized outcomes criteria, adults in good general health yet substantially disabled by single-level diskogenic low back pain (although a few two-level cases were performed), with or without herniated disks, and often with substantial accompanying leg pain, were selected. Basically, they were candidates for consideration of an interbody fusion or a diskectomy, being not quite so symptomatically advanced in back pain as to require a fusion but more advanced than for a simple diskectomy.

The primary function of the PDN implant in replacing the diseased, surgically removed central nucleus is to swell through postimplantation hygroscopic expansion, lifting the disk space, tightening the annulus fibers, and restoring essentially normal function.[6] It was known that annular stretch through intradiskal lifting pressure keeps the fibers tight, providing ~80% of the normal stability of the segment. The initial design of the PDN device required a dual prosthesis implant because the perforation of the annulus was kept small, and yet the footprint requirement of the final implant replacing the original diskal nucleus was wider than that which a single implant at the time could provide. Thus two smaller devices were implanted side by side and then tethered together inside the nucleus cavity to prevent dislodgment. Nonetheless, the dislodgment rate was initially ~24% and clearly unacceptable. After two additional shape changes and more recently formulation and fabrication changes, the present, singular implant, the PDN-SOLO, was developed. The singular PDN-SOLO implant, made of a modification of the original, remarkably biostable copolymer formulation, described later, was molded and dehydrated using a new production method. When inside the disk cavity, the device rehydrates and swells to the initial size through its polymeric memory, resulting in both height and width increases. This combined swelling behavior both tightens the annular fibers and widens the footprint. By accomplishing both of these expansion modes the stability and natural functions of the disk are painlessly restored.

◆ Materials and Methods

In brief introduction here, the PDN devices have been constructed of two components: an inner copolymer hydrogel pellet and an outer, superstrong woven jacket of high molecular weight polyethylene (HMWPE) fibers (**Fig. 14–1**). The PDN-SOLO pellets are formed of a physiologically inert proprietary copolymer of polyacrylonitrile and polyacrylamide, pressure molded into predetermined sizes and shapes, and dehydrated. This controlled dehydration reduces both size and volume while preserving the PDN-SOLO

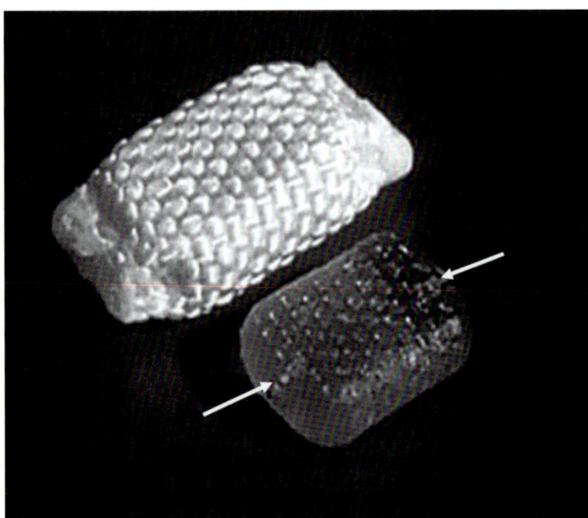

Figure 14–1 Photograph of the PDN-SOLO implant showing the internal copolymeric pellet (lower figure) and the intact implant with its woven jacket of high molecular weight polyethylene. The arrows at the ends of the pellet indicate the internal location of the x-ray-visible platinum-iridium wire stubs.

implant's expansion memory so that when rehydrated inside the prepared, evacuated nucleus cavity, the implant properly fills the cavity (**Fig. 14–2**). The outer, loosely woven, remarkably strong constraining jacket of HMWPE limits expansion of the pellet thus preventing unrestrained overexpansion that could fracture the end plate. The jacket also makes the insert far easier to surgically manipulate. The presently developed polymer formulation permits the PDN-SOLO device to absorb up to 80% of its dry weight in water, providing a softer, more conformal device while maintaining the important expansion and lifting forces. No other water-soluble hydrogel polymer, among several tested, was found to have these needed abilities. This rehydration-expansion, beginning immediately after insertion and slowing exponentially over 7 to 10 days, restores height and mechanical stability to the disk while maintaining reasonable segmental flexibility. Small, short, platinum-iridium wires are inserted into each end of the pellets or jackets rendering visible the position of an implant by ordinary C-arm fluoroscopic or plain x-ray views (**Fig. 14–3**).

Extensive bench and animal testing were performed on the polymer formulations and jackets using established scientific test methods and in keeping with FDA guidelines for implant materials.[7] No intact polymeric device has ever been approved for permanent human intradiskal use; therefore, considerable fundamental investigations were required. The PDN devices and individual components passed all FDA- and ISO-required animal, cytological, and toxicity testing. Extensive bench testing was performed at the Raymedica, Inc., facility, and in vitro biomechanical testing using human cadaver spines adhering to standard procedures has been repeatedly performed at two U.S. and two European academic centers.[8,9] These test outcomes certified biological safety and mechanical durability and also guided subsequent prototype improvements. Normal or abnormal human disk nucleus tissue specimens, removed at surgery, were found to be unsuitable models for developing nucleus replacement components because this tissue has hydration and mechanical behaviors unlike any of the several experimental hydrogel polymers tested. The natural hygroscopic glycosaminoglycan tissue of the natural nucleus cannot be physically or chemically reproduced. In addition, for testing purposes, no suitable animal model exists for reasonable investigation of any spinal implant other than for studies of tissue acceptance, carcinogenicity, and biocompatibility. Nonetheless, animal studies were ethically performed in standard, approved experiments using large mongrel dogs, large goats, and transgenic mice as well as in tissue culture preparations. However, as is somehow notwithstanding required by the FDA, a baboon study has also been done. None of these tests showed an adverse response to the components, the pellets and jackets, or intact miniaturized implants (the animal disk space is a fraction of the human in diameter and height). The author implanted two of these animal-sized PDN devices into his own intercostal muscle and after 3 years, on removal, they were found to have caused no reactions or deteriorations.

The pellet and jacket were subjected to standard mechanical testing for up to 50 million normal range compression cycles and to 10 million compression-translation cycles;

Increase in Height =
6.0 mm   ☉   9.2 mm

Increase in Width =
11.5 mm   ☉   15.0

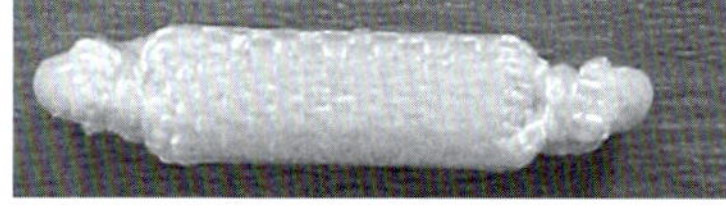

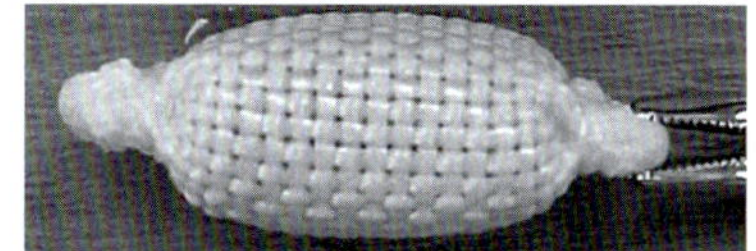
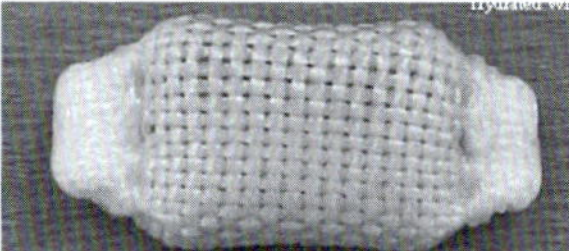

All Implants ~ 29 mm In Length

Figure 14–2   Composite photograph of PDN-SOLOs showing their dehydrated form (for implant facilitation) and fully hydrated form (after implantation), indicating the substantial rise in both height and width. These dimensions vary with the particular model/size of device implanted.

neither method showed deterioration of the pellets or jackets. Following prolonged cyclic tests the terminal burst strength of intact implants exceeded the 6 kN limit of the test machine. Thus structural and biological prolonged-term safety was confirmed. Additionally, in cadaver segment biomechanical studies, enucleated segments showed loss of normal stiffness and, therefore, decreased stability as compared with initially intact segments, but when the PDN-SOLO was inserted and hydrated, normal stiffness-stabilization was reestablished. Clinically, the exclusive use of the PDN-SOLO device version began in 2002 and has clearly demonstrated that this new single implant can perform as well as the initial dual implants but with marked simplification of the procedure and marked reduction in dislodgments. The PDN-SOLO implants are 5,7, or 9 mm in dehydrated heights and each is ~29 mm in length; furthermore, the corners of the jackets are now more rounded than were the dual devices. Importantly, although several artificial disk devices have been proposed and actually patented, few have ever been appropriately studied or applied clinically.[10–13]

◆ Patient Selection

As already indicated, and in accordance with the original FDA-agreed protocol, the initial subjects were adults in good health and substantially disabled by diskogenic low back pain. Degeneration at the target level was at least 10%, by height and magnetic resonance imaging (MRI) changes, as compared with adjacent lumbar disk spaces, with or without herniation; cases commonly had additional leg pain. Cases had essentially intact facet joints, minimal osteophyte formation, and were without notable central or lateral stenosis. All patients had a minimum of 6 months of unrewarding conservative trial. The clear majority of cases were those with single-level degenerations, with an exceptional two-level case. A minority of the cases had provocative preoperative diskography performed for segment selection because in many countries provocative diskography is not performed or is not routine. Using the initial dual PDN implants, ~1400 cases were performed in 36 countries. A select group of surgeons were asked to participate in a prospective study on the device. Each surgeon underwent training consisting of lectures, demonstrations, videos, and spine model mock surgery, and the majority also attended one or more cadaver surgery training workshops. Further, experienced surgeons were appointed in most countries to provide subsequent surgical participation for trainee colleagues. All surgeons were nationally certified, practicing orthopedists or neurosurgeons. Each target space was required to have greater than 5 mm in central height and no prior surgery at that level. Questionnaires of clinical history, symptoms, preoperative and follow-up Oswestry and Prolo scales, and visual analog pain scales were translated into native tongues to improve comprehension and informed consent.[14,15] All data were requested to be recorded and sent for processing at the Raymedica, Inc., office in Minneapolis, Minnesota. Further, all pre- and postoperative x-ray films and scan images were reviewed by a single neuroradiologist in Minnesota.

Figure 14–3   A lumbar vertebral segment showing the PDN-SOLO implant in excellent position and with its marker wires highlighted.

◆ Posterior Approach

Patients were given a suitable prophylactic antibiotic (e.g., Ancef 1 g IV) 1 to 2 hours preoperatively. General anesthesia was primarily used, but a few cases were performed using an epidural anesthetic technique. For a posterior approach, standard diskectomy positioning, preparation, drapery, and incision were used. The posterior approach was employed both in the original paired and frequently in the new PDN-SOLO implants. The appropriately cut lamina was spread open using a modified Cloward-type distractor; the dura and nerve structures were visualized and protected. The annulus was cleaned of loose tissue and a small horizontal stab incision was made on one side. This incision was then instrument-dilated creating access to the nucleus cavity. As much as possible of the old nucleus was then evacuated while being flooded with saline (**Fig. 14–4**). During the nearly total removal of the nucleus, caution was taken not to damage the end plates by curettage or trauma. Removing adequate contralateral nucleus tissue was ordinarily the only challenge in the procedure. The completeness of nucleus removal was estimated with probes and the injection of radiocontrast medium for intraoperative diskography (**Figs. 14–5 and 14–6**). The latter method proved to be the best means to visualize remaining tissue so that additional nuclectomy was often needed. The largest PDN device that could be passed without overdistraction was chosen using special sizing instruments, similar to the initial annulus dilators. A thin, flexible guide was inserted into the annulus opening and placed deeply in the nucleus cavity (**Fig. 14–7**). For cases with tight cavitary space, a strong no. 0 or 1 suture or cord was often temporarily sewn through the leading end of the PDN jacket and kept as a loop with an identifying knot tied in the

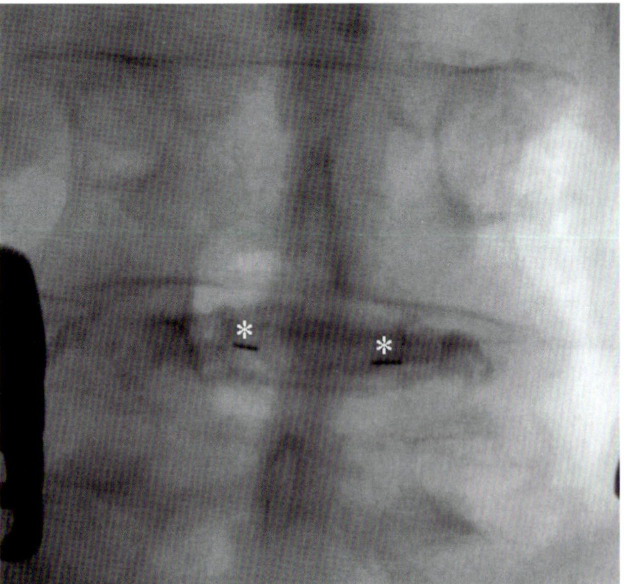

Figure 14–5 On-table fluoroscopic x-ray image showing the PDN-SOLO surrounded by contrast medium (injected prior to PDN implantation) to determine adequacy of the nucleus evacuation. The x-ray markers (at asterisks) are clearly visible in this excellently positioned device.

free ends (**Fig. 14–8**). The dehydrated jacketed polymer implant, compressed into a slim form, was inserted, often by impaction, through the small dilated annular incision and along the flexible guide, and when used, the traction suture was pulled firmly and dorsally, elevating the leading end of the PDN inside the nucleus cavity (**Fig. 14–9**). With the implant apparently in proper transverse position the flexible guide was removed (**Fig. 14–10**) and the position confirmed

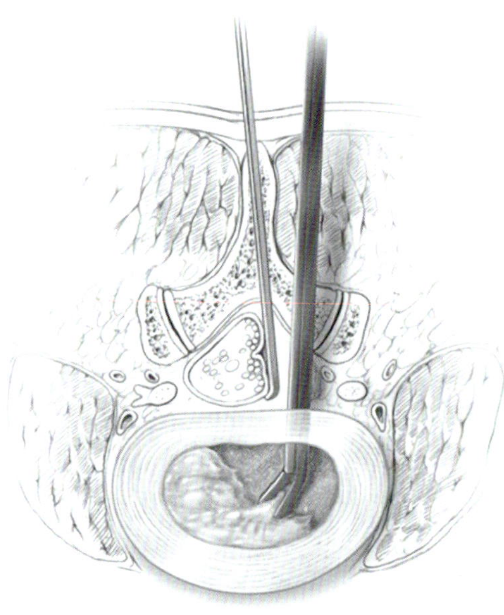

Figure 14–4 Removal of deep and nucleus tissues using an offset or angulated rongeur to cross to the side opposite the annulotomy entrance.

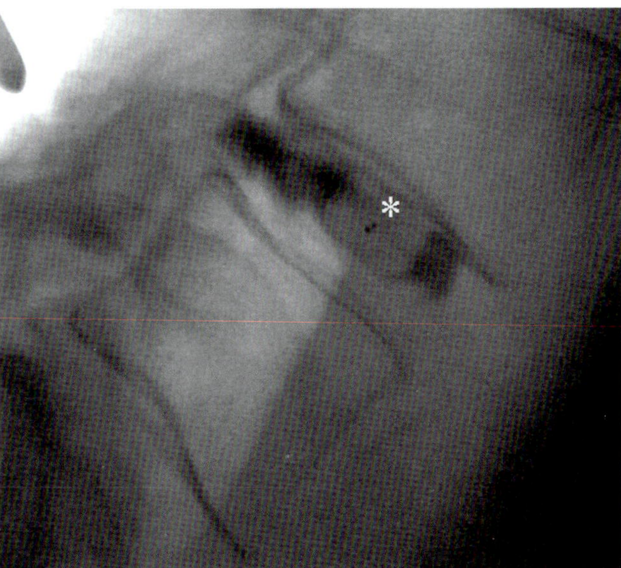

Figure 14–6 Lateral fluoroscopic view of the same case as shown in **Fig. 14–5** again showing the intradiskal contrast medium, the more transparent shadow of the PDN-SOLO implant and the excellent alignment of the two marker wires (at the arrow) appearing almost as a single dot.

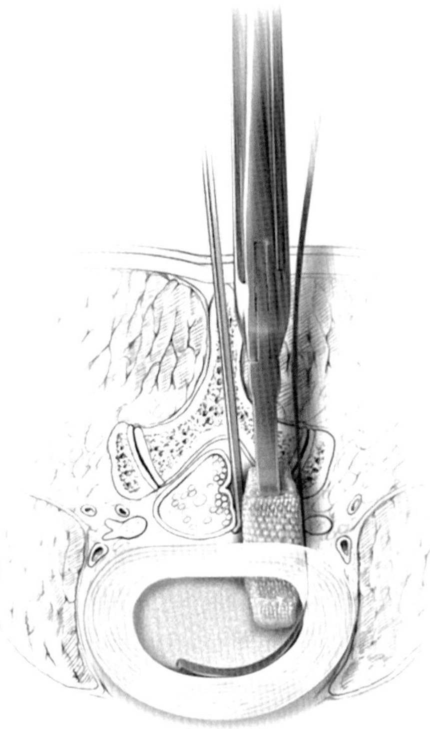

Figure 14–7   The forced insertion of a PDN-SOLO implant along a flexible guide into the empty nucleus cavity.

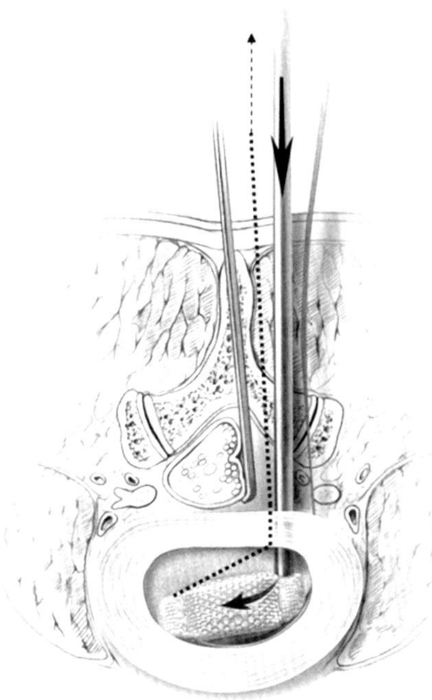

Figure 14–9   Forcing the implant along the guide surface using a small impactor as the traction suture (dashed line) is firmly pulled. The traction causes the implant to deflect more dorsally into the preferred final transverse position.

using the C-arm fluoroscope; the platinum wire markers in each end of the implant showed the implant positioning, as seen in **Figs. 14–5 and 14–6**. Needed positional corrections were made by pressing or impacting an appropriate area of the PDN or by using the pull suture, somewhat as seen in **Fig. 14–9**. With the SOLO device's transverse position confirmed, it was flooded with saline to begin expansion. At present there appears to be no satisfactory or reliable method for closing the annular opening; however, none appears needed when the SOLO implant surgical protocol, in particular a complete nucleectomy, is carefully followed. The cut and stretched annular fibers rapidly swell, effectively closing the access tract. The final position was permanently x-ray imaged. Routine tissue layer closure was achieved without drainage.

The larger PDN-SOLO XL implant version expanded even further after implantation, more fully distributing the load over the larger end plate surfaces; however, the increased profile limited its use to L5–S1 in most cases.

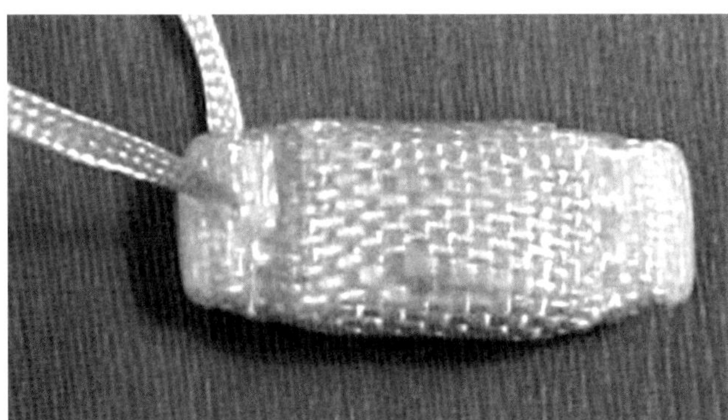

Figure 14–8   A strong traction suture or cord has been temporarily sewn through the distal (leading end) of the jacket to be used as an aid in transverse positioning of the implant.

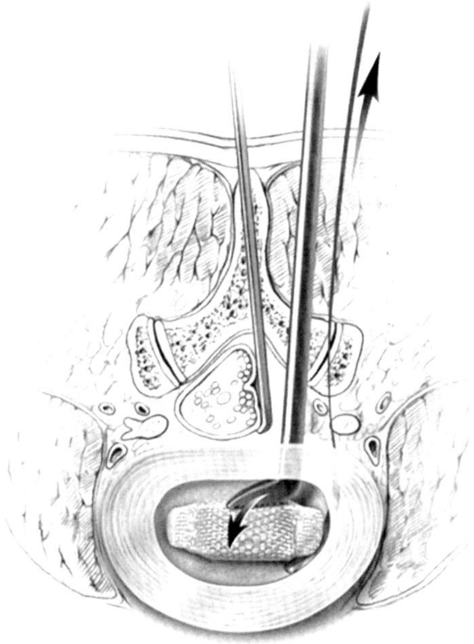

Figure 14–10   Pressing and holding the implant ventrally by a footed impactor as the flexible guide is removed.

◆ Anterior, Lateral, and Posterolateral Approaches

Basically, these alternative approaches are quite similar to the standard posterior method already given, although obviously not utilizing a laminotomy (**Fig. 14–11**). A standard retroperitoneal approach is employed for anterior or posterolateral implants; however, the cleared portion of annulus was incised and turned as a small closable flap. This small annular entrance was distracted and the nucleus cleared out under direct vision, using caution not to damage the end plates. Again the adequacy of the cleared nucleus cavity was estimated, probed, or measured and usually diskographed. The largest sizing instrument that would pass determined the PDN or PDN-SOLO implant size to be used. Implant insertion was performed by impaction on the device but without the flexible guide or traction suture, with the final position determined by direct vision or by using the C-arm fluoroscope to visualize the platinum markers. The flap was sewn shut and the incision closed routinely without drainage. Routine follow-up MRI scans in many patients demonstrated excellent appearance of the implants (**Fig. 14–12**).

The far lateral retroperitoneal approach passed just anterior to or through the iliopsoas muscle. The direct lateral dissection was blunt in the direction of the fibers, simple, and almost bloodless and could be performed using local or epidural anesthesia with mild sedation. A lateral 3 to 5 cm skin incision was placed using lateral fluoroscopy, and the transmuscular dissection done primarily with a finger, passing anterior to the transverse process and with caution not to encounter nerve or vascular structures. A Steinmann pin was often passed into the disk space with its position confirmed on fluoroscopy. Only ~3 to 4 cm of the annulus was exposed and incised as a short flap, discussed earlier. The remaining technique was also the same as already given, with the

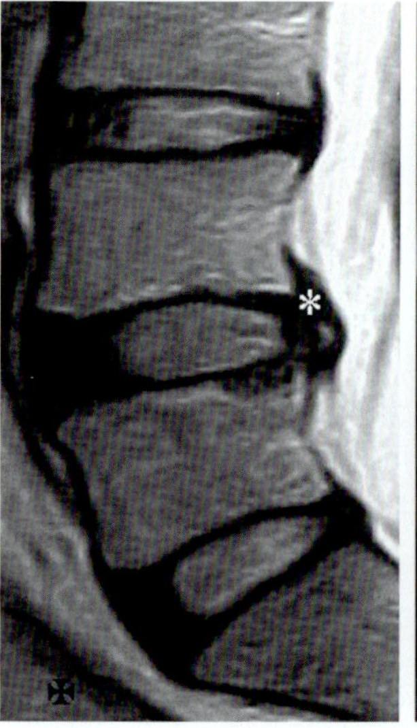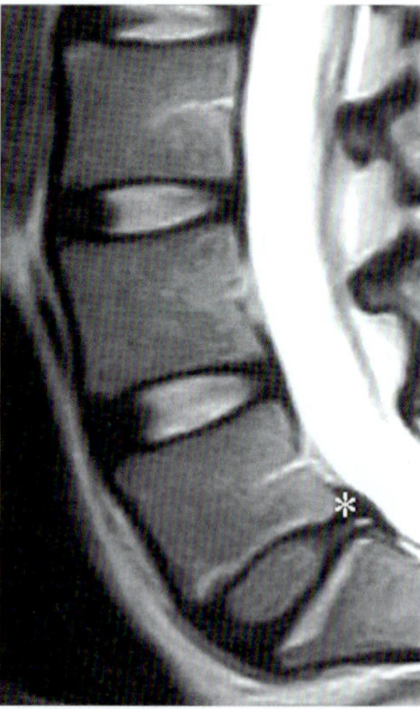

Figure 14–12 Lateral T2-weighted magnetic resonance imaging of the lumbar spine of two cases (male left and female right) 6 months after PDN SOLO implantation. The nucleus cavities appear remarkably like normal ones although the preoperative scans showed marked darkening of the painful disks, now asymptomatic. The healing entry tracts have developed fibrous plugs (asterisks) appearing similar to high-intensity zones of annular tears. Minimal Modic changes are seen in the adjacent vertebral bodies.

exception that with the direct insertion of the device, there was no manipulation needed to position the device transversely. The earlier paired PDN or later the PDN-SOLO implant was driven inside and the flap and fascial layers closed without drainage.

Dr. Luiz Pimenta of Brazil (personal communication) performed 40 cases using an endoscopic approach under local anesthesia using a 12 mm cannula without turning a flap.[16]

◆ Postoperative Care

Routine, ordinary postdiskectomy care and medications were used. With posterior approaches, patients remained in bed for 24 hours and then arose to wear a corset (reminding them to limit flexion and torsion). They resumed physical activity after 6 weeks of restrictions. The anterolateral or posterolateral patients were discharged after a short or overnight stay. The corset, and in a few less stable cases a brace, was worn for about 6 weeks. Routine follow-ups with anteroposterior (AP) and lateral x-ray films occurred at 6 weeks, and 3, 6, and 12 months. A separate, smaller, controlled, investigational cohort has been followed for several years.

◆ Results

The first case, using the dual implant version, was performed in January 1996 by the author and Prof. Robert Schönmayr in his practice in Wiesbaden, Germany. This case and the nine subsequent cases were operated and followed by Prof. Schönmayr 9 years before this report. Outcomes were measured using the visual analog pain scale and the Prolo

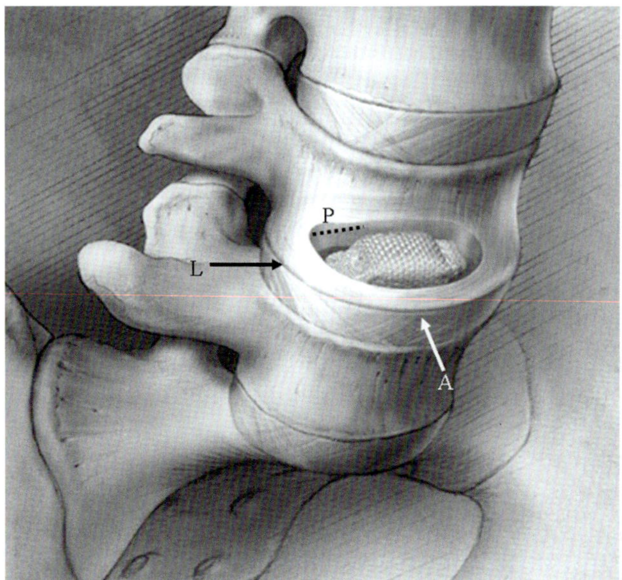

Figure 14–11 The lumber spine with an implant at the lumbosacral level. Indicated are the three potential implantation approaches. A, anterior; L, lateral (anterolateral or posterolateral); P, posterior (dotted line on the posterior annular wall).

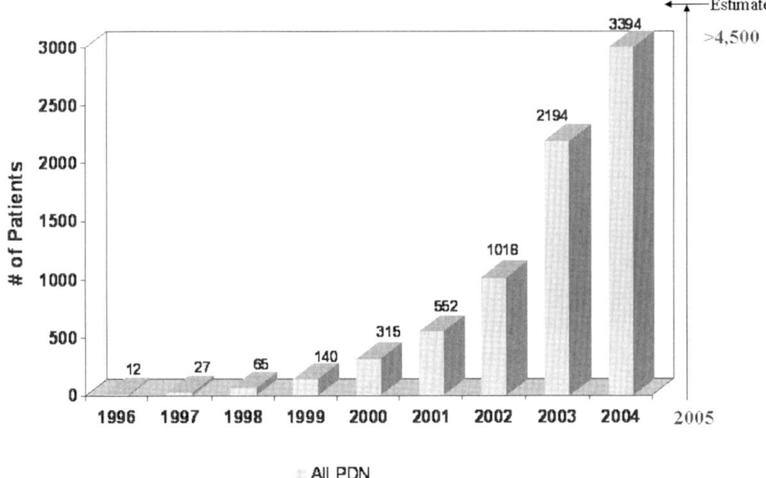

Figure 14–13   The increasing employment of the PDN-SOLO device by surgical consultants in 38 nations worldwide. Also indicated is the anticipated total number of cases (3700) at year end 2005.

and Oswestry function or disability scales, as well as by physical reexaminations and x-ray films as mentioned earlier and as summarized in **Figs. 14–13, 14–14, and 14–15.** General activity of the patients and medication usage were also recorded. Mobility of the spaces was estimated using flexion-extension in many but not all patients. The initial cohort of 65 patients implanted between 1996 and 1998 was observed for 6 months before resuming further implantations. They had a surgical success rate of 77% (50 of 65 patients; the remaining 15 patients required revision or explantation of the device). Based on indications of displacement of the implants, several changes in the devices and instruments for implantation and surgical technique were made, and the next cohort of 488 patients, implanted from 1999 through 2001, enjoyed a surgical success rate of 84%. However, after further developments, patients implanted in 2002 and 2003 enjoyed a success rate of 90%; this

rate is still improving. By the time this book is published, it is anticipated that well over 4500 patients worldwide will have been implanted exclusively with PDN-SOLO devices. The overall success rates, in terms of the aforementioned measures, has showed excellent progress in overall patient outcomes over the past 9 years, particularly during the last 3 years.

In a few cases, believed to have had intraoperative damage to the end plates, Modic changes were seen in T2-weighted MRI scans. This appears to improve over time in the majority of those cases, nonetheless. In a small 1-year follow-up comparing the success rate for the simpler SOLO technique with that of posterior fusion cages as reported to the FDA, the PDN-SOLO implant clinical results were equal or better (unpublished data). Regarding dislocations among the earlier cases, before the PDN-SOLO device was employed, it is noteworthy that none of these cases had a neurological catastrophe or permanent damage; as far as is known and

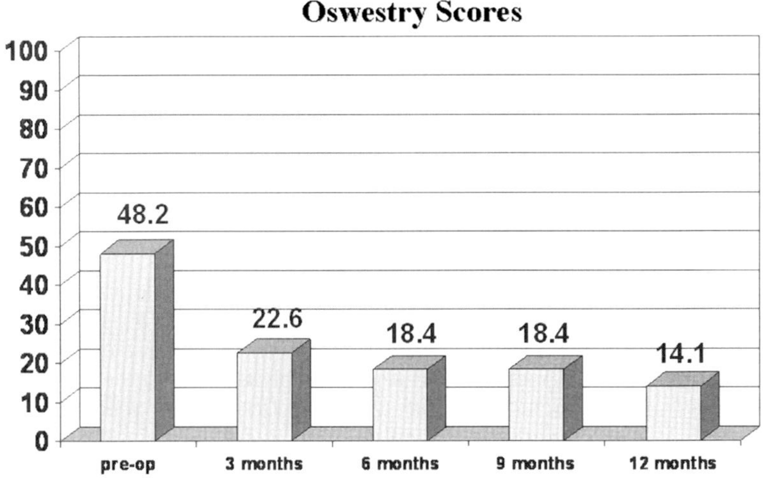

Figure 14–14   Improvement in disability rating over time, as indicated by the Oswestry scale. Follow-up data extended to 24 months are essentially unchanged from 12 months, shown.

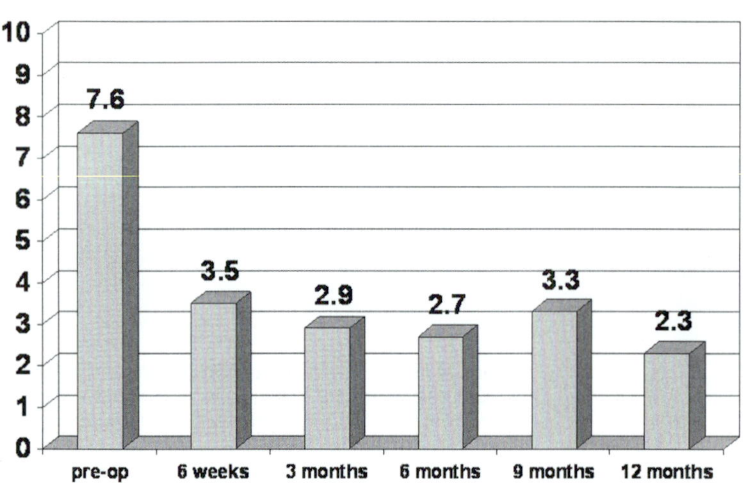

Figure 14–15   Reduction in the visual analog pain scale VAS for the low back following implantation surgeries. As with **Fig. 14–14,** small and large cohorts of patients demonstrate significantly the same response patterns as shown in these two graphs. Follow-up data extended to 24 months are essentially unchanged from 12 months.

reported, a temporary partial drop foot was seen in only one patient of the international cohort of nearly 500 cases. Implant dislodgment has been seen at a range of 2.5 to 16% in a retrospective analysis of ~300 recent PDN-SOLO implants but the rate is being reduced along with surgeons' improved experiences. Two typical cases having postoperative T2-weighted MRI scans of two patients at 6 months postimplant are shown in **Fig. 14–12**. The patient had severe preoperative back pain with a black disk but postoperatively became essentially asymptomatic. The nearly normal appearing, hydrated PDN-SOLO device and the healing of the annulus tract are quite striking in this MRI view. [The white spot seen dorsal in the insertion tract is not a high-intensity zone (HIZ), as is often seen in an unhealed radial annular tear, but rather the edema and normal healing seen in a fibrous tract.] When care was taken not to injure the end plates, the procedure reduced or eliminated vertebral body type 1 Modic changes.

The implanted SOLO device performs ~90% of the desirable behavior of the original dual implant while greatly simplifying the procedure and, very importantly, markedly reducing the tendency for dislodgment as documented above. Indeed, good to excellent results using the single PDN-SOLO device show considerable improvement over the initial paired PDN devices and methods of implantation. In a sample of the earliest clinical cases, now at more than 9 years postoperative, the range of motion in the operated segment had been preserved between 5 to 8 degrees in flexion-extension, very close to or slightly better than the initial preoperative range.

◆ Comments

In that abnormalities or deterioration of the end plate and associated nutrient transport mechanisms appear to be irreversible and because these changes are the most probable cause of nucleus dehydration with disk degeneration, any successfully surviving intradiskal implant or tissue graft must be biologically inert. The implant cannot require active bidirectional nutrient and metabolic by-product transport, otherwise it will fail to thrive. The PDN device is inert and does not depend on trans-end plate nutritional or by-product transport. The relative differential values of the PDN device as compared with the more technically challenging and expensive total artificial disk device are apparent but are yet to be confirmed. Further, should implant revision be required, the PDN-SOLO presents a far less challenging procedure than would a total artificial disk.

◆ Conclusion

Recent worldwide data regarding PDN-SOLO implants show a rising number of cases being performed, the potential complications and displacements are falling (now ~10%), and the measured clinical improvements over time are improving, fulfilling hopes for a successful implant that might become a standard worldwide device for nucleus replacement in selected cases.

◆ Acknowledgments

This long-term multidisciplinary project has been performed by broad teams of biomechanical, biochemical, tissue pathological, engineering, clinical, and business personnel, far too many to denote here. However the author expresses personal appreciation for their contributions to this successful project by the engineering development and test personnel, including Britt Norton, Sinead Kavanagh, Dr. William Hutton, Dr. Hans Wilke, Gene Dickhudt, and Robert Assell. Appreciation is also given abundantly to the clinical team, including: spine surgeons Drs. Robert Schönmayr, Bjorn Branth, Christian Brinkman, Rudolf Bertagnoli, Khalid Batterjee, Jin Dadi, Sang Ho Lee, Alejandro Reyes-Sanchez,

Felix Pino, Luiz Pimenta, Peter Klara, Richard Salib, Kevin Gill, and others internationally. The surgical backup team of Dr. Magdy Osman and O. James May, PA-C; then the business team, making the product available: Steve Van Tyle, John Halliday, Bjorn Linde, and Dr. Kamal Shazly. Raymedica, Inc., is an early-stage company funded by private capital investors, initially including Gary Stoltz of Pathfinder, Inc.

FULL DISCLOSURE

Although the author is the inventor of the PDN and a consultant, lecturer for, and shareholder of Raymedica, Inc., the manufacturer of the device and associated instruments, he receives no royalties from device sales.

References

1. Ray CD. The artificial disc: introduction, history and socioeconomics. In: Weinstein JN, ed. Clinical Efficacy and Outcome in the Diagnosis and Treatment of Low Back Pain. New York: Raven; 1992:205–225
2. Ray CD. The PDN prosthetic disc-nucleus device. Eur Spine J 2002;11 (Suppl 2):S137–S142
3. Pappas CTE, Harrington T, Sonntag VKH. Outcome analysis in 654 surgically treated lumbar disc herniations. Neurosurgery 1992; 30:862–866
4. Ray CD. The Raymedica prosthetic disc nucleus: an update. In: Kaech DL, Jinkins JR, eds. Spinal Restabilization Procedures. Amsterdam: Elsevier Science; 2002:273–282
5. Ray CD, Sachs BL, Norton BK, Mikkelson ES, Clausen NA. Prosthetic disc nucleus implants: an update. In: Szpalski M, Gunzburg R, eds. Lumbar Disc Herniation, pp. 222–233. Philadelphia: Lippincott, Williams, and Wilkins; 2001.
6. Eysel P, Rompe JD, Schoenmayr R, et al. Biomechanical behavior of a prosthetic lumbar nucleus. Acta Neurochir (Wien) 1999;141: 1083–1087
7. Norton BK. Polyethylene Wear Debris: Is It Relevant to the PDN Prosthetic Disc Nucleus? Internal research publication. Bloomington, MN: Raymedica, Inc.; 1998
8. Meakin JR, Redpath TW, Hukins DW. The effect of partial removal of the nucleus pulposus from the intervertebral disc on the response of the human annulus fibrosus to compression. Clin Biomech (Bristol, Avon) 2001;16:121–128
9. Wilke HJ, Kavanagh S, Neller S, et al. Effect of a prosthetic disc nucleus on the mobility and disc height of the L4–5 intervertebral disc postnucleotomy. J Neurosurg 2001;95(Suppl 2):208–214
10. Edeland HG. Some additional suggestions for an intervertebral disc prosthesis. J Biomed Eng 1985;7:57–62
11. Hedman TP, Kostuik JP, Fernie GR, et al. Design of an intervertebral disc prosthesis. Spine 1991;16(Suppl 6):S256–S260
12. Lee CK, Langrana NA, Parsons JR, et al. Development of a prosthetic intervertebral disc. Spine 1991;16(Suppl 6):S253–S255
13. Fernstrom U. Arthroplasty with intercorporal endoprosthesis in herniated disc and in painful disc. Acta Chir Scand Suppl 1966; 357:154–159
14. Fairbank JC, Couper J, Davies J, et al. The Oswestry low back pain disability questionnaire. Physiotherapy 1980;66:271–273
15. Prolo DJ, Oklund SA, Butcher M. Toward uniformity in evaluating results of lumbar spine operations: a paradigm applied to posterior lumbar interbody fusion. Spine 1986;11:601–606
16. Pimenta LHM, Ray CD: The lateral endoscopic transpsoas retroperitoneal approach (LETRA) for implants in the lumbar spine. (abstr) proc. World Spine II, Chicago, Aug 12, 1003, pp. 120–1–9.

15

Functional Lumbar Artificial Nucleus Replacement: The DASCOR System

John Emery Sherman and Bruce Randall Bowman

◆ **Principles and Expectations of Nucleus Replacements**

    Surgical Approaches

    Post Operative Results

    Design Implications

    Clinical Assessments

◆ **The DASCOR Disc Arthroplasty System**

◆ **Conclusions**

The intervertebral disk consists of two primary structures: the nucleus pulposus and the annulus fibrosus. Annular tearing and disruption are associated with decreased proteoglycan synthesis, with dehydration of the nucleus leading to degeneration of the disk. If this becomes symptomatic, traditional surgical treatment consisting of diskectomy or arthrodesis can be performed. Acceptable clinical outcomes have been reported with arthrodesis, using many surgical approaches.[1,2] Eliminating motion of the functional spinal motion segment, however, is clearly a nonphysiological approach to the symptomatic spinal motion segment. Alternatives to arthrodesis have been offered by total disk arthroplasty (TDA), with devices such as the Charité Artificial Disc (DePuy Spine, Raynham, MA) and ProDisc Total Disc Replacement (Synthes, Inc., West Chester PA).[3–5] Two metal-on-metal prostheses have recently concluded clinical enrollment in U.S. Investigational Device Exemption (IDE) studies. However, total disk replacement requires an extensive surgical exposure with mobilization of the great vessels, near complete resection of the nucleus and annulus, and fixation to the bony end plates. Additionally, revision of TDA is likely to be extremely difficult technically.

Potentially, to address the clinical situation of degenerative disk disease, replacement of only the dehydrated nucleus in a less surgically invasive approach is appealing.[6–9] Disk nucleus replacement presents different anatomical, biochemical, and biomechanical challenges than TDA. The goal of either treatment is to relieve pain, restore disk kinematic function, restore or maintain disk height, limit progression of adjacent level disease, and improve long-term outcomes. This chapter addresses some of the preclinical research and early clinical results of disk arthroplasty by replacing the nucleus pulposus with an in situ curable polymer injected and contained in an expandable balloon.

◆ Principles and Expectations of Nucleus Replacements

Biomechanically, normal disk structure allows both stability and flexibility within each individual spinal motion segment. Normal load carried by the nucleus diminishes with increasing load on the annulus as the disk degenerates. Increased load will accelerate annular incompetence with diminished disk height. This may lead to bulging or herniation of the nucleus pulposus with nerve root compression or, with time, spinal stenosis. Diskogenic low back pain is another clinical manifestation of this process. Increased stimulation of nociceptors within the outer aspect of the annulus and vertebral end plates secondary to the increased loads likely contributes to the underlying pain syndrome of diskogenic back pain.[10,11] If a diskectomy is performed for herniated nucleus pulposus, this can further disrupt the load-sharing function of the nucleus, with increasing compressive load requirements on the annulus and facet joints accompanied by an increase in the degenerative cascade.[12]

Whereas a biological replacement of the nucleus is appealing, a more practical biomechanical solution could achieve these goals. Mechanical replacement of the disk nucleus could be performed to reestablish the normal load on the nucleus and annulus and restore disk height. This would help to restore the overall normal disk function of stability as well as allow motion.[13,14] There may be an advantage for the remaining nucleus or implant to hydrate, mimicking the biophysical function of diurnal variation in normal disks.[8] Theoretically, less adjacent level disease than seen with other treatment methods could be realized if normal height and function of the disk could be restored. Ideally, greater long-term clinical outcomes would be achieved.

The ideal artificial nucleus has several basic requirements.[13] Multiple surgical techniques should be possible for any given nucleus replacement procedure based on specific patient indications. Ideally, the procedure should involve a small annular incision, decreasing the risk of migration of the implant, even when large annular defects are present. The implant should have good conformity to the superior and inferior end plates, improving the loading characteristics. The procedure should allow for a minimally invasive or percutaneous-type technique to be implemented and at the same time be technically practical. In the face of a postoperative clinical failure, the revision strategy should be safe and reliable and should allow for different surgical solutions, such as total disk arthroplasty or arthrodesis.

Surgical Approaches

Current surgical approaches to the lumbar disk include posterior laminotomy, anterior retroperitoneal, trans-psoatic, extraforaminal, open, and percutaneous. Each approach has its own clinical indications and advantages. The technique of prosthetic implantation should be adaptable to the clinical need to address the patient's pathology. If the patient has a typical posterolateral extruded herniation requiring excision, the prosthetic nucleus would ideally be implanted by a posterior laminotomy approach while limiting further disruption of the annular defect. Anatomically, the area for placement is more constrained in the posterior or percutaneous application than in the anterior retroperitoneal. This limitation makes the nuclectomy as well as implantation more difficult. It is difficult to envision that a preformed nucleus replacement device of a fixed geometry would prove to be successful as a stand-alone device because placement requires a commensurate annular opening. If this were inserted without bony fixation, it is quite likely that the preformed device would extrude through the annulotomy defect. The annulotomy defect created for placement of a device or a preexisting large annular defect may be associated with extrusion. Certain prostheses may have the additional requirement of repair of the annular defect for them to be safely applied.

Postoperative Results

Revision surgery of a nucleus replacement prosthesis will be driven by the surgical approach of the index procedure. Epidural scarring during repeat posterior surgery will be challenging. Although technically demanding, revision could be accomplished by an experienced surgeon without undue patient morbidity. It may require the prosthesis to be fragmented within the disk space to avoid undo neural retraction during explantation. Repeat anterior surgery may require mobilization of the great vessels. However, if the initial retroperitoneal approach did not require mobilization of the great vessels, such as would occur with a small annulotomy, this revision could be accomplished with less risk than after a total disk arthroplasty. The potential for catastrophic bleeding in this approach needs to be considered.[15,16] At some point in time, clinical failure may occur and whether a disk prosthesis could remain in situ as an anterior spacer while pain relief is achieved by adding a posterior fusion or other posterior stabilization remains unknown.

Restoration of the nuclear load is a basic principle of nucleoplasty.[8,13] This load is created by the interface of the nucleus implant with the vertebral end plates and annulus. A device with greater conformity to the end plates with large surface area coverage should result in more balanced, even loading. This likely will result in less bony reaction and postoperative modic changes. This is best accomplished by forming the implant in situ or allowing a preformed device to deform in situ under the influence of load, as with certain hydrogel prostheses.

Design Implications

There are additional biomechanical and biomaterial issues that arise with respect to artificial nucleus prostheses. Implants utilized to achieve an arthrodesis need to withstand load without failure until an arthrodesis is solidly achieved.[17] At that time the device becomes partially off-loaded as the fusion mass begins to share the load. However, when the goal is to maintain motion, there will be ongoing, continued load and shear across the device. This creates unique biomechanical requirements for the nucleus prosthesis. The ideal nucleus replacement should have a similar modulus of elasticity as the intact nucleus. A prosthesis with a modulus that is too low will have a high incidence of extrusion and may not reestablish normal biomechanical loading. A nucleus replacement with a relatively high modulus of elasticity would be associated with increased load on the end plates and could lead to subsidence or other untoward effects. Fernström reported this issue with the use of the stainless steel ball endoprosthesis.[18] In this study, he demonstrated that 88% of the implants were found to have loss of vertebral disk height over time.

The interface between the implant and the end plates is critically influenced not only by the modulus and contouring of the device but by the contact area and by the coefficient of friction between the device and the end plates. The goal of minimal end plate wear would be enhanced if the ideal prosthesis distributed the forces evenly over a large percentage of the surface area of the end plates. Likewise, a lower coefficient of friction between the implant and the end plates would be expected to lead to less end plate or prosthetic wear. An additional benefit of improved implant end plate conformity is likely a diminished risk of implant extrusion.

Clinical Assessments

Nucleus replacement devices will require clinical studies with standard outcome measures, including visual analog pain scales, Oswestry disability scores, and the short form (SF)-36. The patients will need to be followed for some time to assess the long-term clinical outcome and potential late complications. In addition to clinical evaluation of patients, it will be equally important to follow individuals with appropriate imaging. Because end plate changes are most readily seen on magnetic resonance imaging (MRI), this documentation should be included in the routine follow-up. It is likely that the U.S. IDE studies will be randomized against total disk arthroplasty. Unfortunately, the MRI implant device artifact associated with total disk replacement is such that postoperative MRI will not allow for this comparison in prospective studies. Whether postoperative Modic changes correlate with any clinical outcomes will be an interesting question. Ideally, an implanted prosthesis should not lead to MRI observations of end plate changes.

One of the most challenging components of clinically studying a nucleus replacement prosthesis is the proper selection of the comparative control group. Because the nucleus replacement would ideally be placed in a less invasive fashion than TDA or arthrodesis, the control group should not inherently have an experimental bias of dramatically greater surgical morbidity. Anterior stand-alone interbody cages can potentially be implanted with less morbidity than, for example, arthrodesis of both the anterior column and the posterior elements (a so-called 360 degree fusion). In earlier disk degeneration with a relatively tall disk space, reliability and clinical outcomes of stand-alone interbody cages are somewhat questionable. In the United States, randomization against a device not approved by the Food and Drug Administration (FDA) is not likely to receive approval. Currently the Charité total disk arthroplasty device (DePuy Spine, Raynham, MA) is commercially available. However, it is still early in its clinical application in the United States, and long-term outcomes in well-controlled populations are not available. Thus randomization against a total disk arthroplasty device could also be problematic.

Other potential randomization protocols could include diskectomy alone or other nonsurgical, minimally invasive intradiskal therapies.[19] Some have suggested a nucleus replacement prosthesis could be studied in the context of a population primarily with lumbar radiculopathy who have received routine excision of a disk herniation. It is well known that the disk space postdiskectomy can narrow and in a certain percentage of patients lead to chronic back pain. If the primary indication for surgery is radiculopathy, both the study group (microdiskectomy) and the control group will likely demonstrate good early outcomes. Longer-term follow-up would be necessary to establish statistical improvement in back pain. In the design of a clinical investigation with randomization to microdiskectomy with or without a prosthetic nucleus, it may be appropriate to allow crossover of the control group of patients to a nucleus replacement should an individual go on to develop either a recurrent disk herniation or significant diskogenic back pain. However, it is more likely that further surgical intervention would be required to adhere to current FDA-approved methods. This situation may, in fact, represent an ideal patient for which a nucleus replacement could be applied either in the index diskectomy or as a late secondary procedure.[20–22]

The appropriate patient indication needs to be established to enhance the study's value.[23,24] Currently, it is thought that the relevant patients would have mechanical back pain that is "diskogenic" in origin. The individual must have failed standard nonsurgical management and have single-, or potentially two-level, disease.

◆ The DASCOR Disc Arthroplasty System

Disc Dynamics, Inc. (Eden Prairie, MN) has developed an injectable in situ curable polyurethane nucleus replacement device called the DASCOR Disc Arthroplasty System[25]

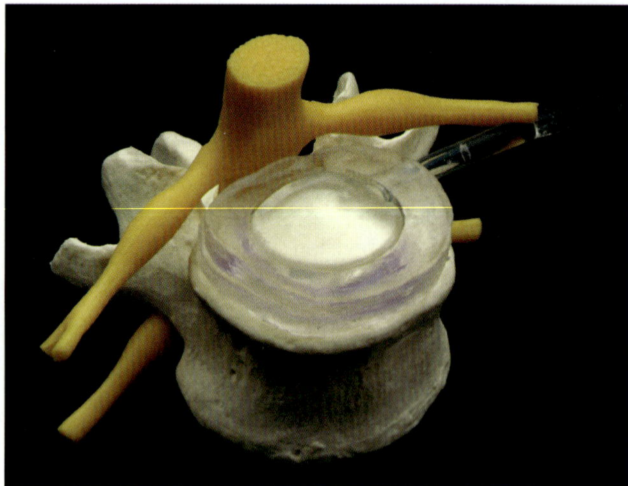

Figure 15–1   DASCOR Disc Arthroplasty Replacement System shown in a spine model. The in situ curable polymer is injected into a polyurethane balloon placed in the disk space. The balloon expands to fill any void that has been created during the diskectomy. The polymer cures in a matter of minutes from a liquid to a firm but pliable state. (From: Disc Dynamics, Inc., reprinted with permission.)

(**Fig. 15–1**). The DASCOR device is made by mixing two parts of liquid polymer while delivering it through a catheter to an expandable polyurethane balloon that is placed in the disk space (**Fig. 15–2**).

The polymer cures in a matter of minutes, changing state from a liquid to a firm but pliable solid device. After 15 minutes, the delivery catheter is removed, leaving the final implant device.

There are several features to this system. The balloon catheter has a low profile and can be inserted into the disk space through only a 5.5 mm annulotomy. The mixed liquid polymer is delivered to the balloon under controlled pressure, causing the balloon to expand to contour and fill the entire disk space left by the nuclectomy procedure. This allows the ability to implant a large-footprint, large-volume device through a small annulotomy, thus making migration unlikely. In addition, the system creates an implant of variable size that conforms to the nuclectomy. The deployment of a large, pliable, end plate—contouring prosthesis can help balance associated load transfer between the annulus and the artificial nucleus while minimizing end plate disruption. The DASCOR device also has the ability to distract the disk space. Therefore, the implantation of the device not only offers the ability to fill any given space established by nuclectomy but also the potential to distract and restore a collapsed intervertebral disk.

The DASCOR prosthesis can be implanted using multiple surgical approaches (i.e., posterior laminotomy, extraforaminal, anterior, and lateral), with minimal variation in surgical technique. Key to any approach, however, is achieving total nucleus removal. The implantation of a nucleus prosthesis should not be perceived to be a simple adjunct to a standard diskectomy for herniated nucleus pulposus. To create a prosthesis with maximal size, end plate conformity, and optimal biomechanical loading, complete removal of the nucleus must be conducted while preserving the annulus and end plates. Because traditional diskectomy typically removes

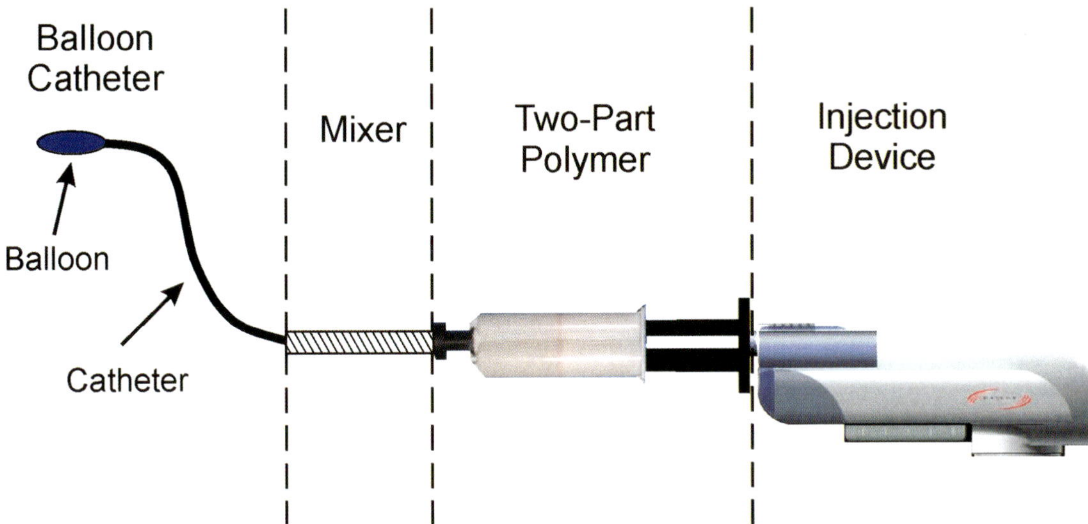

Figure 15–2   DASCOR Disc Arthroplasty System. The two-part liquid polymer is packaged in a dual-barrel syringe cartridge. A custom-injection device drives the liquid polymer through an inline mixer and into the delivery catheter. The mixed, pressurized polymer then enters the containment balloon, which has been placed in the disk space, expanding the balloon to fill the entire space. (From: Disc Dynamics, Inc., reprinted with permission.)

only herniated fragments or bulging tissue creating nerve impingement, a new procedure for total nucleus removal (TNR)[26] was developed. Human cadaveric studies identified that standard diskectomy instruments did not allow TNR to be adequately performed through a 5.5 mm annulotomy. A set of standard pituitary rongeurs were chosen and customized pituitary rongeurs were developed according to each instrument's ability to reach a particular mapped region of the nucleus (**Fig. 15–3**). When specific instruments are utilized and coupled with detailed intraoperative fluoroscopic imaging, TNR can be reliably accomplished. Different templates have been developed for TNR when approaching the disk from different anatomical entry sites.

Final evaluation with an imaging balloon further characterizes the geometric location of the prosthesis as well as the anticipated volume of the final implant (**Fig. 15–4**) prior to implanting the final device.

The initial annulotomy is created by using a 5.5 mm trephine. Particular care is taken to avoid damage to the remaining annulus and the cartilaginous end plates (**Fig. 15–5A**). Following TNR, an imaging balloon is inserted into the disk space and contrast media is injected under pressure, filling the balloon and disk cavity created by TNR. Fluoroscopic

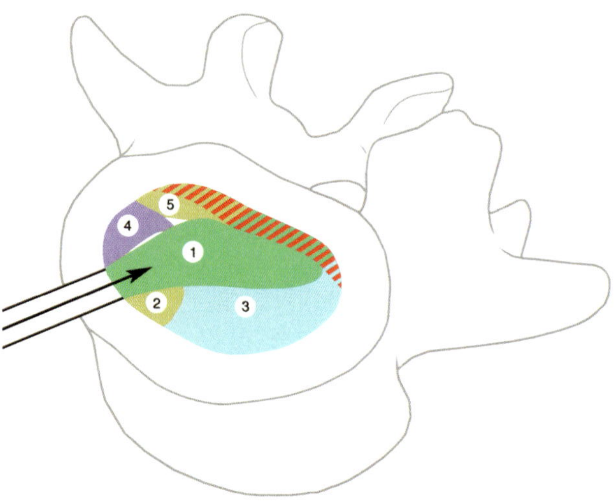

Figure 15–3   Five-zone anterolateral total nucleus removal approach. Instruments are specifically chosen according to their ability to reach and remove nucleus material from each of the five zones shown. The step-by-step approach to nucleus removal one zone at a time results in total nucleus removal. (From: Disc Dynamics, Inc., reprinted with permission.)

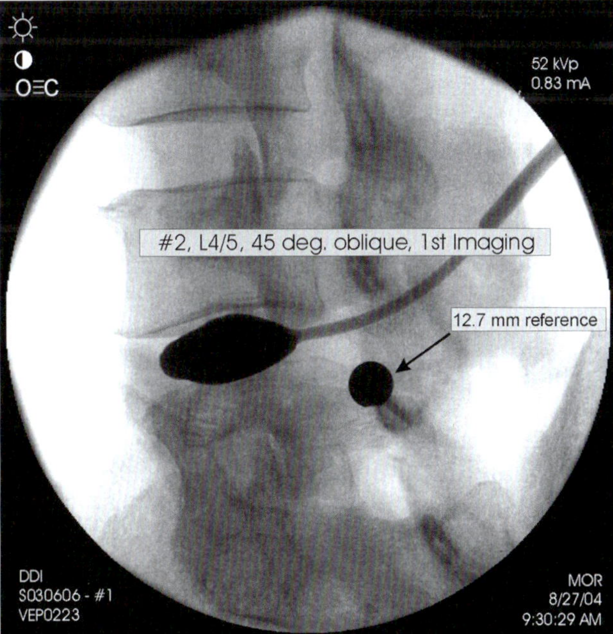

Figure 15–4   Radiograph of the imaging step prior to DASCOR device implantation. An imaging balloon is placed through the annulotomy and into the disk space. Contrast solution is injected and images are taken from multiple directions to assess the completeness of total nucleus removal. (From: Disc Dynamics, Inc., reprinted with permission.)

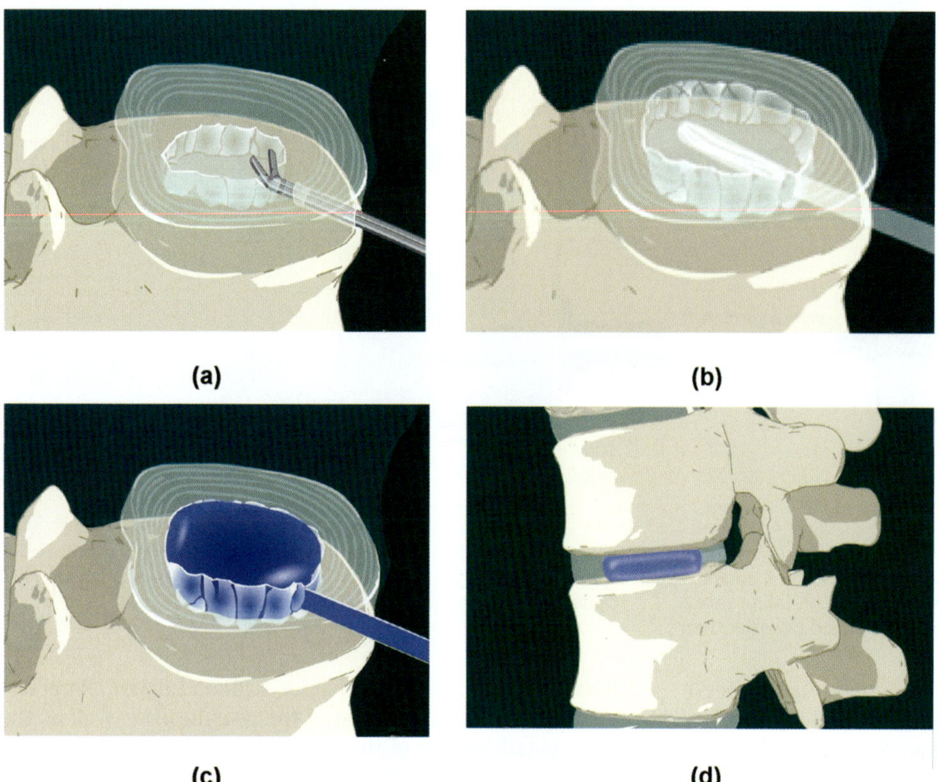

Figure 15–5   Technique for the implantation of DASCOR Disc Arthroplasty device. **(A)** A series of rongeurs are used to perform total nucleus removal (TNR). Confirmation of TNR is made by injecting contrast solution into an expandable balloon placed in the disk space and taking multiple fluoroscopic images. **(B)** Following TNR, the implant balloon is inserted into the disk space. **(C)** The two-part liquid polymer is mixed as it is being injected under pressure through the catheter, filling the balloon and the disk space and allowing for disk height restoration. The device cures to form a firm but pliable implant that conforms to the individual's anatomy. **(D)** The delivery catheter is then cut off at the edge of the implant using a special tool, and the catheter is removed. (From: Disc Dynamics, Inc., reprinted with permission.)

images are then taken in multiple planes, and an assessment is made as to the completeness and symmetry of the nuclectomy. If the cavity is not symmetrical and centrally located, additional steps of nucleus removal and fluoroscopic imaging are conducted. The contrast media and imaging balloon are then removed, and the implant balloon is inserted (**Fig. 15–5B**). The liquid polymer is then injected under controlled pressure into the balloon, filling the cavity (**Fig. 15–5C**). After 15 minutes, the delivery catheter is cut off and removed (**Fig. 15–5D**). The patients are gradually mobilized postoperatively, allowing for soft tissue healing.

Extensive preclinical testing of the DASCOR device has been conducted, including component and device characterization, biodurability bench testing, biomechanical testing,[27] and biocompatibility confirmation. Several biocompatibility tests were conducted, including the extended ISO 10993 battery of 12 tests, with successful outcomes. Because this prosthesis differs from others on the market by virtue of the device being in situ cured, the risk of the device leaching certain monomeric chemicals exists. Studies have therefore included safety assessment of key toxicological chemicals that have potential for leaching out of the device both during the polymerization period and long-term. In vivo testing in sheep under both typical use and worst-case scenarios has been conducted. In addition, both typical and worst-case in vitro exhaustive extraction studies have been conducted to determine the maximum potential dose of key chemicals a

patient could ever be exposed to. These studies have shown that the maximum potential dose of these chemicals, even under worst-case scenarios, is far below those currently estimated for Occupational Safety and Health Administration (OSHA) occupational exposure safety limits.

The biodurability of the device was investigated in a custom-made, six-station, mechanical testing apparatus using unconstrained device conditions to create a worst-case test construct. Cyclic axial compression was combined with cyclic ± 5.5 degree flexion-extension to represent high-end daily activity loads of 1.8 MPa peak stresses. None of the six samples tested for 25 million cycles showed signs of device degradation. Wear rate was measured for devices tested during the first 10 million cycles. Average wear rate was only 0.26 mg/million cycles, and no significant permanent set was observed.[27]

Biomechanical tests have also been conducted in both a porcine and a human cadaveric model. The fatigue response to cyclic compression—shear loads was investigated in a porcine model. Ten porcine lumbar functional spine units were implanted with a DASCOR device, and five other porcine motion segments were tested intact to serve as controls. Extreme cyclic axial compressive loads of 100 to 5000 N with 35 to 350 N shear were applied for 2000 cycles to both experimental groups. Dynamic stiffness, creep, deformation, and hysteresis of all instrumented segments demonstrated device stability, and implanted constructs did not

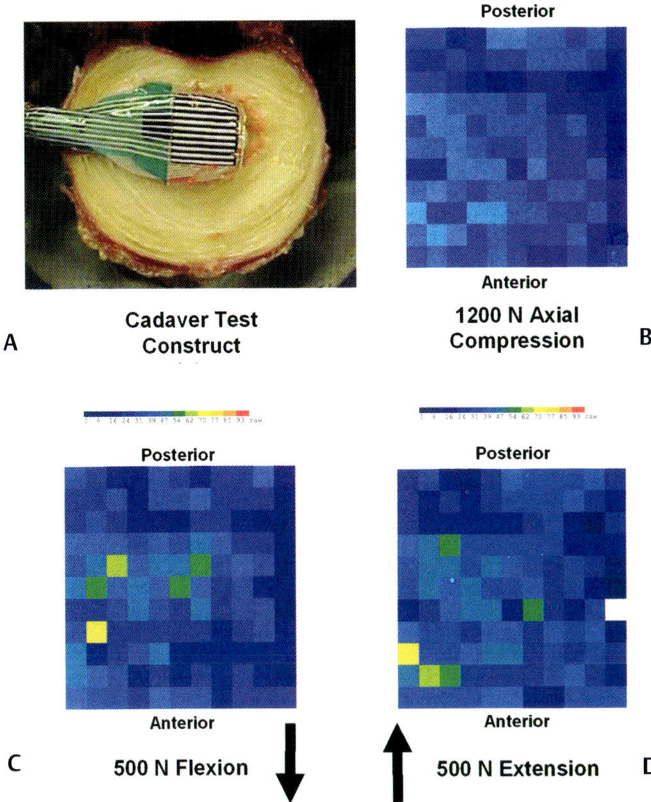

Figure 15–6 Contact stress evaluation in human cadaver using Tekscan 121 Element Array Sensor. **(A)** Tekscan sensor is shown in position over implant device following transection of the Functional Spine Unit. Sensor was placed between the implant and the end plate and monitored during axial, flexion, and extension loadings. Each element color is related to stress with darker colors representing low stress and light colors (orange, red) representing high stress (uncalibrated). **(B)** Array showing color distribution related to stress distribution during 1200 N axial loading. **(C)** Array showing color distribution related to stress distribution during 500 N flexion. **(D)** Array showing color distribution related to stress during 500 N extension. The relatively even distribution in color demonstrates a relatively even distribution in contact stress. (From: Disc Dynamics, Inc., reprinted with permission.)

differ from controls. None of the implants showed signs of failure.[27]

Segmental flexibility using a human cadaveric model was studied by comparing intact, nuclectomy, and instrumented constructs. It was demonstrated that the device was able to restore the segmental flexibility lost after a nuclectomy while still preserving segmental level biomechanics to within ±5% of the intact motion segment behavior.[28] In a similar study, human cadaveric specimens were instrumented with a 121 element Tekscan sensor (Tekscan, Inc., South Boston, MA) placed between the implant and end plates (**Fig. 15–6A**). Contact stress was evaluated during segmental flexibility testing. A typical stress distribution at 1200 N axial compressive load is shown in **Fig. 15–6B**. Similarly, **Figs. 15–6C** and **15–6D** show stress distribution during 500 N flexion and extension loads, respectively. A relatively uniform contact stress distribution was observed during all segmental flexibility loads applied.[27]

The initial clinical experience of the DASCOR system evaluating safety and effectiveness is being investigated in a multicenter, prospective, nonrandomized European study.[29,30] Inclusion criteria include patients with symptomatic single-level lumbar degenerative disk disease diagnosed by MRI and a positive diskogram with a minimum disk height of 5.5 mm. They must have failed 6-month nonoperative care and have had no prior fusion. A standardized retroperitoneal midline or lateral approach was used to perform a TNR and implant the DASCOR device in this study.

As of early 2005, 17 patients (eight female, nine male) with an average age of 38.1 years were implanted at the L5–S1 ($n = 10$) or L4–L5 ($n = 7$) levels. Eleven patients have been followed up to 1 year. The mean operating time was 78.1 minutes with an average blood loss of 59.1 mL. A 6-week postoperative MRI of the DASCOR device in a patient is shown in **Fig. 15–7**. The implant is centrally located and fills the former nucleus space. Outcome measures have been tracked from preoperative measures through 12 months. Average Oswestry results showed a 64% reduction from a preoperative average of 52.2 (**Fig. 15–8**). Average visual analog scale (VAS) back pain scores showed a 60% reduction from a preoperative average of 7.3 (**Fig. 15–9**), whereas VAS leg pain scores showed a 68% reduction from a preoperative average of 5.3. Analgesic use based on a three-point scale decreased 89% from a preoperative average of 1.8. In addition, MRI evaluations showed that the DASCOR device had not led to any significant Modic changes, bone edema, subsidence, or migration. Anteroposterior and lateral radiographic films showed that disk height and range of motion were maintained.[29,30] Although clinical experience has been limited at this time, early results were very encouraging. Study subjects demonstrated pain reduction and functional improvement allowing a considerable early clinical success with the DASCOR Disc Arthroplasty System. The DASCOR system has received CE marking and further studies are being initiated, with long-term data to be accumulated.

◆ Conclusions

The concept of being able to achieve pain relief and disk function restoration using an easy to use nucleus replacement procedure is quite appealing. The ideal implant will allow for reestablishment of disk height as well as reestablishing the normal biomechanics of the motion segment. The ultimate goal remains achieving significant clinical improvement with diminished morbidity over current techniques. However, many questions still need to be addressed with respect to nucleus replacement technologies. Although, no "perfect" material has been identified for replacing the nucleus, the DASCOR device design currently under study does address many of the perceived needs of nucleus replacement.

There are significant differences in design features between the DASCOR device and other nucleus devices, which may influence clinical results. The injectable, contained DASCOR device results in a large cross-sectional area that contours to the end plates as well as having a

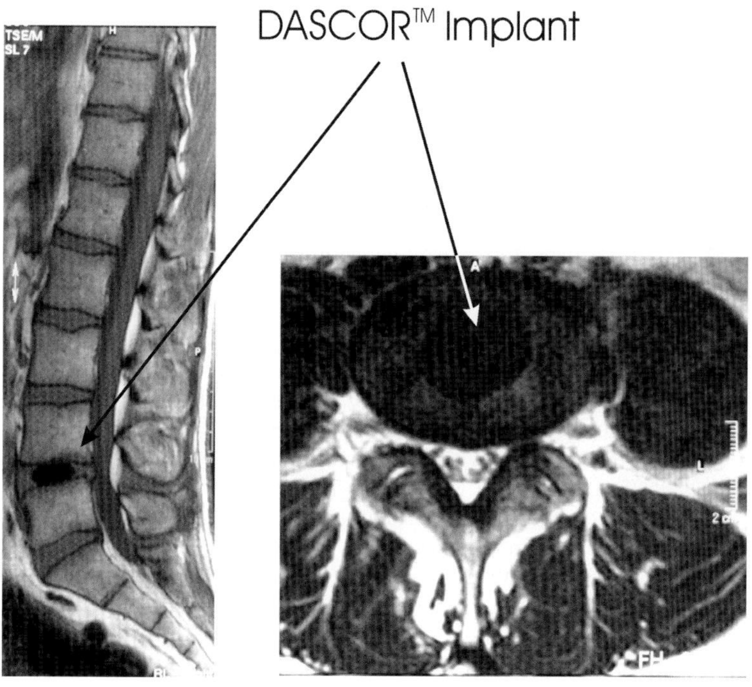

Figure 15–7   Magnetic resonance imaging of DASCOR device 6 weeks postimplantation. Images show the implant device centrally located without any signs of modic changes or inflammatory reaction. (From: Disc Dynamics, Inc., reprinted with permission.)

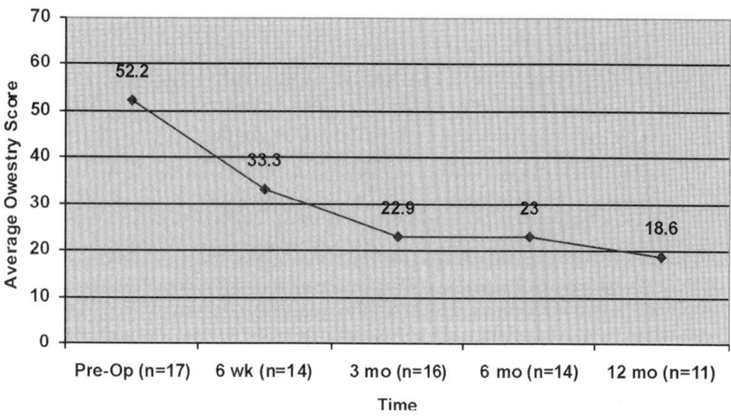

Figure 15–8   Oswestry low back pain score results. Seventeen patients had an average Oswestry preop pain score of 52.2. Eleven patients have been followed to 12 months and showed a 64% drop in pain score to 18.6.

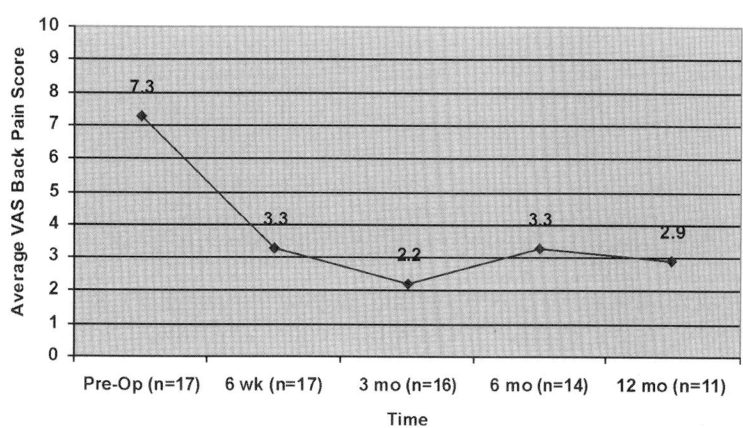

Figure 15–9   Visual analog scale (VAS) low back pain score results. Seventeen patients had an average VAS preop back pain score of 7.3. Eleven patients have been followed to 12 months and showed a 60% drop in pain score to 2.9.

favorable modulus of elasticity. This contributes to a more uniform distribution of pressure on the vertebral end plates and potentially may contribute to the lack of end plate reaction seen in early studies, in contrast to other nucleus replacement devices reported. Enhanced load sharing between the annulus and implant is consistent with the biomechanical results of returned motion segment stability and functional performance following DASCOR device implantation. Lastly, although it has a large footprint and volume, the DASCOR device is implanted through a small annulotomy, making migration unlikely, which has not been the case for preformed devices that require large annulotomies.

Nucleus arthroplasty does require rigorous clinical studies to be performed with appropriate control groups to access this emerging technology. However, as with any technology, selecting the appropriate patient and applying precise surgical technique will enhance the possibility for successful long-term clinical outcome. Given the early state of this technology, it will be some time before data are available to identify the ideal patient for the DASCOR system and also to identify the value of selected surgical approaches and multilevel application. This does not diminish the potential enthusiasm for successful clinical introduction of nucleus replacement arthroplasty in general and the DASCOR system technology specifically.

References

1. Kuslich SD, Danielson G, Dowdle JD, et al. Four-year follow-up results of lumbar spine arthrodesis using the Bagby and Kuslich lumbar fusion cage. Spine 2000;25:2656–2662

2. Zdeblick TA, Phillips FM. Interbody cage devices. Spine 2003;28 (Suppl 15):S2–S7

3. Guyer RD, Ohnmeiss DD. Intervertebral disc prosthesis. Spine 2003;28 (Suppl 15):S15–S23

4. McAfee PC, Fedder IL, Saiedy S, Shucosky EM, Cunningham BW. SB Charité disc replacement: report of 60 prospective randomized cases in a US center. J Spinal Disord Tech 2003;16:424–433

5. Zigler JE, Burd TA, Vialle EN, Sachs BL, Rashbaum RF, Ohnmeiss DD. Lumbar spine arthroplasty: early results using the ProDisc II: a prospective randomized trial of arthroplasty versus fusion. J Spinal Disord Tech 2003;16:352–361

6. Bao QB, Yuan HA. New technologies in spine. Nucleus Replacement. Spine 2002;27:1245–1247

7. Carl A, Ledet E, Yuan H, Sharan A. New developments in nucleus pulposus replacement technology. Spine J 2004;4(Suppl 6):325S–329S

8. Klara PM, Ray CD. Artificial nucleus replacement: clinical experience. Spine 2002;27:1374–1377

9. Sieber AN, Kostuik JP. Concepts in nuclear replacement. Spine J 2004; 4(Suppl 6):322S–324S

10. Kuslich SD, Ulstrom CL, Michael CJ. The tissue origin of low back pain and sciatica: a report of pain response to tissue stimulation during operations on the lumbar spine using local anesthesia. Orthop Clin North Am 1991;22:181–187

11. Yamashita T, Minaki Y, Oota I, Yokugushi K, Ishii S. Mechanosensitive afferent units in the lumbar intervertebral disc and adjacent muscle. Spine 1993;18:2252–2256

12. Goel VK, Nishiyama K, Weinstein JN, Liu YK. Mechanical properties of lumbar spinal motion segments as affected by partial disc removal. Spine 1986;11:1008–1012

13. Bao QB, McCullen GM, Higham PA, Dumbleton JH, Yuan HA. The artificial disc: theory, design and materials. Biomaterials 1996;17: 1157–1167

14. Eysel P, Rompe J, Schoeymayer R, Zoellner J. Biomechanical behavior of a prosthetic lumbar nucleus. Acta Neurochir (Wien) 1999;141: 1083–1087

15. Brau SA. Mini-open approach to the spine for anterior lumbar interbody fusion: description of the procedure, results and complications. Spine J 2002;2:216–223

16. Brau SA, Delamarter RB, Schiffman ML, Williams LA, Watkins RG. Vascular injury during anterior lumbar surgery. Spine J 2004;4:409–412

17. Martz EO, Goel VK, Pope MH, Park JB. Materials and design of spinal implants—a review. J Biomed Mater Res 1997;38:267–288

18. Fernström U. Arthroplasty with intercorporal endoprosthesis in herniated disc and in painful disc. Acta Chir Scand Suppl 1966;357:154–159

19. Biyani A, Andersson GB, Chaudhary H, An HS. Intradiscal electrothermal therapy: a treatment option in patients with internal disc disruption. Spine 2003;28(Suppl 15):S8–14

20. Hanley EN Jr, Shapiro DE. The development of low-back pain after excision of lumbar disc. J Bone Joint Surgery 1989:71:719–721

21. Keskimaki I, Seitsalo S, Osterman H, Rissanen P. Reoperations after lumbar disc surgery: a population-based study of regional and interspecialty variations. Spine 2000;25:1500–1508

22. Loupasis GA, Stamos K, Katonis PG, Sapkas G, Korres DS, Hartofilakidis G. Seven- to 20-year outcome of lumbar discectomy. Spine 1999;24: 2313–2317

23. Bao QB, Yuan HA. Prosthetic disc replacement: the future? Clin Orthop Relat Res 2002;394:139–145

24. Lemaire JP, Skalli W, Lavaste F, et al. Intervertebral disc prosthesis: results and prospects for the year 2000. Clin Orthop Relat Res 1997; 337:64–76

25. Yuan HA, Hudgins G, Bao QB, Bowman B. Early experience with a new and novel approach to disc nucleus arthroplasty. Presented at the Third Annual Meeting of the Spine Arthroplasty Society, Phoenix, Arizona, May 1–4, 2003

26. Ahrens M, Halm H, Liljenqvist U, et al. An innovative surgical approach for total nucleus removal from a posterior approach for use with a nucleus replacement device. Presented at the Annual Meeting of the Spine Society of Europe, Barcelona, Spain, September 21–24, 2005

27. Sherman J, Bowman B, Tsantrizos A, Yuan H. Preclinical testing of the DASCOR™ nucleus replacement device. Presented at the Fifth Annual Meeting of the Spine Arthroplasty Society, New York, NY, May 4–7, 2005

28. Ordway N, Tsantrizos A, Yuan H, Bowman B. Restoration of segmental kinematics following nucleus replacement with an in situ curable balloon contained polymer. Presented at the 20th Annual Meeting of the North American Spine Society, Philadelphia, Pennsylvania, September 27–October 1, 2005

29. Yuan H, Halm H, Le Huec JC, Sherman J, Ahrens M, Yeung C. Nucleus replacement using the DASCOR™ device: one-year follow up results of a prospective non-randomized multi-center clinical study. Presented at the Eighteenth Annual International Intradiscal Therapy Society Meeting, San Diego, California, May 25–28, 2005

30. Halm H, Le Huec JC, Ahrens M, et al. Early clinical experience with an in situ curable nucleus replacement implant one year follow-up of a prospective nonrandomized multicenter clinical study. Presented at the 20th Annual Meeting of the North American Spine Society, Philadelphia, Pennsylvania, September 27–October 1, 2005

16

NeuDisc

Rudolf Bertagnoli, Ann Prewett, James J. Yue, and Christopher Sabatino

◆ **Device Design**

◆ **Biocompatibility Testing**

◆ **Mechanical Testing**
   Endurance Testing
   Range of Motion Testing

Expulsion Testing
Human Cadaver Fatigue Testing

◆ **Clinical Studies**

◆ **Conclusion**

Degenerative disk disease (DDD) and low back pain are the leading causes of lost wages in the United States with nearly 700,000 surgical procedures per year.[1] When surgical intervention is deemed necessary, the most common method of treatment is fusion of the adjacent vertebral bodies. In certain patients, fusion is successful in treating pain associated with DDD but may lead to undesirable consequences such as degenerative changes in adjacent segments due to the altered biomechanics and loss of flexibility.[2,3] Clearly, an unmet need exists for a nonfusion treatment of back pain that would restore function, maintain motion, and eliminate the pain associated with DDD. According to the new, defined-step algorithm for treatment of DDD, nucleus arthroplasty has its predefined role between simple disk degeneration and total disk replacement.[4,5]

The concept of replacing the degenerating nucleus of the spine with a hydrogel or other synthetic material has been explored with varying degrees of success.[6–13] Early attempts at replacing the nucleus with materials ranging from metallic spheres[14] to silicone gels have been plagued with several problems. Complications including extrusion from the disk space and subsidence into the vertebral end plate have been experienced in both animal models and human clinical testing.[6,7] Among the large number of materials explored, synthetic hydrogels hold considerable promise. Like the nucleus itself, these materials can absorb and desorb fluid in relation to applied load. Hydrogels can be prepared from several polymer sources, including polyvinyl alcohols, polyurethanes, and hydrolyzed polyacrylonitriles. In particular, the hydrolyzed polyacrylonitrile-based hydrogel holds considerable promise. In addition to the hydrogel chemistry, the form in which the hydrogel is introduced is particularly important. The implant must present with a small insertion geometry to minimize damage to the annulus created by the large incision. After insertion, the implant must swell or otherwise change shape such that it may fill the space previously occupied by the nucleus. Homogeneous, isotropic hydrogels will have a

tendency to expand during swelling or deform in all directions or both under axial load. This is particularly true for the direction of least resistance, which may be in the direction of the defect created in the annulus fibrosus (AF) for implant insertion. There may also be portions of the AF that are weakened or otherwise damaged. The result may be either or both extrusion and reherniation.

New generations of nucleus arthroplasty devices like the NeuDisc™ device (Replication Medical, Inc., New Brunswick, NJ) have been designed to bypass these general problems. The NeuDisc comprises a proprietary hydrolyzed polyacrylonitrile hydrogel, Aquacryl. It is highly resistant to mechanical failure even at high water content. In the absence of mechanical restrictions, the hydrogel may contain 90% volume as a liquid. One of the properties of this novel implant is the capability to swell anisotropically (axial direction principally). When implanted in a dehydrated state, this hydrogel implant is substantially smaller than the volume of nucleotomy space and is easily placed through an incision in the annulus; however, it is substantially larger than the annular incision following hydration. The potential for extrusion is, therefore, greatly decreased over other designs. Furthermore, the implant has a "stacked" configuration, which includes layers of a medical-grade polyester fiber mesh within the hydrogel. These mesh layers act to restrict radial deformability ("bulging") so that the device will not "creep" through a defect in the AF.

The device replaces the overall function of the native nucleus pulposus (NP), which has been compromised as a result of the disease process. The design of the NeuDisc takes into account the physical, mechanical, and physiological properties of the NP. Clinical considerations, including ease of insertion, fatigue life, wear characteristics, and device biocompatibility were also considered. The NeuDisc has been the subject of extensive preclinical in vivo and in vitro testing, biocompatibility testing, and rigorous mechanical characterizations to ensure its utility as a nucleus replacement.

◆ Device Design

The NeuDisc is designed to simulate the essential properties of the native NP and has been developed to reproduce as closely as possible its elastic modulus, yield strength, and energy-absorptive properties. Mechanical studies suggest that compressive loads across the L3 disk of a 70 kg subject vary from 400 N to as much as 1400 N in different sitting postures and lifting activities.[15] Based on the simplistic assumption that the load sharing between the nucleus and annulus is roughly proportional to the ratio of their respective cross-sectional areas,[15] one might expect the nucleus to support maximal loads of ~200 to 700 N. Nucleus loads of this magnitude are in agreement with recent in vivo disk pressure measurements.[16]

The NeuDisc is also designed to resist extrusion during normal loading. The addition of the mesh layers to the device helps prevent radial deformability or "bulging." The stiffness of the gel layers combined with the constraint added by the mesh layers prevents the NeuDisc from blebbing through defects in the AF.

The native NP has biological functions other than maintaining the mechanical properties of the intervertebral disk. The native NP continually absorbs and desorbs fluid during normal activity in a diurnal rhythm. This fluid action delivers the nutrients contained within the fluid to the cartilaginous end plates. The ability to absorb fluid and transport nutrients depends on the health of the end plates. It is arguable that a successful nucleus replacement must have the capability to perform this same biological function. The NeuDisc like the native NP is capable of absorbing and desorbing fluid under load. The NeuDisc is permeable to molecules as large as 60 to 100 kilodaltons (kDa) as the fluid component of the device reaches equilibrium with the surrounding in vivo intradiskal fluids. The osmotic gradient and fluid transfer ability allow the NeuDisc to perform the same function as the native NP.

The NeuDisc is designed to be inserted in a nearly dehydrated state, which allows a smaller incision to be used for insertion. The ability of the NeuDisc to hydrate anisotropically greatly decreases the chance of the device extruding from the relatively small insertion incision. The NeuDisc is similar in size to the native NP, which ranges between 25 and 50% of the cross-sectional area of the entire intervertebral disk. The hydrated volume of the NeuDisc must be closely similar to the volume of the native NP, which restores normal spinal function by transferring pressure to the surrounding annulus fibers, preloading these fibers physiologically while it strengthens the whole segment mechanically.

◆ Biocompatibility Testing

A primary concern with any implantable medical device is its ability to function without eliciting an adverse biological response. Tests for pyrogenicity, cytotoxicity, irritability, toxicity, and mutagenicity were performed as per International Standards Organization (ISO) 10993 standards.

Reverse mutation assays using *Escherichia coli* and *Salmoella typhimurium* showed no significant increase in revertant colonies. Additional mutagenicity testing was performed using a rodent bone marrow micronucleus assay. Extracts of Aquacryl did not induce a significant increase in micronucleated cells as compared with negative controls at 24 and 48 hours. The NeuDisc was tested to determine its potential to increase the number of mutants in the L5178Y mouse lymphoma cell line when compared with the background rate. There was not a significant increase in number of mutant L5178Y cells. The results of these tests identified Aquacryl as nonmutagenic.

Aquacryl was analyzed using a mammalian cell culture media (MEM) Elution test in L929 mouse fibroblast cells and showed no biological activity, grade 0, and was classified as noncytotoxic. The implantation of particulate hydrolyzed polyacrylonitrile in rabbit epidural and intradiskal space did not exhibit an inflammatory response and the material is considered nonpyrogenic.

Systemic and intracutaneous injection testing is used to analyze the possibility that the material is an irritant. Results showed that Aquacryl did not elicit a greater biological response than control materials. Short-term and long-term implantation tests in rabbits demonstrated that Aquacryl was both nontoxic and biocompatible. The long-term and chronic toxicity of the material was analyzed by implantation in rat paravertebral muscles. The results were similar to control implantations and showed no chronic cytotoxicity.

◆ Mechanical Testing

The NeuDisc has also undergone extensive mechanical testing to verify that its mechanical properties closely match those of the native NP and to ensure that the NeuDisc would survive long-term implantation and use. The testing included endurance testing in multiple motions, range of motion studies, expulsion testing, and fatigue testing in a cadaveric model.

Endurance Testing

The endurance testing was performed on implants in compression, flexion and extension combined with compression, lateral bending combined with compression, and axial torsion combined with compression. All endurance testing was performed in an unconfined state, simulating a situation where the AF does not provide support of the device, and in displacement control with concave platens to mimic the shape of native end plates. The NeuDisc was tested for 10 million cycles, representing a 10-year lifetime, in each of the motions. All testing was performed in 37°C Hanks' Balanced Salt Solution (HBSS) (Krackeler Scientific, Inc., Albany, NY). Following each endurance test, the fluid was collected and analyzed for wear debris and monomer elution.

The NeuDisc samples were tested in axial compression to a simulated life of 10 years with no delaminations, tears, cracks, or surface defects evident after testing. All compressive endurance tests tested samples still hydrated to levels similar to controls when unconfined and the hydration percentage of the compressive endurance tested implants and controls were comparable. The mean compressive modulus of the endurance tested samples was equivalent to the mean

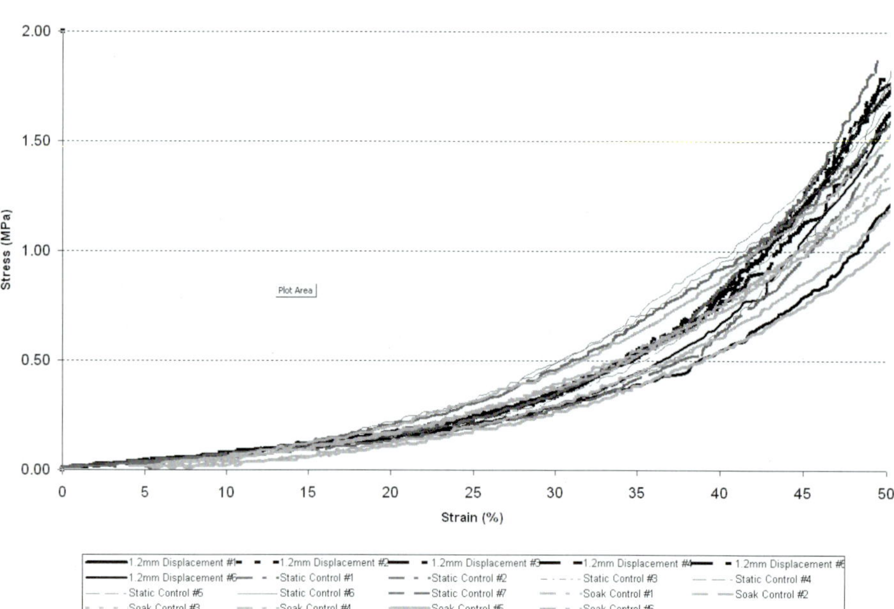

Figure 16–1   Stress-strain graphs of endurance-tested samples.

compressive modulus of control samples. Stress-strain graphs are included in **Fig. 16–1**. Analysis of the fluid collected during compressive endurance testing did not show evidence of monomer elution and the samples had a mean wear rate of 0.25 mg/million cycles.

Flexion and extension motions about the major axis of the NeuDisc were performed to a simulated life of 10 years. Three of the flexion-extension samples were removed from endurance testing to be evaluated against controls. The remaining three samples proceeded to lateral bending testing. The three flexion-extension endurance samples removed for evaluation showed no signs of delaminations, tears, cracks, or major surface defects. All three samples had small wear lines oriented radially from the major axis (**Fig. 16–2**).

Lateral bending motions about the minor axis of the NeuDisc were performed on six samples, three of which had first been tested to a simulated 10-year lifespan in flexion-extension.

All six samples survived the simulated 10 years of testing in lateral bending without evidence of delaminations, tears, cracks, or major surface defects. All samples had small wear lines oriented radially from the minor axis similar to the wear lines seen from flexion-extension testing. The three samples that underwent flexion-extension and lateral bending testing continued onto axial torsion endurance testing.

Six samples, three of which had first been tested to a simulated 10-year lifespan in both flexion-extension and lateral bending, were tested in axial torsion. All six samples survived the simulated 10 years of testing in axial torsion without evidence of delaminations, tears, cracks, or major surface defects.

The samples that were endurance tested in combined loading modes underwent post-testing evaluations to determine hydration levels, mechanical properties, monomer elution, and wear analysis. All samples had hydration percentages equivalent to controls. The hydration of samples was also measured after subjecting the implants at an isotropic pressure of 600 kPa for 24 hours, simulating normal intradiskal pressures, and was equivalent to controls. Static compressive modulus of endurance-tested implants was determined through static axial testing of the implants. All samples tested in combined loading modes had compressive moduli equivalent to controls. No monomer elution was evident in the fluid gathered from any of the endurance-tested samples. Wear analysis for samples from the combined mode endurance testing had wear rates similar to the devices endurance tested in unconfined compression.

The extensive endurance testing performed on the NeuDisc spinal nucleus implant (SNI) demonstrated the device's ability to survive long-term strenuous use in multiple loading modes. The three implants that underwent sequential testing in flexion-extension, lateral bending, and axial torsion survived a simulated 30-year lifetime, 30 million cycles, of use. The endurance testing also established the chemical and mechanical

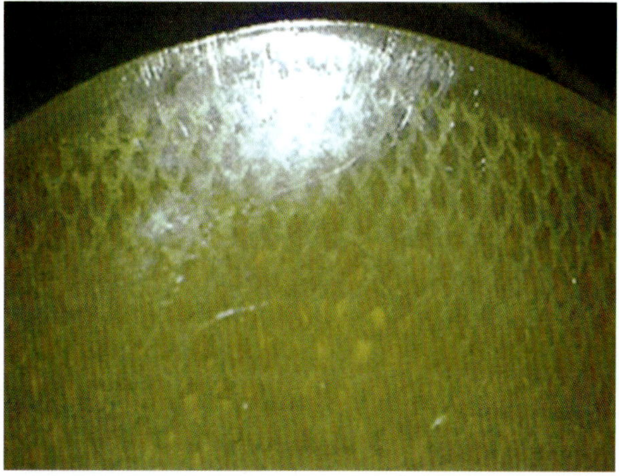

Figure 16–2   Image of radial wear lines observed in bending testing.

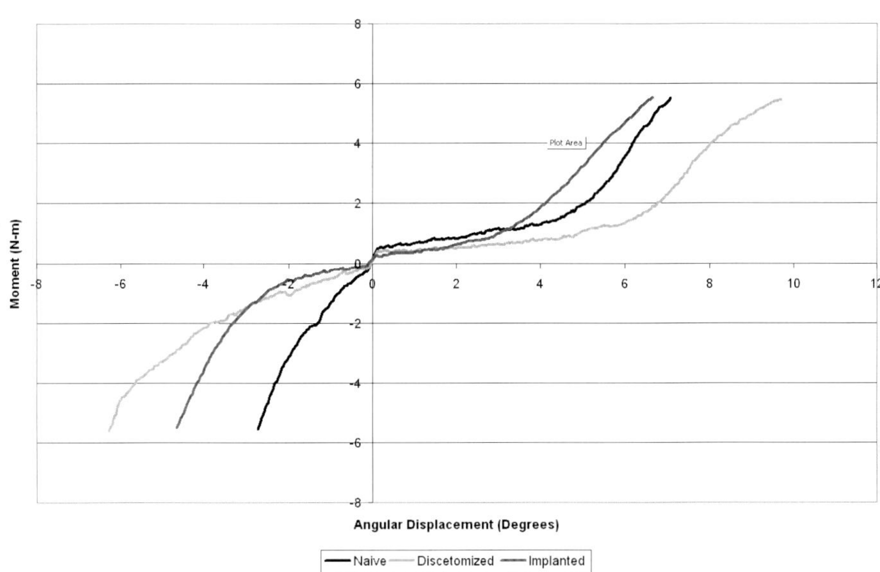

Figure 16–3 Flexion-extension range of motion for cadaver testing.

stability of the device after long-term use. Analysis of the fluid from all the endurance testing found no evidence of monomer elution and that the implants had a wear rate of 0.25 mg/million cycles or less in all loading modes. Mechanical testing of all endurance-tested samples showed that the mechanical properties of the device do not deteriorate beyond acceptable clinical levels after a simulated 10-year lifespan.

Range of Motion Testing

The ability of a nucleus replacement device to restore or preserve spinal motion is its primary function. Mechanical evaluation of a device to restore spinal motion would therefore not be complete without investigating the device's function during normal range of motion in functional spinal units (FSUs). Normal spinal motion stress/strain curves have a distinctive shape with a neutral zone, where changes in displacement are not accompanied by changes in force, and an elastic zone, where conventional Hookean motion occurs. An increase of the size of the neutral zone is seen after diskectomy with only minor changes in elastic zone stiffness. It is therefore important during range of motion testing of a nucleus replacement implant to restore the neutral zone to the naive condition when compared with the diskectomized samples. This method of testing presents certain difficulties; namely, variability of biological samples, fixed order of testing, and long-term testing of a biological specimen.

Range of motion testing was performed on a total of 36 FSUs. Specimens were tested under the following conditions: flexion-extension, 8 degrees or 10 Nm, lateral bending, 6 degrees or 10 Nm, and axial torsion, 2.5 degrees or 10 Nm. All testing was performed with a compressive preload of 400 N and at a frequency of 0.33 Hz. Two preconditioning trials were executed for each sample followed by a third trial. Angular displacement versus moment graphs were generated for all tests from the third trial. Analyses were made of neutral zone size, overall range of motion, and construct stiffness in the elastic zone. Small but not significant differences were seen during testing in neutral zone size, overall range of motion, and construct stiffness between naive, diskectomized, and implanted specimens. Neutral zone size and range of motion increased from naive to diskectomized and returned toward naive once implanted in most specimens (**Fig. 16–3**). The construct stiffness showed a great deal of variability from specimen to specimen but implanted specimens generally had stiffness values close to the values of naive specimens. The NeuDisc did not expulse or extrude from any of the 36 FSUs.

Range of motion testing confirmed the efficacy of the NeuDisc in restoring normal spinal motion characteristics. Additionally, the testing demonstrated that the NeuDisc did not extrude or expulse during activity through a normal range of motion.

Expulsion Testing

Following range of motion testing, 32 implanted FSUs were tested to failure. Twelve specimens were failed in compression, eight specimens were failed in flexion, and 12 specimens were failed in lateral bending. The 12 specimens failed in compression were loaded at a rate of 100 N/s until failure. The eight specimens failed in flexion were loaded at a rate of 0.4 Deg/s. The 12 specimens failed in lateral bending were all loaded in the direction opposite insertion at a rate of 0.4 Deg/s until failure occurred. The most common mode of failure in compression was end plate fracture, occurring in 10 of the 12 specimens. One specimen with an extremely thin annulus had complete reduction in height of the implant and in one specimen the implant expulsed. The average force at failure was 3533 N, which agrees with literature values for failure force,[17,18] and the implant expulsion occurred at 4100 N. The eight flexion specimens failed by end plate fractures and ligament ruptures. The failures in the flexion specimens occurred at an average moment of failure of 52.2 Nm. The 12 specimens failed in lateral bending had five different failure modes. One specimen had an end plate fracture, three had fractures of the facet joint, six had ligament rupture, one had an annulus tear, and one implant expulsed. The average moment at failure was 24.8 Nm and the implant expulsion occurred at 47.9 Nm. The failure strengths in bending also agree with published values.[19]

Expulsion testing further demonstrated that the NeuDisc is unlikely to expulse during normal activity. Both expulsions that were observed occurred at extremely high loads.

Human Cadaver Fatigue Testing

Further evaluation of the endurance characteristics of the NeuDisc SNI were performed in an in situ biomechanical model. Implanted FSUs were compressively loaded for a simulated implant lifetime of 10 years in sealed vinyl containers filled with HBSS. Environmental control devices were also placed in the vinyl containers. Fluid from the vinyl containers was collected and determined to have a protein concentration of 8%. Compression and hydration testing was performed on all explanted NeuDiscs.

All implanted devices survived the in situ fatigue testing. The explanted devices all showed little or no wear after the simulated 10 years of implantation. When the explanted devices were compared with shelf and environmental controls it was observed that hydration percentages were lower, but on average still near 80% hydration, and mechanical properties were comparable to controls.

Cadaver fatigue testing demonstrated the ability of the NeuDisc to endure a 10-year lifetime of in situ use. Cadaver fatigue testing also showed that the device was still able to hydrate in a proteinaceous medium and maintain its mechanical properties after 10 years of in situ loading.

The mechanical testing performed on the NeuDisc addressed many of the clinical concerns that have been raised in regard to nucleus replacement devices. The NeuDisc was endurance tested in multiple modes and survived to a simulated life of 30 years. The wear characteristics of the NeuDisc during mechanical testing were found to be on average less than 0.25 mg/million cycles, which is equivalent to 0.02% mass loss of the implant per year of life. The mechanical properties of the NeuDisc were found to decrease slightly after endurance and fatigue testing, but were still within clinically acceptable levels.

◆ Clinical Studies

The NeuDisc radially anisotropic bullet is the subject of a clinical investigation under way in Germany. The study inclusion criteria are single-level DDD, disk height > 7 mm, intact facets, and unrelenting back pain nonresponsive to conservative care for 6 months. The postoperative follow-up is performed at 6 weeks, 12 weeks, and 6 months. Preoperative and postoperative Oswestry scores and visual analog scale (VAS) scores are used to evaluate the success of the treatment with NeuDisc. Follow-up NeuDisc is designed to treat patients with back and leg pain but not leg pain exclusively. The NeuDisc may be inserted endoscopically or through an open approach with direct visualization. If inserted through a cannula, an endoscope can be used to visualize the placement postinsertion. Surgical access to the disk space can be achieved using several approaches, including posterior, posterolateral, or anterolateral.[20] The early-stage evaluation of patients receiving the NeuDisc implant are encouraging. At 6 months postoperative, the implant is hydrated and well positioned within the nuclear cavity. The results of the first patient to receive a NeuDisc radially anisotropic bullet implant show excellent early reduction in pain on both VAS and Oswestry tests. The first recipient of the current format of the NeuDisc implant was a 39-year-old female presenting with severe back and leg pain at L4–L5 as evidenced by magnetic resonance imaging and confirmed with provocative diskography. The patient had pain scores of 8 for VAS and 44 for Oswestry evaluations. At 6 weeks postoperatively, the VAS for NeuDisc radially anisotropic bullet patient no. 1 was 0 and the Oswestry had declined to a value of 6, resulting in an 86% reduction in pain. An increase in disk height of greater than 2 mm was observed radiographically (**Figs. 16–4A,B and 16–5A,B**).

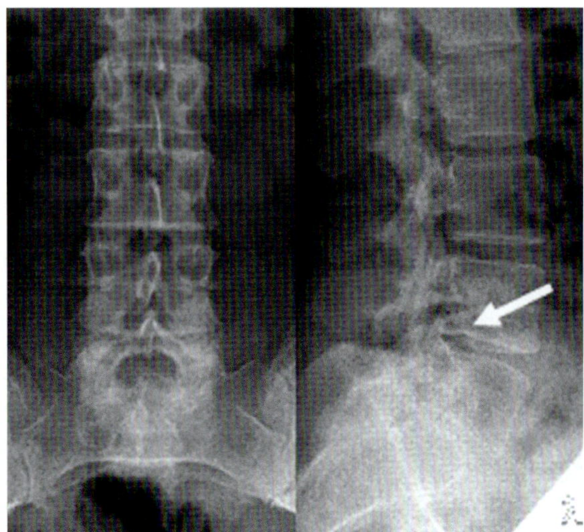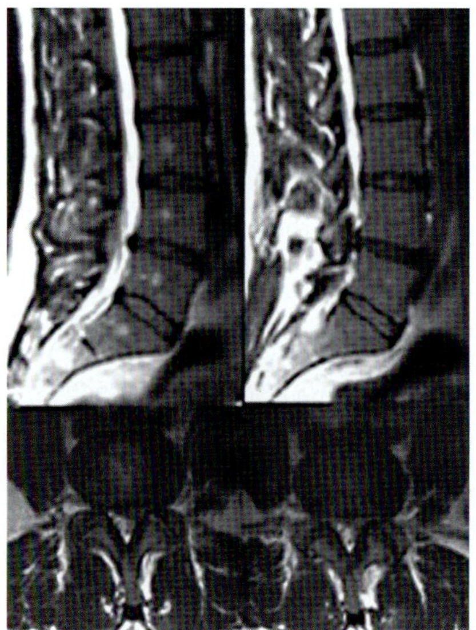

Figure 16–4   **(A)** Preoperative x-ray images of patient (arrow: loss of disk height). **(B)** Preoperative magnetic resonance imaging of patient.

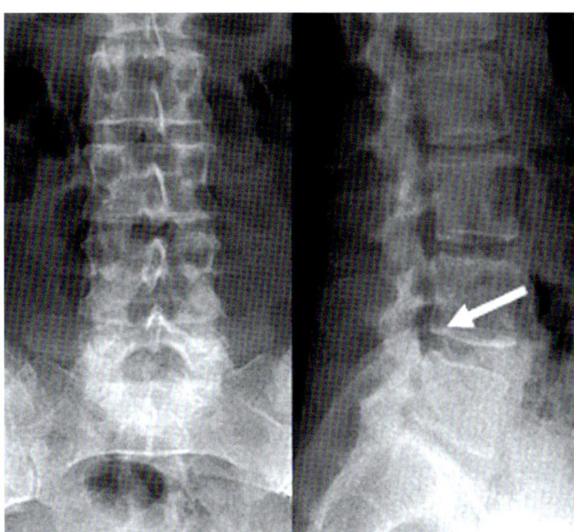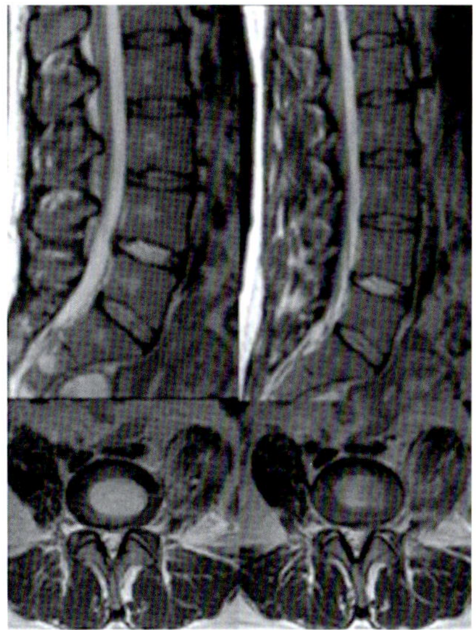

Figure 16–5   (A) Postoperative x-ray images of patient (arrow: restoration of disk height). **(B)** Postoperative magnetic resonance imaging of patient.

◆ Conclusion

The NeuDisc Spinal Nucleus Implant was carefully designed and thoroughly tested to ensure its efficacy as a nucleus replacement device. Biocompatibility testing performed in accordance with ISO 10993 guidelines demonstrated that the NeuDisc is nontoxic and biocompatible. Mechanical testing of the NeuDisc demonstrated that the device possesses mechanical and physical properties closely similar to the native NP. Early clinical results demonstrate that the NeuDisc hydrates following insertion and resists migration or dislodgment. The end plate surface in contact with the implant remains unaltered, with no evidence of remodeling or modic changes at up to 6-month follow-up. Although early results suggest that the NeuDisc has the potential to reduce low back pain associated with the degenerative process, long-term clinical evaluation is under way to confirm these findings.

References

1. Praemer A, Furner S, Rice DP. Musculoskeletal Conditions in the United States. Rosemont, IL: American Academy of Orthopaedic Surgeons; 1999
2. Lee CK. Accelerated degeneration of the segment adjacent to a lumbar fusion. Spine 1988;13:375–377
3. Yang SW, Langrana NA, Lee CK. Biomechanics of the lumbosacral spinal fusion in combined compression-torsion loads. Spine 1986;11:937–941
4. Bertagnoli R. Disc surgery in motion. Spine Line 2004;11/12:23–28
5. Bertagnoli R. Review of modern treatment options for degenerative disc disease. In: Kaech DL, Jinkins JR, eds. Spinal restabilization procedures. Elsevier, Amsterdam, NY; 2002:365–375
6. Allen MJ, Schoonmaker JE, Ordway NR, et al. Preclinical testing of a poly (vinyl alcohol) hydrogel nucleus in baboons. In: Proceedings of the 13th Annual Meeting of the North American Spine Society, New Orleans, LA, October 25–28, 2000, Rosemont, IL: North American Spine Society, 2000:1
7. Ray CD, Schönmayr R, Kliniken HS. Two-year follow-up on PDN device disc replacement patients. In: Proceedings of the 15th Annual Meeting of the North American Spine Society, San Francisco, CA, October 28–31, 1998, Rosemont, IL: North American Spine Society, 1998:34
8. Ray CD. The PDN® prosthetic disc-nucleus device. Eur Spine J 2002;11 (Suppl 2):S137–S142
9. Bertagnoli R, Schönmayr R. Surgical and clinical results with the PDN® prosthetic disc-nucleus device. Eur Spine J 2002;11(Suppl 2): S143–S148
10. Eysel P, Rompe JD, Schoemayr R, Zoellner J. Biomechanical behaviour of a prosthetic lumbar nucleus. Acta Neurochir (Wien) 1999;141: 1083–1087
11. Meakin JR, Reid JE, Hukins DW. Replacing the nucleus pulposus of the intervertebral disc. Clin Biomech (Bristol, Avon) 2001;16: 560–565
12. Thomas J, Lowman A, Marcolongo M. Novel associated hydrogels for nucleus pulposus replacement. J Biomed Mater Res A 2003;67: 1329–1337
13. Ordway NR, Han ZH, Bao QB, et al. Restoration of biomechanical function with a hydrogel intervertebral disc implant. In: Proceedings of the 21st Annual Meeting of the International Society of the Study of the Lumbar Spine, Seattle, WA, 1994:8
14. Fernström U. Arthroplasty with intercorporal endoprosthesis in herniated disc and in painful disc. Acta Chir Scand Suppl 1966; 357:154–159
15. Nachemson A. Lumbar intradiscal pressure. In: Jayson MIV, ed. The Lumbar Spine and Back Pain. London: Churchill Livingstone; 1987:191
16. Wilke HJ, Neef P, Caimi M, Hoogland T, Claes L. New in vivo measurements of pressures in the intervertebral disc. Spine 1999; 24: 755–762
17. Tencer AF, Johnson KD. Biomechanics in Orthopaedic Trauma. Philadelphia: Lippincott; 1994:31
18. White AA, Panjabi MM. Clinical Biomechanics of the Spine. Philadelphia: Lippincott; 1978:36
19. Adams MA, Green TP, Dolan P. The strength in anterior bending of lumbar intervertebral discs. Spine 1994;19:2197–2203
20. Bertagnoli R, Vazquez RJ. The anterolateral transpsoatic approach (ALPA): a new technique for implanting prosthetic disc-nucleus devices. J Spinal Disord Tech 2003;16:398–404

17

Pioneer Surgical Technology NUBAC Artificial Nucleus

Qi-Bin Bao, Hansen A. Yuan, and Matthew N. Songer

◆ **Pioneer Surgical Technology NUBAC Nucleus Device Design Rationale**

◆ **Summary of the NUBAC Preclinical Studies**

  Biocompatibility and Biodurability

  Biomechanical Assessment and Fatigue and Extrusion Characteristics of the NUBAC Nucleus Implant

Multidirectional Flexibility and Load to Failure Analysis of the Pioneer Surgical Nucleus Pulposus Replacement: An In Vitro Cadaveric Model

Wear and Fatigue Studies

◆ **NUBAC Nucleus Implant Indication and Surgical Technique**

◆ **Conclusion**

For diskogenic back pain, fusion is no longer being considered the gold standard of treatment due to the concern of adjacent disk disease. After more than 40 years of relentless effort, disk arthroplasty is finally becoming a clinically viable option for the treatment of diskogenic back pain. Disk arthroplasty can be divided into total disk replacement and nucleus replacement. Although the goals of these two arthroplasty treatments are the same (i.e., relieving back pain through removing the pain source and restoring or maintaining disk anatomy and function), each approaches the problem from a different perspective. For total disk replacement, almost all of the disk tissue is removed and, therefore, functional restoration depends completely on the device itself. However, for a nucleus replacement, only the nucleus is removed and functional restoration relies on the device and the remaining annulus and ligaments. Although total disk technology has been narrowed to two basic designs (ball and socket and metal-elastomer-metal), there are more variations in nucleus designs, from metal ball to in situ curable elastomer.

To design an effective prosthesis, it is important to understand the functions played by the original tissue and the prosthesis. Biologically, the nucleus pulposus functions as a fluid pump that facilitates fluid diffusion, carrying nutrients to and removing metabolites from the avascular disk.[1] Biomechanically, although the nucleus presents as a loose gel and has little resistance to physiological loads by itself, it inflates the annulus and shares about one half to two thirds of the compressive load on the disk.[2] In most nucleus replacements, because the majority of the natural nucleus is replaced with a nonbiological material, the biological function of fluid diffusion might no longer be important for the implanted disk, although conceptually it might still bring the benefit of preventing degeneration of the remaining nucleus and annulus. Therefore, for most nonbiological nucleus devices, the main objective would be to restore or maintain the disk height, sagittal balance, and biomechanical function of the index disk.

Many past and current nucleus replacements are made of elastic materials, either preformed or in situ cured, probably due to the viscoelastic nature of the nucleus. However, there is a major limitation in using a material that attempts to mimic the exact properties of the natural nucleus for a nucleus replacement device because of the change in boundary conditions. As mentioned earlier, the mechanical function of the nucleus is largely achieved by the total encasement and resulting constraint of the annulus, just like air is encased and constrained by a tire. If there is a rupture in the annulus, the nucleus will immediately leak through this defect with a drastic reduction of intradiskal pressure which compromises its load-sharing capability. Before the technology of repairing the annulus becomes available, a nucleus prosthesis will always be used with some annular defect, which can either exist prior to the surgery or be created during the surgery. Therefore, most elastic nucleus replacement devices use materials with a modulus much higher than the natural nucleus so they will not deform easily and can be readily extruded through the annular defect.

Several nonelastic nucleus devices have also been attempted. In fact, the two nucleus implants first used in humans were made of nonelastic materials. The first nucleus implant used in a human was polymethyl methacrylate (PMMA), which is a plastic material. The clinical data on this device are limited. Although the initial data on 14 patients appeared to be encouraging,[3] a subsequent small randomized study using diskectomy as a control found that the PMMA nucleus device provided no obvious clinical advantages over the control.[4] The second nucleus implant used in a human was the Fernström ball, a stainless steel ball bearing, which was even stiffer than PMMA. Although the Fernström ball design seems simple, the concept showed clinical evidence of being fairly sound. Based on biomechanical data that suggested the plane of intervertebral movement could be described by the movement of a contiguous vertebra over a small ball located in the nucleus pulposus recess,[5] Fernström believed a ball nucleus device would best restore the articulation of the adjacent vertebrae and prevent anterior or posterior slippage of the neighboring vertebrae. The Fernström ball has been implanted in many more patients than the PMMA nucleus, and all the published clinical data on this device appeared to be fairly favorable. Fernström reported his own series of a total of 125 patients with 191 nucleus implants with a follow-up of 6 months to $2\frac{1}{2}$ years.[6] He divided his patients into two groups; group 1 with disk herniation and group 2 with only diskogenic back pain. For comparison purposes, he also analyzed 100 control patients with similar indications who were treated with diskectomy only. He found that low back pain occurred in only 12% of group 1 patients, which compared very favorably with the control group of 60%. For patients with only diskogenic back pain (group 2), low back pain occurred in 40% of patients, which also compared favorably with the 88% occurrence rate in the control group. Roentgen examination performed on 30 lumbar implanted segments every 6 months for $2\frac{1}{2}$ years revealed preservation of bending motion in the index segment. In a separate study, McKenzie implanted a total of 155 Fernström Balls in 103 patients. He also divided his patients into two groups based on the indications in the same way as Fernström. In a short-term study of 40 patients, half of whom had acute disk herniation and half of whom had disabling degenerative disk disease, he reported excellent and good results in 85% of patients.[7] Many years later, McKenzie reported the long-term follow-up data with an average follow-up time of 17 years on 69 of his 103 patients.[8] Results in group 1 (herniated disk) patients and group 2 (diskogenic back pain only) in the long-term series were graded excellent and good in 83% and 75%, respectively. Ninety-five percent of all patients returned to work. McKenzie's results, even by today's standards, would be considered a success. Like almost any clinical study, there were certainly some limitations with these studies. Foremost, it can be argued that these were retrospective, nonrandomized, controlled studies. However, it should be realized that the vast majority of clinical studies on spinal implants, especially for those started in the 1960s, were retrospective, nonrandomized, and controlled.

If one is to judge the clinical success of the Fernström Ball from the published data, the Fernström Ball should be a clinically viable device, even compared with the clinical results of many other modern disk arthroplasty devices.[9–11] However, for whatever reasons, the Fernström Ball was not further commercialized beyond its initial use in the 1960s. Most of the negative criticism on the Fernström nucleus device has been focused on its subsidence. From the design of the Fernström Ball, it is obvious that some subsidence is inevitable due to the initial small or nearly point contact area, resulting in a high initial contact stress. As a matter of fact, some initial subsidence was the intention of Fernström. Fernström instructed users to utilize an implant at least

1 mm taller than the disk height.[6] The initial subsidence seated the implant in the disk space and prevented the implant from extrusion in almost all cases. Most subsidence for the Fernström Ball stopped after 1 to 3 mm per end plate.[6]

◆ Pioneer Surgical Technology NUBAC Nucleus Device Design Rationale

The design of the Pioneer Surgical Technology (PST) (Marquette, MI) NUBAC nucleus device was largely based on the lessons learned from other previous nucleus devices, with the intention to capture the features that contributed to the success of previous devices and to address pitfalls that existed in the previous devices. From the clinical experience of the Fernström Ball, it is clear that a nonelastic nucleus device design works well in relieving diskogenic back pain and maintaining the index disk anatomy and function. It is more encouraging to note that the effectiveness in relieving diskogenic back pain was maintained over a long time with almost no major safety issue. The Fernström Ball forms two articulating surfaces with the adjacent vertebrae and allows the rotational motion of the index disk, which has become a key design requirement for any disk arthroplasty device. The major deficiency of the Fernström nucleus is the small initial contact area, which inevitably led to some degree of subsidence.

The PST NUBAC is a two-piece implant consisting of a top and a bottom plate, with a ball and socket inner articulation joint allowing rotational motions along all three major axes within the physiological ranges. The motion of the device in axial rotation is unconstrained, whereas the motions in flexion-extension and lateral bending are semiconstrained slightly beyond the physiological ranges of motion in these directions. Unlike a total disk, the NUBAC device's range of motion is largely dependent upon the constraints from the adjacent tissues. The device is designed to restore or maintain the load-sharing capabilities of the index disk. By selecting the proper wedge angle of the device it can restore the normal sagittal balance. There are several size configurations to ensure that individual differences in anatomy can be accommodated. Both the top and bottom plates are in the shape of a racetrack, similar to the shape of a typical nucleus cavity. This will ensure sufficient implant/cavity conformity and adequate stress distribution on the end plates. The outer surfaces of the implant are either flat or slightly convex to approximate the flat or slight concavity of the end plates (refs).[12] The device is manufactured from polyetheretherketone (PEEK), an exceptionally strong engineering thermoplastic. The elastic modulus of PEEK is close to that of the underlying bone. The device is radiolucent and will not interfere with any images. It is more important for a nucleus device than a total disk device to be radiolucent so it does not interfere magnetic resonance imaging (MRI) for evaluation of potential pathology at the index disk. Tantalum markers are used to facilitate the visualization of implant location using x-ray radiography. PEEK is one of the top medical thermoplastics with a well-documented biocompatibility and biostability history, along with an excellent track record of being used as a permanent implant, including spinal implants.[13] Biostability is

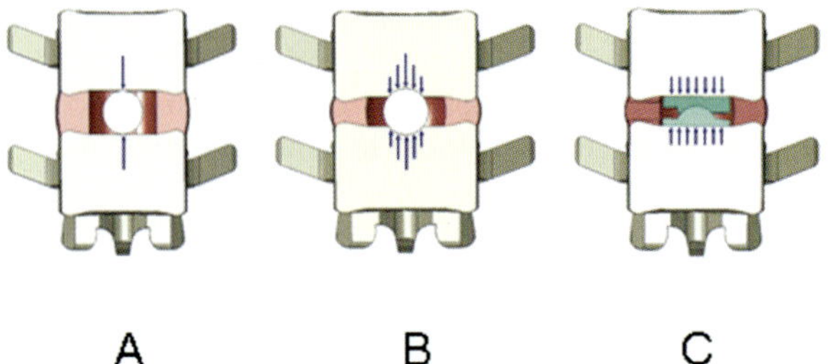

Figure 17–1 Schematic drawings of contact stress distribution. **(A)** Initial contact stress of the Fernström Ball. **(B)** Contact stress of the Fernström ball after some subsidence. **(C)** Contact stress of the NUBAC™ nucleus implant.

extremely important for load-bearing disk arthroplasty devices because of the long life expectation for the device. In general, the biostability for biomaterials follows the order of metal > plastic > elastomer. Biodegradation of a biomaterial can be affected by many different factors, such as stress, biological environment, and oxidation, and may be difficult to evaluate using in vitro studies. For example, the Acroflex (DePuy-Acromed, Inc., Raynham, MA) total disk replacement device, which has a hexane-based polyolefin elastomer core, had passed vigorous in vitro fatigue tests under various compression and shear conditions.[14] However, in a pilot study of 28 patients, fracture on the elastomer core was found in 10 out of 28 implants within 2 years.[15] It is likely this failure was due to the biodegradation occurring in the body, which was not assessed during the fatigue test. Therefore, unless the biomaterial has an established clinical history of biostability, there will always be some uncertainties on the biostability of the material for disk arthroplasty applications, especially for elastomers. The chemical structure of PEEK ensures extreme stability against hydrolysis, even at elevated temperature. PEEK can be steam or gamma sterilized repeatedly without deterioration in its bulk mechanical properties.

As reported by Fernström, most of the subsidence related to the Fernström Ball stopped after 1 to 3 mm per end plate.[6] This phenomenon can easily be explained with the contact stress and the ultimate compressive strength (UCS) of the end plate. If the initial contact stress is above the UCS of the end plate, the implant will experience subsidence and lead to an increase in the contact area, which in turn leads to a decrease in contact stress. The subsidence will eventually stop when the contact stress is below the UCS. Lowe et al reported that the static end plate UCS was around 17 to 20 MPa for lumbar vertebrae when compressed with a circular indenter.[16] However, Tan et al, in a more recent study, found that the UCS was only ~2.7 MPa when compressed with an elliptical indenter.[17] The low UCS reported by Tan et al is likely due to the much older samples (mean age of 77 years) used in this study than the samples (age range, 40–50 years) used in Lowe et al's study. It is likely that the vertebral fatigue fracture strength will be less than the static UCS. When the Fernström Ball nucleus was first implanted, it had a near point contact with the end plates (**Fig. 17–1A**). This point contact leads to a contact stress much higher than the UCS of the end plate and, therefore, inevitably causes the implant subsiding into the end plate. As the Fernström ball subsides, the contact area increases and the contact stress decreases. The subsidence eventually stops as the contact area increases to a point at which the contact stress gets to below the UCS. To better understand the contact area and contact stress between the NUBAC artificial nucleus and the Fernström Ball (range, 10–16 mm diameter), the calculations in **Table 17–1** and **Fig. 17–1** illustrate the contact area and stress difference between the Fernström Ball and the NUBAC nucleus implant. If the load on the nucleus implant is 400 N, assuming the nucleus implant shares 50% of a total load on the disk of 800 N, the contact stress for a 12 mm diameter Fernström ball would be 11.6 MPa and 4.7 MPa with 1 mm and 3 mm subsidence, respectively. Because most Fernström Balls had a subsidence of 1 to 3 mm per end plate, the fatigue compressive strength for most end plates should be in the range of 4.7 to 11.6 MPa, which is not much off from the static UCS reported by Lowe et al.

To address the subsidence problem of the Fernström ball nucleus, the design of the NUBAC nucleus implant provides a much larger initial contact area than the Fernström ball. As illustrated in **Fig. 17–2**, the large contact surface of the NUBAC nucleus device leads to a much lower contact stress. The calculations in **Table 17–1** show that even after 3 mm subsidence of a 12 mm diameter Fernström ball the contact stress is still 2.2 times the contact stress of a medium-sized NUBAC nucleus implant. Therefore, the subsidence risk of the NUBAC nucleus device should be significantly reduced.

Table 17–1 Contact Area and Contact Stress Comparison between Fernström Ball Nucleus Implant and NUBAC Nucleus Implant

	Contact Area	Average Contact Stress (under 400 N)	Stress Difference from Pioneer Nucleus
NUBAC nucleus (medium)	191 mm²	2.1 MPa	1
12 mm Fernström ball with 1 mm subsidence on each side	35 mm²	11.6 MPa	5.5 ×
12 mm Fernström ball with 2 mm subsidence on each side	62.8 mm²	6.4 MPa	3 ×
12 mm Fernström ball with 3 mm subsidence on each side	84.8 mm²	4.7 MPa	2.2 ×

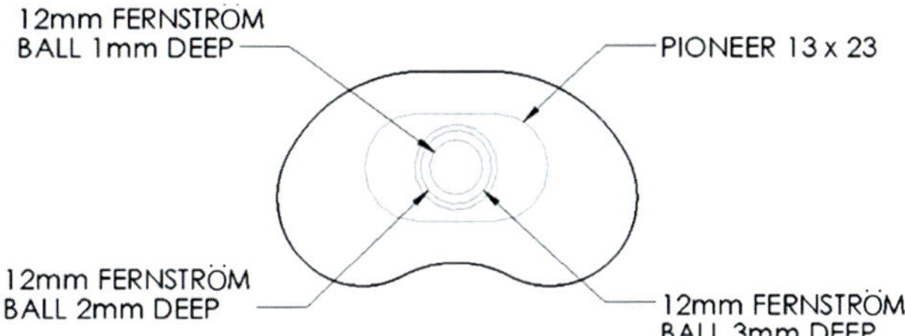

Figure 17–2   Contact areas of a 12 mm Fernström Ball with 1, 2, and 3 mm subsidence and a medium-sized NUBAC nucleus device.

Unlike a total disk replacement, a nucleus implant is not designed to be fixed to the vertebrae. Therefore, in general, it has a higher risk of implant extrusion than a total disk replacement. If the major deficiency of the Fernström Ball is its initial small contact area, which led to some degree of subsidence, one of the benefits of this ball design is its low migration rate due to the implant settling into the end plates. Combining the Fernström series of 191 implants and the McKenzie series of 155 implants, only one implant extruded (< 0.3%). This stunningly low implant extrusion rate is comparable or even better than any total disks and has set a high bar for any subsequent nucleus devices. Since the Fernström Ball nucleus device, only one nucleus device, the PDN (Raymedica, Inc., Minneapolis, MN), has reached the clinical scale of the Fernström Ball device. The PDN is composed of a bulky hydrogel pellet encased in a polyethylene jacket. This device has faced a clinical implant extrusion rate between 8 and 36% but appears to be effective in relieving diskogenic back pain if the implant stays in the disk space.[18,19] The high extrusion rate for a bulky pellet-shaped implant such as the PDN could be due to the uneven load distribution on the implant and the inability to adjust the dimensions of the implant during bending (**Fig. 17–3**). In pure compression, the load on the PDN, or any other bulky implant with surface contours matching with the end plates, would be fairly even. The rim of the vertebra will form a bump to prevent the implant from extrusion. Because it is known that the annular window, which is necessary to insert the nucleus implant, does not structurally heal over time,[20] a bending motion opposite to the annular window will increase its dimension. Given that the dimension of the proximal end (the end near the annular window) of any bulky implant remains the same, the implant can then easily pass through the vertebral rim and extrude through this window. As shown in **Fig. 17–3B**, the bending will also shift the shear load toward the distal side of the implant (opposite to the annular window) and will start to push the implant toward this window (**Fig. 17–3C**). This is similar to the phenomenon that occurs when a watermelon seed is squeezed between a finger and thumb. Under pure compression, the watermelon seed will tend to stay between two fingers. However, a shift in your finger or thumb toward the edge of watermelon seed will result in the watermelon seed being ejected. The ball and socket design of the NUBAC will eliminate this uneven loading during bending because the two plates will always rotate with the vertebrae due to the inner ball and socket articulation. As the disk bends opposite to the annular window, the dimension of the proximal end (the end near the annular window) of the NUBAC nucleus increases to match that of the disk space, and the edge of the two plates will stay behind the rim of the vertebra (**Figs. 17–3D,E**). Therefore, the articulating plate feature may significantly reduce the risk of implant extrusion during any bending motion.

The even load distribution of the NUBAC under various bending motions is another advantage over other bulk nucleus devices. Most bulk nucleus devices are designed to have end plate contact surfaces that match the geometry of the end plate for even pressure distribution. However, this even pressure distribution can be achieved only under a pure compressive loading condition. It is well-known that during daily activities several bending motions can take place, with flexion-extension angles over 10 degrees or more.[21] Due to the lack of an articulating feature of these bulk nucleus devices, the load distribution becomes uneven under these bending motions as shown in **Fig. 17–3**. This uneven loading distribution not only contributes to the high risk of implant extrusion as discussed here but can also cause high local stresses on the end plate, which may lead to end plate edema or even end plate fracture. The inner articulation feature of the NUBAC nucleus device always allows the implant plates to rotate and stay in contact with the vertebral end plates and therefore maintain an even stress distribution under all loading conditions.

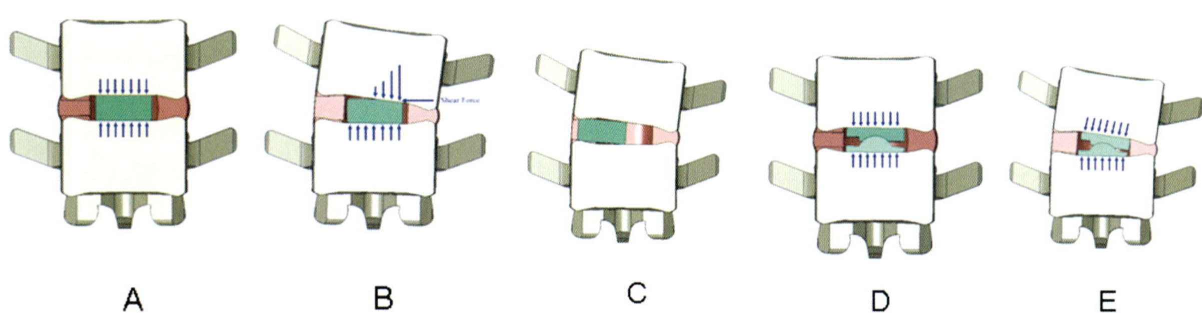

Figure 17–3   Schematic drawings of stress distribution under compression and bending. **(A)** Bulk polymer nucleus implant under compression. **(B)** Bulk polymer nucleus implant under bending. **(C)** Partial extrusion of bulk polymer nucleus implant under bending. **(D)** NUBAC nucleus device under compression. **(E)** NUBAC nucleus device under bending.

◆ Summary of the NUBAC Preclinical Studies

Biocompatibility and Biodurability

In addition to its superb mechanical properties, PEEK-OPTIMA polymer (Invibio, Greenville, SC) was chosen for the NUBAC artificial nucleus because of its established biocompatibility and biodurability. Since its introduction to the medical market in 1999, PEEK-OPTIMA has quickly gained the confidence and acceptance of the medical community as a highly reliable implantable material. Independent laboratories have performed biocompatibility and biostability testing on PEEK-OPTIMA relevant to International Standards Organization ISO 10993 and United States Pharmacopeia (USP) Class VI procedures, which have shown excellent results. Device (MAF) and drug (DMF) Master Files are on file with the U.S. Food and Drug Administration (FDA) containing these results, as well as additional testing and extensive data concerning the polymer and its manufacturing methods.

The biodurability requirement for a permanent implantable device is largely dependent on its application. For implants primarily used for older patients, such as total joints, a biodurability of 15 years would most likely be adequate, although with an increasing life expectancy and a progressively younger age group receiving these implants, the biodurability requirements for these implants are likely to increase as well. However, for disk arthroplasty devices, such as the artificial disk and artificial nucleus, which are used for much younger patients, the biodurability requirement should be much higher than that for total joints. Invibio, the manufacturer of PEEK-OPTIMA, has conducted extensive biodurability studies. In a study subjecting PEEK-OPTIMA to 200 kGy gamma irradiation and then followed with accelerated aging in oxygen (40 days at 5 bar at 70-C), it was found that there was no significant change in material mechanical properties, Fourier transform infrared spectroscopy (FTIR), gel permeation chromatography (GPC), and differential scanning calorimetry (DSC).[22] In an in vivo biodurability study, samples of PEEK-OPTIMA extruded rod were gamma sterilized with a dose of 73.2 kGy and then incubated in physiological saline for 3 months at 90°C (simulation of 10 years real-time aging at 37°C). The PEEK-OPTIMA samples were implanted in an animal model for a period of 12 months and subjected to cytotoxicity testing (ISO 10993–5), chemical analysis (ISO 10993–18), and histopathological examination. These tests confirmed the material to be noncytotoxic, and histopathology found no muscle degradations, necroses or marked inflammatory responses, or any significant changes.[22]

Biomechanical Assessment and Fatigue and Extrusion Characteristics of the NUBAC Nucleus Implant

Objectives of this study (performed by Nathanial Ordway at State University of New York-Syracuse, NY) were to evaluate the biomechanical function of the NUBAC nucleus device and to assess the risk of implant extrusion and potential adverse effects of the NUBAC artificial nucleus on the vertebral end plate under physiological loading conditions for 100,000 cycles.

Twelve functional spinal units (FSUs) from fresh frozen human cadaver lumbar spines were used in this study. Each test specimen consisted of a pair of FSUs with a total of six specimens used. One FSU of each specimen was left intact and served as a control level, whereas the second FSU served as the test level. To mimic the normal surgical procedure, a 6–10 mm box window was cut on the right side of the disk. A nucleotomy was performed followed by the implantation of the NUBAC nucleus device via a right lateral approach. Specimens were tested at three different stages: intact, post-diskectomy, and post–nucleus implant, under the physiological loading conditions of compression, flexion-compression, extension-compression, lateral bending–compression (right and left), and torsion (right and left). A maximal load of 1200 N was applied for the compression test and a maximum moment of 7.5 Nm was applied for the flexion-, extension-, bending-, and torsion-loading modes. Range of motion and stiffness were measured during the biomechanical testing and were used to assess the biomechanical function.

Implantation of the NUBAC nucleus implant significantly increased the FSU height under load in comparison with the diskectomy condition. **Fig. 17–4** displays the mean loss in disk height for the various conditions tested. Increasing the disk height at the surgical level is important for maintaining normal anatomy and sustaining the biomechanical characteristics of the intervertebral disk. It should be noted that disk height changes measured in this study are the summary of disk height changes of two disks. These disk height changes for different testing stages (intact, diskectomy, and implant) reported in **Fig. 17–4** assumed that the control disk maintained its disk height during the entire testing period. In reality, it is likely that there would be some permanent creep over the extended testing period for both the control disk and the index disk. If this creep effect is taken into account, it is likely the height restoration effect of the NUBAC nucleus device would be slightly better than the data in **Fig. 17–4.**

The range of motion (ROM) at the surgical levels showed increased flexion motion following diskectomy, but this was not statistically significant. For extension, the motion was significantly reduced ($p < .05$) following diskectomy. The ROM was restored back to intact status following insertion of the implant. There were no significant changes in left or right bending after diskectomy or following insertion of the implant. There were no significant differences in torsional motion for any disk condition as well.

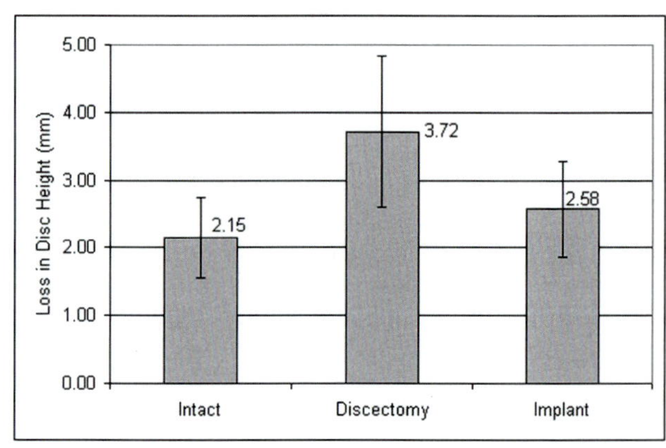

Figure 17–4   Mean loss in disk height (mm) at peak compressive load.

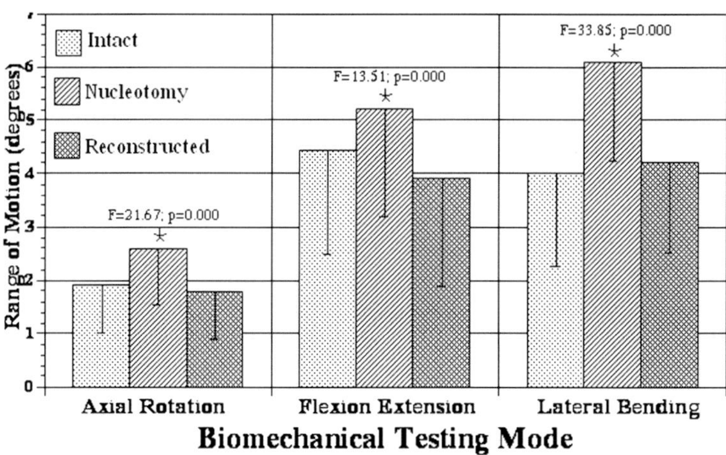

Figure 17–5   Range of segmental motion: Repeated measures analysis of variance demonstrates significance under each loading mode. *Indicates statistical difference between the nucleotomy condition versus the intact and reconstructed conditions at $p < .05$. No other differences were observed. Error bars indicate one standard deviation.

The only significant stiffness change was in the extension test mode on the surgical levels. Following diskectomy there was a significant increase ($p < .05$) in stiffness in comparison with the intact condition. With the implant in place, the stiffness was restored and was not significantly different from the intact condition. There were no significant changes in compressive and torsional stiffness between the three testing conditions.

Following the initial biomechanical tests, each specimen was tested under cyclic load to assess the risk of implant extrusion as well as the risk of end plate fracture. The bending moment ranged from 2.5 to 7.5 Nm (500 N offset 5–15 mm) for 100,000 cycles at 2 Hz. The left lateral bending mode represented a "worst-case" scenario with regard to implant extrusion. The risk of implant extrusion was evaluated through direct observation. Five of the six specimens completed 100,000 cycles of left lateral bend fatigue testing. The specimen that didn't complete the testing had to be stopped due to a specimen failure (disk/end plate separation from the vertebra at the intact level). All implants completed the testing without any implant extrusions. Following the fatigue test, gross examination, plain x-ray, and micro-computed tomographic (micro-CT) images showed no end plate and vertebral fracture, even though two of the three spines used in this study were osteopenic.

Multidirectional Flexibility and Load to Failure Analysis of the Pioneer Surgical Nucleus Pulposus Replacement: An In Vitro Cadaveric Model

The objectives of this study (performed by Bryan Cunningham at Union Memory Hospital, Baltimore, MD) were to quantify the multidirectional flexibility and destructive load-to-failure properties of the NUBAC nuclear device.

A total of eight fresh-frozen human lumbar functional spinal units (L2–L3 and L4–L5) were harvested en bloc and utilized in this investigation. Prior to biomechanical analysis, standard anteroposterior and lateral plain films were obtained to exclude specimens demonstrating intervertebral disk or osseous pathology. Bone mineral density (BMD) scans using dual-energy x-ray absorptiometry (DEXA) were performed to exclude specimens demonstrating BMDs less than 0.9 g/cm^3.

To determine the multidirectional flexibility, six pure moments (flexion and extension, left and right lateral bending, and left and right torsion) were applied to the superior end of the vertically oriented specimen while the caudal portion of the specimen remained fixed to a testing platform. A maximum applied moment of ± 7 Nm was used for each loading mode. For the six main motions corresponding to the moments applied, the operative level vertebral rotations (degrees) were quantified in terms of ROM and neutral zone (NZ).

Following the intact analysis, an annulotomy defect (1 cm–1 cm) was created on the anatomical left, followed by a midline annulotomy and complete nucleotomy. After biomechanical testing of the destabilized condition, the NUBAC nucleus device was implanted and the operative motion segment retested. As a final test, the reconstructed specimen was destructively evaluated under axial compression.

Biomechanical data were normalized to the intact condition and expressed as mean $\pm$ one standard deviation, with statistical analyses including descriptives, repeated measures analysis of variance (ANOVA) and Student-Newman-Keuls test to determine differences among individual groups. Statistical results at $p < .05$ were considered to be significant. **Figs. 17–5 and 17–6** show the ROM and NZ comparisons between the three treatment groups. Multidirectional flexibility testing indicated significant increases in the segmental ROM and NZ secondary to the annulotomy/nucleotomy procedures after the implantation of the NUBAC nuclear device. For both calculated parameters, the segmental rotation increased for the destabilized condition versus the intact and reconstructed specimens ($p < .05$). Importantly, the NZ (an indicator of spinal stability) of the reconstructed segment returned to levels not statistically different from the intact condition.

As a final test, the reconstructed specimens were destructively evaluated under axial compression. In all specimens except one, the observed failure mechanism was fracture of the vertebral body, without significant disruption of the vertebral end plate. The mean failure load was 3340 $\pm$ 2029 N. This average fracture load of 3340 N is comparable to the compressive failure load for an intact lumbar segment.[23,24] The primary mode of fracture was through the vertebral bodies above and below the operative disk level.

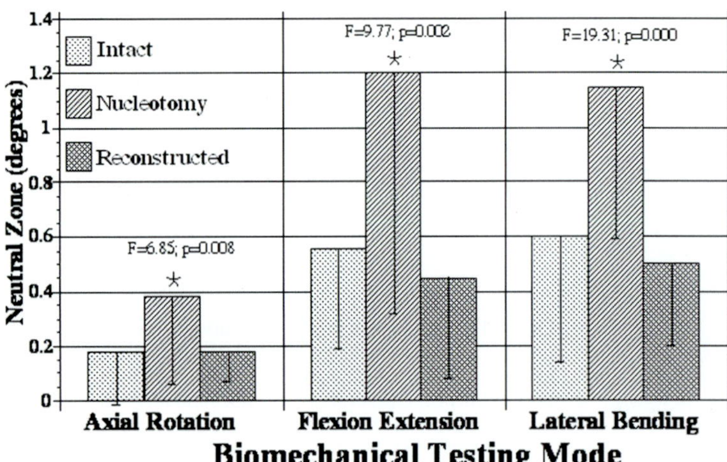

Figure 17–6   Neutral zone: Repeated measures analysis of variance demonstrates significance under each loading mode. *Indicates statistical difference between the nucleotomy condition versus the intact and reconstructed conditions at $p < .05$. No other differences were observed. Error bars indicate one standard deviation.

Wear and Fatigue Studies

Wear and durability are important characteristics for any permanent joint prosthesis. For total joints, such as hip and knee joints, implant wear, which can lead to osteolysis and ultimately late aseptic loosening, has been and remains a clinical concern today. To adequately assess the wear on hip prostheses, American Society for Testing and Materials (ASTM) guidelines have been established since 1996.[25] Because disk arthroplasty is a relatively new technology as compared with hip and knee joints, disk arthroplasty wear test standards per ASTM and ISO have not yet been established. For total disk replacement devices, currently there is one ASTM and one ISO working draft that suggest testing parameters to be used to evaluate the wear and durability of these devices.[26,27] Both of these draft standards clearly state that the proposed methodologies are only applicable to total disk prostheses, not nucleus prostheses. Due to the lack of a complete understanding of lumbar segmental kinematics and limited clinical data, especially the wear data from clinically retrieved total disk explants, both draft standards also recognize that the proposed testing conditions do not reproduce the complex in vivo loading conditions.

As compared with the total disk prostheses, there is even less clinical experience for nucleus prostheses. Currently, there is no ASTM or ISO standard for wear testing of nucleus prostheses. The Raymedica PDN, which has been used clinically since 1996 and has been implanted in more than 3500 patients, has by far the most clinical experience among any nucleus prostheses. The only published PDN fatigue and wear data were tested under pure compressive load between 397 and 1589 N.[28] More recently, Disc Dynamics, Inc. (Eden Prairie, MN) published its rationale and methodology on wear test for the DASCOR nucleus implant.[29] It incorporates a flexion-extension motion in addition to compressive loading into its wear test. The total range of motion in the wear test was 5.9 degrees. Although there are many other nucleus prostheses under development lumnt, public disclosure of associated methodologies is limited.

Pioneer Surgical Technology has conducted a wear test on its NUBAC nucleus implant using loading conditions more severe than other published wear test methods used for nucleus prostheses. The loading conditions consisted of cyclic compressive loads of 223 to 1024 N with ±7.5 degrees of flexion and extension at a frequency of 2.0 Hz. The rationale for the loading and kinematic testing conditions used was determined after a rigorous literature review. The compressive load and the ROM were represented by sine waves in phase with each other. To mimic a physiological environment, the samples were tested in newborn calf serum solutions with a protein content of 20 g/L at 37°C. A total of six samples were tested to 10 million cycles in accordance with established FDA Investigational Device Exemption (IDE) guidelines. Three unloaded soak controls were used to account for fluid absorption. A measurement of weight loss along with a test fluid change was performed every 0.5 million cycles, and a gravimetric method was used (ASTM F2025–00) to determine the wear rate and mass loss of the specimens. After 10 million cycles of wear testing, the average total wear was 2.8 mg, with a corresponding wear rate of 0.28 mg/million cycles (**Fig. 17–7**). The preliminary wear particle analysis showed that wear particle size and morphology were similar to what was found in the Charité (DePuy Spine, Raynham, MA) wear test.

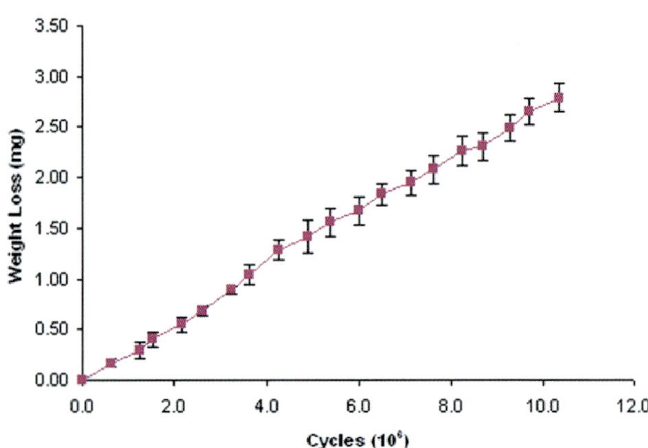

Figure 17–7   The NUBAC nucleus implant weight loss (mg) over 10 M cycles.

In light of the ISO and ASTM drafts, which call for coupled motions to determine their effect on the wear rates and to better understand the wear characteristics of the NUBAC device under coupled motions, 10 million cycles of lateral bending with the same loading and motion as used in flexion and extension were applied to these previously tested (under flexion-extension) samples. The average wear in the 10 million cycles of lateral bending on the remaining four samples was 2.7 mg, and the wear rate stayed fairly consistent over the entire testing period. The average of total mass loss at the end of 20 million cycles was 5.5 mg.

Despite the lack of a standard for wear testing of nucleus prostheses, a relatively severe loading condition was used as compared with the published wear tests used by other nucleus devices. The total wear rate compares favorably with the wear rate on total joints and is comparable with other disk arthroplasty devices.[29–31] Considering the fact that simulated wear rates of disk arthroplasty devices may be five to 10 times higher than the clinical wear of explanted devices,[32] the risk of device failure due to wear of the NUBAC device is relatively low.

Static and fatigue testing were also performed to determine the axial static compressive strength and axial dynamic fatigue failure load of the NUBAC. The test specimens used in this study consisted of the worst-case scenario for contact stress distribution. The specimens tested were representative of the smallest true contact stress area for all current designs. In the axial static compressive test, the results showed that the specimens failed at a static load of 10427 N, which is well beyond the static failure strength of the human vertebral body or end plate.[23,24] The primary mode of failure in tested constructs was excessive plastic deformation. The results of the dynamic axial fatigue test showed that the device has excellent fatigue strength under the testing conditions utilized. There was no specimen failure at 80% (8342 N) of the average static offset yield load of 10427 N. Vertebral compression fractures can occur from cyclic loads of up to 3995 N in as little as 200 cycles to a maximum of 1.25 million cycles,[33] and the fatigue strength can range from ~600 N to ~950 N when normalized to age and disk degeneration, respectively.[34] These results from the static and fatigue testing are well beyond those of the expected physiological loads the device would be subject to. Therefore, in vivo compressive failure of the NUBAC device in either static axial compression or dynamic axial compression is not expected to occur.

◆ NUBAC Nucleus Implant Indication and Surgical Technique

The main indication for the NUBAC artificial nucleus or any artificial nucleus device is diskogenic low back pain caused by degenerative disk disease (DDD). Although an artificial total disk has a similar indication, the coverage of these two technologies in the spectrum of DDD is different, with the artificial nucleus more for early to moderate DDD and artificial disk more for late stage DDD. In the late stage of DDD, the disk might already have lost a majority of its height with significant changes of the annulus structure and morphology. Therefore it might be difficult for a nucleus device to distract the disk height to a normal level without the nucleus device bearing a very high load, which could lead to a high risk of implant subsidence. Although an artificial disk can be used for early to moderate DDD, it would be difficult to justify using an artificial disk for early and moderate DDD due to the inherited high risks and more traumatic surgery associated with a total disk procedure. The benefit:risk ratio would therefore be low, especially when an option that is less invasive and poses less risk, such as an artificial nucleus, becomes available.

◆ Conclusion

Implantation of the NUBAC nucleus implant is relatively easy compared with that of a total disk. It starts with a nuclectomy. The cavity location and size are assessed with a custom-designed trial and verified with fluoroscopic images. A proper-sized implant is then selected and loaded to the implant inserter. The implant can be inserted via posterior or anterior or lateral approach.

References

1. Urban JPG, Smith S, Fairbank CT. Nutrition of the intervertebral disc. Spine 2004;29:2700–2709

2. Nachemson A. The load on lumbar disks in different positions of the body. Clin Orthop Relat Res 1966;45:107–122

3. Cleveland DA. The use of methyl acrylic for spinal stabilization after disc operations. Marquette Med Rev 1955;20:62–64

4. Hamby WB, Glaser HT. Replacement of spinal intervertebral discs with locally polymerizing methyl methacrylate. J Neurosurg 1959;16:311–313

5. Armstrong JR. Lumbar Disc Lesions. Edinburgh and Landon: E & S Livingstone Ltd; 1965:24–34

6. Fernström U. Arthroplasty with intercorporal endoprosthesis in herniated disc and in painful disc. Acta Chir Scand Suppl 1966;357:154–159

7. McKenzie AH. Steel ball arthroplasty of lumbar intervertebral discs: a preliminary report. J Bone Joint Surg Br 1971;54:766

8. McKenzie AH. Fernström intervertebral disc arthroplasty: a long-term evaluation. Ortho Int Ed 1995;3:313–324

9. Griffith SL, Shelokov AP, Büttner-Janz K, Lemaire LP, Zeegers WS. A multicenter retrospective study of the clinical results of the LINK SB Charité intervertebral prosthesis: the initial European experience. Spine 1994;19:1842–1849

10. Zeegers WS, Bohnen LM, Laaper M, Verhaegen MJ. Artificial disc replacement with the modular type SB Charité III: 2-year results in 50 prospectively studied patients. Eur Spine J 1999;8:210–217

11. Tropiano P, Huang RC, Girardi FP, Cammisa FP Jr, Marnay T. Lumbar total disc replacement: seven to eleven-year follow-up. J Bone Joint Surg Am 2005;87:490–496

12. Eijkelkamp MF, Hayen J, Veldhuizen AG, van Hom JR, Verkerke GJ. Improving the fixation of an artificial intervertebral disc. Int J Artif Organs 2002;25:327–333

13. Green S. Using implantable-grade PEEK for in vivo devices. Medical Device & Diagnostic Industry 2005:May

14. Serhan H, Ross ER, Lowery GL, et al. Biomechanical characterization of a new lumbar disc prosthesis. International Society for the Study of the Lumbar Spine. Edinburgh, 2001:June 19–23

15. Fraser RD, Ross ER, Lowery GL, Freeman BJ, Dolan M. AcroFlex design and results. Spine J 2004;4(Suppl 6):245S–251S

16. Lowe TG, Hashim S, Wilson LA, et al. A biomechanical study of regional endplate strength and cage morphology as it relates to structural interbody support. Spine 2004;29:2389–2394

17. Tan JS, Bailey CS, Dvorak MF. Interbody device shape and size are important to strengthen the vertebra-implant interface. Spine 2005; 30:638–644

18. Klara P, Ray C. Artificial nucleus replacement: clinical experience. Spine 2002;27:1374–1377

19. Shim CS, Lee SH, Park CW, et al. Partial disc replacement with the PDN prosthetic disc nucleus device. J Spinal Disord Tech 2003;16:324–330

20. Hampton D, Laros G, McCarron R, Franks D. Healing potential of the anulus fibrosus. Spine 1989;14:398–401

21. White AA, Panjabi MM. Kinematics of the spine. In: White AA, Panjabi MM, eds. Clinical Biomechanics of the Spine. Philadelphia: Lippincott Williams & Wilkins;1990:85–126

22. Cartwright K, Devine J. Investigation into the Effect of Gamma Sterilization (200 kGy) and Accelerated Aging on the Properties of PEEK-OPTIMA. Invibio Technical Report. Greenville, SC: Invibio; 2005

23. Bell GH, Dunbar O, Beck JS, Gibb A. Variations in strength of vertebrae with age and their relation to osteoporosis. Calcif Tissue Res 1967;1:75-86

24. Perry O. Fracture of the vertebral end-plate in the lumbar spine. Acta Orthop Scand 1957;(Suppl):25

25. ASTM F 1714–96. Standard guide for gravimetric wear assessment of prosthetic hip-designs in simulator devices. West Conshohocken, PA: American Society for Testing and Materials; 1996

26. ASTM WK454, Draft 5. Standard Test Method for the Functional and Kinematic Wear Assessment for Total Disc Prostheses. West Conshohocken, PA: American Society for Testing and Materials; 2004

27. ISO/Dros Inf Serv 18192–1. Implant for Surgery: Wear of Total Intervertebral Spinal Disc Prostheses, Part1: Loading and Displacement Parameters for Wear Testing and Corresponding Environmental Conditions for Tests. Geneva: International Standards Organization; 2005

28. http://www.raymedica.com/abstracts3.htm#A%20Prosthetic%20 Lumbar%20Nucleus%20"Artificial%20Disc

29. Hudgins RG, Bao QB. Durability Test Method for a Prosthetic Nucleus (PN), Spinal Implants: Are We Evaluating Them Appropriately? ASTM STP 1431. Melkerson MN, Griffith SL, Kirkpatrick JS, eds. West Conshohocken, PA: American Society for Testing and Materials; 2002

30. Anderson PA, Rouleau JP, Bryan VE, Carlson CS. Wear analysis of the Bryan Cervical Disc prosthesis. Spine 2003;28:S186–S194

31. FDA Charité Panel Transcript, 2004

32. Anderson PA, Rouleau JP, Toth JM, Riew KD. A comparison of simulator-tested and -retrieved cervical disc prostheses: invited submission from the Joint Section Meeting on Disorders of the Spine and Peripheral Nerves. J Neurosurg Spine 2004;1:202–210

33. Hardy W, Lissner H, Webster J, Gurdijian E. Repeated loading tests of the lumbar spine. Surg Forum 1958;9:690–695

34. Hansson TH, Keller TS, Spengler DM. Mechanical behavior of the human lumbar spine, II: Fatigue strength during dynamic compressive loading. J Orthop Res 1987;5:479–487

18

SINUX (Sinitec)

Jan Zoellner

◆ **Methodology**

◆ **In Vitro Investigation of Lumbar
  Disk Implants (SINUX)**

◆ **Conclusion**

Degenerative changes to the spinal column and disk-related disorders of human beings were described in antiquity by Hippocrates (460–377 B.C.) as hip pain. Even before the age of 30 people begin to suffer degenerative changes of the intervertebral disks, and four out of five people suffer from back pain at some time in their lives. However, 80 to 90% of all cases of acute backache clear up within 6 weeks regardless of whether they are treated or of the type of therapy received. The disk is the largest unvascularized structure in the body. In children, disks have a water content of up to 90%, but as age increases, this figure falls to less than 70%. The solid constituents of the disk, such as proteoglycans, form up to 50% of its dry weight. The water is not free, rather being bound to structural components of the macromolecules. In vivo, the pressure in the nucleus pulposus is generated via the osmotic gradients of the proteoglycans and the water-binding molecule hyaluronic acid. With the exception of organ pain, pain syndrome in the lumbar spine region is generally due to premature disk deterioration, particularly at L4–L5 and L5–S1. Atrophy and compression of the disk lead to loosening of the vertebral motor segments. Degeneration involves the disturbance of fluid transfer due to sclerosis of the end plates and basal plates. As a result, the disk loses more and more water and the intradiskal pressure falls, leading to reduction in the intervertebral space. Kolditz et al[1] were able to show that the disk loses water under increasing strain, and in consequence the osmotic gradient increases until equilibrium between osmotic and mechanical pressure is reached. When the strain on the disk is relieved there is a corresponding influx of fluid. The normal intradiskal pressure (L5–S1), without any additional external load, has been put at up to 5 atm (500 kPa).[2] In their paper, Wilke et al[3] showed that, under unfavorable load when lifting heavy weights, the intradiskal pressure in segment L4–L5 can rise as high as 2300 kPa.

In an intact segment the outer fibers are aligned with the longitudinal ligaments, whereas the fibers in internal layers are arranged at a 60 degree angle.[4] This orientation is the principal factor producing torsional strength.[5] An important element in the degenerative process is the microsystem for transporting matter via the end plates. As the disk becomes drier, the end plates transform into a sclerotic barrier. The segment reduces in height, with attendant parallelization of the type I collagen fibers in the region of the external annulus fibrosus. This parallelization causes the segment to lose torsion resistance.

This process may be regarded as a vicious circle. The degeneration of the nucleus pulposus leads to reduction in segmental height and accompanying loss of torsion resistance. This, in turn, entails an increase in the segment's physiological mobility and accelerated degeneration. Degeneration involving radial fissures in the annulus fibrosus can lead to a prolapsed disk and a subsequent need for nucleotomy. In this vicious circle the segmental degeneration and the nucleotomy are intimately linked because the nucleotomy has a similar effect to the degeneration just described. However, unlike that process, the changes after nucleotomy can proceed at a significantly faster rate, so that mobility compensation mechanisms such as osteophytic bone spurs, which produce a secondary reduction in mobility, do not cut in until later. The removal of disk tissue reduces the intradiskal pressure and the intervertebral space, thus increasing segmental mobility. This process causes considerable wear of the vertebral arch joints, which can lead in turn to significant symptoms. The pain caused by these degenerative symptoms, such as narrowing of the spinal canal, is often difficult to distinguish from pain resulting from disk problems. Furthermore, if age leads to a natural stiffening of the segment the symptoms will rapidly diminish. However, all too often this process takes many years and is not complete until advanced old age, or indeed it may not occur at all. Meanwhile, as long as mobility is retained the accompanying pain can be expected to persist.

In the presence of the relevant indications, lumbar nucleotomy may be performed. However, the procedure is associated with a significant rate of postoperative problems. A meta-analysis of the literature conducted by Schulitz et al,[6] involving a total of 20,148 patients, found rates of poor postoperative outcomes ranging from 7 to 27%. These postoperative problems in connection with disk surgery are often described either as postdiskectomy syndrome (PDS) or as failed back surgery syndrome (FBSS). Two major causes of these problems are postoperative instability and postoperative recidivism, although they may also be due to

"

narrowness of the recessus lateralis, epidural fibrosis, arachnoiditis, facet syndrome, operating on the wrong segment, or poor surgical technique. The changed postoperative mobility of the vertebral motor segment is a significant causative factor for the occurrence of postoperative pain.[7] Increasingly, diskectomy was found to lead to decreased height of the intervertebral space and reduced intradiskal pressure. White and Panjabi[8] describe a variable pivot in the dorsal region of the segment. Increasing instability can lead to a displacement and widening of this pivot, which means in turn that this increase causes complex changes in the overall biomechanical structure. Because there is no precise definition of the term *instability* in relation to the vertebral motor segment, this state of affairs is better described as "abnormal mobility" or "increasing mobility," and most closely resembles the situation after a nucleotomy. Others, though, describe the postnucleotomy situation as an increased range of motion (ROM) between adjacent vertebral bodies.

The field of spinal surgery, and in particular the surgical treatment of degenerative disease of the lumbar spine, is currently undergoing a paradigm shift. Both disk operations in their technical variants and fusion methods are being viewed in an increasingly critical light. In a leading article for *Scientific American* entitled "New Thinking about Back Pain," the author notes the minimal correlation of pathological findings and imaging techniques, of the simultaneous frequency of back pain syndrome and the consequent problems in determining whether surgical or conservative therapy is indicated.[9] A new "old" concept involves the development of a flexible disk implant, which aims to stabilize the affected segment while also reconstructing the physiological mobility of the vertebral motor segment. The principal requirements of a disk implant are well-functioning biomechanical reconstruction of the intervertebral space, good biocompatibility, and long-term load resistance coupled with ease of handling conducive to implantation via minimally invasive methods of surgical access.

◆ Methodology

The three-dimensional (3D) study was performed under the leadership of Professor F. Lavaste in connection with a cooperation agreement with ENSAM (Ecole Nationale Supérieure d'Arts et Métiers), University of Paris, and also the biomechanics laboratory located there [Laboratoire de biomécanique (LBM)]. The research setup developed there[10] allowed us to conduct a 3D study of the lumbar motor segments. Two segments plus three vertebrae were required to conduct each study. The adjacent musculature was removed but the bony and ligament structures were retained. The vertebral motor segment under investigation, together with its lower vertebral body, was fixed to a special metal with a low boiling point (70°C) to avoid damaging the bony and ligamentous structures (**Fig. 18–1**).

The test receptacle was attached to the adjacent, central vertebral body, and to ensure that it interfered as little as possible with the application of force, the force transducer was attached to the upper vertebral body. As a result it was possible to take measurements of even large ranges of

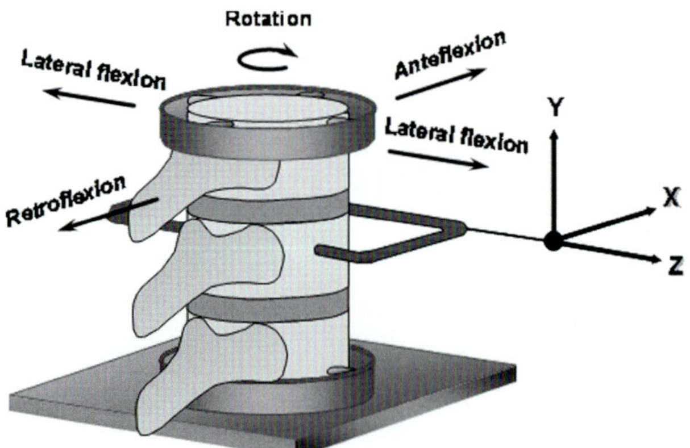

Figure 18–1   Three-dimensional experimental setup.

motion. The force applied was limited to a physiologically nondestructive 7 Nm. In investigating anteflexion, retroflexion, lateral flexion, and torsion in the three directions of movement (**Fig. 18–2**), rotation was measured in degrees and translation in millimeters over each of the three spatial axes (X, Y, Z). The rotation and translation could be directly recorded and processed digitally via the electromechanical resistors (**Fig. 18–2**). Test values were always recorded from maximum amplitude to maximum amplitude and back, thus ruling out errors in determining the neutral point or neutral zone.

To evaluate the stability of the motor segment, the degree of movement relative to the force applied was calculated, and the value for the maximum experimental force of 7 Nm was used as the measure of maximum segmental stability. The results were then shown as percentage increases or decreases in the ROM as compared with the zero measurement for the intact disk segment (the relative extent of motion). For anteflexion and retroflexion the rotation Az and translation Dx were recorded, whereas for lateral flexion Ax and Dz were calculated and for torsion Ay and Dy (**Fig. 18–3**).

Human spinal segments L2–L3 and L3–L4 were selected for experimental purposes because these are subject to less degenerative changes than the lower segments of the lumbar spine. The mean time of removal was 12 hours postmortem. Immediately after removal, the segments were frozen to –20°C, and the maximum preservation duration was limited to 3 months.[11,12] The exclusion criteria applied were bone-destroying processes or injury to the annulus fibrosus, and in particular a prolapsed disk.

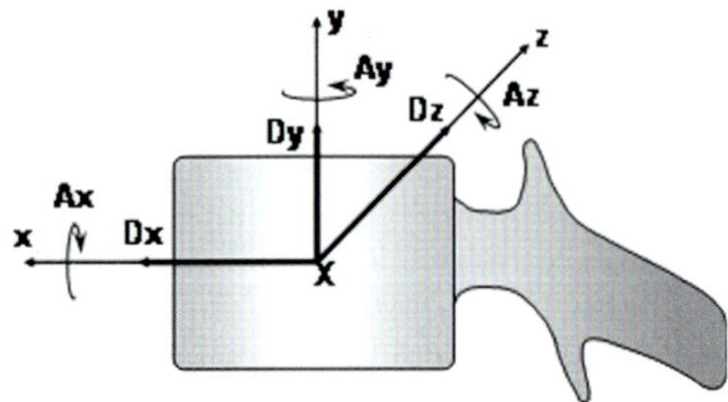

Figure 18–2   Three-dimensional measurement axes. Dx, Dy, and Dz directions of translation. Ax, Ay, and Az directions of rotation.

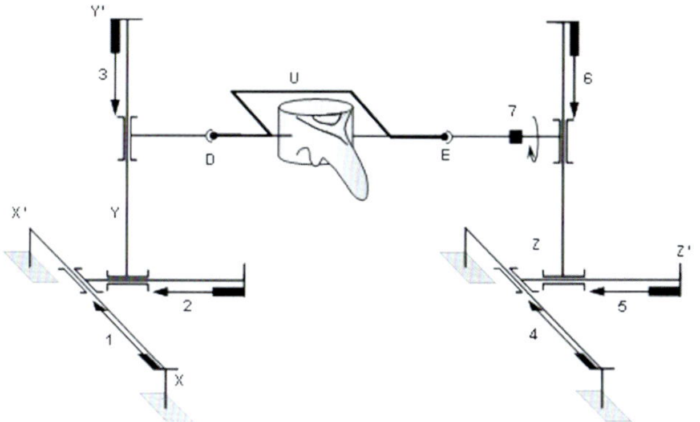

Figure 18–3 Recording and spatial layout of the electromechanical resistors.

◆ In Vitro Investigation of Lumbar Disk Implants (SINUX)

Apart from their biomechanical and toxicological properties, the most important criteria for disk implants are their intraoperative manageability and the size of the surgical access route. The suitability of a variety of different autopolymerizing plastics has been tested. Aryl- and vinyl-based compounds were found to be unsuitable because the chemical softeners that are added to these materials lead to severe wear and breakage under long-term load. Accordingly, the only option was to use a silicon-based plastic because its strength is controlled by intramolecular cross-linking. The plastic chosen was a polymethylsiloxane polymer. This was processed using a twin-cartridge system and applied using a mixing attachment. The polymer is initially a viscous liquid, but within 15 minutes it hardens without heat treatment into a dimensionally stable and permanently elastic solid.

Before testing the material's biomechanical suitability any possible tissue incompatibility had to be ruled out. Sterilization with both ultraviolet (UV) and gamma radiation led to material destruction, and the only possible means of sterilizing the polymer was through the use of ethylene oxide gas. It was found that sterilization did not lead to any changes in the plastic's physical properties because a variety of experimental setups uncovered no differences compared with the unsterilized material. Cytotoxicity was investigated in accordance with the International Standards Organization (ISO) 10993–5 standard. An important finding was that both the fully polymerized plastic and the two individual components did not cause any incompatibility reactions. Both the polymer and its two components were tested in direct and indirect contact. The tests were performed using HeLa cells, a line of human carcinoma cells. Tissue culture polystyrene (TCPS) was used as the negatively cytotoxic material and the metals tin and nickel as positively cytotoxic materials. In direct cell contact, the morphology, cell count, proliferation after the Ki-67 test,[13] and cytoskeleton after immunostaining were investigated microscopically. None of these tests revealed any cytotoxic reactions under direct cell contact. The morphology was then examined microscopically in indirect (extract) contact. The metabolism after the 3-[4,5-dimethylthiazol-2-yl]-2,5-diphenyltetrazoliumbromide (MTT) test, proliferation after the Ki-67 test, and cell count after crystal violet dyeing were recorded using an enzyme-linked immunosorbent assay (ELISA) reader, and no cytotoxic reactions were found under indirect contact either.

Finally, long-term stress testing was performed. Using sterile materials, six elliptical test pieces were manufactured, each with a diameter of 31–20 mm and 3.5 mm thick. These dimensions represent those of an idealized nucleus pulposus. In an experimental setup using glass ceramic contact surfaces, the test pieces were subjected to long-term load at 37°C in a culture medium with an antibiotic additive. The components were then either autoclaved at 131°C for 20 minutes or disinfected using a 70% alcohol solution in the case of non-heat-resistant parts. Over the planned ~6-day period for the long-term load test, the medium in which each test piece was immersed was changed each day to examine the fluid for abrasion particles and possible cytotoxic reactions. The load profile was determined following a recent paper by Wilke et al.[3] This involved a self-experiment conducted by a colleague in orthopedics who had a pressure sensor implanted in his L4–L5 intervertebral space to measure the pressure exerted under a variety of different load situations. The figures recorded were compared with those from the seminal study,[14] to a large extent confirming these earlier findings. In our experimental setup the lowest pressure was fixed at 0.1 MPa (1 bar), equivalent to lying on one's back, and the maximum long-term load was set at 0.8 MPa, which is equivalent to the load exerted when jogging, and thus covering any normal load likely to be exerted during everyday life. Coughing, for instance, increases intradiskal pressure to only 0.38 MPa. Each test piece was subjected to a total of 5 million load cycles (LCs) at a frequency of 10 Hz. After each million LCs the load was raised to 1.7 MPa for 1000 LCs, a load equivalent to lifting 20 kg from the knees following back school recommendations. This load pattern was designed to test the demands placed on an implant over a 5-year lifetime. The varying load profile produced five load blocks for each of the six test pieces.

First, the dynamic modulus (**Fig. 18–4**) was evaluated. In the first block there was a significant increase in the modulus and thus of the test piece's rigidity, but in each subsequent block the rigidity leveled out at a stable value.

The mean plastic strain changed in similar fashion (**Fig. 18–5**). Initially, the load caused pronounced creep in the test piece, leading to reduced mean strain, but subsequently this leveled out at a stable value.

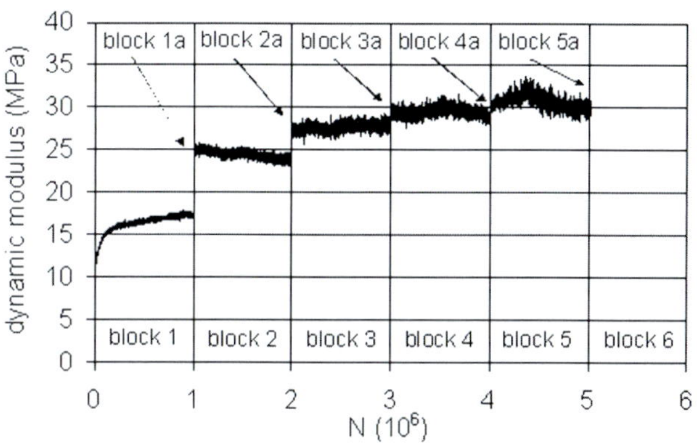

Figure 18–4 Dynamic modulus changes during the experiment.

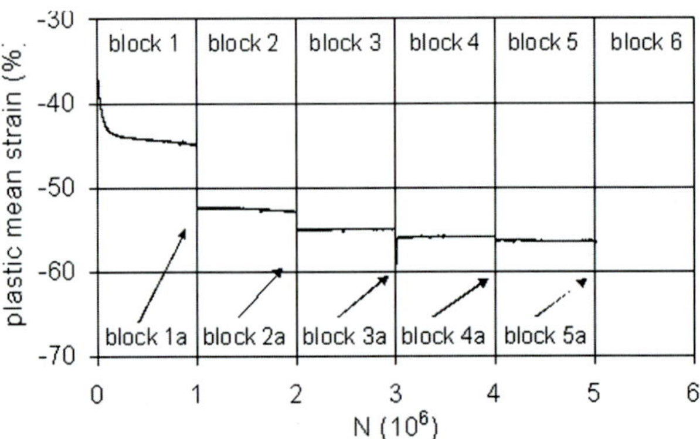

Figure 18–5   Mean plastic strain changes during the experiment.

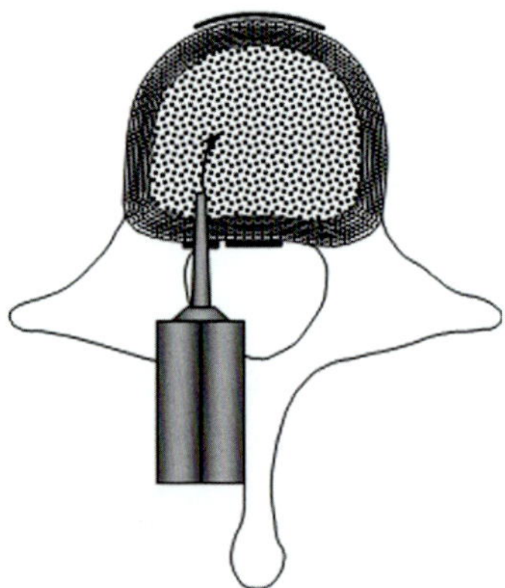

Figure 18–7   Application of the polymer in line with standard nucleotomy with left mediolateral access.

Tests of damping (**Fig. 18–6**) as both a measure of work performed and of plastic damage to the test piece showed stable readings with little change throughout the load cycle. All three parameters indicate that the test pieces withstood the load cycle undamaged, and there is no reason to expect material failure under further sustained load.

In a second experimental approach, one test piece was subjected to a high long-term load of 1.7 MPa for 3.6 million LCs with just five brief respites of 0.1 MPa for 1000 LCs. In this test the dynamic modulus and plastic mean strain both approximated constant values, and all in all the readings confirmed the polymer's good long-term load capabilities. Meanwhile, initial research findings on the culture medium have revealed no significant abrasion particles or indications of cytotoxicity.

The aim next was to reproduce these findings in the 3D experiment described earlier. To this end seven human L3–L4 vertebral segments were investigated. The ages of the vertebral segments ranged from 66 to 78 years with a mean age of 72 years; four were female and three male. First, the intact motor segment was measured again. Then, after virtually complete removal of the nucleus pulposus (mean wet weight 6 g) via a left mediolateral access point in line with standard nucleotomy, new readings were taken. Final readings were then taken after inserting the implant (**Fig. 18–7**).

The polymer was inserted in the intervertebral space using the mixer attachment. The pre-load pressure applied by the mixing gun is sustained by a locking ring for a period of

15 minutes until the material hardens to a dimensionally stable and permanently elastic form. After removal of the mixer attachment, no dislocation of the material was observed. There was no significant increase ($p = .0156$) in segmental mobility, as compared with an intact vertebral motor segment, in terms either of translation or of rotation ($p = .0156$ to $p = .0313$) of the measuring point in any of the planes examined. Furthermore, despite the nucleotomy, no significant loss of height along Dy was observed ($p = .3281$). After implantation of the polymer, mobility was reconstructed for all parameters tested with no significant difference ($p = .1563$ to $p = 1.0$). The only reduction in mobility as compared with the intact segment was found in the flexion-extension, yielding a difference here of $p = .0156$. The 3D research thus confirmed the good stabilization of the entire motor segment for all directions of motion investigated.

◆ Conclusion

In conclusion, the 3D research setup revealed good stabilization of the motor segment after implantation of the SINUX in both the human and calf lumbar spine models. After dorsal insertion good alignment of the segment was observed. Without any suturing of the annulus fibrosus, the plastic's dimensionally stable polymerization meant that no tendency to dislocation was found during the experiment.

In collaboration with an independent test laboratory (RCC Cytotest Cell Research GmbH), corresponding tests of acute cytotoxicity were performed. Among the tests conducted were the Ames test of genetic toxicity, tests of acute systemic toxicity, and experimental implantations in six rabbits. The overall assessment in accordance with ISO 10993 is that the polymer displays neither cytotoxicity, genetic toxicity, nor acute systemic toxicity, and there were no negative findings impacting on the requirements for CE licensing as laid down in the ISO standard.

The first clinical study began in November 2000, and a license for use in the CE followed in January 2004. Currently the implant is being used in Europe in an extended study entitled "A multi-centre, prospective, non-comparative, open, post-marketing surveillance study to obtain clinical outcome data on the use of the SINUX Nucleus Replacement device for degenerative disk disease."

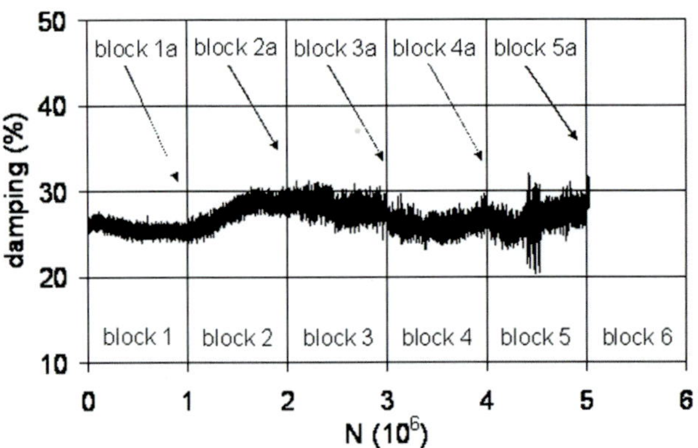

Figure 18–6   Damping changes during the experiment.

References

1. Kolditz D, Krämer J, Gowin R. Water and electrolyte content of human intervertebral disc under variable load. Spine 1985;10:69–71

2. Ghosh P. The Biology of the Intervertebral Disc. Vols 1 and 2. Boca Raton, FL: CRC Press; 1989:152–161

3. Wilke HJ, Neef P, Caimi M, Hoogland T, Claes LE. New in vivo measurements of pressures in the intervertebral disc in daily life. Spine 1999;24:755–762

4. Marchand F, Ahmed AM. Investigation of the laminate structure of lumbar disc anulus fibrosus. Spine 1990;15:402–410

5. Krismer M, Haid C, Rabl W. The contribution of anulus fibers to torque resistance. Spine 1996;21:2551–2557

6. Schultz K-P, Abel R, Schöppe K, Assheuer J. Der Bandscheibenvorfall. Dt Ärztebl 1999;96:B424–B428

7. Krämer J. Bandscheibenbedingte Erkrankungen. Stuttgart; New York: Georg Thieme Verlag; 1994, 1997

8. White AA, Panjabi MM. Clinical Biomechanics of the Spine. 2nd ed. Philadelphia: Lippincott; 1990

9. Deyo RA. Low back pain. Sci Am 1998;279:48–53

10. Lavaste F, Asselineau A, Diop A, et al. Experimental procedure for mechanical evaluation of dorso-lumbar segments and osteosynthesis devices. Rachis 1990;6:435–446

11. Panjabi MM, Krug MH, Summers D, Videmann T. Biomechanical time tolerance of fresh cadaveric human spine specimens. J Orthop Res 1985;3:292–296

12. Flynn JC, Rudert MJ, Olson E, Baratz M, Hanley E. The effects of freezing or freeze-drying on biomechanical properties of the canine intervertebral disc. Spine 1990;15:567–570

13. Klein CL, Wagner M, Kirkpatrick CJ, van Kooten TG. A new quantitative test method for cell proliferation based on the detection of the Ki-67 protein. J Mater Sci Mater Med 2000;11:125–132

14. Nachemson A. The load on lumbar disks in different positions of the body. Clin Orthop Relat Res 1966;45:107–122

19

NuCore Injectable Disk Nucleus

Scott H. Kitchel, Lawrence M. Boyd, and Andrew J. Carter

◆ **Injectable Biomaterials for Nucleus Pulposus Augmentation**

NuCore Injectable Nucleus

◆ **Conclusion**

The use of an injectable material for nucleus replacement gives the flexibility of allowing treatment of partial nucleotomies such as are found following microdiskectomy treatment of disk herniation, as well as indications such as early stage degenerative disk disease (DDD), where complete nucleus removal and replacement are required.

Clinical symptoms resulting from a protruding or painful intervertebral disk (IVD) are commonly treated by the surgical removal of all or part of the intradiskal structure (diskectomy). Diskectomy is the most common spinal surgical treatment, frequently used to treat radicular pain resulting from nerve impingement. Approximately 350,000 diskectomies were performed in 2003 in the United States. During a total diskectomy, a substantial amount (and usually all) of the volume of the nucleus pulposus and inner annulus fibrosus is removed and immediate loss of disk height and volume can result. Even with a partial diskectomy, loss of disk height can ensue. The sudden decrease in disk volume caused by the surgical removal of the disk or disk nucleus results in both local and global effects on the IVD and spinal segment, as will be discussed later.

This procedure is typically performed in a relatively young patient population, with a mean age reported in the literature of between 25 and 40 years.[1–3] However, the impact of altered biomechanics and long-term sequelae in this young patient population may be significant. Specifically, the local and global effects of reduced disk height following diskectomy may be important.

Substantial disk height reduction following diskectomy may occur and is evident soon following the diskectomy procedure. Disk height loss has been found to be proportional to the amount of nucleus removed in an in vitro study.[4] Clinically, the operated disk spaces of patients postoperatively are significantly narrower following diskectomy ($p = .01$) than controls.[5] Scoville and Corkill[6] found a 50% incidence of narrowing following surgery at the 3-month follow-up. In another study, Tibrewal and Pearcy[7] found disk space narrowing evident within 3 months following surgery as compared with nonoperated controls.

Proper disk height is necessary to ensure proper functioning of the intervertebral disk and spinal column. On the local (or cellular) level, decreased disk height results in increased pressure in the nucleus pulposus, which can lead to a decrease in cell matrix synthesis and an increase in cell necrosis and apoptosis. It has been shown in other cartilaginous tissues that increased static loading decreases matrix protein biosynthesis.[8–10] Animal models have shown that overloading of the intervertebral disk can initiate disk degeneration.[11,12] In addition, an increase in intradiskal pressure creates an unfavorable environment for fluid transfer into the disk, which can cause a further decrease in disk height.

Decreased disk height also results in significant changes in the global mechanical stability of the spine, which may result in further degeneration of the spinal segment. With decreasing height of the disk, the facet joints bear increasing loads and may undergo hypertrophy and degeneration, which may act as a source of pain over time.[13,14] Decreased stiffness of the spinal column and increased range of motion resulting from loss of disk height can lead to further instability of the spine.[14] Excessive motion can manifest itself in abnormal muscle, ligament, and tendon loading, which can ultimately be a source of back pain.

Radicular pain may result from a decrease in foraminal volume caused by decreased disk height. Specifically, as disk height decreases, the volume of the foraminal canal, through which the spinal nerve roots pass, decreases. This decrease may lead to spinal nerve impingement, with associated radiating pain and dysfunction. Finally, adjacent segment loading increases as the disk height decreases at a given level.[14,15] The disks that must bear additional loading are now susceptible to accelerated degeneration and compromise, which may eventually propagate along the destabilized spinal column.

A further issue with microdiskectomy surgery is the occurrence of reherniation. Atlas et al[16] reported a reoperation rate of 25% at 10-year follow-up of a study of patients with lumbar disk herniation, with the median time to reoperation 24 months. Carragee et al[17] reported an 11.5% reherniation rate, with 6.5% reoperation at 5 years.

The objectives of augmentation of the nucleus pulposus following disk removal are to prevent disk height loss and the associated biomechanical and biochemical changes resulting from reduced disk height and volume. Use of an injectable biomaterial to restore disk volume and prevent loss of disk height is currently being evaluated. The ability of an injectable material to seal the disk and prevent or reduce the incidence of reherniation is also being studied.

◆ Injectable Biomaterials for Nucleus Pulposus Augmentation

An injectable biomaterial is ideal for restoration of disk volume removed during diskectomy and for preventing loss of disk height. Flowable materials may be injected via a small incision, allowing minimally invasive access to the disk space. Fluids can interdigitate with the irregular surgical defects and may, depending on the material used, physically bond to the adjacent tissue. The use of an injectable material allows for complete filling of the disk, a task that is not possible with preformed implants. Complete filling allows pressurization of the annulus ensuring load transfer, and load sharing between the annulus and nucleus. Injectable biomaterials may also allow for incorporation and uniform dispersion of either or both cells and therapeutic agents. Growth factors, such as members of the bone morphogenetic protein (BMP), transforming growth factor (TGF), and insulin-like growth factor (IGF) families, may be valuable in enhancing the repair process. Inhibitors of inflammatory cytokines (e.g., interleukins, tumor necrosis factors) and proteases (e.g., matrix metalloproteinases) may act to retard matrix degradation and the potential effects of these cytokines on surrounding tissue and neural (especially nociceptive) structures.

Generally, the candidate biomaterials are injected as viscous fluids and then cured through methods such as thermosensitive cross-linking, pH-sensitive cross-linking, photopolymerization, or addition of a solidifying agent to form a gel-like substance. It is important to consider the amount of time it takes for the material to set. The setting time should be long enough to allow for accurate placement during the procedure yet short enough so as not to prolong the surgical procedure. If the material experiences a temperature change while curing, the increase in temperature should be small. Heat generated during this process should not cause harm to surrounding tissue. The viscosity or fluidity of the material should balance the need for the substance to remain at the site of its introduction into the disk, with the ability of the surgeon to manipulate its placement, and with the need to assure complete filling of the intradiskal space or voids. Ease in accessing the disk space also needs to be considered. For example, polymers that cure through a photopolymerization procedure could pose a problem due to a limited ability to access the small cavities of the disk space with light needed to initiate cross-linking.

Injectable biomaterials have been considered as an augment to a diskectomy for over 40 years. As early as 1962, Nachemson suggested the injection of room temperature vulcanizing silicone into a degenerated disk using an ordinary syringe.[18] In 1974, Schneider and Oyen studied the use of silicone elastomer in the intervertebral disk.[19,20] Since then, injectable biomaterials or scaffolds have been developed that may act as a substitute for the disk nucleus pulposus, such as hyaluronic acid, fibrin glue, alginate, elastin-like polypeptides, collagen type 1 gel, and others. Several patents and publications have been issued concerning various injectable biomaterials that may have utility for nucleus augmentation, including cross-linkable silk elastin copolymer,[21–26] polyurethane-filled balloons,[27,28] collagen-polyethylene glycol (PEG),[29–31] chitosan,[32–34] various injectable synthetic polymers,[35] recombinant bioelastic materials,[36–38] light-curable PEG polymers,[39] and other multicomponent precursor systems.[40] Several groups are actively pursuing the development of an injectable biomaterial for use in the intervertebral disk.[41,42]

Recent efforts have focused on the evaluation of a recombinant protein copolymer consisting of amino acid sequence blocks derived from silk and elastin structural proteins as an injectable biomaterial for augmentation of the nucleus pulposus. These proteins have been well-characterized over more than a decade of intensive research and development. The material appears to have ideal characteristics for the augmentation of the nucleus pulposus following diskectomy procedures. Cappello and coworkers have reported on the development and characterization of structural protein polymers, especially those derived from the structural proteins silk and elastin.[43,44] This implant, the NuCore Injectable Disc Nucleus, is being developed by Spine Wave, Inc. (Shelton, CT).

NuCore Injectable Nucleus

Protein Polymer Technologies, Inc. (San Diego, CA) has developed a technology for the production of synthetically designed protein polymers consisting of repeated blocks of amino acid sequence. Through a combination of biological and chemical methods, block polymers are produced using gene template-directed synthesis. Using this method, the design and polymerization of a new polymer occurs once during the synthesis of the gene template. Through the construction of synthetic genes, it is possible to specify the sequence of protein blocks (the unit of repetition of a protein polymer) several hundred amino acids in length, manyfold greater than the limit of sequence control of chemical synthesis.

Molecular architecture is critical to biological systems. Proteins fold into precisely controlled, three-dimensional conformations of single chains or assemblies of chains that are determined by the sequence of the 20 amino acid building blocks from which they are assembled. This three-dimensional structure not only influences the properties of the specific protein but also the properties of other proteins with which it may associate. Although different proteins perform very different functions, they share common structural elements. The four most common elements of secondary structure are α helices, β sheets, reverse turns, and collagen helices. Nearly 85% of the structures of most proteins can be described in terms of these four elements of secondary structure.

Beta sheets form the primary structural element of the silk fibroin protein. Silk fiber is composed of highly oriented and densely packed protein chains that are configured into β sheets. Laterally, β sheets are hydrogen bonded between the peptide CO and NH groups, alternately linking one strand with its neighboring strands on both sides. Because of this closely packed bonding and limited flexibility, protein domains consisting of β sheets can serve as reinforcing scaffolds for the surrounding protein. The β sheets of the silk fiber pack with each other through van der Waals associations between their ordered faces. To maximize close packing, silk fibroin protein consists almost exclusively of the three amino acids with the smallest side chains: glycine,

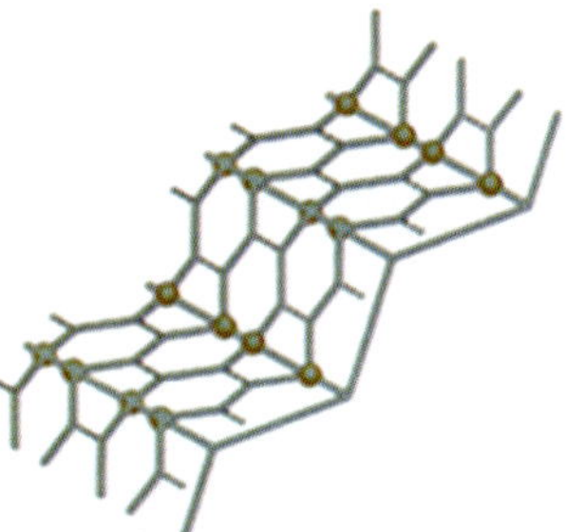

Figure 19–1   Beta sheet secondary structure.

Table 19–1   Comparison of Properties

Property	NuCore Injectable Nucleus	Natural Nucleus
Protein Content	19.4%	13.6–21.9%[*]
Water Content	79.1%	74–81%
pH	7.1	6.7–7.1
Complex Shear Modulus (G^*)	26 kPa	7–21 kPa[†]

[*]Data from Kitano T, Zerwekh JE, Usui Y, Edwards ML, Fuzker PL, Mooney V. Biomedical changes associated with the symptomatic human intervertebral disk. Clin Orthop Relat Res 1993;(293):372–377.

[†]Data from Iatridis JC, Weidenbaum M, Setton LA, Mow VC. Is the nucleus pulposus a solid or a fluid? Mechanized behaviors of the nucleus pulposus of the human intervertebral disc. Spine 1996;21(10):1174–1184.

alanine, and serine. **Fig. 19–1** shows a β sheet structure like that found in the silk fibroin protein.

Globular proteins composed of one or more structural elements contain flexible segments throughout the polypeptide chain that allow the chain to abruptly change direction. These reverse turns often contain amino acids with low propensity for the secondary structure elements on either side of the turn and most often contain the amino acids proline and glycine. A good example of a protein structure that utilizes the flexibility created by reverse turns (**Fig. 19–2**) is elastin. Tropoelastin is the protein monomer that assembles to form elastic fibers in the body and its sequence reveals that it contains tandem repetitions of several oligopeptide blocks four to nine amino acids in length. Urry and coworkers have shown that the pentapeptide valine-proline-glycine-valine-glycine forms a reverse turn (type II β turn) around the proline-glycine dipeptide and that when linked in numbers greater than three, the turns of the polypeptide wind into a spiral that functions as a flexible molecular spring and functions as a nearly ideal rubber.[45]

The protein polymer used in the NuCore Injectable Nucleus is a sequential block copolymer of silk and elastin, with two silk blocks and eight elastin blocks per polymer sequence repeat. One of the elastin blocks is modified to provide for chemical cross-linking. The protein polymer is synthesized using recombinant DNA techniques via *Escherichia coli* strain K12, a nonpathogenic strain of bacterium and the workhorse of recombinant protein expression. Following batch fermentation, the cells are ruptured by homogenization and the protein polymer is purified from the lysate using precipitation and a series of filtration and adsorption purification steps. The identity and purity of the polymer are confirmed using amino acid composition, amino acid terminal sequencing, mass spectroscopy, and other biochemical tests.

The NuCore material is composed of a solution of the protein polymer and a polyfunctional cross-linking agent and is formulated to closely match the properties of the human nucleus pulposus as shown in **Table 19–1**.

The material closely mimics the protein content, water content, pH, and complex modulus of the natural nucleus pulposus. The material is injected following mixing with a very low concentration of a diisocyanate-based cross-linking agent and has an approximately 90-second working time following addition of the cross-linking agent before it becomes a viscous gel. The material reaches near final mechanical strength ~30 minutes following addition of the cross-linker but is sufficiently gelled after 5 minutes to allow the surgery to be completed. As a consequence of the very low concentration of cross-linker used there is no measurable temperature rise during the curing process.

Testing of cadaver functional spinal units was done to determine how well the NuCore material restores stability and function to a spinal unit.[46] Anterior column units were tested in compression, first in the intact condition, then with annulotomy, then with a partial nucleotomy, and finally with NuCore material injected. Statistical analysis using repeated measured analysis of variance (ANOVA) and post hoc Tukey comparisons showed that the diskectomy caused a significant loss of height during the test ($p < .05$). However, the NuCore material injection caused a restoration such that there was no significant difference ($P > .05$) between the displacement of the intact condition (1.28 mm) and the NuCore material-treated condition (1.22 mm). Specimens were also tested in flexion-extension, right and left lateral bending, and right and left axial rotation. Testing evaluated first the intact condition, then after a partial nucleotomy, and finally after NuCore material injection. Statistical analysis using repeated measures ANOVA and post hoc Tukey pairwise comparisons showed that in all degrees of freedom, the diskectomy condition caused a destabilization of the unit ($p < .05$), whereas once the NuCore material was injected, in no cases were there significant differences between the intact or NuCore material conditions ($P > .05$). This analysis indicates that the NuCore Injectable Nucleus restores function and stability to the spine after a destabilizing diskectomy procedure.

Extensive biocompatibility and toxicology testing following the International Standards Organization (ISO) 10993 guidelines has been performed on the NuCore material.

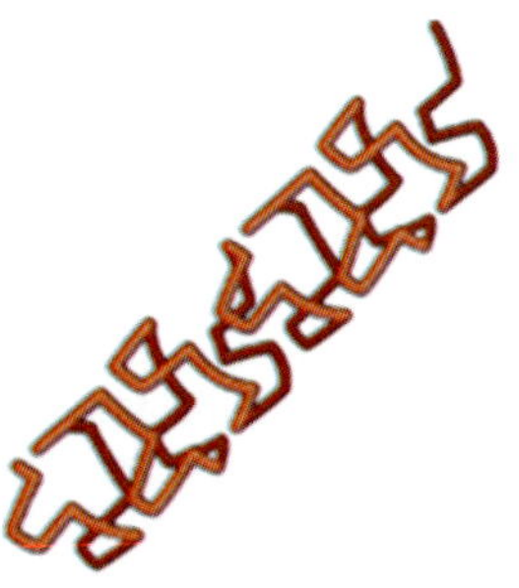

Figure 19–2   Beta turn secondary structure.

Acute tests include cytotoxicity, sensitization (guinea pig), intracutaneous reactivity (rabbit), systemic toxicity (mouse), pyrogenicity, muscle implant evaluation, and genotoxicity testing. The material is noncytotoxic, nonirritating, and nontoxic in all of these test evaluations.

Chronic toxicity testing has been conducted in a rat model, with material placed subcutaneously and evaluated at time points to 1 year and beyond, with no toxicity seen. Neurofunctional testing in a rat showed no neurotoxicity of the material when placed adjacent to spinal nerve roots. A sheep model has been used to assess the NuCore material placed within the intervertebral disk following diskectomy.

To evaluate mechanical performance in vivo, testing has been done in a cadaver model. To simulate dynamic loading over long periods of time, testing has been performed in a synthetic disk model. The annulus fibrosus of the disk was simulated with a molded silicone elastomer. This silicone annulus was injected with NuCore material, and the model was subjected to cyclic loading up to 10 million cycles with no failure of the NuCore material or test model. This testing indicates the NuCore material to be fatigue resistant and durable, capable of withstanding in vivo loads for an extended period of time.

Testing of cadaver anterior column units was done to determine how well the NuCore material resists forces to cause extrusion. Segments were tested in axial compression in both a neutral posture and hyperflexion. In all cases, there was no extrusion prior to bony failure or end plate failure. The average failure load of the spinal segments was 3555 N in the neutral position, and 2637 N in the hyperflexed position.

Results demonstrated that the NuCore material integrated extensively with the surrounding disk tissue and did not extrude during any of the testing (**Fig. 19–3**).

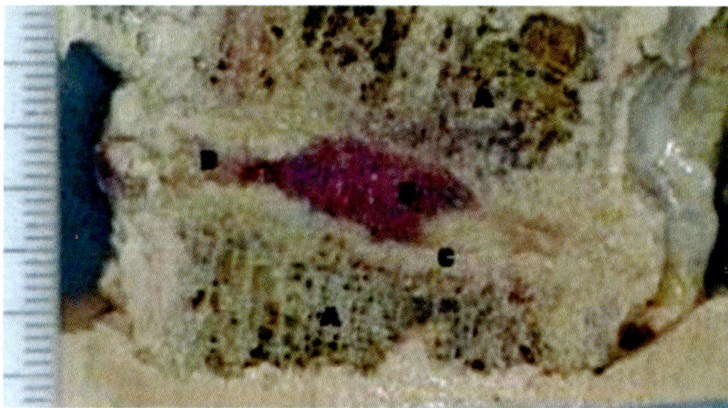

Figure 19–3   Lateral image of NuCore material filling nuclear cavity.

◆ Conclusion

In conclusion, characterization studies indicate that the NuCore Injectable Nucleus is able to restore the biomechanics of the disk following a microdiskectomy. Extensive biomaterial characterization shows the material to be nontoxic and biocompatible. The mechanical properties of the material mimic those of the natural nucleus pulposus. Thus NuCore Injectable Nucleus is suitable to replace the natural nucleus pulposus following a diskectomy procedure. Human clinical evaluation is under way in a multicenter clinical study on the use of the material as an adjunct to microdiskectomy. Further clinical studies of the use of the NuCore Injectable Nucleus for treatment of early-stage degenerative disk disease are due to start imminently. Ongoing efforts are characterizing the use of the material as a cell delivery vehicle for disk repair and reconstruction, as well as the use of the material for repair of articular cartilage defects.

References

1. Hermantin FU, Peters T, Quartararo L, Kambin P. A prospective, randomized study comparing the results of open discectomy with those of video-assisted arthroscopic microdiscectomy. J Bone Joint Surg Am 1999;81:958–965

2. Mochida J, Toh E, Nomura T, Nishimura K. The risks and benefits of percutaneous nucleotomy for lumbar disc herniation: a 10-year longitudinal study. J Bone Joint Surg Br 2001;83:501–505

3. Yorimitsu E, Chiba K, Toyama Y, Hirabayashi K. Long-term outcomes of standard discectomy for lumbar disc herniation: a follow-up study of more than 10 years. Spine 2001;26:652–657

4. Brinckmann P, Frobin W, Hierholzer E, Horst M. Deformation of the vertebral endplate under axial loading of the spine. Spine 1983;8:851–856

5. Frymoyer JW, Hanley EN, Howe J, Kuhlmann D, Matteri RE. A comparison of radiographic findings in fusion and nonfusion patients ten and more years following disc surgery. Spine 1979;4:435–440

6. Scoville WB, Corkill G. Lumbar disc surgery: technique of radical removal and early mobilization. J Neurosurg 1973;39:265–269

7. Tibrewal SB, Pearcy MJ. Lumbar intervertebral disc heights in normal subjects and patients with disc herniation. Spine 1985;10:452–454

8. Buschmann MD, Gluzband YA, Grodzinsky AJ, Huziker EJ. Mechanical compression modulates matrix biosynthesis in chondrocyte/agarose culture. J Cell Sci 1995;108(Pt 4):1497–1508

9. Ohshima H, Urban JPG, Bergel DH. Effect of static load on matrix synthesis rates in the intervertebral disc measured in vitro by a new perfusion technique. J Orthop Res 1995;13:22–29

10. Rand N, Juliao S, Spengler D, Dawson J. Static Hydrostatic Loading Induces In Vitro Apoptosis in Human Intervertebral Disc Cells. Orlando: Orthopaedic Research Society; 2000

11. Iatridis JC, Mente PL, Stokes AF, Aronsson DD, Alini M. Compression-induced changes in intervertebral disc properties in a rat tail model. Spine 1999;24:996–1002

12. Lotz JC, Colliou OK, Chin JR, Duncan NA, Liebenberg E. Compression-induced degeneration of the intervertebral disc: an in vivo mouse model and finite element study. Spine 1998;23:2493–2506

13. Gotfried Y, Bradford DS, Oegema TR. Facet joint changes after chemonucleolysis-induced disc space narrowing. Spine 1986;11: 944–950

14. Panjabi MM, Krag MH, Chung TQ. Effects of disc injury on mechanical behavior of the human spine. Spine 1984;9:707–713

15. Natarajan RN, Ke JH, Andersson GBJ. A model to study the disc degeneration process. Spine 1994;19:259–265

16. Atlas SJ, Keller RB, Wu YA, Deyo RA, Singer DE. Long-term outcomes of surgical and nonsurgical management of sciatica secondary to a lumbar disc herniation: 10 year results from the Maine lumbar spine study. Spine 2005;30:927–935

17. Carragee EJ, Han MY, Yang B, Kim DH, Kraemer H, Billys J. Activity restrictions after posterior lumbar discectomy: a prospective study of outcomes in 152 cases with no postoperative restrictions. Spine 1999;24:2346–2351

18. Nachemson A. Some mechanical properties of the lumbar intervertebral disc. Bull Hosp Joint Dis 1962;23:130–132

19. Schneider PG, Oyen R. Intervertebral disc replacement, experimental studies, clinical consequences. Zeitschrift Orthopaedics 1974;112: 791–792

20. Schneider PG, Oyen R. Plastic surgery on intervertebral disc, I: Intervertebral disc replacement in the lumbar regions with silicone rubber: theoretical and experimental studies. Zeitschrift Orthopeadic 1974;112:1078–1086

21. Betre H, Setton LA, Meyer DE, Chilkoti A. Characterization of a genetically engineered elastin-like polypeptide for cartilaginous tissue repair. Biomacromolecules 2002;3:910–916

22. Cappello J, Stedronsky ER. Synthetic proteins for in vivo drug delivery and tissue augmentation. Patent 6,380,154. 2002

23. Ferrari FA, Richardson C, Chambers J, et al. Peptides comprising repetitive units of amino acids and DNA sequences encoding the same. Patent 6,355,776. 2002

24. Nettles DL, Vail TP, Morgan MT, Grinstaff MW, Setton LA. Photocrosslinkable hyaluronan as a scaffold for articular cartilage repair. Ann Biomed Eng 2004;32:391–397

25. Stedronsky ER. Methods of using primer molecules for enhancing the mechanical performance of tissue adhesives and sealants. Patent 6,258,872. 2001

26. Stedronsky ER, Cappello J. Sealing or filling tissue defects using polyfunctional crosslinking agents and protein polymers. Patent 6,423,333. 2002

27. Bao Q-B, Yuan HA. Implantable tissue repair device. Patent 6,224,630. 2001

28. Felt JC, Rydell MA, Zdrahala RJ, Arsenyev A. Biomaterial for in situ tissue repair. Patent 6,306,177. 2001

29. Olsen DR, Chang R, McMullin H, Hitzeman RA, Chisholm G. Methods for the production of gelatin and full-length triple helical collagen in recombinant cells. Patent 6,428,978. 2002

30. Olsen DR, Chang R, McMullin H, Hitzeman RA, Chisholm G. Recombinant gelatin and full-length triple helical collagen. Patent 6,413,742. 2002

31. Rhee WM, DeLustro FA, Berg RA. Method of making crosslinked polymer matrices in tissue treatment applications. Patent 6,323,278. 2001

32. Alini M, Roughley PJ, Antoniou J, Stoll T, Aebi M. A biological approach to treating disc degeneration: not for today, but maybe for tomorrow. Eur Spine J 2002;11(Suppl 2):S215–S220

33. Chenite A, Chaput C, Combes C, Selmani A, Jalal F. Temperature-controlled pH-dependent formation of ionic polysaccharide gels. Patent 6,344,488. 2002

34. Chenite A, Chaput C, Wang D, et al. Novel injectable neutral solutions of chitosan form biodegradable gels in situ. Biomaterials 2000;21:2155–2161

35. Milner R, Arrowsmith P, Millan EJ. Intervertebral disc implant. Patent 6,187,048. 2001

36. Daniell H, McPherson DT, Urry DW, Xu J. Hyper-expression of bioelastic polypeptides. Patent 6,004,782. 1999

37. Urry DW. Polynanopeptide bioelastomers having an increased elastic modulus. Patent 5,064,430. 1991

38. Urry DW. Polymers capable of baromechanical and barochemical transduction. Patent 5,226,292. 1993

39. Hubbell JA, Pathak CP, Sawhney AS, Desai NP, Hill JL. Photopolymerizable biodegradable hydrogels as tissue contacting materials and controlled-release microcarriers. Patent 5,626,863. 1997

40. Hubbell JA, Wetering PVD, Cowling DSP. Novel polymer compounds. Patent 2002/0177680. 2002

41. Bao Q-B, Yuan HA. New technologies in spine: nucleus replacement. Spine 2002;27:1245–1247

42. Yuksel U, Walsh S, Curd D, Black K. Fatigue durability of a novel disc nucleus repair system: in vitro studies in a calf spine model. Spine J 2002;2:103S–104S

43. Cappello J. Genetically engineered protein polymers. In: Domb AJ, Kost J, Wiseman D, eds. Handbook of Degradable Polymers. Amsterdam: Harwood Academic; 1996:387–414

44. Cappello J, Ferrari F. Microbial product of structural protein polymers. In: Mobley DP, ed. Plastics from Microbes. Munich: Carl Hanser Verlag; 1994:35–92

45. Urry DW, Hugel T, Seitz M, et al. Elastin: a representative ideal protein elastomer. Philos Trans R Soc Lond B Biol Sci 2002;357:169–184

46. Mahar AT, Oka R, Whitledge J, Cappello JR, Powell J, McArthur T. Biomechanical efficacy of a protein polymer hydrogel for intervertebral nucleus augmentation and replacement. In: World Congress on Biomechanics. 2002. Calgary, Canada

Section III

**Restoration of Lumbar Motion Segment
B. Lumbar Total Disk Replacement**

20

Biomechanical Considerations for Total Lumbar Disk Replacement

Jean-Charles Le Huec, S. Aunoble, Y. Basso, C. Tournier, and K. Yamada

◆ **Why Perform Total Disk Replacement Rather than Fusion?**

◆ **Biomechanical Analysis of the Normal Lumbar Disk**

◆ **Biomechanical Analysis of Degenerative Lumbar Disk**

◆ **Why Use a Total Disk Prosthesis?**
   Disk Height Reestablishment
   Height Recovery
   Ideal Equilibrium

◆ **Conclusion**

Total lumbar disk replacement with a prosthesis is a challenge involving many factors. The primary hypothesis is that the disk is the first element to degenerate in lumbar spine aging, and that this induces most of the other problems associated with spinal degeneration. This point of view is held by Fujiwara et al[1] and Butler et al,[2] who note that lumbar disk degeneration is the primordial factor of any spinal disk pathology. If this opinion is accepted, then total disk replacement becomes an interesting concept, providing that an almost anatomical function can be restored. For this reason, it is essential to examine the biomechanics of the normal and pathological lumbar spine before performing replacement.

◆ Why Perform Total Disk Replacement Rather than Fusion?

Among the numerous reasons that total disk replacement has gained ground, we should first look at the less than satisfactory results obtained by O'Beirne et al[3] and Bono and Lee[4] with the usual fusion techniques. The customary discrepancy between the high radiological success rates of fusion[4] and the residual pain felt by patients is the primary reason for trying to find a therapeutic alternative. Even if fusion has led to a decrease or disappearance in back pain, it is now recognized that there is an increased short- or medium-term risk of involving the adjacent disk, as pointed out by Gertzbein and Hollopeter[5] and Etebar and Cahill.[6] The initial studies had already demonstrated adjacent level disease after posterolateral fusion without instrumentation, and the use of rigid instrumentation, which has led to high fusion rates, seems to have increased the risk of this complication.[7,8]

The question is whether these less than satisfactory results obtained with lumbar fusion should lead to developing an alternative technique for disk arthroplasty.[9] Disk arthroplasty first involves removing the disk tissue that has apparently been causing pain.[10] This is the case when performing an intersomatic arthrodesis by anterior or posterior approach in posterior lumbar interbody fusion (PLIF). Only posterolateral grafts are unable to remove this painful tissue. The second role of disk arthroplasty is to restore the height of the disk, thereby restoring the height of the foramen,[11] freeing the canal and allowing sagittal realignment of the spine while decreasing the stress on the posterior facets.[12] Third, the technique restores or maintains the mobility of the disk space. It is now widely accepted that mobility is one of the main advantages of total disk replacement,[13] thus underlining the value of disk replacement in adjacent level disease, as confirmed by the long-term follow-up reported by Tropiano et al[14] and Lemaire et al.[15]

◆ Biomechanical Analysis of the Normal Lumbar Disk

The human lumbar disk is endowed with a mechanical structure allowing it to resist very large stresses.[16] Indeed, it can resist stresses greater than those on the bone, which is frequently where fractures occur before the disk itself becomes involved.[17] Experimental studies have shown the lumbar disk to withstand stress as great as 17,000 N during lifting tasks.[18] To do so, the disk converts a compressive force into tensile stress at the annulus by way of hydrostatic pressure transmitted by interstitial fluids inside the disk. This tensile property varies according to the region of the annulus, thereby leading to two distinct phases during lifting. Because the external fibers of the annulus are more rigid than those inside, the former convert the compression into hoop stresses while the others absorb the shock.[19]

The high tensile modulus of the normal annulus helps to prevent disk bulging in the degenerating disk. The swelling pressure of the nucleus pulposus decreases and the stiffness of the annulus fibrosis increases,[20,21] resulting in poor load dissipation and increased stress transfer to the bony elements of the spine.[20]

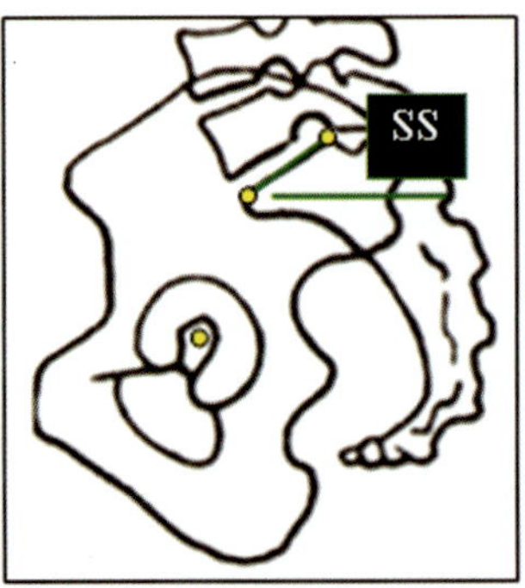

Figure 20–1   Sacral slope.

Many studies have shown that pathological loading of the spine could play a role in disk degeneration.[22,23] Twisting while lifting induces degeneration and rapid changes to the disk, including an increase in phospholipases A2 and a decrease in volume of the nucleus pulposus.[24] Once this process has set in, concentrations of calcitonin gene-related peptide and vasoactive intestinal peptide increase at the level of the adjacent spinal ganglion, thus accounting for the relationship between degeneration and pain. One must be aware of these biomechanical and biochemical processes when replacing an intervertebral disk. Persistent chemical irritation may be the underlying cause of the poor functional results obtained by patients who have received prostheses. Hadjipavlou et al[24] and Ching et al[25] demonstrated in animal models that statically loaded disks had a greater tendency to degenerate compared with cyclically loaded disks. MacLean et al[26] demonstrated that pathological loading of disks seemed to decrease the disk metabolism and lead to the production of catabolic enzymes, according to how the load was administered. As shown by Mimura et al,[27] disk mobility temporarily increases at the onset of degeneration, leading to an increase in stress exerted on the disk cell and to decreased disk capacity, a finding confirmed by Krismer et al.[28]

When considering the overall biomechanics of the lumbar spine, one should consider not only the intervertebral disk but also the equilibrium of the lumbar spine in the frontal and sagittal planes. A normal spinal column is absolutely straight in the frontal plane. However, the curvature of the lumbar column or lordosis is an important parameter impacting on the overall equilibrium and leading to considerable modifications of the stresses applied to the various lumbar disks. The sagittal equilibrium of the spine should be assessed on coronal

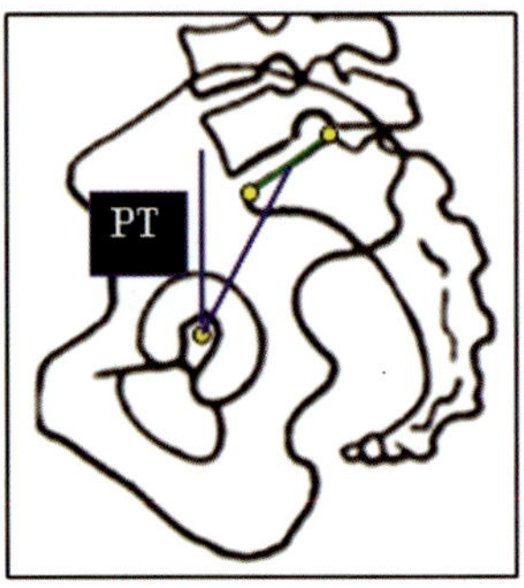

Figure 20–2   Pelvic tilt.

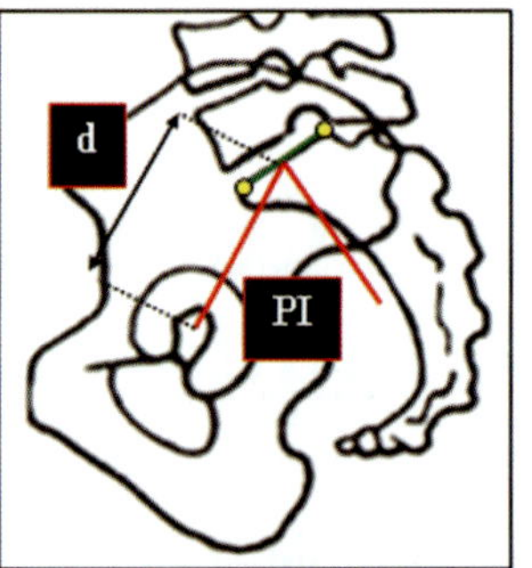

Figure 20–3   Pelvic incidence.

images while the spine is subjected to a load and, if possible, with projection of the center of gravity by using a "force plate." It is also essential to examine the center of the femoral heads and the pelvis. If there is no anomaly in the lower members, this type of sagittal view provides a detailed analysis of the lumbar spine. An initial study was performed by Roussouly et al[29] on healthy volunteers in whom various criteria of equilibrium were analyzed: sacral slope (**Fig. 20–1**), pelvic tilt (**Fig. 20–2**) and angle of incidence (**Fig. 20–3**), the latter being obtained by summing the other two. Roussouly et al[29] found that there was a direct correlation between sagittal equilibrium, lumbar lordosis, and sacral slope, and that it was possible to subdivide the spine into four categories. Therefore, it is essential to analyze spinal equilibrium biomechanically before attempting any prosthetic intervention. The work by Kroeber et al[22] and Sandover[23] demonstrated the harmful effects of asymmetric stress on disks, and it is clear that any disk prosthesis must be able to withstand such stresses if spinal equilibrium has not been restored.

◆ Biomechanical Analysis of Degenerative Lumbar Disk

To date, the exact cause of disk degeneration is not clear but one of the main factors is a decrease in the nutrition the disk receives.[8] This largely depends on the vertebral end plates that ensure nutrition of the vertebral disk, as demonstrated by Langrana and Lee[30] and Akamaru et al.[31] As degeneration sets in, fissures, fractures, and clefts are formed in the vertebral end plates, thus making them thinner as reported by Shono et al[32] and Benneker et al.[33] Loss of hydrous matter in the nucleus pulposus results in a drop in pressure within the disk and a decrease in disk height.[8] The final stages of degeneration are characterized by a fibrous nucleus and a fibrous annulus with numerous fissures and clefts, with the result that the internal part of the annulus and the bonds between it and the nucleus pulposus become much less distinct. In the beginning, the healthy disk has a fluidlike capacity, whereas a degenerated disk is much more solid as shown by Horst and Brinckmann.[34]

The analysis of load transmission in the disk is a highly important element of disk biomechanics because stresses at this level will have a bearing on the quality of prostheses that may subsequently be used. The lumbar disk transmits the load between the vertebrae by way of the intervertebral disk and the two posterior articular facets. Many studies have demonstrated that under compression, the load is first transmitted through the anterior column while the posterior facets are subjected to only 18% of the compression load.[17] The amount of load transmitted through the posterior elements is highly dependent upon the sagittal equilibrium of the spine[35] and also upon the degree of disk degeneration, as demonstrated by Pollintine et al.[36] Nachemson[3] found that the load on the intervertebral disk also depends on posture: the portion of the body situated above L3 receives 60% of the body weight, whereas if the subject leans forward 20%, the load increases to 250% of body weight. When a 20 kg weight is lifted in an upright position, the load on the spine is equivalent to 300% of body weight. The study also demonstrated that the load exerted on the lumbar spine during daily activity can reach maximal values.

Hydrostatic pressure in the nucleus pulposus is a key factor in the behavior of the intervertebral disk. The annulus fibrosus and the vertebral end plates must be able to withstand very high pressure. It would be inappropriate here to describe in detail the studies of Shirazi-Adl et al[37] and McNally and colleagues.[38,39] Suffice it to say that the compression load in a degenerated disk is transmitted over the surface of the disk by way of the annulus, thus intensifying the stress. The load on the posterior elements also increases as degeneration sets in. In fact, a significant change in load transmission becomes apparent through the degenerated segment and especially for shear forces. Under compression, the symmetry of stress distribution increases as the load moves off center and the disk degenerates, thus explaining why degeneration has already begun to affect adjacent areas when a patient presents with lumbar pain originating in a disk.[39] The aim of disk replacement is therefore to replace the deficient disk and to exert a protective effect on adjacent areas that have already begun to suffer from the harmful effects of the more or less long-term loss of disk function already under way.

Gertzbein et al[40] demonstrated the variation in instantaneous axis of rotation (IAR) between degenerated disks and normal ones. In disks showing the least degeneration, it was difficult to localize the IAR, whereas in those with considerable degeneration, the IAR could easily be found at the level of the lower vertebral end plate. This means that the cinematic behavior of a highly degenerated disk is not significantly different in flexibility compared with that of a normal one. The disk has increased mobility when the disk segment begins to degenerate, then less flexibility as degeneration continues to evolve and finally reaches a stage of disk stability. The latter may indirectly cause pain owing to changes in spinal equilibrium and their consequences on the muscles, ligaments, and articular facets. Such secondary effects may be corrected by replacing the disk, but long-standing lesions will not regress and must be repaired by compensation.

In summary, degeneration in the intervertebral disk modifies load transmission and the cinematic behavior of the lumbar spine. Under compression, it decreases load transmission through the nucleus and increases it through the annulus fibrosus. However, few changes occur in shear force. The proportion of load transmitted through the posterior elements also increases as degeneration worsens, as demonstrated by Pollintine et al.[36] Long-standing degeneration can lead to disk restabilization, sometimes with considerable loss of height, and to changes in spinal biomechanics. When performing disk restoration with a device, surgeons must take these changes into account because replacement does not simply mean a return to the initial state for the adjacent stabilizing structures.

◆ Why Use a Total Disk Prosthesis?

Disk Height Reestablishment

Total disk replacement should aim at reestablishing the height of the disk. This has several consequences. First, by recovering disk height, it becomes possible to put the posterior articular facets back into a more anatomical position. Opening the disk space in turn opens up the foramina, as described by Chen et al.[11] This has a beneficial impact on some radicular pain. When height is recovered, the peripheral annular structures are placed under tension, especially the mechanical receptors situated on the outer part of the annulus. In this way, the proprioceptive capacity of these receptors can once again transmit pertinent information about spinal equilibrium. Care must be taken, however, to restore only the natural anatomical height. The height of the L5–S1 disk is particularly variable, with a mean of 8.5 mm in its posterior part.[41] Because the anterior part of L5–S1 may be very high and exceed the height of the L4–L5 disk, restoring its height may create considerable shear forces on the device. For this reason, the sacral slope is an essential factor to be examined on radiographic views taken with the patient standing and under load before any surgery is envisaged. When the slope is too steep, an attempt should be made to decrease it to reduce the resulting shear forces on the device.[29] At the level of the adjacent level L4–L5 and beyond, restoration of disk height is easier because the lordosis is less pronounced and the disks are more rectangular in shape.

Height Recovery

The device should allow height to be recovered. As shown by Kirkaldy-Willis and Farfan,[42] the onset of disk degeneration is accompanied by increased mobility, then by reduced mobility, and finally by disk ankylosis. Total disk replacement should not result in increased mobility because hypermobility is often associated with pain, as in the minor intervertebral disturbance described by Maigne.[43] Mobility should be recovered but not more than is natural anatomically. The center of rotation of the disk and the IAR are the factors most frequently considered as important by the manufacturers of lumbar disk devices.[13] However, the IAR has little mobility, as demonstrated by Gertzbein et al.[40] It is useful in practice to position the rotational center of the device just behind the median line of the vertebral body on sagittal views and below the superior end plate of the inferior vertebra, as described previously.[13] The IAR is situated on an ellipse so taking it to be just one point is too simplistic to solve the issue. Nevertheless, reproducing this variability of the IAR does not seem to have any major consequence on the clinical outcome, as shown by Tournier et al.[44] Any disk prosthesis should allow flexion, extension, lateral inclination, and rotation. All of these movements are controlled by the surrounding muscles and ligaments, the proprioceptive nervous system, and the posterior articular facets. The flexion, extension, and lateral inclination provided by the device are physically limited by its end-stop, unlike a physiological disk with its elastic tissue. Disk devices are only rarely limited in their rotational movement, an exception being the FlexiCore (Stryker Spine, Allendale, NJ),[13] but the rotation of intervertebral disks is in effect limited by their elastic properties and the orientation of the annular fibers. Movement limitation thus assists considerably in stabilizing the disk when it is replaced by a prosthesis. However, when inserting a device, most surgeons[14,15] prefer to leave in place part of the annulus as well as the lateral ligaments and the muscle structures, thus enabling mobility to be controlled. The potential pitfall of this approach is to leave degenerated disk tissue behind that may cause subsequent pain. Ideally, the objective is that a device ensures compression and dilation movements, thereby providing a shock-absorbing effect.[45] However, although the currently available devices cannot absorb shocks, the actual physical impact of this drawback on the adjacent lumbar structures remains to be demonstrated clinically. Indeed, the cancellous bone of the vertebral structures provides excellent shock absorption and the intervertebral disk acts as a slow shock absorber.

Ideal Equilibrium

Disk replacement allows the patient to adopt the ideal frontal and sagittal equilibrium. This choice depends on sacral slope and pelvis tilt and, therefore, on incidence. The relationship between spine and pelvis is established on the basis of criteria decided upon by patients themselves and especially by their ability to compensate their hip movements and to contract their muscles, particularly in the region of the psoas. As shown by Le Huec et al,[46] sagittal equilibrium is regulated by disk replacement, the patient then being able to choose the best coronal and sagittal equilibrium. When performing replacement, it is essential not to create an imbalance between the coronal and sagittal planes because this could lead to iatrogenic complications. Replacement of a degenerated disk results in recovery of the initial height of the physiological disk and the lordosis but also in a significant loss of lordosis at the supra-adjacent level as demonstrated by Le Huec et al.[47]

Total lumbar disk replacement requires ablation of the anterior part of the annulus and frequently also the posterior part, which in turn means ablation of the central part. On the other hand, this eliminates numerous inflammatory structures responsible for painful diskopathies arising in the disk. Ablation of this damaged inflammatory tissue makes it possible to remove the nociceptive nerve terminations involved in the vascular invasion of degenerated disks.[48] An antalgic effect is therefore obtained by the mandatory cleaning that the disk space undergoes before total disk replacement. However, the lateral part of the annulus containing the proprioceptive receptors must be resected, so the risk exists of leaving nerve terminations behind that may induce pain in the long run. It would therefore be useful to determine preoperatively the quantity of disk matter to be removed so that resection only concerns the affected region. In this way, painful sequelae could be avoided.

The fixation of devices to the vertebrae is an important factor governing their longevity. In a study of the osteointegration of the Acroflex (DePuy Spine, DePuy-Acromed, Inc., Raynham, MA) devices, Cunningham et al[49] found very good bone growth at the bone-implant interface. However, the initial stability that is essential for obtaining excellent bone integration is best ensured by a keel system.[14,46] Devices that do not have this function must be positioned in such a way that contact is optimal between the metal end plates of the device and the vertebral end plates. However, current devices do not mimic the natural physiological contours so certain abutting points are subjected to excessive load. This accounts in part for the failure of some vertebral end plates at points where there is insufficient contact between the device and end plate as reported by Putzier et al in a long-term follow-up.[50] The use of keels allows better load distribution but requires the etching of a groove in the vertebral body that may cause subsequent fractures.

◆ Conclusion

The ideal total lumbar disk replacement should allow disk height to be reestablished, the peripheral proprioceptive receptors of the annulus to be conserved; the extreme movements of flexion, extension, lateral inclination, and rotation to be limited; and shocks to be absorbed. Moreover, the mobility offered by the device should resemble that of the physiological structure as much as possible and should allow central movement to avoid overloading the articular facets. However, when performing disk replacement for back pain, it is essential to treat the adjacent structures if they have been affected over time and have engendered loss of optimal function. These biomechanical considerations should be taken into account, as demonstrated by recent work[51] showing that a limited amount of arthrosis of the facets is not a contraindication for total lumbar disk replacement as the quality of the posterior muscles.

References

1. Fujiwara A, Lim TH, An HS, et al. The effect of disc degeneration and facet joint osteoarthritis on the segmental flexibility of the lumbar spine. Spine 2000;25:3036–3044
2. Butler D, Trafimow JH, Andersson GBJ, McNeill TW, Huckman MS. Discs degenerate before facets. Spine 1990;15:111–113
3. O'Beime J, O'Neill D, Williams DH. Spinal fusion for back pain: a clinical and radiological review. J Spinal Disord 1992;5:32–38
4. Bono C, Lee C. Critical analysis of trends in fusion for degenerative disc disease over the last twenty years: influence of technique on fusion rate and clinical outcome. Spine 2004;29:455–463
5. Gertzbein SD, Hollopeter MR. Disc herniation after lumbar fusion. Spine 2002;27:E373–E376
6. Etebar S, Cahill DW. Risk factor for adjacent-segment failure following lumbar fixation with rigid instrumentation for degenerative instability. J Neurosurg 1999;90(Suppl 2):163–169
7. Ghiselli G, Wang JC, Bhatia NN, Hsu WK, Dawson EG. Adjacent segment degeneration in the lumbar spine. J Bone Joint Surg Am 2004;86-A: 1497–1503
8. Lee CK. Accelerated degeneration of the segment adjacent to a lumbar fusion. Spine 1988;13:375–377

9. Shuff C, An HS. Artificial disc replacement: the new solution for discogenic low back pain? Am J Orthop 2005;34:8–12
10. Frymoyer JW, Hanley E, Howe J, Kuhlmann D, Matteri R. Disc excision and spine fusion in the management of lumbar disc disease: a minimum ten-year follow-up. Spine 1978;3:1–6
11. Chen D, Fay LA, Lok J, Yuan P, Edwards WT, Yuan HA. Increasing neuroforaminal volume by anterior interbody distraction in degenerative lumbar spine. Spine 1995;20:74–79
12. Dooris AP, Goel VK, Grosland NM, Gilbertson LG, Wilder DG. Load sharing between anterior and posterior elements in a lumbar motion segment implanted with an artificial disc. Spine 2001;26:E122–E129
13. Errico TJ. Lumbar disc arthroplasty. Clin Orthop Relat Res 2005;435:106–117
14. Tropiano P, Huang RC, Girardi FP, Cammisa FP, Marnay T. Lumbar total disc replacement: seven to eleven year follow-up. J Bone Joint Surg Am 2005;87:490–496
15. Lemaire JP, Skalli W, Lavaste F, et al. Intervertebral disc prosthesis: results and prospects for the year 2000. Clin Orthop Relat Res 1997;337:64–76
16. Nachemson A. The load on lumbar discs in different positions of the body. Clin Orthop Relat Res 1966;45:107–122
17. Nachemson A. Lumbar intradiscal pressure: Experimental studies in post-mortem material. Acta Orthop Scand 1960; (Suppl 43):1–104
18. Cholewicki J, Van Vliet JJ IV. Relative contribution of trunk muscles to the stability of the lumbar spine during isometric exertions. Clin Biomech (Bristol, Avon) 2002;17:99–105
19. Buckwalter JA, Mow VC, Boden SD, Eyre DR, Weidenbaum M. Intervertebral disc structure, composition and mechanical function. In: Buckwalter JA, Ainhorn TA, Simon SR, eds. Orthopaedic Basic Science Biology and Biomechanics for the Musculoskeletal System. 2nd ed. Rosemont, IL: American Academy of Orthopaedic Surgeons; 2000:548–555.
20. Acaroglu ER, Iatridis JC, Setton LA, Foster RJ, Mow WC, Weidenbaum M. Degeneration and aging affect the tensile behavior of human lumbar annulus fibrosus. Spine 1995;20:2690–2701
21. Panagiotacopulos ND, Knauss WG, Bloch R. On the mechanical properties of human intervertebral disc material. Biorheology 1979;16:317–330
22. Kroeber MW, Unglaub F, Wang H, et al. New in vivo animal model to create intervertebral disc degeneration and to investigate the effects of therapeutic strategies to stimulate disc regeneration. Spine 2002;27:2684–2690
23. Sandover J. Dynamic loading as a possible source of low back disorders. Spine 1983;8:652–658
24. Hadjipavlou AG, Simmons JW, Yang JP, Bi LX, Simmons DJ. Torsional injury resulting in disc degeneration, I: An in vivo rabbit model, II: Associative changes in dorsal root ganglion and spinal cord neurotransmitter production. J Spinal Disord 1998;11:312–321
25. Ching CT, Chow DH, Yao FY, Holmes AD. The effect of cyclic compression on the mechanical properties of the intervertebral disc: an in vivo study in a rat model. Clin Biomech (Bristol, Avon) 2003;18:182–189
26. MacLean JJ, Lee CR, Grad S, Ito K, Alini M, Iatridis JC. Effects of immobilization and dynamic compression on intervertebral disc cell gene expression in vivo. Spine 2003;28:973–981
27. Mimura M, Panjabi MM, Oxland TR, Crisco JJ, Yamamoto I, Vasavada A. Disc degeneration affects the multidirectional flexibility of the lumbar spine. Spine 1994;19:1371–1380
28. Krismer M, Haid C, Behensky H, Kapfinger P, Landauer F, Rachbauer R. Motion in lumbar functional spine units during side bending and axial rotation moments depending on the degree of degeneration. Spine 2000;25:2020–2027
29. Roussouly P, Gollogly S, Berthonnaud E, Dimnet J. Classification of the normal variation in the sagittal alignment of the human lumbar spine and pelvis in the standing position. Spine 2005;30:346–353
30. Langrana NA, Lee CK. Lumbosacral spinal fusion: biomechanical and clinical considerations. In: Pope M, ed. Seminars in Spine Surgery. Philadelphia: WB Saunders; 1993:81–87
31. Akamaru T, Kawahara N, Yoon ST, et al. Adjacent segment motion after a simulated lumbar fusion in different sagittal alignments: a biomechanical analysis. Spine 2003;28:1560–1566
32. Shono Y, Kaneida K, Abumi K. Stability of posterior spinal instrumentation and its effects on adjacent motion segments in the lumbosacral spine. Spine 1998;23:1550–1558
33. Benneker LM, Heini PF, Alini M, Anderson SE, Ito K. 2004 Young Investigator Award winner: vertebral endplate marrow contact channel occlusions and intervertebral disc degeneration. Spine 2005;30:167–173
34. Horst M, Brinckmann P. Measurement of the distribution of axial stress on the end-plate of the vertebral body. Spine 1981;6:217–232
35. Yang KH, King AI. Mechanism of facet load transmission as a hypothesis for low-back pain. Spine 1984;9:557–565
36. Pollintine P, Dolan P, Tobias JH, Adams MA. Intervertebral disc degeneration can lead to "stress-shielding" of the anterior vertebral body: a cause of osteoporotic vertebral fracture? Spine 2004;29:774–782
37. Shirazi-Adl A, Ahmed AM, Shrivastava SC. A finite element study of a lumbar motion segment subjected to pure sagittal plane moments. J Biomech 1986;19:331–350
38. McNally DS, Adams MA. Internal disc mechanics as revealed by stress profilometry. Spine 1992;17:66–73
39. McNally DS, Shackleford IM, Goodship AE, Mulholland RC. In vivo stress measurement can predict pain on discography. Spine 1996;21:2580–2587
40. Gertzbein SD, Seligman J, Holtby R, et al. Centrode patterns and segmental instability in degenerative disc disease. Spine 1985;10:257–261
41. Zhou SH, McCarthy ID, McGregor AH, Coombs RR, Hughes SP. Geometrical dimensions of the lower lumbar vertebrae—analysis of data from digitised CT images. Eur Spine J 2000;9:242–248
42. Kirkaldy-Willis WH, Farfan HF. Instability of the lumbar spine. Clin Orthop Relat Res 1982;165:110–123
43. Maigne R. Pain syndromes of the thoracolumbar junction. Phys Med Rehab Clin North Am 1997;8:87–100
44. Tournier C, Le Huec JC, Aunoble S, Lemaire JP, Tropiano P, Skalli W. Total disc arthroplasty, consequences for sagittal balance and lumbar spine movement. Eur Spine J In press
45. LeHuec JC, Kiaer T, Friesem T, Mathews H, Liu M, Eisermann L. Shock absorption in lumbar disc prosthesis: a preliminary mechanical study. J Spinal Disord Tech 2003;16:346–351
46. Le Huec JC, Mathews H, Basso Y, et al. Clinical results of Maverick lumbar total disc replacement: two-year prospective follow-up. Orthop Clin North Am 2005;36:315–322
47. Le Huec JC, Basso Y, Mathews H, et al. The effect of single level total disc arthroplasty on sagittal balance parameters: a prospective study. Eur Spine J 2005;14:480–486
48. Freemont AJ, Peacock TE, Goupille P, Hoyland JA, O'Brien J, Jayson MI. Nerve ingrowth into diseased intervertebral disc in chronic back pain. Lancet 1997;350:178–181
49. Cunningham BW, Dmitriev AE, Hu N, McAfee PC. Total disc replacement arthroplasty using the Acroflex lumbar disc: a nonhuman primate model. Eur Spine J 2002;11:S115–S123
50. Putzier P, Funk JF, Schneider SV et al. Charité total disc replacement: clinical and radiographical results after an average follow-up of 17 years. Eur Spine J 2005
51. Le Huec JC, Basso Y, Aunoble S, Friesem T, Brayda BM. Influence of facet and posterior muscle degeneration on clinical results of lumbar total disc replacement: two year follow-up. J Spinal Disord Tech 2005;18:219–233

21

Indications for Total Lumbar Disk Replacement

Rudolf Bertagnoli

◆ **Artificial Disk Prosthesis**

◆ **Indications**

◆ **Contraindications**

◆ **Case Studies**

Group I: "Ideal" Indications
Group II: "Good" Indications
Group III: "Expanded" Indications

◆ **Conclusion**

Chronic back pain and musculoskeletal diseases are among the most common reasons for consultations worldwide. Back pain is a result of alterations in the natural mechanics of the lumbar spine associated with degeneration of the intervertebral disk. Even though disk degeneration is a normal aging process of the lumbar spine[1] younger people are also affected. This results from a change in lifestyle, the tendency to sedentary work, and other unhealthy factors that promote degenerative disk disease (DDD).[2] This fact leads to an increasing number of people worldwide who suffer from back pain and therefore to a greater necessity for better treatment options on the spinal market.

Primarily many of patients' back ailments can be treated with conservative therapy. But the number of cases that have failed conservative treatment is growing,[3] and consequently the need for surgical intervention rises.

Potential pain sources in the lumbar spine are the disks, the facet joints, and the spine muscles. Conservative therapy is the first step to relieve pain. There are different surgical options for patients who have failed conservative treatment and still suffer from back pain. Due to the fact that fusion and nucleotomies are not optimal solutions for every patient, total disk replacement (TDR) has become more important in recent years. Fusion surgery achieves no restoration of the natural disk function and also eliminates the motion of the affected segment. This may lead to "fusion diseases," such as facet hypertrophy, spinal stenosis, or adjacent level disk degeneration.[2] Nucleus replacement technologies (nucleus arthroplasty) are still under investigation and at this time there is no standard definition as to which degree of annulus degeneration and disk height loss will achieve a successful implantation.[4] Nucleotomies are not indicated for patients with multilevel degenerative disk disease.[4]

The ideal goals of any low back pain surgery should be decompression of neurogenic structures, pain relief, preserving the range of motion, and achieving segmental motion. All of these requirements can be reached in a TDR surgery where the whole damaged disk is replaced by an artificial disk.

◆ Artificial Disk Prosthesis

Artificial disk prostheses replace the disk completely and, opposite to nucleus replacement devices, they are biomechanically independent of the disk tissue.[5] An ideal artificial disk should restore the disk height and segmental motion, generate kinetics at the spinal triple joint complex, and absorb shocks.[6] The goal is to mimic the loading and motion characteristics of the natural intervertebral disk whereby degeneration of the adjacent levels will be not accelerated. Due to the fact that more and more younger people are affected by DDD a TDR prosthesis should work properly for many decades.[7]

In search of better possibilities to treat degenerative disk disease, the development of total disk replacement has increased over the last several years. Various prostheses are under clinical trial or have already entered the market. The lumbar devices with the longest experience are the SB Charité (DePuy Spine, Raynham, MA) and the ProDisc-L (Synthes, Inc., West Chester, PA).

The SB Charité was the first total disk device that entered clinical trials (in 1984). The most unconstrained of all prostheses consists of two cobalt-chromium-molybdenum (CoCrMo) alloy end plates that surround a biconvex polyethylene core. The latest version has a hydroxyapatite coating.

The ProDisc-L, designed in the late 1980s, is a semiconstrained prosthesis consisting of a monoconvex polyethylene core and two CoCrMo end plates coated with a titanium plasmapore surface.

Two other devices that have been in clinical trials over the last few years are the Maverick Artificial Disc (Medtronic Sofamor Danek, Memphis, TN), and more recently the FlexiCore prosthesis (Stryker Spine, Kalamazoo, MI).

According to the design and the function total lumbar disk prostheses can be classified into three groups: unconstrained prostheses (e.g., Charité), semiconstrained devices (e.g., ProDisc-L, Maverick), and constrained prostheses (e.g., FlexiCore). At this point there are basic types to classify the kinematics of the prosthesis:

1. Clinical classification (unconstrained, semiconstrained, constrained) defines the behavior compared with the physiological motion pattern; for example, the unconstrained Charité most closely imitates the natural motion pattern by having a changing center of rotation (COR) during flexion-extension and lateral bending motion. ProDisc-L or Maverick has a fixed COR and forces the segment to run in a predefined motion pattern.

2. Biomechanical classification defines the mechanical stop of the prosthesis. Constrained devices have a mechanical stop within the normal physiological range of motion, semiconstrained devices have the mechanical stop outside the range of normal physiological motion. In contrast, unconstrained devices are without mechanical stop. Depending on these kinematics, the condition of the facets plays a more (unconstrained devices) or less (semiconstrained and constrained devices) important role.

◆ Indications

In most of the randomized and prospective trials total lumbar disk replacement can be performed in male and female patients aged 18 to 60 years with single- or double-level intervertebral disk disease.[8] Before indicating a total disk replacement surgery the patients should undergo at least 6 months of failed conservative or nonoperative treatments.[8]

To receive an optimal treatment outcome some critical factors for a total lumbar disk replacement surgery should be considered previous to surgery, including the mobility of the segment (depending on degree of degeneration), the condition of posterior elements (facets), the profile, the distance, the type and kinematics of prosthesis, as well as the surgeon's experience. Sizing, positioning, and anticipated kinematics of the implant are essential to achieve a good surgical result.[9] Aside from these factors it is vital to adhere the indications properly[5] and select the patients carefully.

In a simple clinical classification that has been related to outcome success [clinical success related classification (CSRC)] for total disk replacement with the ProDisc-L, three groups of indications can be classified: ideal, good, and expanded indications.

Group I represents the "ideal" indications group with the best clinical outcome. The group includes patients with dominant low back pain with monosegmental lumbar symptomatic DDD with or without herniation or patients with large central herniation. The patients should not have had previous surgeries (**Table 21–1**).

Patients with less disk height loss ($>$ 5 mm) do have the tendency to reach better results than patients with a more significant loss of disk height ($<$ 5 mm).

Studies with the full prosthesis ProDisc-L in this indications group have shown the effectiveness and safety of this treatment method.[10]

Table 21–1 Indication Groups and Criteria for Total Lumbar Disk Replacement

Indication Group	Criteria	Success Rate (%)
Ideal	Monosegmental lumbar symptomatic degenerative disk disease (DDD) with or without herniation Large central herniation No previous surgery	98
Good	Bisegmental lumbar symptomatic DDD with or without herniation Failed disk surgery syndrome without laminectomy or severe facet alteration	94
Expanded	Postfusion adjacent level instabilities Instabilities at more than two levels Degenerative scoliosis Degenerative spondylolisthesis (grade I and II)	83

Group II represents patients with "good" indications. Patients with the existence of bisegmental lumbar symptomatic DDD with or without herniation, or failed disk surgery syndromes without laminectomy or severe facet alteration are indicated as "good" for TDR.

In these groups of patients clinical success rates typically reach the higher 80% range (**Table 21–1**).

Group III, the "expanded indications group," includes patients with multilevel disk degeneration (more than two levels), patients with postfusion adjacent level instabilities, and patients with mild or moderate degenerative scoliosis ($<$ 25 degree Cobb angle) or degenerative self-reducible spondylolisthesis (grade I and II) (**Table 21–1**).

In this group of patients we can also achieve very good clinical success rates similar to those of group II. Due to the lack of long-term outcomes and the relatively small cohort of patients who have been treated so far, these indications cannot be recommended at this point for regenerative treatment modality. A larger number of patients as well as more studies on this group are necessary.

◆ Contraindications

Total disk replacement is contraindicated in patients who have inherently reduced load-bearing capacities of the end plates and vertebral bodies due to major underlying bone pathology such as osteoporosis, osteopathy, or bone metabolism diseases. Patients with primarily posterior-element pathologies such as lytic spondylolisthesis, canal stenosis, hypertrophic spondylarthrosis, significant facet joint changes (grade III–IV), and nerve root compression should be excluded from receiving TDR surgeries, as well as patients with segmental defects due to spondylitis, tumors, or fractures.[8] The use of TDR devices in patients with predominantly psychosocial factors and patients with severe obesity (body mass index $>$ 35) are also contraindicated.

Segments with severe end plate irregularities that make the positioning of the devices difficult should also be excluded in

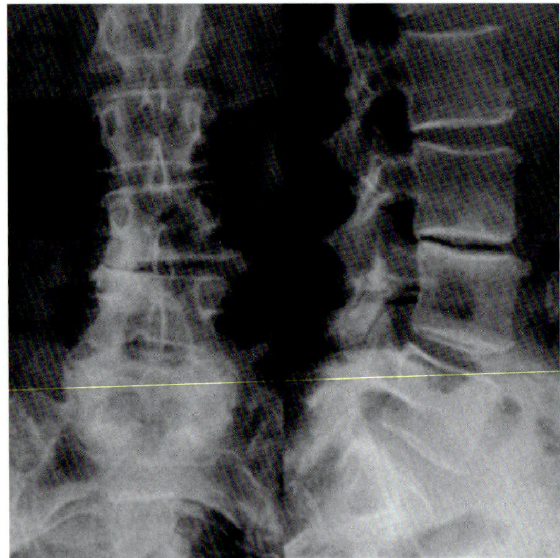 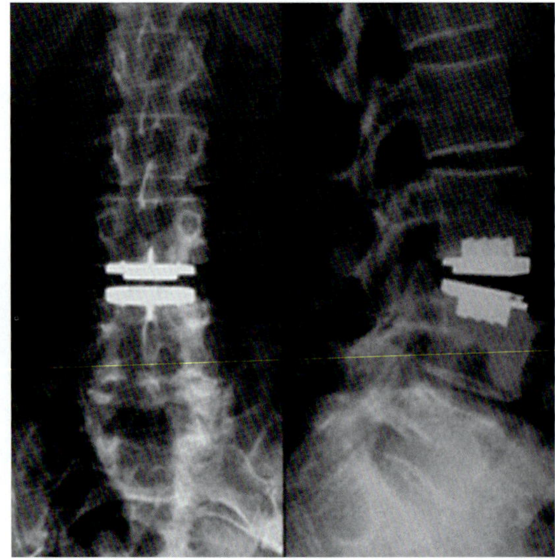

A   B

Figure 21–1   (A) Preoperative radiographs (anteroposterior, lateral). **(B)** Postoperative radiographs (anteroposterior, lateral).

the first application because the risk of either or both malposition and subsidence in these cases is relatively high.

◆ Case Studies

Group I: "Ideal" Indications

- ◆ Monosegmental lumbar symptomatic DDD with or without herniation
- ◆ Large central herniation
- ◆ No previous surgery

Case Study 1

A 42-year-old female patient with severe vertical segmental instability and severe increasing low back pain for 2 years. All conservative treatment failed. The patient was treated with a total disk replacement surgery in level L3–L4 using the ProDisc-L device (**Fig. 21–1A,B**).

Case Study 2

A 57-year-old female patient with vertical segmental instabilities (VISs) L4–L5, diskopathy L3–L4, and severe low back pain had had no previous surgery. Conservative treatment was unsuccessful (**Fig. 21–2A,B**).

Group II: "Good" Indications

- ◆ Bisegmental lumbar symptomatic DDD with or without herniation
- ◆ Failed disk surgery syndrome without laminectomy or severe facet alteration

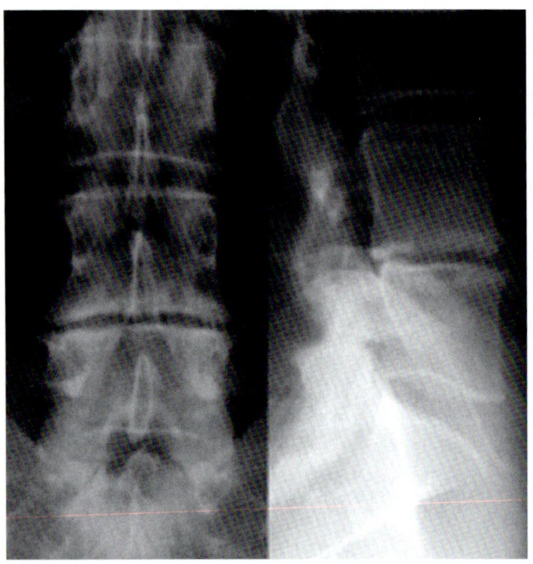 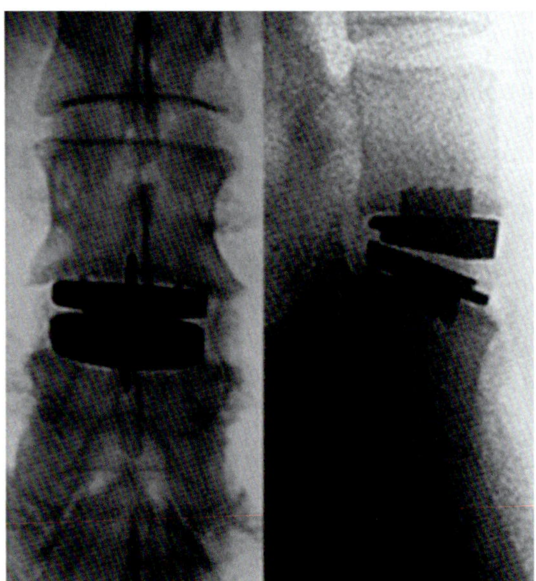

A   B

Figure 21–2   (A) Preoperative radiographs (anteroposterior, lateral). **(B)** Postoperative radiographs (anteroposterior, lateral).

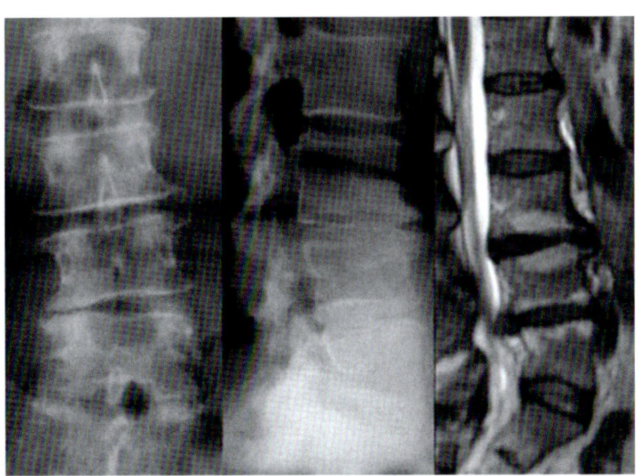

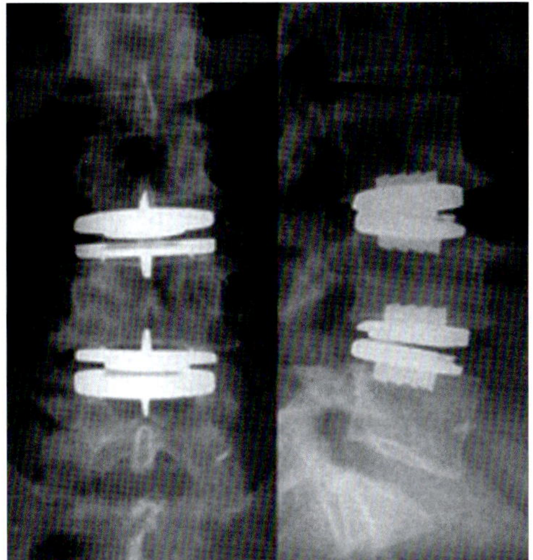

Figure 21–3   **(A)** Preoperative radiographs (anteroposterior, lateral) and magnetic resonance imaging. **(B)** Postoperative radiographs (anteroposterior, lateral).

Case Study 1

A 52-year-old female patient with VSIs in L3–L5, fixed kyphosis in L3–L4, fixed scoliosis in L4–L5 with herniation, severe low back pain, and rotated dorsal position L5. The patient was treated with a ProDisc-L full prosthesis at levels L3–L5 (**Fig. 21–3A,B**).

Case Study 2

A 48-year-old female patient with VSIs, severe low back pain, and more than 2 years of unsuccessful conservative treatment (**Fig. 21–4A,B**).

Group III: "Expanded" Indications

- Postfusion adjacent level instabilities
- Instabilities at more than two levels
- Degenerative scoliosis
- Degenerative spondylolisthesis (grade I and II)

Case Study 1

A 34-year-old male with 360 degree fusion of L4–S1 in 1996 due to failed back syndrome in 1995. Progression of adjacent instability L3–L4, severe low back pain, and unsuccessful conservative treatment followed. The affected level L3–L5 was treated with an implantation of a ProDisc-L full prosthesis (**Fig. 21–5A–C**).

Case Study 2

A 56-year-old female with VSI at L1–S1, degenerative scoliosis at L3–L5, lateral slip at L3–L4 who suffered from severe low back pain (**Fig. 21–6A,B**).

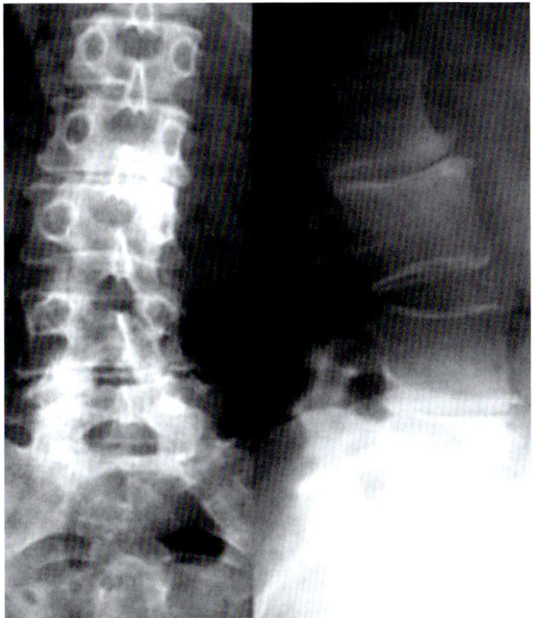

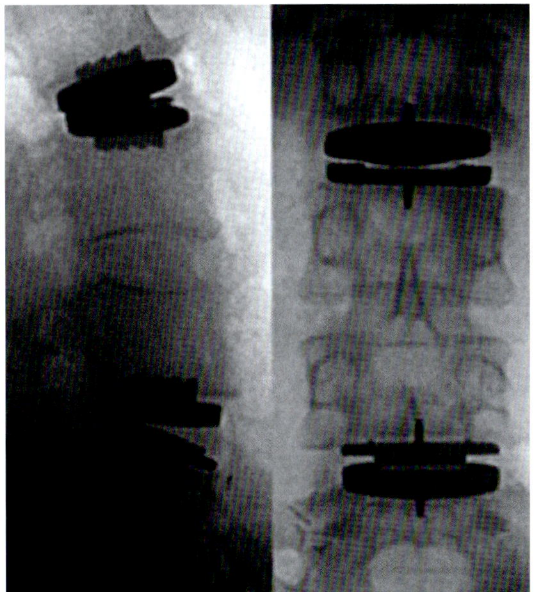

Figure 21–4   **(A)** Preoperative radiographs (anteroposterior, lateral). **(B)** Postoperative radiographs (anteroposterior, lateral).

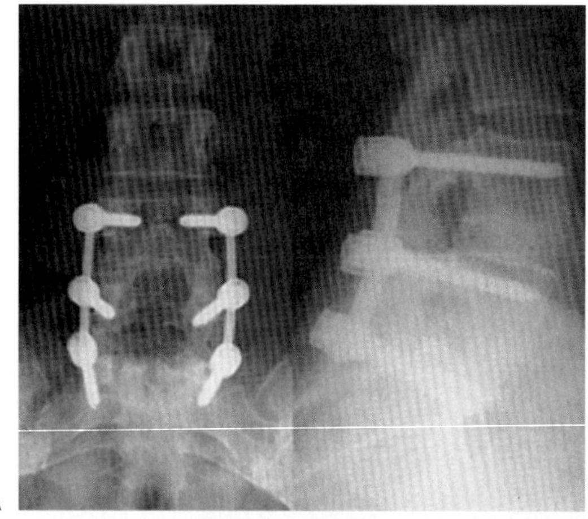

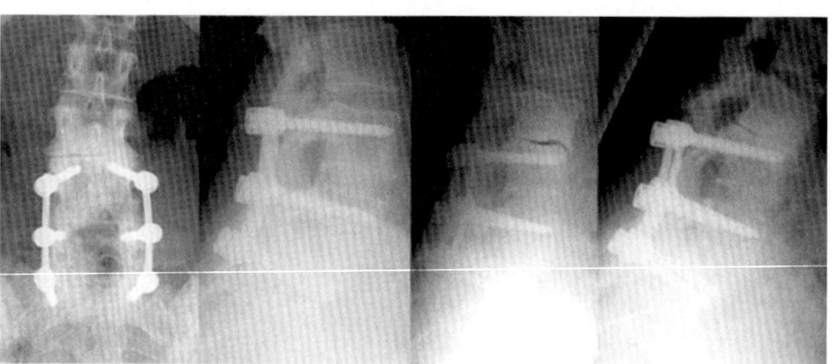

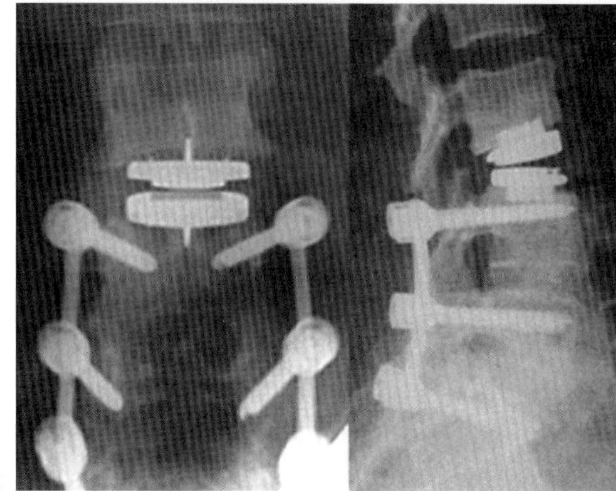

Figure 21–5   **(A)** Postoperative radiographs 36 months after fusion (anteroposterior, lateral). **(B)** Postoperative radiographs 60 months after fusion (anteroposterior, lateral, flexion, extension). **(C)** Postoperative radiographs after total disk replacement (anteroposterior, lateral).

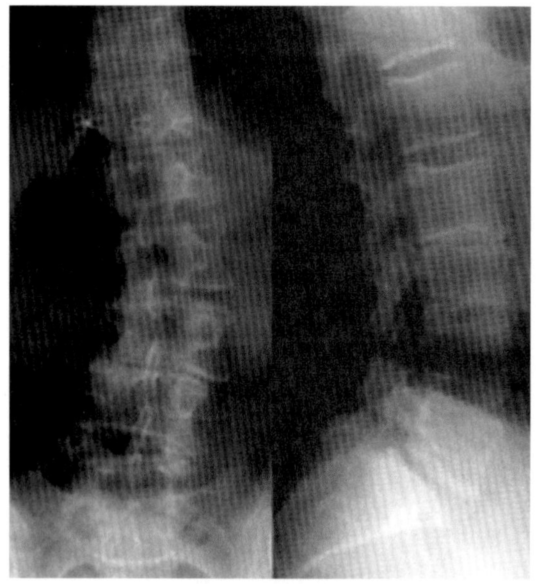

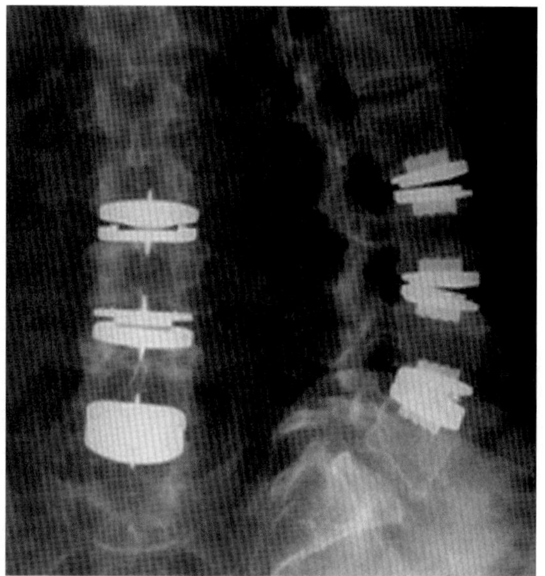

Figure 21–6   **(A)** Preoperative radiographs (anteroposterior, lateral). **(B)** Postoperative radiographs (anteroposterior, lateral).

◆ Conclusion

Accurate indications and precise implantation are necessary to achieve good success rates in motion-preserving treatments.[9] Various studies with the total disk prosthesis ProDisc-L have shown the efficacy and safety of the implant and good clinical outcome rates.[10–13]

According to the success outcomes in total lumbar disk replacement, the three indication groups can be classified using CSRC as ideal, good, and expanded indications. The clinical outcome for all three groups is very satisfactory. Compared with the experiences of patients within the ideal and good indications group, there is a lack of clinical experience for the expanded indications group. Long-term follow-up and an adequate number of patients are required to make statements about the clinical success rate for patients of this group. Further investigations are necessary to receive long-term follow-up for every indications group.

References

1. Delamarter RB, Fribourg DM, Kanim LE, Bae H. ProDisc artificial total lumbar disc replacement: introduction and early results from the United States Clinical Trial. Spine 2003;28:S167–S175
2. Bertagnoli R. Disc surgery in motion. SpineLine 2004;Nov/Dec: 23–28
3. Bertagnoli R, Kumar S. Indications for full prosthetic disc arthroplasty: a correlation of clinical outcome against a variety of indications. Eur Spine J 2002;11(Suppl. 2):S131–S136
4. Bertagnoli R, Karg A, Voigt S. Lumbar partial disc replacement. Orthop Clin North Am 2005;36:341–347
5. Bertagnoli R. Review of modern treatment options for degenerative disc disease. In: Kaech DL, Jinkins JR, eds. Spinal Restabilization Procedures. Amsterdam: Elsevier Science; 2002:B.V:365–375
6. Tropiano P, Huang RC, Girardi FP, Marnay T. Lumbar disc replacement. preliminary results with the ProDisc II after a minimum follow-up period of 1 year. J Spinal Disord Tech 2003;16:362–368
7. Huang RC, Girardi F, Cammisa FP Jr, Wright TM. The implications of constraint in lumbar total disc replacement. J Spinal Disord Tech 2003;16:412–417
8. McAfee PC. The indications for lumbar and cervical disc replacement. Spine J 2004;4(Suppl 6):177S–181S
9. Bertagnoli R, Zigler J, Karg A, Voigt S. Complications and strategies for revision surgery in total lumbar disc replacement. Orthop Clin North Am 2005;36:389–395
10. Bertagnoli R, Yue JJ, Sha RV, et al. The treatment of disabling single-level lumbar discogenic low back pain with total disc arthroplasty utilizing the ProDisc prosthesis. a prospective study with 2-year minimum follow-up. Spine 2005;30:2192–2199
11. Bertagnoli R, Marnay T, Mayer HM. Total Disc Replacement for Degenerative Disc Disease in the Lumbar Spine. Tüttlingen: Spine Solutions GmbH;2003
12. Bertagnoli R, Yue JJ, Sha RV, et al. The treatment of disabling multi-level lumbar discogenic low back pain with total disc arthroplasty utilizing the ProDisc prosthesis. a prospective study with 2-year minimum follow-up. Spine 2005;30:9;2230–2236
13. Bertagnoli R, Yue JJ, Kershaw T, et al. lumbar total disc arthroplasty utilizing the ProDisc prosthesis in smokers versus non-smokers: a prospective study with 2-year minimum follow-up. In process.

22

CHARITÉ Artificial Disc

Fred H. Geisler

- ◆ **Rationale for an Artificial Disk**
- ◆ **History**
- ◆ **The CHARITÉ Artificial Disc**
- ◆ **Clinical History of the CHARITÉ Artificial Disc**
- ◆ **Surgical Treatment**

- ◆ **The FDA IDE Multicenter Trial of the CHARITÉ Artificial Disc**
- ◆ **Revision Techniques**
- ◆ **Outcomes**
- ◆ **Conclusion**

The etiology of low back pain is widely variable and largely unknown. However, degenerative disk disease (DDD) can lead to disk dehydration, annular tears, and loss of disk height or collapse, and can result in abnormal motion of the segment and biomechanical instability causing pain.[1] The diagnosis of DDD is determined as a result of radiographic diagnostic testing such as magnetic resonance imaging in conjunction with patient history and symptomatology. In patients suffering from intractable low back pain caused by DDD, nonoperative treatment including physical therapy, therapeutic injections, and management with analgesics often fails. In these cases, surgical intervention may be considered.

Several techniques for lumbar fusion have been developed over the past 50 years that have become the standard of care for these patients, including rigid segmental pedicle screw fixation, titanium and polymer interbody cage fusion, and fusion involving preprocessed allograft interbody spacers. In addition to instrumentation and fusion devices, osteobiological materials have been developed to reduce or eliminate the need for iliac crest autograft while maintaining a high rate of solid arthrodesis. These include demineralized bone matrix, platelet-rich plasma, bone marrow aspirate, stem cell harvesting technology, bone morphogenetic proteins (BMPs), and numerous osteoconductive bone graft extenders.

But while lumbar fusion serves to eliminate abnormal motion and instability at the symptomatic degenerated levels to reduce or eliminate low back pain for patients with DDD, reported clinical outcomes for these procedures vary widely. A recent meta-analysis performed by Geisler et al[2] of clinical outcomes with minimum 2-year follow-up resulting from lumbar fusion procedures for the treatment of DDD showed the elimination of lumbar segmental motion resulted in a significant reduction in pain and subsequent improvement in overall function. However, as demonstrated in a cadaver study by Cunningham et al,[3] lumbar fusion can lead to increased (abnormal) motion at levels similar to a lumbar fusion.

◆ Rationale for an Artificial Disk

Fusion is designed to eliminate the normal motion of one or more lumbar segments. Fusion is successful in many cases because the motion itself is the root cause of pain owing to the inability of the degenerative segment to support the weight of the body comfortably. Thus, when the segment is fused, it no longer moves and therefore cannot cause pain. Solid fusion, however, can result in stress and increased motion in the segments adjacent to the fused level,[3,4] which may initiate or accelerate the degenerative disease process in adjacent segments. Hilibrand and colleagues[5] demonstrated this concept in the cervical spine. The inherent problem with surgical arthrodesis of the degenerative lumbar segment is that it merely masks the true disease process by eliminating the intervertebral motion and its normal physiological function. In using lumbar artificial disk technology, the restoration and maintenance of normal physiological motion are provided rather than the alternative—the elimination of motion.[6–9]

The premise of surgery involving a lumbar artificial disk is fourfold: (1) correct abnormal motion; (2) restore intervertebral lumbar segmental space height, lordosis, and instantaneous axis of rotation; (3) maintain the corrected normal intervertebral motion over time; and (4) relieve pain and restore function. If these goals are achieved, it stands to reason that the segments adjacent to the dynamically stable segment would not be subject to abnormal loads and motions, and therefore, deceleration or elimination of adjacent level disk disease would follow.

◆ History

Numerous artificial disks have been designed during the past 35 years, but most have never been produced.[10] There are four types of dynamic stabilization systems derived

160

from artificial disk technology: (1) nucleus pulposus replacements with a hygroscopic gel or fluid-filled cylindrical sacs (for use after standard diskectomy in which the annulus maintains normal disk space height);[11–13] (2) posterior dynamic stabilization systems (which increase posterior column stiffness);[14–16] and (3) total lumbar joint replacement (which replaces both anterior and posterior lumbar motion segment components). Currently, these total joint replacement devices are not available in any U.S. Food and Drug Administration (FDA) trial, nor are any being used elsewhere in the world. Finally, total disk replacement is used to replace the entire lumbar disk. Because these devices replace only the disk portion of the joint, a partial joint replacement, they require healthy facet joints as well as intact posterior ligaments and muscular structures. An artificial lumbar disk should reproduce the biomechanical functions of a normal disk. Additionally, an artificial disk should reduce the mechanical forces transmitted to the adjacent levels, slowing or halting the degenerative changes. A total diskectomy eliminates the chance of a disk herniation and would probably retard spondylosis, stenosis, and instability at the dynamically stabilized segment. By restoring the disk space height, an artificial disk should restore normal motion, height, and lordosis; decrease the forces on the adjacent level(s); and prevent compression on the existing nerve roots at the stabilized level.

The design of artificial lumbar disks has multiple, very strict requirements. These devices must possess superb mechanical strength and endurance. They are designed to last several decades because many will be implanted in young individuals. The base materials need to be biocompatible without causing significant surrounding inflammatory reaction either due to the base material reaction or secondary to any wear-related debris. The base material or potential debris of these devices must not produce organotoxic or carcinogenic reaction.

The biomechanical functional movement requirements of an artificial lumbar disk are stringent because they need to replicate the full biomechanical functions of a normal disk. The normal motion of a lumbar segment includes independent translation and rotation in all three planes of motion (flexion-extension, lateral bending, and axial rotation). Normal motion is often represented as a factor of coupled motion in two planes. The implant-related geometrical configuration and materials would determine the static configuration, dynamic motion, schematics, and any constrained nature of the motion. The exact placement of the artificial lumbar disk in the disk space is determined by its biomechanical design. Different designs require different degrees of placement accuracy. Fixed pivot devices are believed to require a higher placement precision than devices that include a sliding core or an elastopolymer to decrease forces on the facets.

Potential problems exist with regard to the choice of any base materials with which to construct an artificial disk. There is the possibility of the load-bearing surfaces becoming worn during the clinical lifetime of the device. Broadly, the materials are categorized into three groups: metal-on-metal, metal-ceramic, and metal-plastic designs. Those composed of metal-on-metal material have the potential of either or both metal and metal ionic debris. The ceramic component may shatter in metal/ceramic designs. Plastic wear or cold flow may occur in metal/plastic disks. The plastic components [cobalt-chromium-molybdenum (CoCrMo) and ultra high molecular weight polyethylene] in the current artificial hip and knee designs survive a mean of 10 years before requiring revision.[17,18] If an artificial lumbar disk were made of these same base materials, it may be inferred that the plastic component would also require replacement at a mean of 10 years following implantation. There are, however, three primary differences between total joint replacement and artificial disk replacement. First, with each step the hip and the knee move ~50 degrees, whereas the lumbar spine only tilts a few degrees. This greatly decreases the so-called sandpaper effect by more than one order of magnitude for all base materials. Second, in the CHARITÉ Artificial Disc design (DePuy Spine, Raynham, MA), the high-density polyethylene moves to reduce the stresses, is not constrained, and has two opposite surfaces of contact that share the movement. This is in marked contrast to the hips, where the plastic is constrained in a high-pressure, ball and socket–type metal-plastic joint greatly accelerating wear on the plastic. The unconstrained sliding plastic core in the CHARITÉ lumbar disk has no pressure points. Furthermore, in a report from Europe, the authors noted the absence of plastic wear 10 years after implantation,[19] which implies that the estimation of the lifetime of the material is greater than that used in the hips and knees.

Four artificial disk designs have been the subject of U.S. FDA Investigational Device Exemption (IDE) trials (**Fig. 22–1**). It is notable that these devices do not repair the posterior column degenerative changes, nor do they augment them. In fact, a contraindication to application of any of these devices would be spondylolysis or significant spondylosis, with facet joint hypertrophy and potential for ongoing nerve root compression. These devices have either an unconstrained or a semiconstrained design with a fixed center of rotation.

The original artificial ProDisc (Synthes, Inc., West Chester, PA) was designed by Thierry Marnay in the late 1980s. The current ProDisc design has a spherical articulation with two CoCrMo end plates and an ultra high molecular weight polyethylene core fixed to the lower device end plate, yielding a semiconstrained system. This design provides for a fixed pivot that places the instantaneous axis of rotation within the caudal vertebral body (VB) rather than the disk space. The ProDisc is affixed to the vertebral end plates by a central keel (or fin), which is driven into the vertebral end plates. Enrollment in the ProDisc IDE study has concluded, and the study is expected to be completed by the end of 2004 after a 2-year follow-up period. The FlexiCore artificial disk (Stryker Spine, Allendale, NJ) is a metal-on-metal semiconstrained device with a CoCrMo load-bearing surface with a 13 mm ball and socket joint, which places the stationary center of rotation centrally between the end plates. It has teeth on the outer ring of the implant end plates for fixation to the outer ring of the vertebral end plates. The U.S. FDA IDE trial of the FlexiCore artificial disk began in August 2003. The Maverick artificial disk (Medtronic Sofamor Danek, Memphis, TN) has a

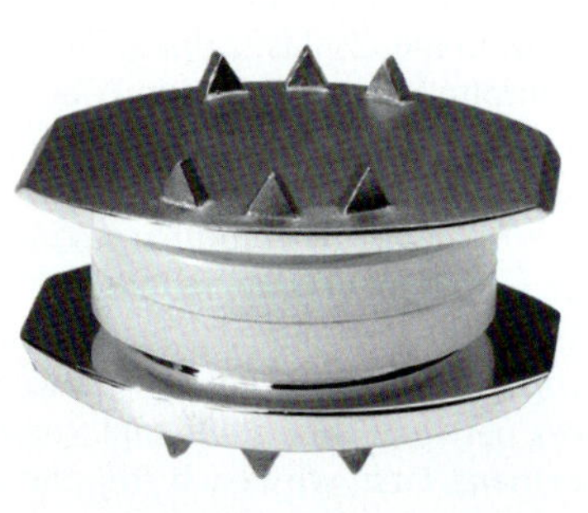

CHARITÉ™ Artificial Disc

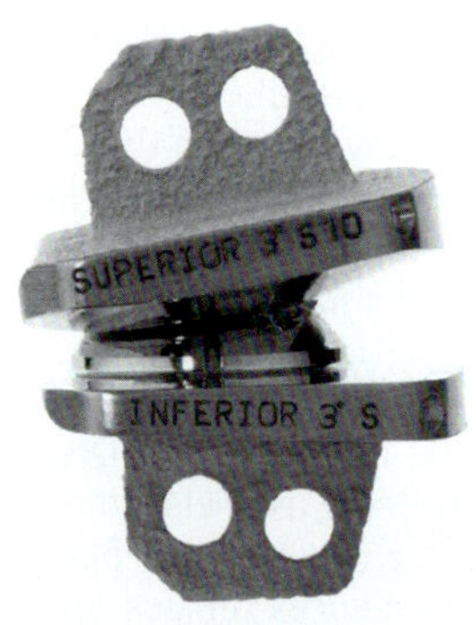

MAVERICK™

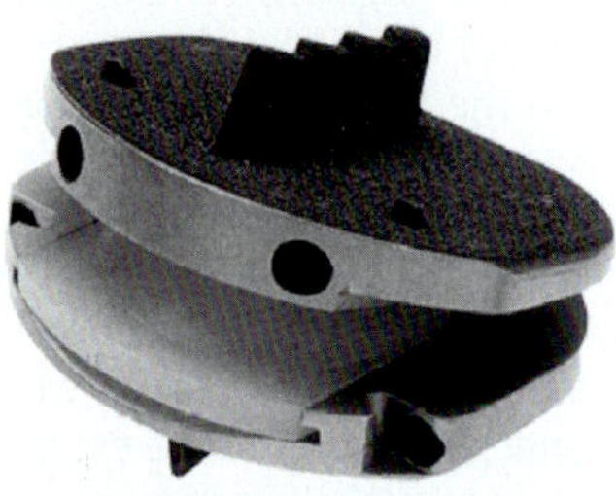

ProDisc®

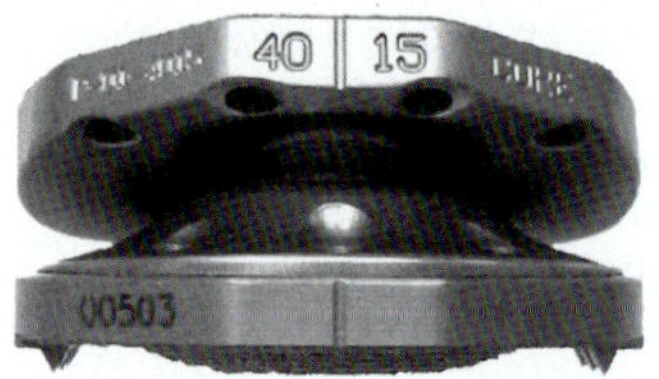

FlexiCore™

Figure 22–1   The four lumbar artificial disks in or finished with U.S. Food and Drug Administration I Investigational Device Exemption clinical trials.

semiconstrained metal-on-metal design. Like the ProDisc, the Maverick implant has central keels that are driven into the vertebral end plates for fixation and stability. Enrollment in the Maverick IDE trial has concluded and FDA approval is expected in 2006.

◆ The CHARITÉ Artificial Disc

The CHARITÉ Artificial Disc (**Fig. 22–2A–D**) was designed to duplicate the kinematics and dynamics of a normal lumbar motion segment[10,20] while restoring disk space height and motion segment flexibility. The CHARITÉ Artificial Disc is composed of two CoCrMo end plates and a free-floating ultra high molecular weight polyethylene core. The primary attachment of the plates is made possible by three anterior and posterior "teeth," which are forcefully implanted into the cranial and caudal vertebral end plates. Layers of plasma-sprayed porous titanium and calcium phosphate were added to the Charité disk in 1998. This coating provides for potential osseous ingrowth and long-term stability of the plates after implantation.[21] The plates are currently available in seven footprint geometrical configurations (including three wide footprints) adaptable to the size of the vertebral end plates, each with four available angles (0, 5, 7.5, and 10 degrees). This allows for built-in lordosis with variations of 0 to 20 degrees. The optimal device placement is 2 mm dorsal of the sagittal vertebral body midline and in the midline from right-left perspective with the metal end plates on the circumferential cortical bone (**Fig. 22–3A,B**).

The unconstrained design allows the core to translate dynamically within the disk space during normal spinal motion, moving posteriorly in flexion and anteriorly in lumbar extension. The mobile sliding core of the Charité disk works in a similar fashion to the mobile knee bearing in many of the contemporary knee implant designs. In essence, this could be considered a second-generation device or an advanced type design over a fixed pivot, much like the mobile core in the knee is considered an advanced design over fixed bearings. The Charité design not only provides unloading of the posterior facet structures during this normal replication of motion but also allows forgiveness for slight off-center positioning of the implant.

In a cadaveric model, Cunningham and associates[3] demonstrated that the center of rotation for Charité closely mimicked that of a normal lumbar disk at the level of implantation and at the superior adjacent level. Fusion, however, greatly distorted the center of rotation at the level of implantation and at the superior adjacent level. In addition, compared with a normal intact segment, the Charité device did not adversely affect the range of motion (ROM) at adjacent levels, whereas fusion caused a "marked increase" in adjacent level motion. The coupled translation with angulation was noted in the normal spine and reproduced at the level with the CHARITÉ Artificial Disc (**Fig. 22–4A,B**). He further noted that the ROM was increased at the adjacent levels fused, in marked contrast to the placement of the CHARITÉ Artificial Disc, which preserved motion at both the level operated and the adjacent levels (**Fig. 22–4C**). This increased range

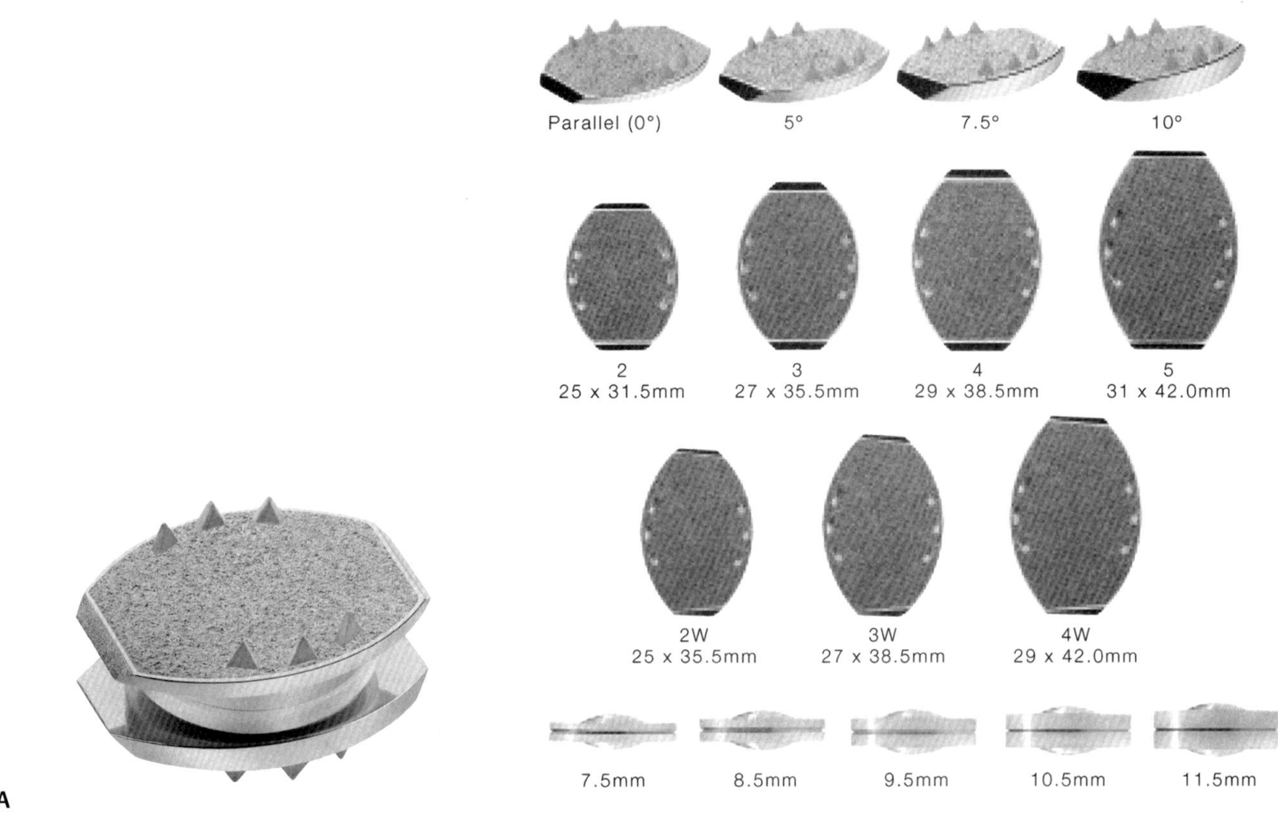

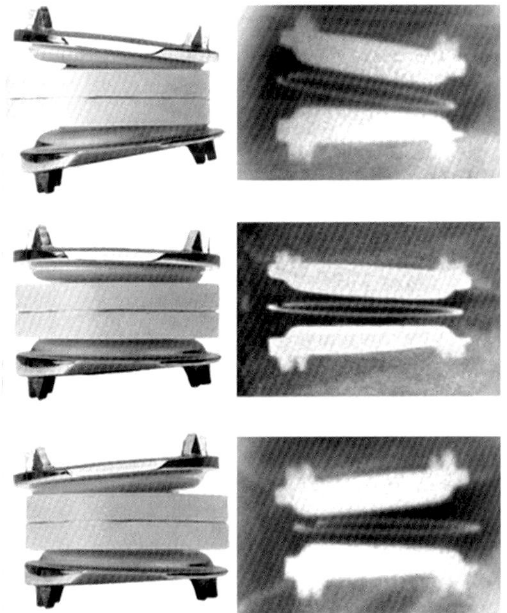

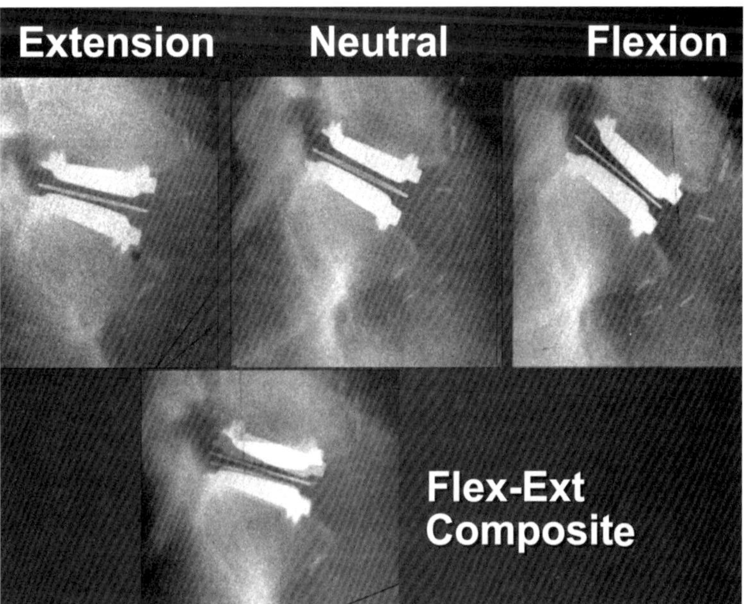

Figure 22–2 **(A)** CHARITÉ Artificial Disc in an assembled form. **(B)** The components of the CHARITÉ Artificial Disc are available in multiple end plate sizes and core heights with four lordotic end plate styles allowing for restoration of lordosis from 0 to 20 degrees. **(C)** The translation provided by the mobile core of the CHARITÉ Artificial Disc, also shown on **(D)** plain flexion-extension radiographs.

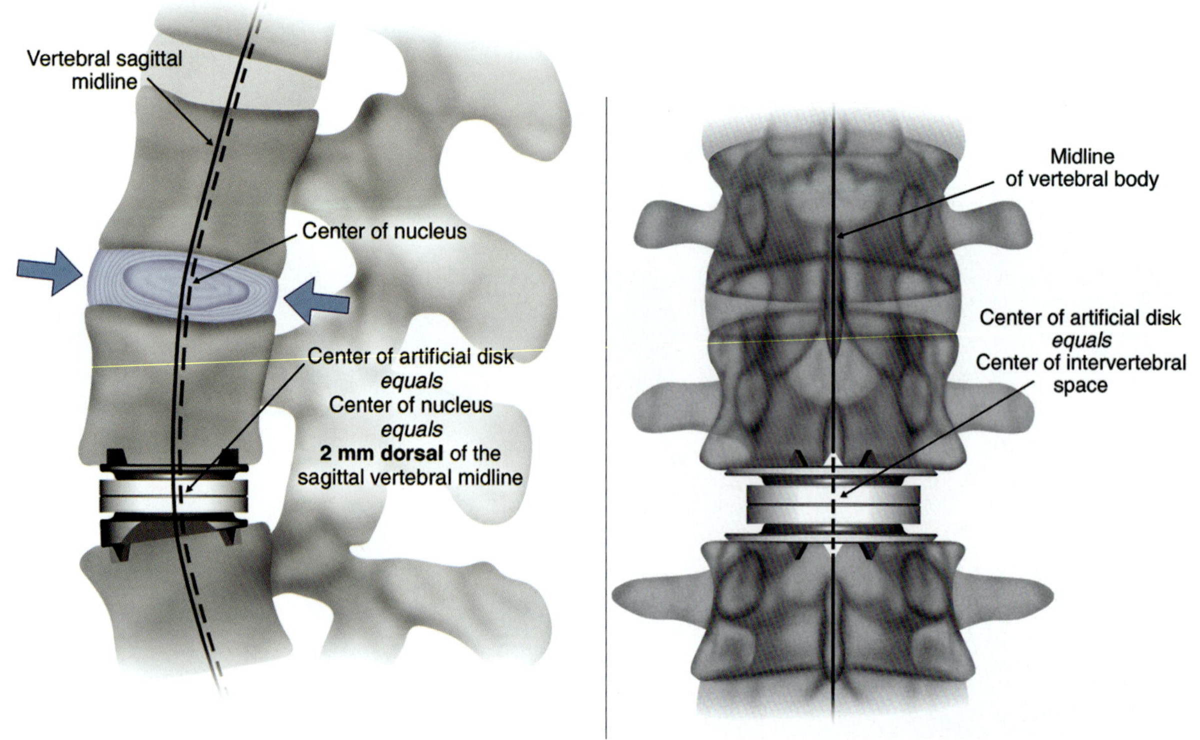

Figure 22–3   To match the location of the floating center of rotation of a normal lumbar disk, the CHARITÉ Artificial Disc should be placed **(A)** 2 mm dorsal to the sagittal midline in the lateral view and **(B)** in the midline in the anteroposterior view.

of motion and hence forces and stress at the adjacent level is hypothesized to be a major contributing factor to accelerating adjacent level degenerative changes. The cortical rim of the vertebral bone is mechanically stronger than the central cancellous portion of the vertebral body. To lessen the chance for subsidence of the body into the bony end plate the largest CHARITÉ metal end plate should be utilized (**Fig. 22–5A–C**).

Finite element analysis supports this concept. In a two-level, three-dimensional, nonlinear, finite element model, Moumene and Geisler[22] described the effect of fusion compared with CHARITÉ disk–related treatment on the facet loading of the adjacent segment. In axial rotation, fusion increased the load on the facet joints at the adjacent level by 96% compared with the normal intact nonoperated segment. The CHARITÉ device decreased the facet joint load at the adjacent level by 50% compared with the normal intact nonoperated segment (**Fig. 22–6A,B**).

◆ Clinical History of the CHARITÉ Artificial Disc

The CHARITÉ Artificial Disc has been used outside the United States since 1987, and in the United States since 2000. Worldwide experience with this unconstrained anatomical replacement disk now comprises more than 11,000 cases. Cinotti and colleagues[23] reported a 70% rate of good or excellent clinical outcome in 46 Italian patients. In 1997, Lemaire and coworkers[24] described a series of 105 Charité disk-treated patients who underwent follow-up

evaluation for 5 years. They reported 84.8% with good or excellent clinical outcome. In 2005, Lemaire[25,26] described 10-year results obtained in 100 patients in whom the CHARITÉ disk was implanted. He reported good or excellent clinical outcome in 90% and a return to work rate of 91%. Lemaire reported no device failures in this or an earlier series. David[27] reported good or excellent clinical outcome in 75% of his series of 92 patients with 5-year follow-up. Zeegers et al[28] reported 50 patients in 1999 in a Dutch series, which showed 70% good results with 2-year follow-up. Recently, Lemaire[25,26] reported long-term follow-up of clinical and radiological outcomes for the CHARITÉ Artificial Disc with a minimum follow-up of 10 years. Of the 107 patients treated with the CHARITÉ Artificial Disc, 100 were followed for a minimum of 10 years (range 10–13.4 years). A total of 147 prostheses were implanted with 54 one-level and 45 two-level procedures and one three-level procedure. Clinically, 62% had an excellent outcome, 28% had a good outcome, and 10% had a poor outcome. Of the 95 eligible to return to work, 88 (91.5%) either returned to the same job as prior to surgery or a different job. Mean flexion-extension motion was 10.3 degrees for all levels (12.0 degrees at L3–L4, 9.6 degrees at L4–L5, 9.2 degrees at L5–S1). Slight subsidence was observed in two patients, but they did not require further surgery. No subluxation of the prostheses and no cases of spontaneous arthrodesis were identified. There was one case of disk height loss of 1 mm. Five patients required a secondary posterior arthrodesis. A good or excellent clinical outcome rate of 90% and a return-to-work rate of 91.5% compare favorably with results described in the literature for fusion for the treatment of lumbar DDD. David concluded that with a minimum follow-up of 10 years, the CHARITÉ Artificial Disc

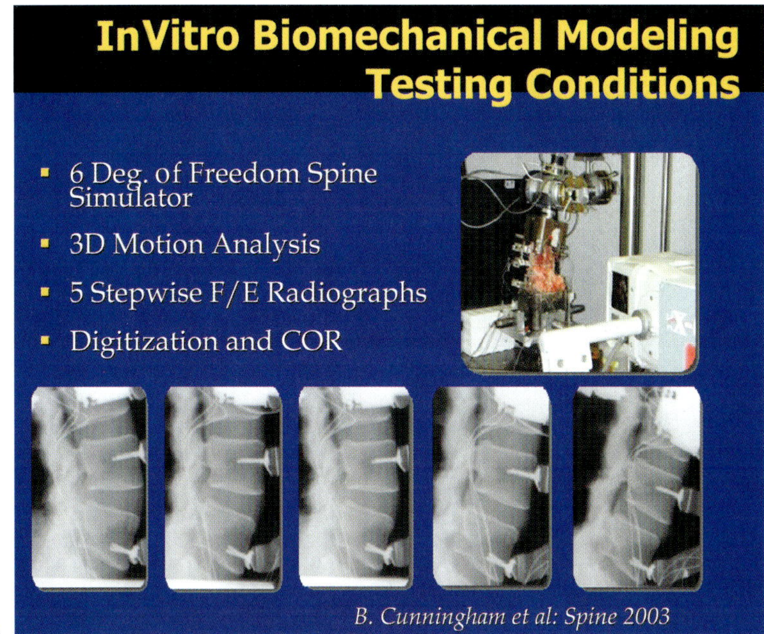

A

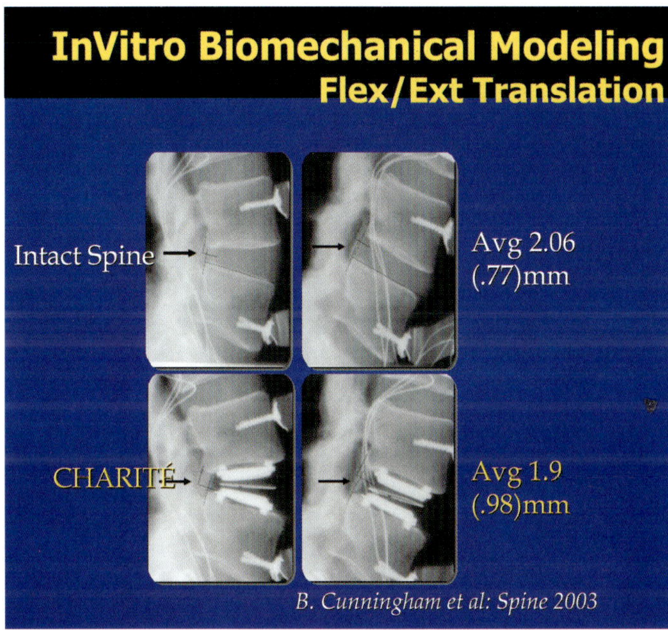

B

Figure 22–4 (*Continued*).

demonstrated excellent flexion/extension and lateral range of motion with no significant complications.

◆ Surgical Treatment

All surgeries were performed via an anterior retro- or transperitoneal approach, which was conducted by a general or vascular surgeon (**Fig. 22–7A,B**). After the direct anterior approach (L4–L5 or L5–S1) to the disk space is completed, the anterior longitudinal ligament is dissected to fit the width of the disk implant (**Fig. 22–7C,D**). A generous (complete) diskectomy is performed, with care taken not to disturb the osseous end plates, although all of the cartilaginous end plates are removed. The diskectomy is enlarged to expose the vertebral body circumferential rim of cortical bone. Posterior osteophytes are removed using a 0.25 in. chisel or a Kerrison punch (**Fig. 22–8A**). Usually the posterior annulus is completely removed but the posterior ligament is left intact. A trial sizer at this stage aids in determining the disk space preparation from the lateral fluoroscopy and also aids in determining the correct implant size (**Fig. 22–8B**). This disk space is prepared in anticipation of accepting the flat metal end plates of the CHARITÉ implant. Care is required during this stage not to damage the osseous end plates because these support the metal plates of the artificial disk. The removal of posterior osteophytes in this flattening of the end plates often allows the use of a larger CHARITÉ end plate (**Fig. 22–9**). Additionally, especially at L5–S1, the anterior longitudinal ligament that is undergoing degenerative

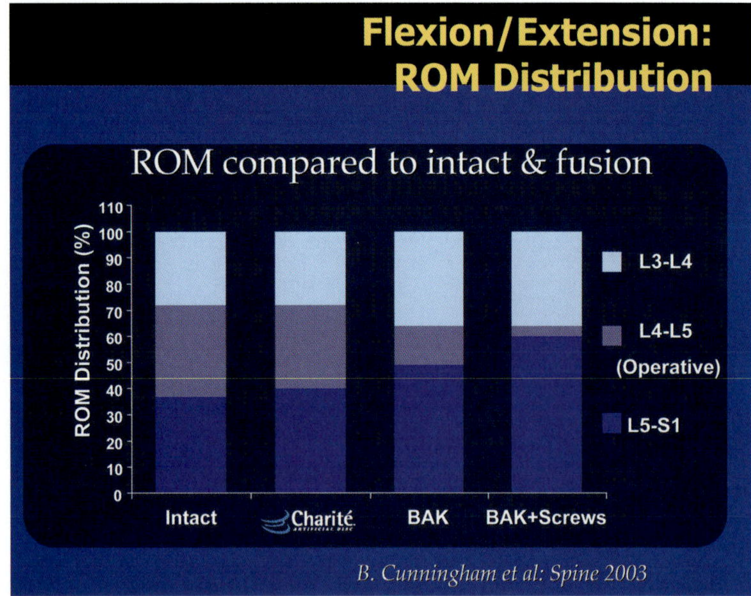

Figure 22–4   (A–C) Postoperative lateral radiographs showing the preservation of angular motion. Note the sliding of the core with the flexion-extension.

C

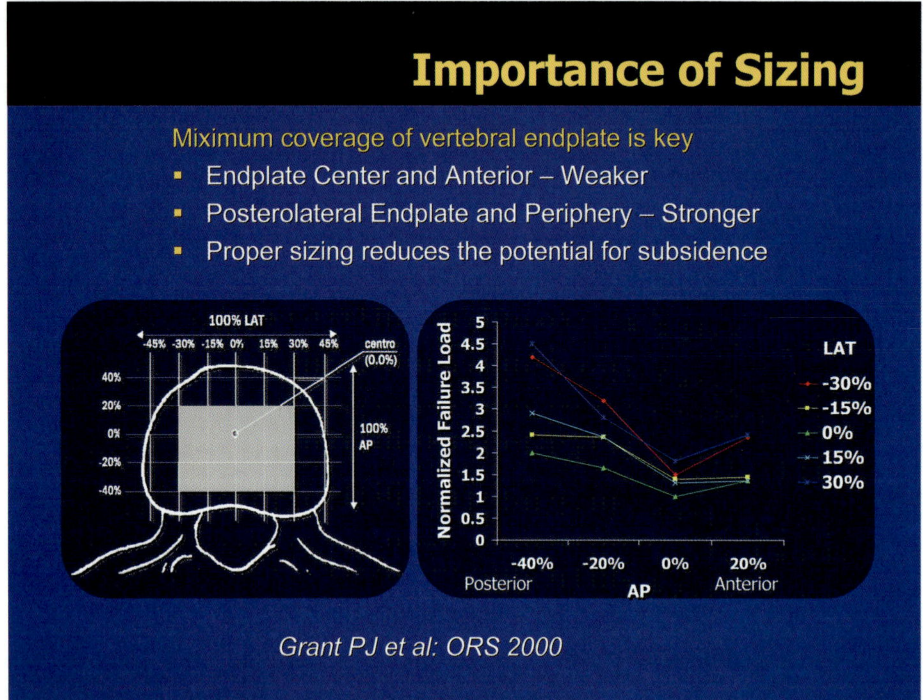

A

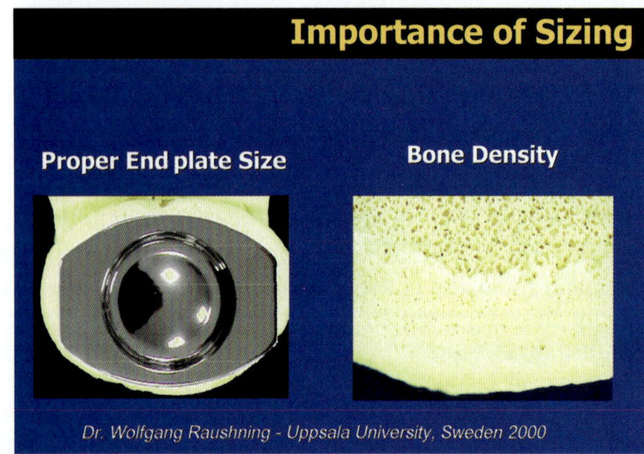

B

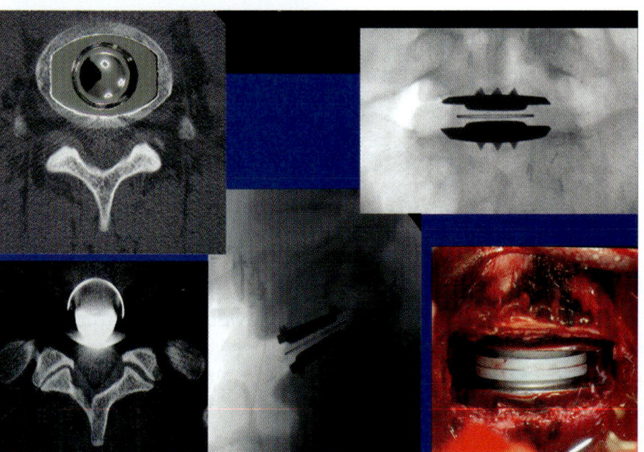

C

Figure 22–5   (A) The importance of end plate sizing is to have the end plate mechanically contact the cortical rim of bone for maximum strength. This increased strength has been demonstrated in both anteroposterior and lateral directions. **(B)** Shows a representative size of the implant relative to the bony end plate rim along with a magnification of the bony rim. **(C)** Intraoperative visualization of the CHARITÉ Artificial Disc and postoperative fluoroscope and computed tomography demonstrating this relationship between the bony rim and the end plate size.

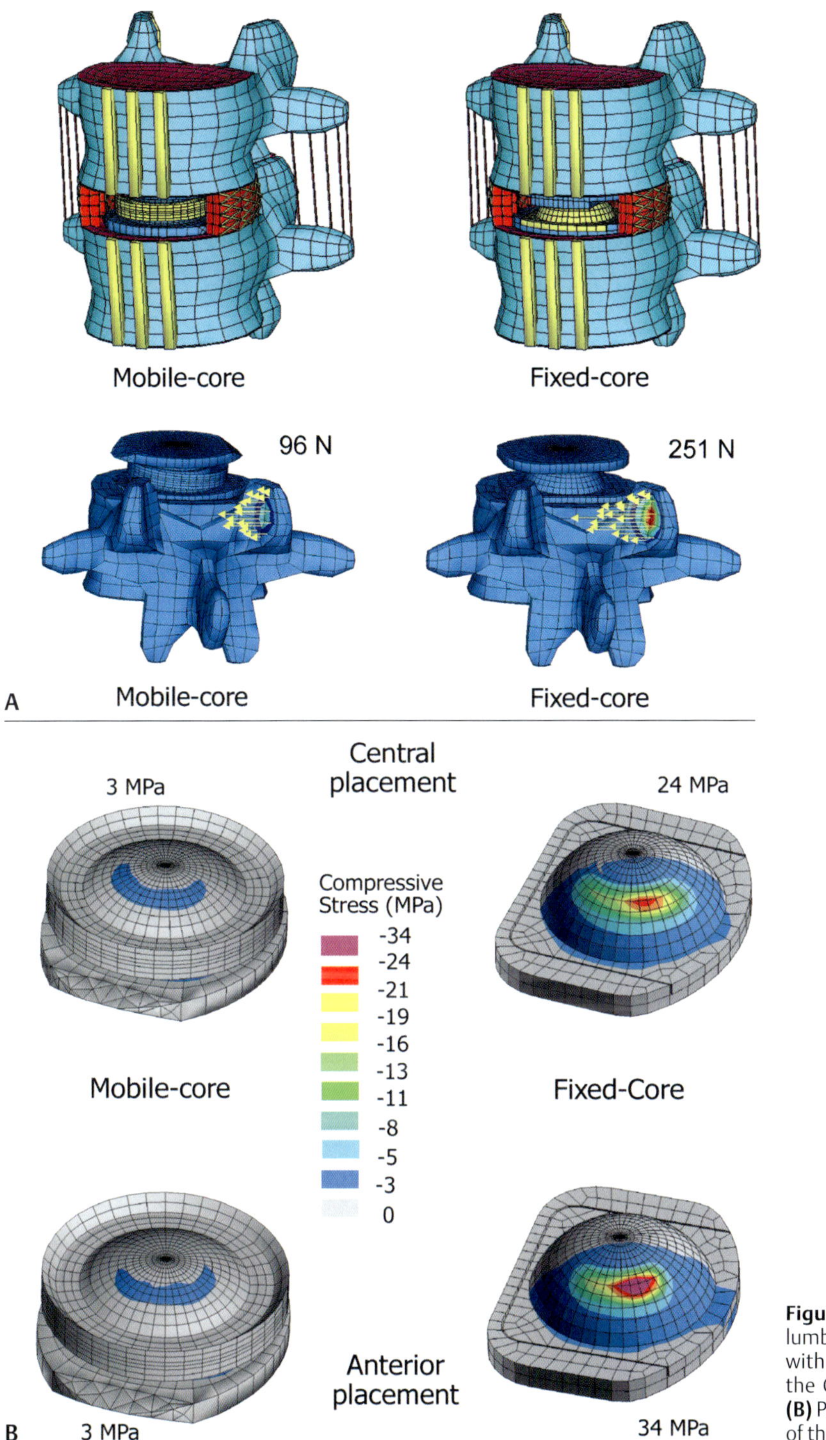

Figure 22–6 Fixed Element Analysis (FEA) model of the lumbar segment demonstrates increased force on the facet with a fixed-core design versus a mobile core such as in the CHARITÉ Artificial Disc. **(A)** Model and the facet views. **(B)** Pressure on the core with central and anterior placement of the center of the two mechanically different devices.

disease progression can be exceptionally thick (sometimes > 1 cm). The anterior longitudinal ligament needs to be removed to define clearly the anterior osseous margin so that after disk placement, its anterior cleats can be confirmed, fluoroscopically and visually, to be below the anterior cortical margin.

Once the disk material and cartilaginous end plates are removed, a sizer is used to measure the disk space fluoroscopically to choose the matching metal end plate footprint. A spreader is then placed into the disk space to produce parallel distraction, which is accomplished using a paint paddle–type instrument placed within the spreader; the posterior ligament is stretched and/or ripped to some extent, increasing the posterior height of the disk space (**Fig. 22–10A–C**). This posterior distraction of the disk space returns the collapsed posterior facets to near normal position. Once the disk space has been distracted, additional disk material that was contained within the buckled ligament within the neural canal is often delivered into the disk space. This is then removed using a Kerrison or biopsy

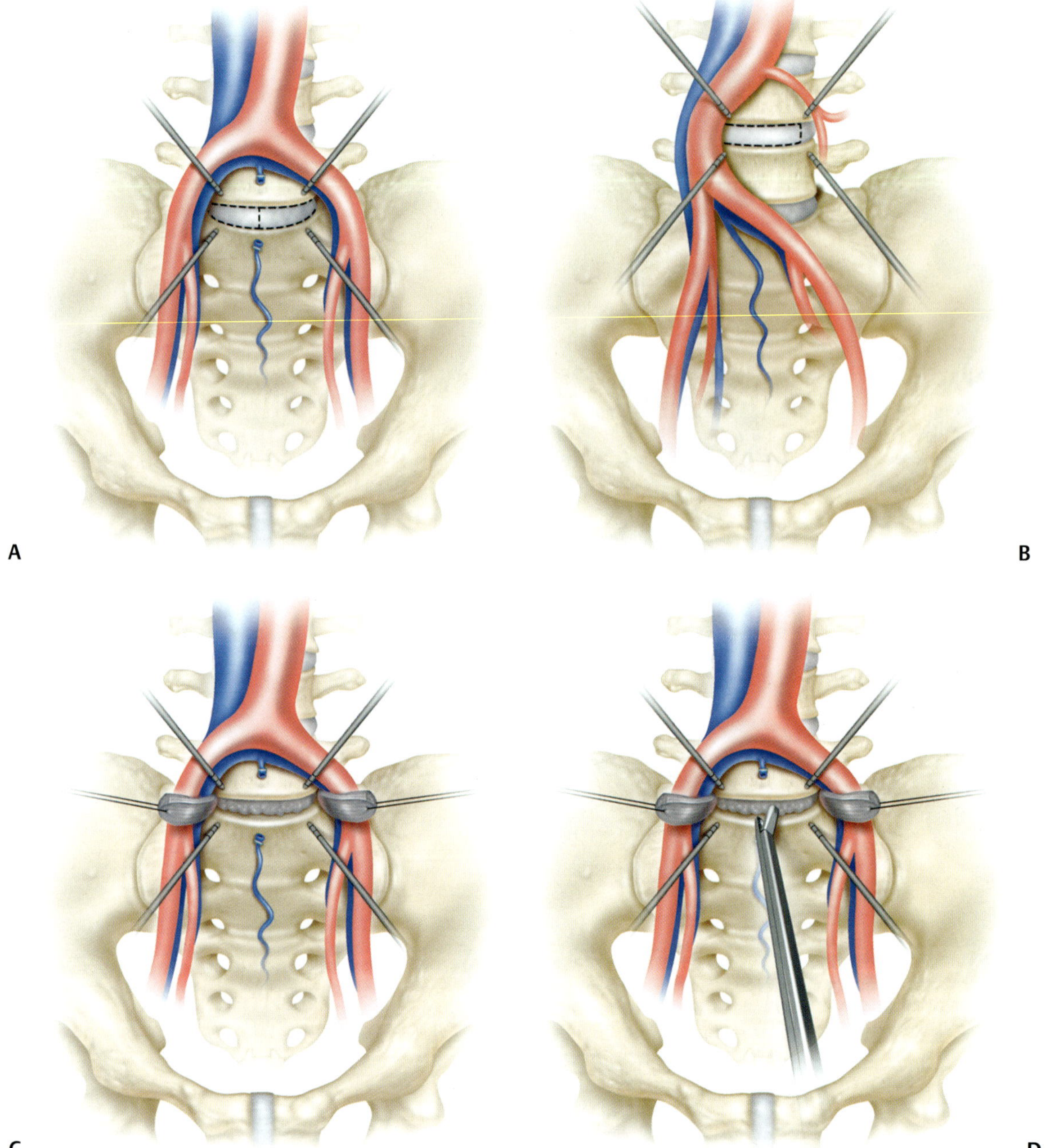

Figure 22–7 **(A)** To prepare the retroperitoneal exposures, carefully impact four retractor pins into the adjacent vertebral bodies or use an appropriate external soft tissue retractor system. Use lateral fluoroscopy to verify the vertebral level. Use a midline incision to open the anterior annulus; the flaps may be used to protect the eccentric vessels. **(B)** To approach L4–L5, move the iliac vein, iliac artery, vena cava, and aorta to the patient's right. Carefully impact four retractor pins into the adjacent vertebral bodies or use an appropriate external soft tissue retractor system. Use lateral fluoroscopy to verify the vertebral level. Use a leftward incision to open the anterior annulus; the flaps may be used to protect the eccentric vessels. **(C)** If desired, hold the annulus fibrosus in position with a suture and mosquito clamp. **(D)** To complete the diskectomy, use rongeurs, curettes and/or the disk elevator.

punch. A trial insertion guide is then inserted into the disk space, which assesses the end plate size, lordotic angle, end plate contact area, and radiographic midline (**Fig. 22–11A–D**). It is often helpful to mark the skin at the contact point of the trial insertion guide handle after radiographic verification of the midline to aid in alignment of the insertion tools with this skin mark and the midline screw on the vertebral body (**Fig. 22–11E**). A broach is then used to scratch the verte-

bral bony end plates at the location of the teeth on the CHARITÉ end plates and verifies the size of the CHARITÉ implant (**Fig. 22–12A,B**).

Next, the metal end plates of the artificial disk are inserted and tapped into position (**Fig. 22–13A,B**). Care is taken to have the center line marked as determined fluoroscopically either using a burn mark or a self-tapping 4.5 mm screw placed within the vertebral body cranially adjacent to the

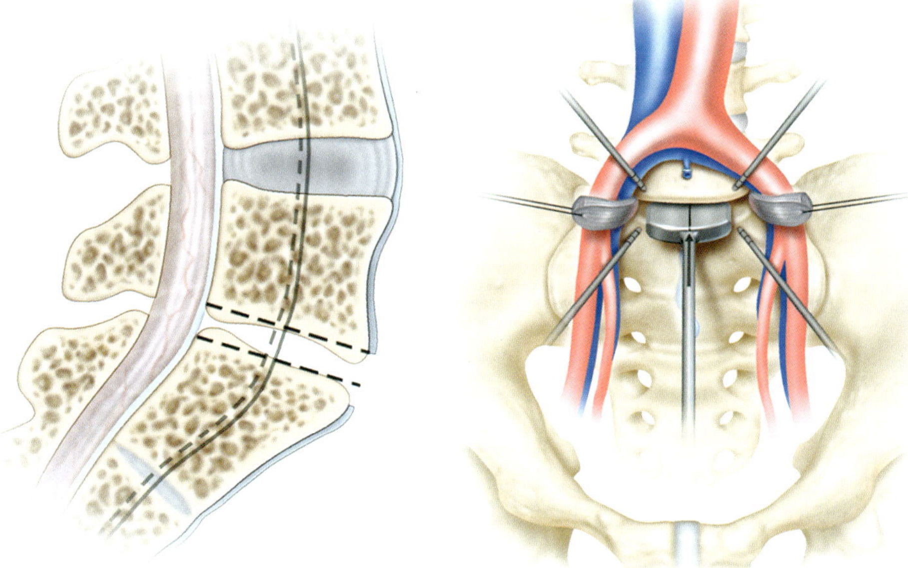

A

B

Figure 22–8   **(A)** To prepare the end plates to accept the CHARITÉ Artificial Disc, remove the cartilaginous end plate with the curettes using a side to side motion. Use great care not to damage the bony end plate. If needed, carefully shape the curved vertebral surfaces by removing dorsal and ventral osteophytes using the curettes and rongeurs or other appropriate instruments. **(B)** Determine the correct footprint size using the sizing gauges, which correspond to end plate footprints; use lateral fluoroscopy to verify accurate size.

Size 3 to 4 with Removal of Posterior Osteophyte

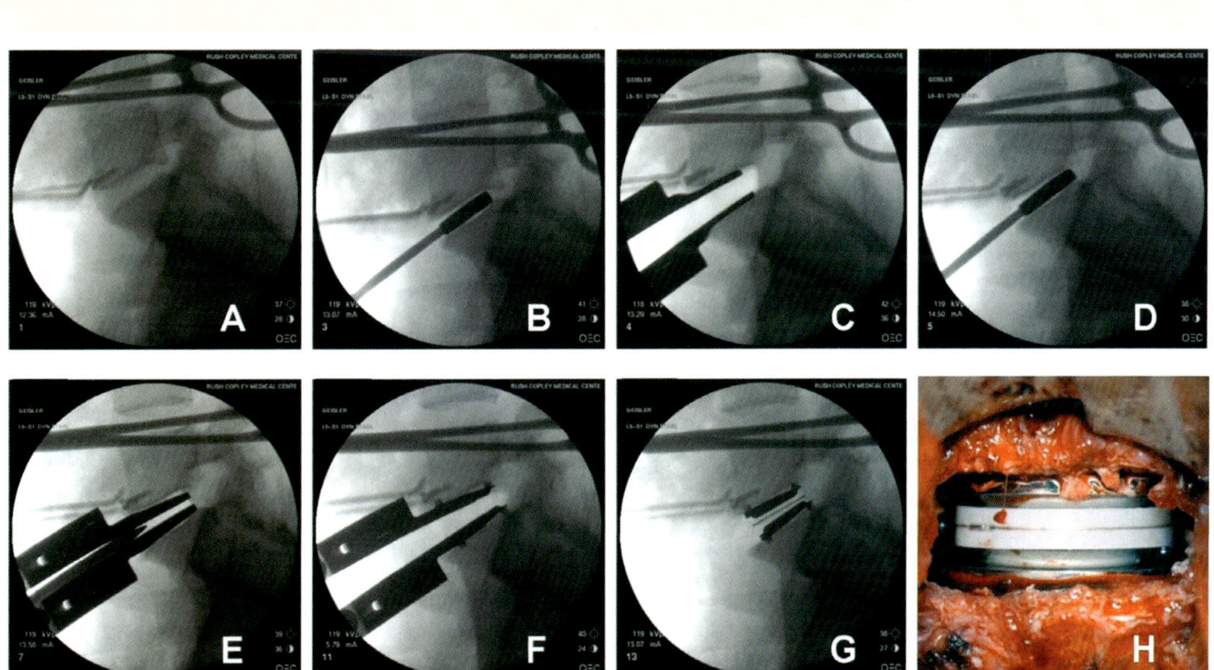

Figure 22–9   An example of the removal of the posterior osteophyte allowing insertion of a larger CHARITÉ implant size. **(A)** Initial lateral fluoroscopy. **(B)** Size 3 sizer intradiskally. **(C)** Disk space distraction. **(D)** Placement of size 4 sizer after posterior osteophyte removal on L5. **(E)** Placement of the CHARITÉ end plates and **(F)** their distraction. **(G)** Final assembly of the CHARITÉ Artificial Disc on lateral fluoroscopy and **(H)** visually intraoperatively.

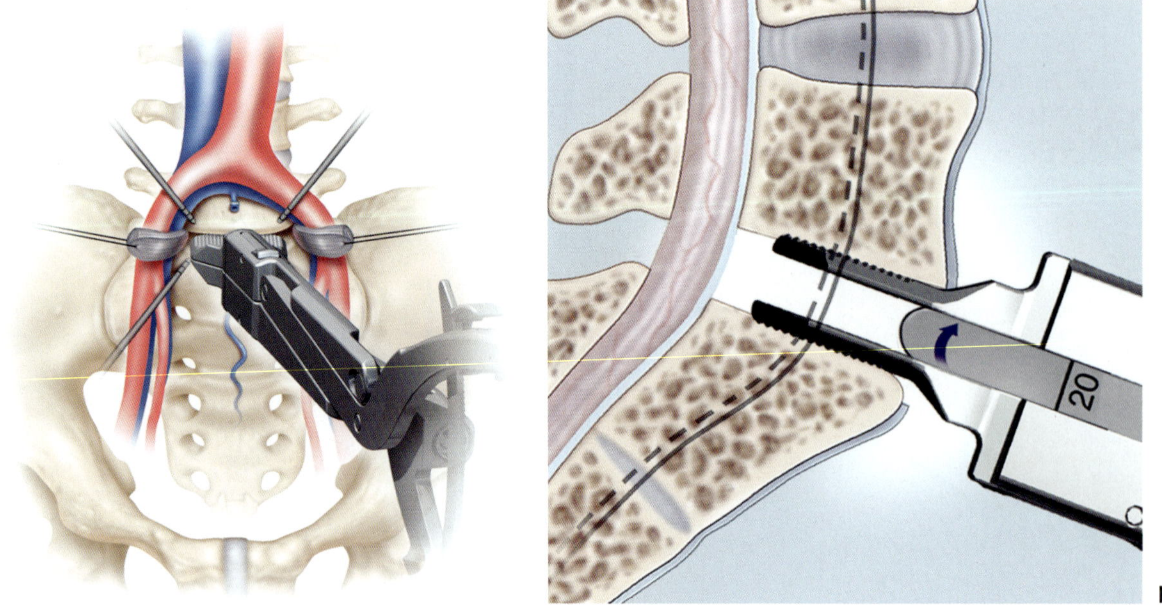

A   B

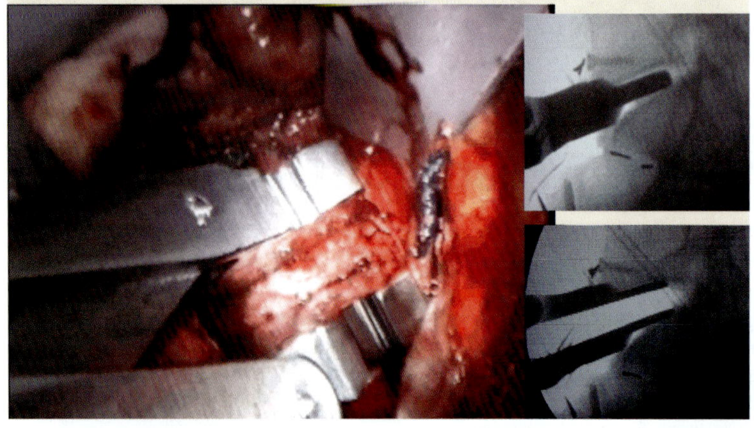

C

Figure 22–10   (A) Apply controlled distraction using the spreading and insertion forceps to visualize and remove the remaining disk tissue, leaving only the lateral annulus. **(B)** Sequentially distract the disk space using the spacers and modular T-handle through the spreading tips. Parallel distraction is critical for restoration of disk height and sufficient opening of the neuroforamen. **(C)** This is a still image of an intraoperative video of the distraction step and the pre- and postdistraction lateral fluoroscopy images.

disk space (**Fig. 22–13C,D**). Because the screw is smooth on the top, it allows the great vessels to slide over if necessary and also provides an unambiguous unique visual and fluoroscopy marker. The metal end plates of the implant are impacted into the disk space, positioned posteriorly within it, and then parallel distraction is performed. During this expansion, it is essential that only the very lateral edges of the implant are touched with the distraction instrumentation to avoid scratching the inside of the cupped metal end plates—this would result in a very significant increase in the amount of plastic wear. Once the metal end plates have been placed, trial cores are used to size the distracted space and the final core is placed (**Fig. 22–14A–D**). The correct position of the plastic core is verified to ensure that it articulates with the cups, and distraction is then fully removed. The slap hammer is then attached to the spreading/insertion implant forceps and with a slight tapping, the insertion device is removed. The screw used for identifying the midline is removed before closure.

In approximately two thirds of the cases during disk space distraction, some epidural bleeding or significant bone bleeding along the posterior edge occurs. This is easily managed by placing strips of Avitene (C.R. Bard, Inc., Murray Hill, NJ) in the disk space and compressing them down against the remaining posterior longitudinal ligament area by using a standard 4 × 4 mm sponge. After allowing it to sit for 2 to 3 minutes, the sponge can be removed, leaving the thin layer of Avitene in place. This is easier to accomplish during the initial diskectomy or after the metal end plates have been inserted than after the core is inserted. Anteroposterior and lateral fluoroscopy is used to aid in positioning the device and to provide final radiological verification. Visual verification is also required in the anterior plane to ascertain that the implant is recessed below the anterior cortical margin. A bone tamp is used on the sides of the metal end plates of the implant to make minor adjustments and also to impact the anterior cleats into the cortical bone of the vertebral body.

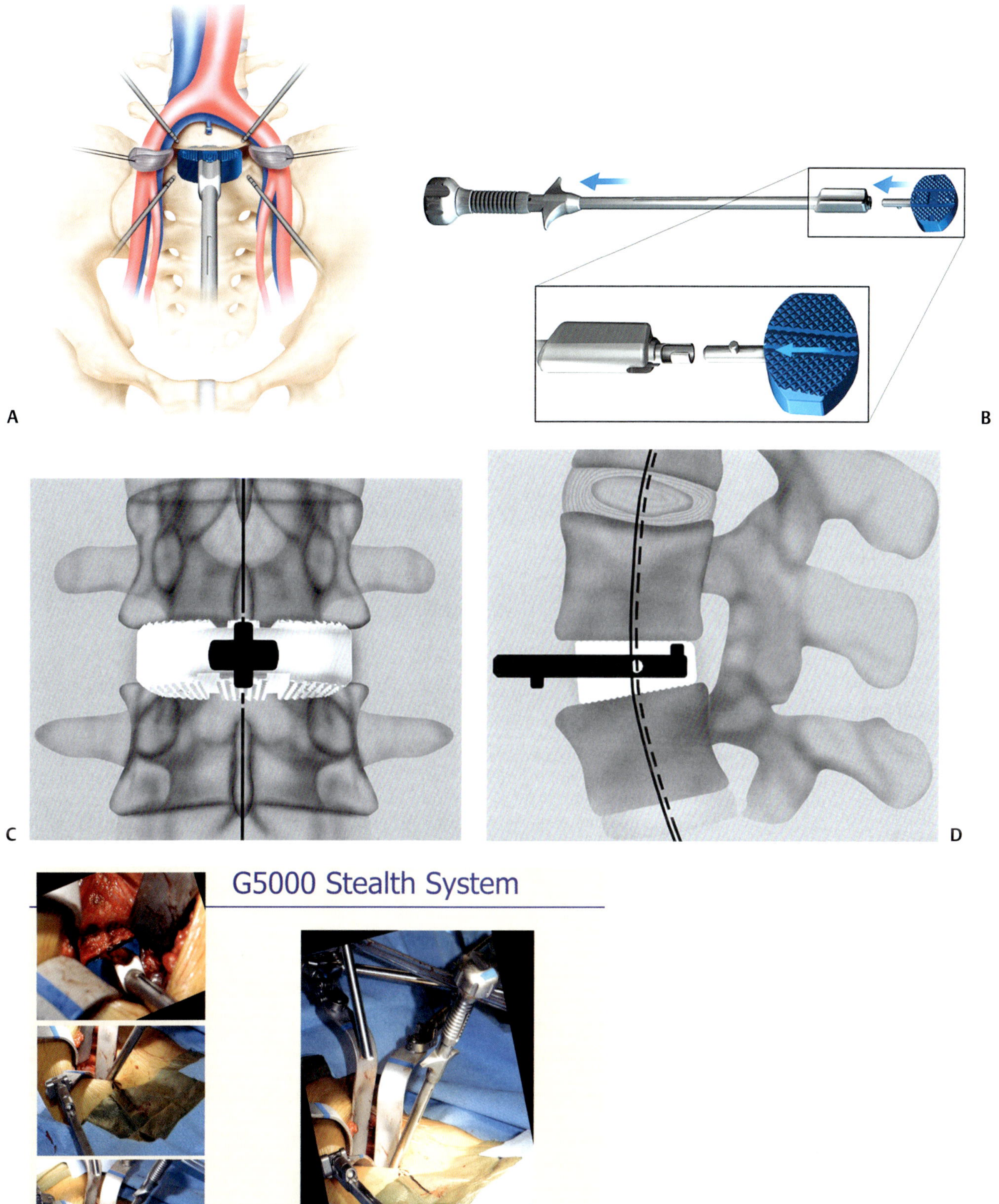

Figure 22–11 **(A)** Insert the Trial Insertion Guide into the disk space. **(B)** Insert the loaded trial insertion instrument through the trial insertion guide to distract and place the trial. **(C)** Verify the correct footprint size, placement, and lordotic angle by anteroposterior (AP) and lateral fluoroscopy. Remove the trial insertion instrument from the trial; leaving the trial in the disk space an AP x-ray is taken. The trial is centered in the AP plane when the AP marker appears as a plus sign aligned with the spinous process. **(D)** Take a lateral x-ray. The hole in the trial represents the center of rotation (COR). To ensure the COR is placed in the optimal location, the COR marker should appear as a full circle 2 mm dorsal to the lateral midline. **(E)** Skin drape mark shows contact location of the radiographic marker/sizer. This line and the screw on the center of the vertebral body are used for the trajectory of the implant insertion.

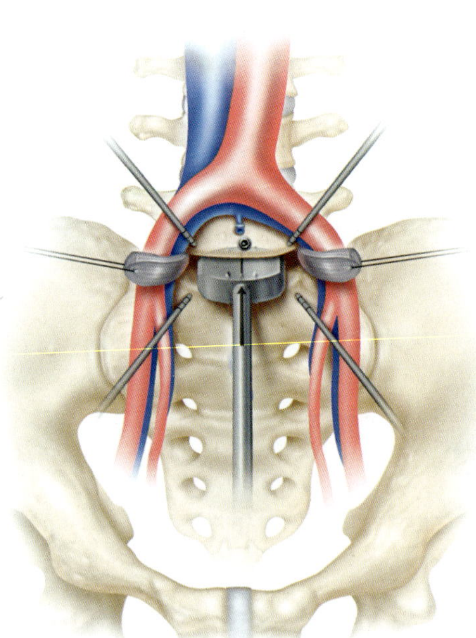

A

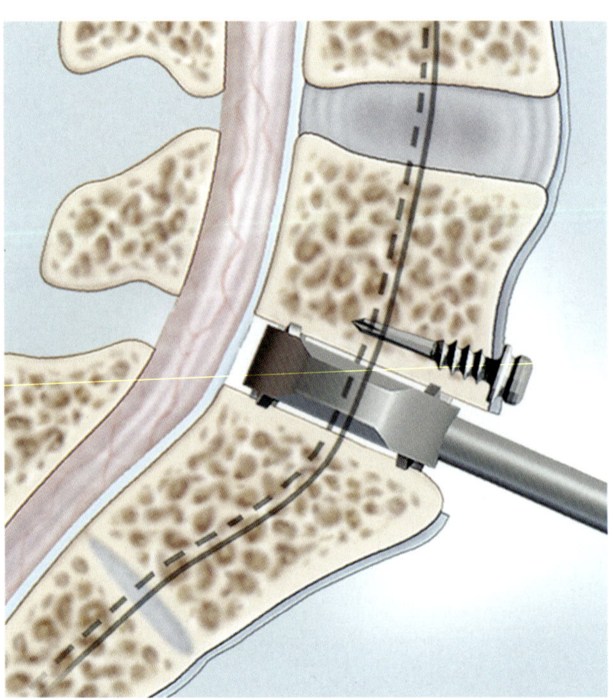

B

Figure 22–12   (A) It is critical to have shaped any curved vertebral surfaces prior to pilot driver impaction to reduce the potential for vertebral body or end plate fracture during pilot driver impaction. **(B)** Accurately align the pilot driver with the midline marker. Carefully impact the pilot driver that corresponds to the chosen footprint to verify the ability to accurately place the end plates into the proper position. The center of the pilot driver should be 2 mm dorsal to the lateral midline.

◆ The FDA IDE Multicenter Trial of the CHARITÉ Artificial Disc

Both short-term and long-term favorable results related to the CHARITÉ Artificial Disc have been reported in the literature.[3,23,29,30] However, until the May 2000 commencement of a U.S. FDA-regulated prospective, randomized, nonblinded, trial, no studies existed that evaluated clinical outcomes with total disk replacement (TDR) compared with lumbar fusion. Between May and April 2002, 304 patients had surgery in this study, which compared the safety and effectiveness of the CHARITÉ Artificial Disc to anterior lumbar interbody fusion (ALIF) using threaded cages filled with bone graft, for the treatment of single-level DDD at L4–L5 or L5–S1. The BAK cages (Zimmer Spine, Inc., Warsaw, IN) were implanted according to the manufacturer's instructions, with two cages packed with iliac crest autograft at each treatment level. This is a similar clinical study design to the FDA BMP study of lumbar fusion, which used an anteriorly placed thread fusion cage with autograft as a control.[31] Patients in the BAK treatment group were required to wear a hard brace for 3 months following surgery; those in the CHARITÉ treatment group did not wear a brace. In both groups patients undertook activities progressively, as tolerated. The hypothesis of the study was that the level of clinical success achieved by patients in the TDR group would be at least as good as the clinical success achieved by patients in the control group, a noninferiority study.

The FDA IDE multicenter trial of the CHARITÉ Artificial Disc was performed at 14 centers across the United States. The primary inclusion criteria included single-level DDD at L4–L5 or L5–S1 confirmed by magnetic resonance imaging (MRI) and provocative diskography, aged 18 to 60 years, Oswestry Disability Index (ODI) score greater than or equal to 30, back pain visual analog scale (VAS) score greater than or equal to 40 with no radicular component (referred leg pain was permitted), and failed nonoperative treatment of at least 6 months' duration. The primary exclusion criteria included previous thoracic or lumbar fusion, multilevel DDD, facet joint arthrosis, noncontained herniated nucleus pulposus, osteoporosis, spondylolisthesis slip greater than 3 mm, scoliosis greater than 11 degrees, and midsagittal stenosis less than 8 mm.

Local institutional review board approval was obtained at each site. The study protocol indicated that participants at each site were to perform five nonrandomized cases prior to beginning the randomization arm; 71 nonrandomized cases were performed to implant the CHARITÉ device. Patients were then randomized into a CHARITÉ group (**Fig. 22–15A**) and a BAK cage group (ALIF and iliac crest autograft) (**Fig. 22–15B**). Two hundred five patients underwent placement of the CHARITÉ disk and 99 underwent BAK cage placement (2:1 ratio). Demographic features were not significantly different between the two groups with respect to age or sex. There was no intergroup difference with respect to levels treated: L4–L5, 61 cases (29.7%) in the CHARITÉ group and 32 (32.3%) in the BAK group; L5–S1, 144 (70.3%) in the CHARITÉ group and 67 (67.7%) in the BAK group.

A typical patient x-ray is shown in **Fig. 22–15C** at L5–S1. The corresponding MRI shows the Modic end plate changes in the collapse of L5–S1, as well as some water loss in L4–L5 in this particular patient (**Fig. 22–15D**). The diskogram would have excluded L4–L5 as the significant pain generator. Another patient is shown in **Fig. 22–15E** in which L4–L5

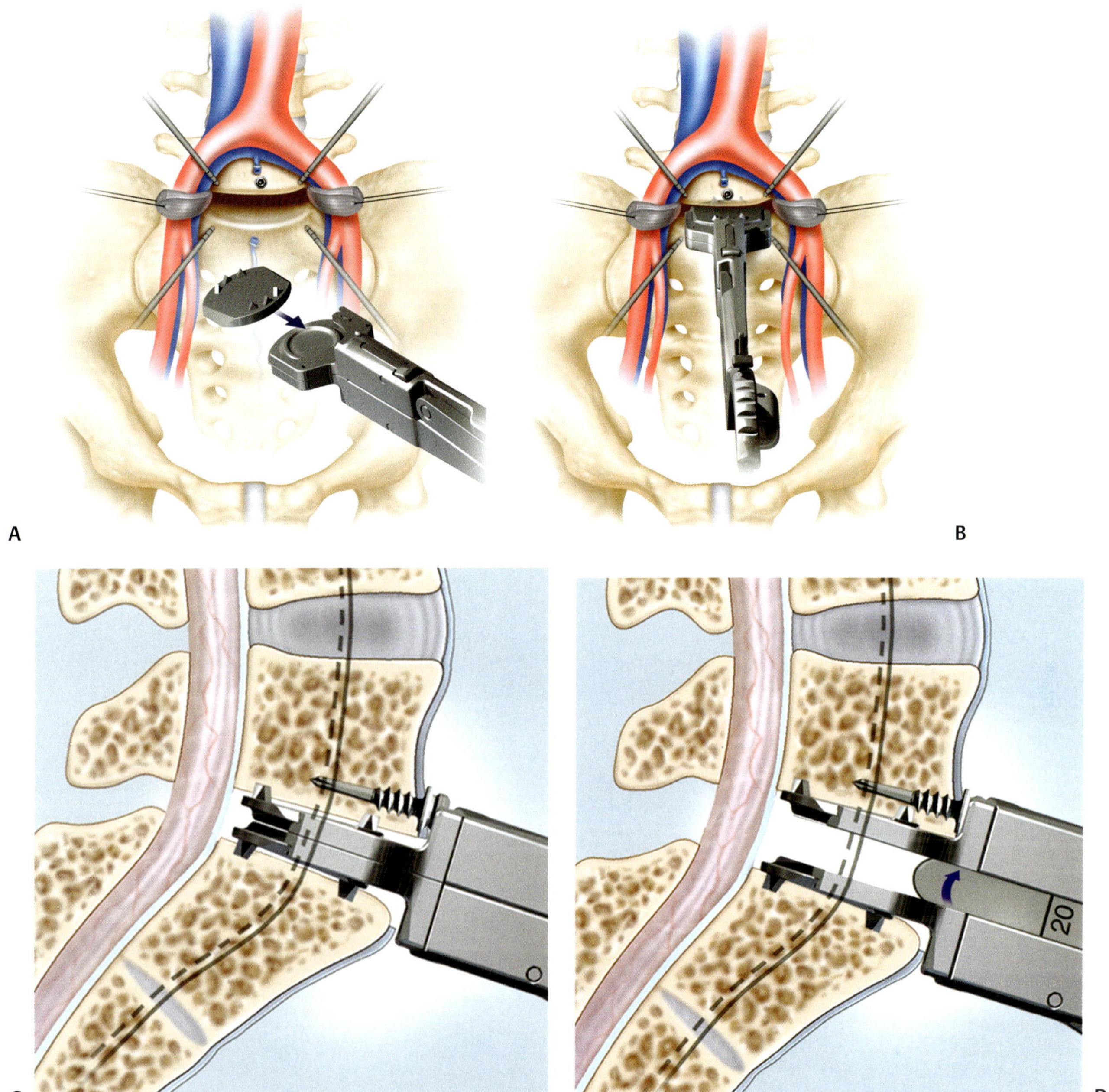

Figure 22–13 **(A)** With the Endplate Insertion Tips attached to the Spreading and Insertion Forceps, the prosthesis endplates are inserted into the tips prior to implantation. **(B)** Direct view of prosthesis endplate insertion. **(C)** Lateral view of prosthesis endplate insertion. **(D)** Lateral view following impaction of the prosthesis endplates into the inferior and superior vertebral bodies.

is the major pain generator with a minor loss of water at L5–S1. In this patient, the L5–S1 disk space would have been excluded as a major pain generator by diskography.

The U.S. FDA IDE of the CHARITÉ Artificial Disc study initiated patient enrollment in May 2000 and all patients were enrolled in the randomized FDA multicenter study with complete 2-year follow-up concluded in December 2003. Following the randomized arm the centers that entered patients into the randomized FDA IDE study had access to the Charité disk on a limited basis as part of a continuing access study. The U.S. FDA granted approval for marketing the

CHARITÉ Artificial Disc in the United States on October 26, 2004. The FDA label states: "The CHARITÉ Artificial Disc is indicated for spinal arthroplasty in skeletally mature patients with degenerative disc disease (DDD) at one level from L4–S1. DDD is defined as diskogenic back pain with degeneration of the disc confirmed by patient history and radiographic studies. These DDD patients should have no more than 3 mm of spondylolisthesis at the involved level. Patients receiving the CHARITÉ Artificial Disc should have failed at least six months of conservative treatment prior to implantation of the CHARITÉ Artificial Disc."[2,32–34]

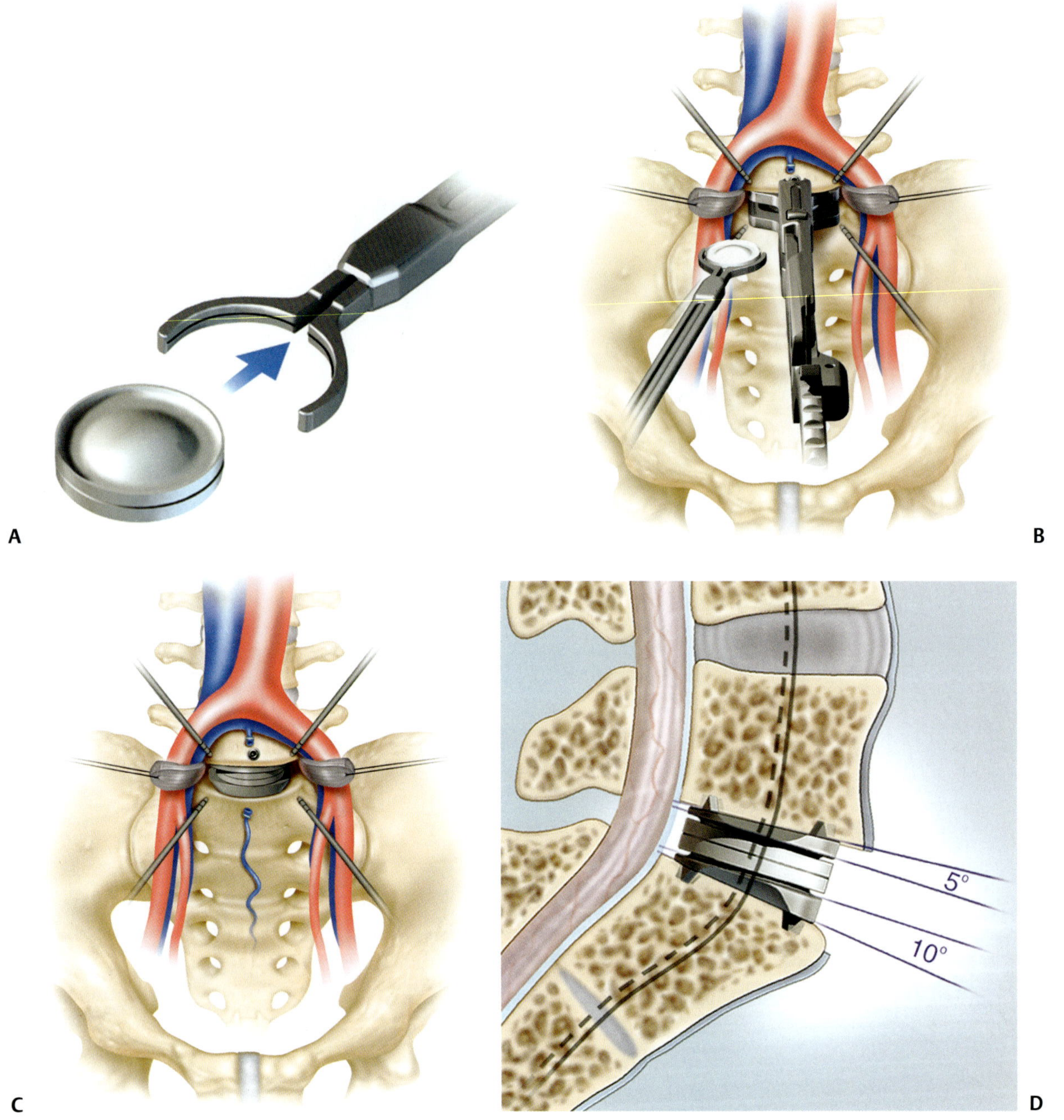

Figure 22–14 **(A)** The appropriate sized Core is loaded into the Core Insertion instrument. **(B)** The Sliding Core is inserted between the prosthesis endplates. If resistance is felt, carefully increase distraction. Release the distraction on the spreading and insertion forceps allowing the end plates to close around and engage the sliding core. Release the sliding core by squeezing the handle of the core insertion instrument. After removing the core insertion instrument, use the slap hammer to safely remove the spreading and insertion forceps. **(C)** Verify the final position of the CHARITÉ Artificial Disc using fluoroscopy in the AP view and **(D)** in the lateral view. It is imperative that the prosthesis is in the correct position in the AP and lateral planes.

◆ Revision Techniques

If the CHARITÉ Artificial Disc were required to be revised, there would be two approaches. One approach would be to redo the anterior surgery. This would involve dissecting the retroperitoneal area and dealing with the postop scarring and hence increased risk of great vessel damage compared with an unoperated case. This would allow removal of the CHARITÉ Artificial Disc. The plastic core would be removed first, and then the metal end plates could be separated from the bony end plates by using a chisel between them and levering away from the bone into the disk space. This would allow the placement of another artificial disk in the disk space because the bony end plates would not be significantly damaged. Alternately, a posterior operation with rod–screw stabilization and posterior lateral fusion could be used to fuse the lumbar segment, which would use the CHARITÉ Artificial Disc as an anterior load share. More important than the exact surgical technique used would be clinically characterizing the pain generator if the patient had recurring or

CHARITÉ Artificial Disc

A

BAK ALIF Fusion Comparison Group

B

Severe L5/S1
Degenerative Disc Disease

C

Severe L5/S1 Degenerative
Disc Disease with
Modic Inflammatory Changes
SAG
FA 90
ETL 16

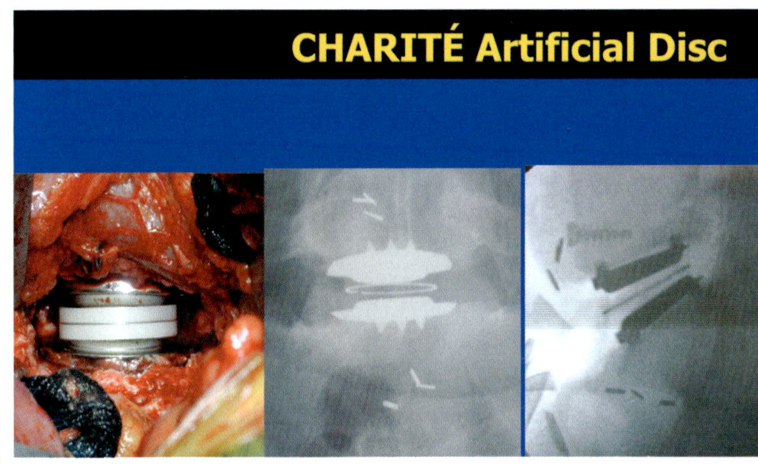

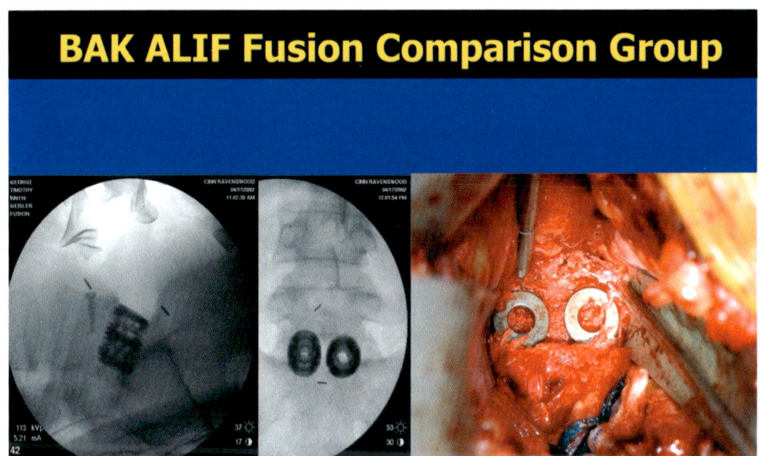

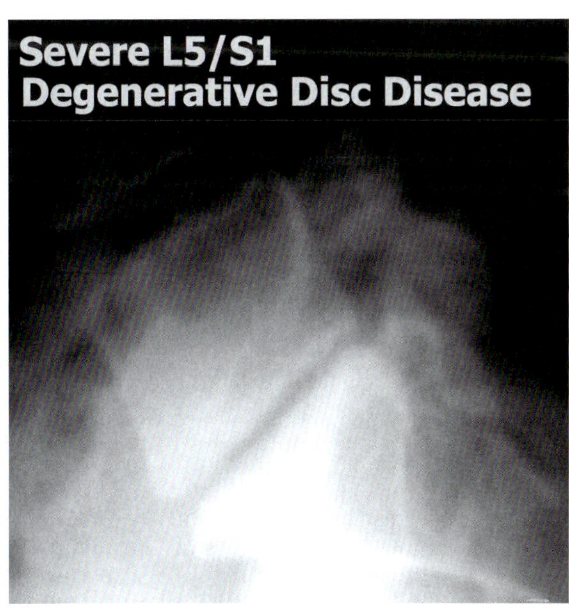

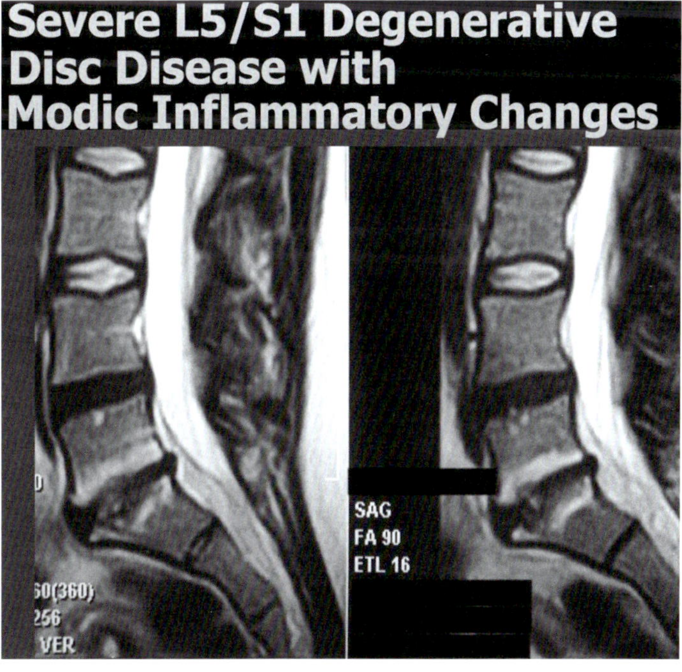

D

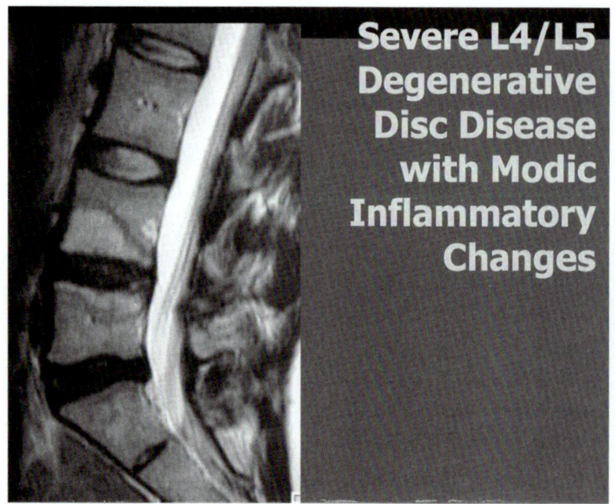

Figure 22–15   **(A)** Example of a Charité Artificial Disc in the U.S. Food and Drug Administration Investigational Device Exemption study. **(B)** Example of a BAK anterior lumbar interbody fusion procedure entered as a control in this study. **(C)** Severe L5–S1 degenerative disk disease typical of patients entered into this study. **(D)** T2-weighted magnetic resonance imaging (MRI) of patient with diskography-verified pain generator at L5–S1. Note Modic changes adjacent to the L5–S1 disk space. **(E)** T2-weighted MRI of patient with diskography-verified pain generator at L4–L5 level.

persistent pain. This would have to be done by a variety of radiological and provocative studies. Diskogram at adjacent levels would be helpful, as would epidural facet injections, and potentially even an anesthetic diskogram at adjacent levels to see if that would remove a majority of the pain.

◆ Outcomes

The pivotal study on the CHARITÉ Artificial Disc was a prospective, randomized, multicenter, FDA-regulated IDE clinical trial. The purpose of this study was to compare the safety and effectiveness of lumbar total disk replacement using the CHARITÉ Artificial Disc with ALIF for the treatment of single-level DDD from L4–S1 unresponsive to nonoperative treatment. Prior to this Class I medical evidence study reported results of lumbar TDR have been favorable, but studies have been limited to retrospective case series or small sample sizes.

In this study, 304 patients were enrolled in the study at 14 centers across the United States and randomized in a 2:1 ratio to treatment with the CHARITÉ Artificial Disc or the control group, instrumented ALIF. Data were collected pre- and perioperatively at 6 weeks and at 3,6,12, and 24 months following surgery. The key clinical outcome measures were a VAS assessing back pain, the ODI questionnaire, and the short form SF-36 Health Survey.

Patients in both treatment groups improved significantly following surgery. Patients in the CHARITÉ Artificial Disc group recovered faster than patients in the control group. Patients in the CHARITÉ Artificial Disc group had lower levels of disability at every time interval from 6 weeks to 24 months, compared with the control group, with statistically lower pain and disability scores at all but the 24-month follow-up ($P \sim .05$). At the 24-month follow-up period, a significantly greater percentage of patients in the CHARITÉ Artificial Disc group expressed satisfaction with their treatment and would have the same treatment again, compared with the fusion group ($p < .05$). The hospital stay was significantly shorter in the CHARITÉ Artificial Disc group ($p < .05$). The complication rate was similar between both groups. When the entire patient population in the study is combined

(training and randomized) and Wilcoxon/Kruskal-Wallis nonparametric test are used, the results of the ODI and the VAS are significant for improvement in the CHARITÉ group at all time points, including the 24-month follow-up time point (**Fig. 22–16A,B**).

This prospective, randomized, multicenter study demonstrated that quantitative clinical outcome measures following lumbar TDR with the CHARITÉ Artificial Disc are at least equivalent to clinical outcomes with ALIF. These results support earlier reports in the literature that TDR with the CHARITÉ Artificial Disc is a safe and effective alternative to fusion for the surgical treatment of symptomatic disk degeneration in properly indicated patients. The CHARITÉ Artificial Disc group demonstrated statistically significant superiority in two major economic areas, a 1-day-shorter hospitalization, and a lower rate of reoperations (5.4% compared with 9.1%). At 24 months, the investigational group had a significantly higher rate of satisfaction (73.7%) than the 53.1% rate of satisfaction in the control group ($p = .0011$). This prospective, randomized, multicenter study also demonstrated an increase in employment of 9.1% in the investigational group and 7.2% in the control group.[2,32–34]

In follow-up x-ray studies, the patients have mobility in both flexion-extension and lateral bending in the level that was dynamically stabilized (**Fig. 22–2C**). X-ray evidence shows clear movement of the core translation with the flexion-extension movement. The author's initial impression is that the clinical outcome results are comparable or better than historical fusion results reported in the literature.

◆ Conclusion

Estimations as to when other devices will be available on the U.S. market vary greatly. At the time of this chapter's writing, the CHARITÉ Artificial Disc is the only artificial disk with U.S. FDA approval. Furthermore, the U.S. FDA trial is the only Class I medical evidence comparing any artificial disk technology with spinal fusion currently available. It is expected that in the coming years ProDisc, FlexiCore, and Maverick will complete their IDE trials and submit their data to the FDA for approval.

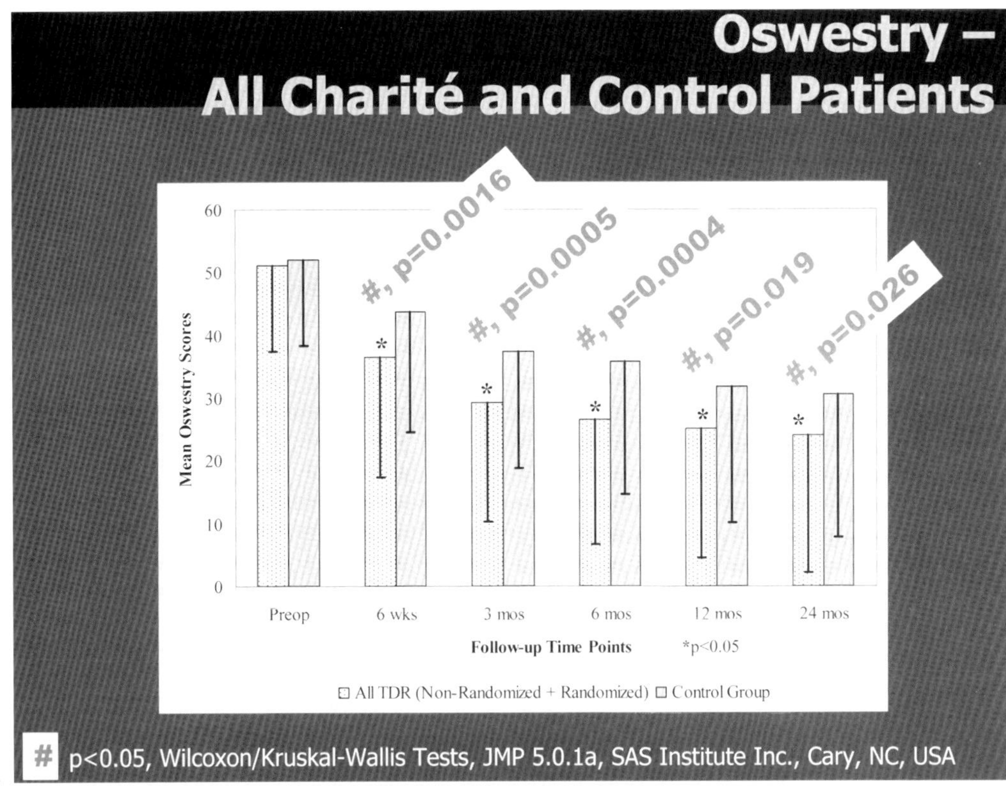

A

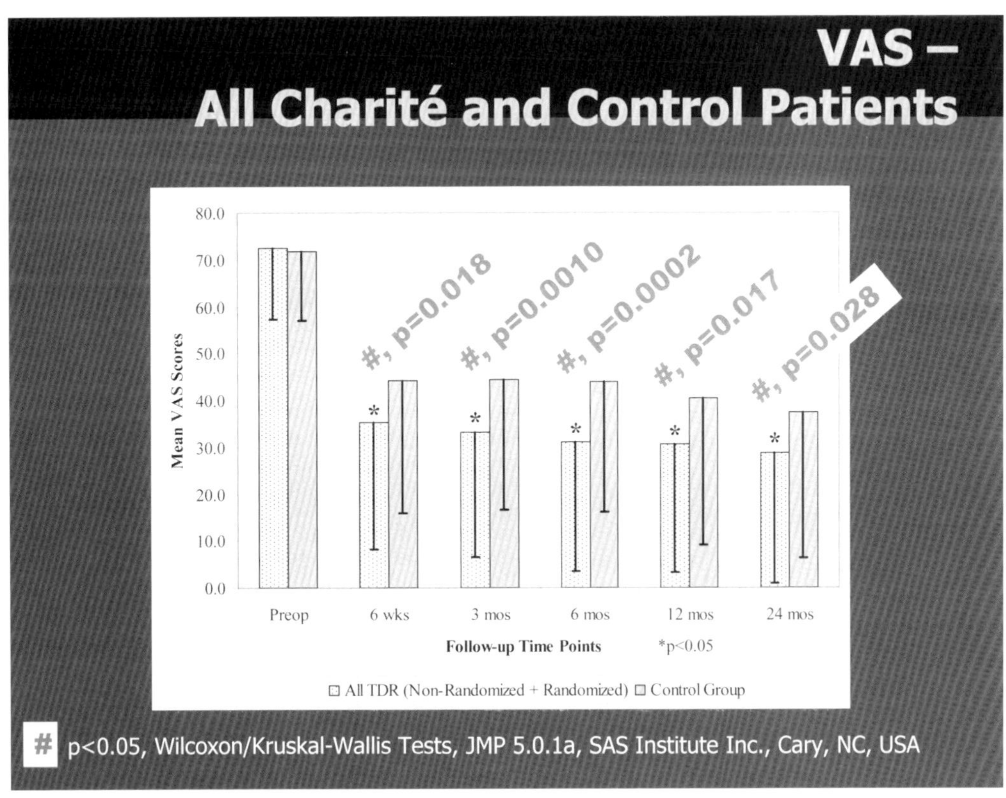

B

Figure 22–16 **(A)** The Oswestry and **(B)** visual analog scale for all patients (nonrandomized and randomized) in the study analyzed with Wilcoxon/Kruskal-Wallis nonparametric test with statistical significance at all time points including the 24-month follow-up. Note that the groups are balanced at baseline and no "baseline correction" was needed or used.

In conclusion, lumbar dynamic stabilization with a CHARITÉ Artificial Disc is a promising treatment modality for axial lumbar pain and preserving joint motion in selected patients. The 2-year clinical outcome after a single-level diskogenic degenerative disk disease appears superior to historical fusion results. Additional research will be done in the coming years to see whether topping off a lumbar fusion will help prevent adjacent level disease, whether this device can be used below a scoliosis when the degenerative changes occur, and whether multilevel disease will have the same good clinical response as the single level appears to be having in this clinical study.

References

1. Hochschuler SH, Ohnmeiss DD, Guyer RD, Blumenthal SL. Artificial disc: preliminary results of a prospective study in the United States. Eur Spine J 2002;11(Suppl 2):S106–S110

2. Geisler FH, Blumenthal SL, Guyer RD, et al. Neurological complications of lumbar artificial disc replacement and comparison of clinical results with those related to lumbar arthrodesis in the literature: results of a multicenter, prospective, randomized investigational device exemption study of CHARITÉ intervertebral disc. Invited submission from the Joint Section Meeting on Disorders of the Spine and Peripheral Nerves, March 2004. J Neurosurg Spine 2004;1:143–154

3. Cunningham BW, Gordon JD, Dmitriev AE, Hu N, McAfee PC. Biomechanical evaluation of total disc replacement arthroplasty: an in vitro human cadaveric model. Spine 2003;28:S110–S117

4. Huang RC, Girardi FP, Cammisa FP Jr, Wright TM. The implications of constraint in lumbar total disc replacement. J Spinal Disord Tech 2003;16:412–417

5. Hilibrand AS, Carlson GD, Palumbo MA, Jones PK, Bohlman HH. Radiculopathy and myelopathy at segments adjacent to the site of a previous anterior cervical arthrodesis. J Bone Joint Surg Am 1999; 81:519–528

6. Bao QB, McCullen GM, Higham PA, Dumbleton JH, Yuan HA. The artificial disc: theory, design and materials. Biomaterials 1996;17: 1157–1167

7. Dooris AP, Goel VK, Grosland NM, Gilbertson LG, Wilder DG. Load-sharing between anterior and posterior elements in a lumbar motion segment implanted with an artificial disc. Spine 2001;26: E122–E129

8. Eijkelkamp MF, van Donkelaar CC, Veldhuizen AG, van Horn JR, Huyghe JM, Verkerke GJ. Requirements for an artificial intervertebral disc. Int J Artif Organs 2001;24:311–321

9. Hedman TP, Kostuik JP, Fernie GR, Hellier WG. Design of an intervertebral disc prosthesis. Spine 1991;16(Suppl 6):S256–S260

10. Link H, Buttner-Janz K, Link SB. CHARITÉ Artificial Disc: history, design, and biomechanics. In: Kaech D, Jinkins J, eds. Spinal Restabilization Procedures: Diagnostic and Therapeutic Aspects of Intervertebral Fusion Cages, Artificial Discs, and Mobile Implants. Amsterdam, the Netherlands: Elsevier Science BV;2002:293–316

11. Klara PM, Ray CD. Artificial nucleus replacement: clinical experience. Spine 2002;27:1374–1377

12. Wilke HJ, Kavanagh S, Neller S, Claes L. Effect of artificial disk nucleus implant on mobility and intervertebral disk high of an L4/5 segment after nucleotomy [in German]. Orthopade 2002;31:434–440

13. Wilke HJ, Kavanagh S, Neller S, Haid C, Claes LE. Effect of a prosthetic disc nucleus on the mobility and disc height of the L4–5 intervertebral disc postnucleotomy. J Neurosurg 2001;95(Suppl 2):208–214

14. Freudiger S, Dubois G, Lorrain M. Dynamic neutralisation of the lumbar spine confirmed on a new lumbar spine simulator in vitro. Arch Orthop Trauma Surg 1999;119:127–132

15. Senegas J. Mechanical supplementation by non-rigid fixation in degenerative intervertebral lumbar segments: the Wallis system. Eur Spine J 2002;11(Suppl 2):S164–S169

16. Stoll TM, Dubois G, Schwarzenbach O. The dynamic neutralization system for the spine: a multi-center study of a novel non-fusion system. Eur Spine J 2002;11(Suppl 2):S170–S178

17. Alsema R, Deutman R, Mulder TJ. Stanmore total hip replacement. A 15- to 16-year clinical and radiographic follow-up. J Bone Joint Surg Br 1994;76:240–244

18. Worland RL, Johnson GV, Alemparte J, Jessup DE, Keenan J, Norambuena N. Ten- to fourteen-year survival and functional analysis of the AGC total knee replacement system. Knee 2002;9:133–137

19. Kuslich SD, Ulstrom CL, Griffith SL, Ahern JW, Dowdle JD. The Bagby and Kuslich method of lumbar interbody fusion: history, techniques, and 2-year follow-up results of a United States prospective, multicenter trial. Spine 1998;23:1267–1278 discussion 1279

20. McAfee P. Artificial disc prosthesis: the Link SB CHARITÉ III. In: Kaech D, Jinkins J, eds. Spinal Restabilization Procedures: Diagnostic and Therapeutic Aspects of Intervertebral Fusion Cages. Amsterdam, the Netherlands: Elsevier Science; 2002:299–310

21. McAfee PC, Cunningham BW, Orbegoso CM, Sefter JC, Dmitriev AE, Fedder IL. Analysis of porous ingrowth in intervertebral disc prostheses: a nonhuman primate model. Spine 2003;28:332–340

22. Moumene M, Geisler FH. Effect of Artifical total disc replacement on facet loading: Unconstrained vs. semi-constrained: 4th Annual Meeting of the Spine Arthoplasty Society, Vienna, Austria, May 4–7, 2004

23. Cinotti G, David T, Postacchini F. Results of disc prosthesis after a minimum follow-up period of 2 years. Spine 1996;21:995–1000

24. Lemaire JP, Skalli W, Lavaste F, et al. Intervertebral disc prosthesis: results and prospects for the year 2000. Clin Orthop Relat Res 1997; 337:64–76

25. Lemaire JP. SB Charité III intervertebral disc prosthesis: biomechanical, clinical, and radiological correlations with a series of 100 cases over a follow-up of more than 10 years. Rachis [Fr] 2002;14: 271–285

26. Lemaire JP, Carrier H, Ali el HS, Skalli W, Lavaste F. Clinical and radiological outcomes with the CHARITÉ Artificial Disc: a 10-year minimum follow-up. J Spinal Disord Tech 2005;18:353–359

27. David T. Lumbar disc prosthesis: five years follow-up study on 96 patients. Paper presented at the 15th Annual Meeting of the North American Spine Society (NASS), 2000; New Orleans, LA

28. Zeegers WS, Bohnen LM, Laaper M, Verhaegen MJ. Artificial disc replacement with the modular type SB CHARITÉ III: 2-year results in 50 prospectively studied patients. Eur Spine J 1999;8:210–217

29. Burkus JK, Heim SE, Gornet MF, Zdeblick TA. Is INFUSE bone graft superior to autograft bone? An integrated analysis of clinical trials using the LT-CAGE lumbar tapered fusion device. J Spinal Disord Tech 2003;16:113–122

30. Burkus JK, Transfeldt EE, Kitchel SH, Watkins RG, Balderston RA. Clinical and radiographic outcomes of anterior lumbar interbody fusion using recombinant human bone morphogenetic protein-2. Spine 2002;27: 2396–2408

31. Burkus JK, Gornet MF, Dickman CA, Zdeblick TA. Anterior lumbar interbody fusion using rhBMP-2 with tapered interbody cages. J Spinal Disord Tech 2002;15:337–349

32. Blumenthal S, McAfee P, Guyer R, et al. A prospective, randomized, multicenter Food and Drug Administration investigational device exemptions study of lumbar total disc replacement with the CHARITÉ Artificial Disc versus lumbar fusion, I: Evaluation of clinical outcomes. Spine 2005;30:1565–1575

33. Geisler FH. Surgical technique of lumbar artificial disc replacement with the CHARITÉ Artificial Disc. Neurosurgery 2005;56(Suppl 1): 46–57

34. McAfee PC, Cunningham B, Holsapple G, et al. A prospective, randomized, multicenter Food and Drug Administration investigational device exemption study of lumbar total disc replacement with the CHARITÉ Artificial Disc versus lumbar fusion, II: Evaluation of radiographic outcomes and correlation of surgical technique accuracy with clinical outcomes. Spine 2005;30:1576–1583

23

ProDisc Lumbar Artificial Disk

Jack E. Zigler and Matthew T. Bennett

◆ Prosthesis Design

◆ Biomechanical Studies

◆ Implantation Technique

◆ European Experience

◆ U.S. Experience

The first-generation ProDisc (Aesculap AG & Co., Tuttlingen, Germany) was developed in 1989 by Thierry Marnay, M.D., at the Clinique du Parc, Montpellier, France. Between March 1990 and September 1993, Marnay and Louis Villett, M.D., (Dunkerque, France) implanted 93 ProDisc I devices into 64 patients at either one or two levels. No further devices were implanted and they waited until the results were evaluated at a mean follow-up of 8.7 years (range, 7–11 years).

After adequate time had elapsed, investigators made an exhaustive effort to locate all patients. From the initial 64 patient cohort, three patients had died and three patients were not found. The remaining 58 patients (95% of all living subjects) were studied. By Marnay's evaluation, all implants were intact and functioning. There was no evidence of subsidence or migration. There was a significant reduction in subjective back and leg pain. In terms of satisfaction, 92.7% of patients were either "satisfied" or "entirely satisfied." There were no differences between the single-level and two-level procedures. Importantly, "there were no device related safety issues, untoward effects, complications or adverse effects."[1]

The second-generation design, ProDisc II (Aesculap AG & Co.), was released to European markets in December 1999. The new device featured several changes in implant design. In 1999, the device had been acquired by Spine Solutions, Inc., which was founded by the Viscogliosi Brothers, LLC. In October 2001, the first ProDiscs were implanted in the United States under a Food and Drug Administration (FDA) Investigational Device Exemption (IDE). In early 2003, ProDisc was acquired by Synthes-Stratec (Oberdorf, Switzerland).

◆ Prosthesis Design

The end plates of the first-generation ProDisc were fashioned entirely of titanium alloy. The ProDisc II end plates are a cobalt-chrome-molybdenum (CoCrMo) alloy coated with a plasmapore titanium alloy that allows for bone growth into the device. The initial ProDisc design had dual keels on each end plate. The second-generation model has a single central keel and two spikes on each end plate that provide immediate rotational stability and allow for bony ingrowth. The cranial end plate has a highly polished concave bearing surface that articulates with the convex polyethylene core. The central core of the device is an ultra high molecular weight polyethylene (UHMWPE) liner that snaps into the caudal end plate, creating a semiconstrained device. The monoconvex design of the liner allows it to be placed without requiring overdistraction of the disk space. The third modification to the first-generation device, the addition of a modular polyethylene, allows the surgeon more options in the reconstruction of the disk space. The resulting motion has been compared with a ball and socket articulation.[2,3] The device allows 13 degrees of flexion, 7 degrees of extension, 10 degrees of lateral bending, and ± 3 degrees of axial rotation[4] (**Fig. 23–1**). The implant was designed to approximate the natural physiological center of rotation that normally exists just inferior to the superior end plate of the caudal vertebra.[5]

◆ Biomechanical Studies

Cadaveric studies comparing instantaneous axes of rotation of the ProDisc II to radiographically normal L5–S1 segments has shown that there is not a significant difference between the paths of motion.[6] During flexion and extension, there was similar vertical motion, whereas with lateral bending, there was comparable horizontal motion (**Fig. 23–2**). In addition, the model showed that there was an increase in the coupled motions of rotation and lateral bending. Of specific interest was the resultant unloading of the facet joints. There was a decrease in facet shear forces by 37%. Although a cadaveric model cannot clearly answer clinical questions, it implies that pristine facet joints may not be a requirement with a semiconstrained device. Current studies are attempting to clarify this clinical question.

Huang et al retrospectively reviewed the radiographs of Marnay's initial cohort.[7] They have shown that 66% of ProDisc I implants had > 2 degree range of motion at a mean follow-up of 8.7 years. Of the two thirds of disks that continued to exhibit measurable motion, the mean range of motion was 5.5 degrees (range, 4.1–7.5 degrees), which was actually less than measured normal ranges of motion in a group of

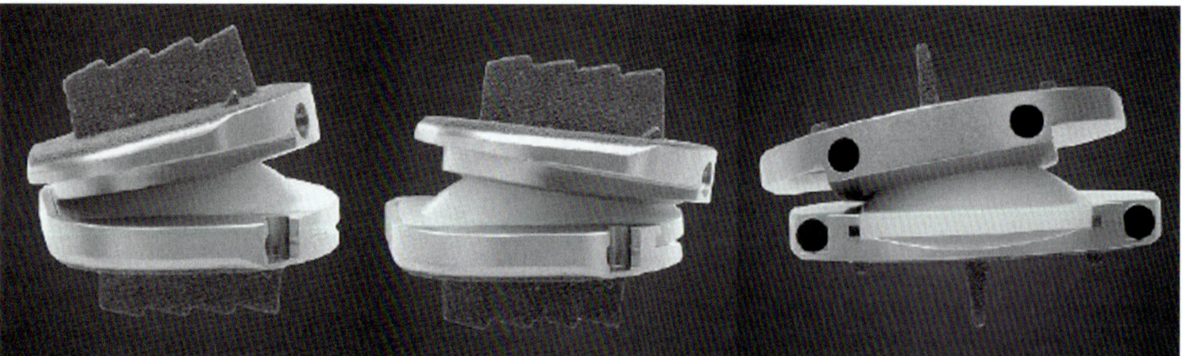

Figure 23–1   The mechanical design of the prosthesis couples forward translation with forward flexion. The device allows 13 degrees of flexion, 7 degrees of extension, 10 degrees of lateral bending, and ±3 degrees of axial rotation.

asymptomatic subjects.[8] Perhaps the most important finding is the correlation between range of motion and adjacent level degeneration. The authors defined degeneration as greater than 2 mm of disk collapse, anterior osteophyte formation, or greater than 3.5 mm of dynamic instability. Patients who maintained at least 5 degrees of motion at their most cephalad ProDisc had a 0% chance of adjacent level degeneration. On the contrary, patients with less than 5 degrees of motion had a 34% prevalence of adjacent segment degeneration. This may be the most compelling evidence that the ProDisc can protect from adjacent segment degeneration with the caveat that a threshold 5 degrees of motion is maintained.[9]

Interestingly, the same authors showed that ranges of motion were greater in the ProDisc II. In the later model, the average range of motion at the L4–L5 level was 10 degrees (range, 8–18 degrees) and at L5–S1 it averaged 8 degrees (range, 2–12 degrees).[3] The second study had a mean follow-up of 1.4 years, so it is unclear whether the improved range of motion reflects improvements based on the second-generation design, better surgical technique, or better patient selection. On the other hand, it is possible that this motion could change with a longer follow-up period.

No clear correlation existed between disk mobility and clinical outcomes. Additionally, no significant correlations were found between lack of motion and age, weight, lumbar level replaced, number of levels, or history of prior surgery. Huang and associates[7] found that female gender was correlated with a higher likelihood of not having measurable motion, even though there was no difference in mean range of motion between male or female patients. Instead, there were more outliers in the female group. None of the radiographs showed signs of instability above or below the level of the disk replacement. However, 24% of patients developed either loss of height or annular traction osteophyte formation adjacent to the replaced level.

One investigator showed that there was an increase in lumbar lordosis after ProDisc arthroplasty.[10] However, a second study showed no difference in sagittal alignment after implant with the ProDisc II prosthesis.[3] This study also showed that there was a significant correlation between lack of motion, poor sagittal plane alignment, and the development of adjacent level breakdown. This may lend credence to the theory that the improved motion allows the spine to "seek" a more desirable lordotic position and may be essential in protecting against adjacent level disease.

Le Huec investigated the role of UHMWPE in dampening vibration and shock transmissibility in the ProDisc's metal-on-poly bearing surface compared with a metal-on-metal design.[11] The shock absorption ratio was measured in a biomechanical testing apparatus. Despite the appreciably lower modulus of elasticity of the UHMWPE (0.8 GPa) versus the chrome-cobalt (235 GPa) there was no difference in load dissipation. Unfortunately, the clinical implications of this finding are not easily decipherable given the lack of information about dynamic loading (shock or vibration) of the human disk in vivo.

◆ Implantation Technique

The ProDisc is typically implanted through a left, mini-anterior retroperitoneal approach (although a transperitoneal approach may be considered under special circumstances). The incision may be transverse for single-level or longitudinal paraumbilical for multilevel reconstructions. The anterior rectus sheath is opened and the rectus abdominis is retracted laterally. The retroperitoneal space is entered inferior to the

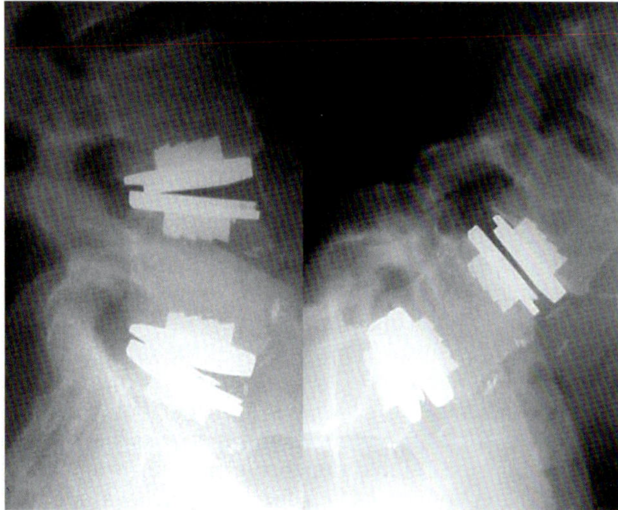

Figure 23–2   L4–L5, L5–S1 two-level ProDisc dynamic radiograph in extension and flexion.

arcuate line. The peritoneum is retracted medially.[12] At our institution, a Balfour self-retaining retractor is utilized longitudinally, and Wiley handheld retractors are used medially and laterally rather than self-retaining retractors. Our access surgeons believe that the great vessels can be more safely handled with the proprioceptive input from a handheld retractor, but table-based self-retaining systems are certainly acceptable. At our institution, the access surgeons remain scrubbed throughout the entire procedure to safely retract and protect the vessels.

Intraoperative fluoroscopy and a Synthes (Paoli, PA) 25 mm × 6.5 mm cancellous screw placed through the anterior annulus are used to verify level and midline. The midlines of the adjacent vertebral bodies are marked with electrocautery. Following a rectangular anterior annulotomy, a complete diskectomy is performed back to the posterior longitudinal ligament. A Cobb elevator is used to separate the disk from the end plates. Combinations of straight and curved curettes as well as various rongeurs complete the removal of the disk material. Oftentimes the posterolateral corners of the disk are the most difficult to fully resect, and special attention is paid to these locations. It is critical to perform a thorough diskectomy to "balance" the often contracted disk space. (Orthopedists can equate this to balancing a varus knee during a total knee arthroplasty.) Recession of the posterior longitudinal ligament from the posterior aspect of the vertebral bodies may also be required for cases where the ligament has become contracted. A herniated nucleus pulposus may also be retrieved at this time. It is useful to position the operative disk space over the break in the table. Intraoperative manipulation of table flexion-extension can give selective exposure to posterior and anterior aspects of the disk space and allow for complete diskectomy. This maneuver can also be extremely useful during implantation of the prosthesis (**Fig. 23–3**).

Distractors and implant trials (along with radiographic templating) determine the appropriate implant size. ProDisc implant trials allow one single instrument to help the surgeon determine footprint size, disk height (allowing for soft tissue balancing), and lordosis angle.[12] A slot for the sagittally oriented central keel is cut into the adjacent vertebral bodies using a chisel guided down the implant trial stem. The ProDisc II implants are assembled by the surgeon and

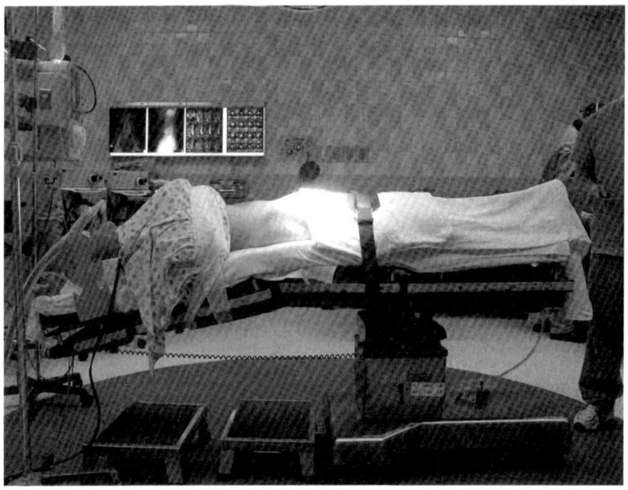

Figure 23–3 Positioning of the patient over the break in the table can assist in opening the disk space for complete diskectomy and in placement of the implant.

impacted in a collapsed, nested position into the disk space using fluoroscopic control (**Fig. 23–4**). Therefore, overdistraction of the disk space is not required. The insertion instrument grasps the metal end plates within their footprint, so the exposure and annulotomy need only accommodate the width of the implant without requiring extra room for the insertion instruments.[13] With use of a sliding distractor to transiently open the disk space, the appropriate-size UHMWPE insert is then snap-fit into the lower end plate. There are two end plate sizes (medium or large), three height selections (10, 12, or 14 mm), and two lordotic angles (6 or 11 degrees) (**Fig. 23–5**).

Postoperatively, the patients are placed in a light corset and ambulate the day of surgery. They are typically maintained on intravenous opioids with a patient-controlled analgesia device the first postoperative night. Mechanical thromboprophylaxis in the form of foot pumps and thigh-high TED hose are utilized. Most patients are ready for discharge on the first or second postoperative day. Patients who require physical therapy undergo a program of standard core strengthening and dynamic stabilization.

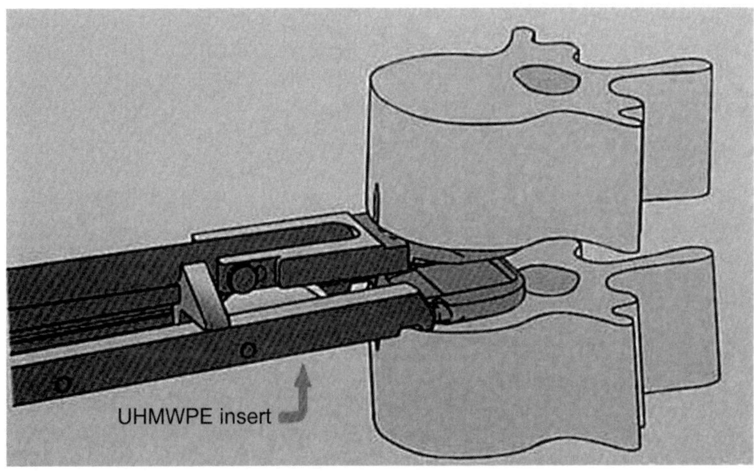

Figure 23–4 The ProDisc is implanted in a nested position within the confines of the insertional device. Note that the ultra high molecular weight polyethylene liner slides down the rails between the end plates without requiring excessive disk space overdistraction.

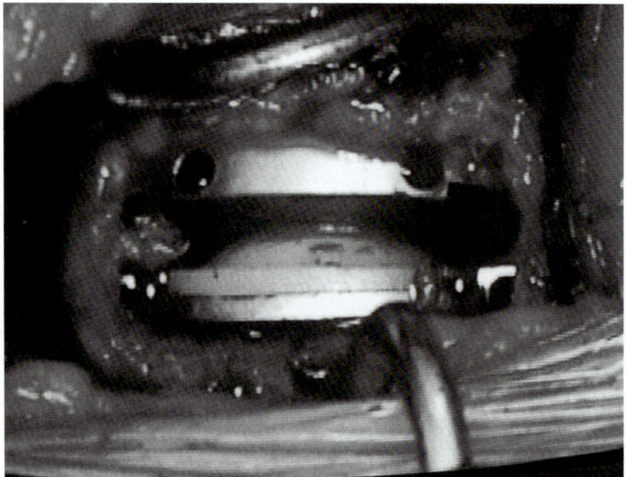

Figure 23–5   Intraoperative photograph of implanted ProDisc.

◆ European Experience

The European experience has been overall quite favorable. Bertagnoli published the results of 134 ProDisc II devices that were implanted in 108 patients with 3- to 36-month follow-ups.[14] One hundred patients had single-level implants. Eleven patients underwent two-level arthroplasty. Two patients had a three-level arthroplasty (**Fig. 23–6**). Patients were not considered appropriate for disk arthroplasty if there was severe osteoporosis, physiological dysfunction, previous infection, severe posterior element pathology, fracture, or tumor. Subjective outcomes were excellent in 90.8%, good in 7.4%, fair in 1.8%, and no patient had a poor result. Nine patients did have residual back or leg pain. Forty-five patients required analgesics for more than 2 weeks. There were 12 patients who required analgesics

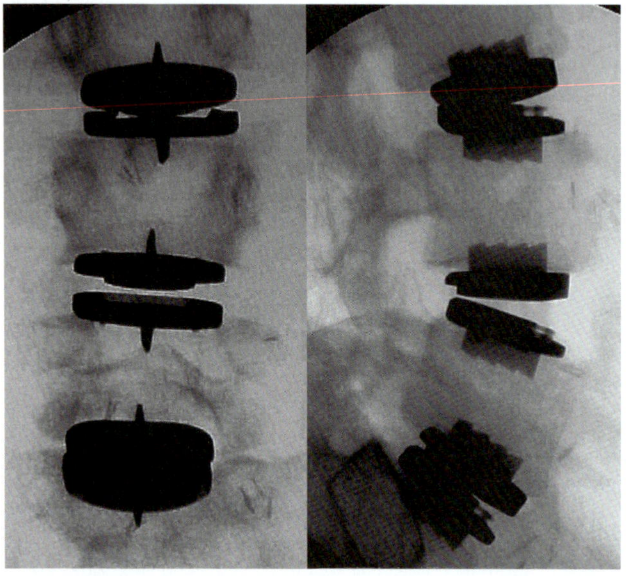

Figure 23–6   Three-level ProDisc implant. Intraoperative fluoroscopic anteroposterior and lateral images.

for 6 months to 1 year. Thirty-three patients used analgesics on an occasional basis. On average, patients were able to independently perform their activities of daily living at 2.3 weeks.

All patients showed an improvement in range of motion at the operated levels. At L5–S1 average motion was 9 degrees (2–13 degrees), at L4–L5 10 degrees (9–13 degrees), at L3–L4 10 degrees (8–15 degrees), at L2–L3 12 degrees (9–15 degrees). Adjacent segment range of motion was also measured. It increased in 86 patients an average of 6 degrees (3–8 degrees). It decreased in six patients an average of 5 degrees (3–8 degrees). In 16 patients, range of motion at adjacent segments did not change postoperatively. Progression of disk degeneration at adjacent segments was noted in five patients (4.6%). These patients all had disk height of < 7 mm prior to surgery. At final follow-up, there was no evidence of loosening or subsidence. There were no structural failures.

The study's primary objective was to examine outcomes in relation to different categories of indication criteria (**Fig. 23–7**). The "prime" indications for surgery were considered single-level disk, > 4 mm remaining disk height, no osteoarthritic (OA) changes in the facet joints, no adjacent level degeneration, and intact posterior elements. "Good" indications were either single-or double-level disks with > 4 mm remaining disk height, no primary OA changes in the facet joints, minimum degeneration of adjacent disks, and minimum posterior segment instability (e.g., postmicrodiskectomy). The "borderline" indications were single, double, or triple disk levels with < 4 mm remaining disk height, primary OA changes in the facet joints, minimum adjacent level degeneration, minimum posterior segment instability, and adjacent to preexisting fusions. Finally, "poor" indications were considered single-, double-, or triple-level disks with gross degeneration of the spine, secondary OA changes to the facet joints, < 4 mm disk height remaining at the adjacent levels, and posterior segment instability.

Bertagnoli's indications were predictive in improving patient satisfaction outcomes. In the "prime" group the average level of satisfaction was 98% (96–99%). In the "good" group it was 93% (89–97%). Finally, in the "borderline" group average level of satisfaction was 83% (79–88%).

Tropiano et al's results with 53 patients implanted with the ProDisc II between December 1999 and December 2001 were reported in 2003.[3] Their results were equally good. Forty patients had single-level implants. Eleven patients had two-level implants, and two patients had three-level implants. There was a mean follow-up of 1.4 years (range, 1–2 years). All patients were subjectively satisfied (87% patients were entirely satisfied, 13% were satisfied). Objectively, 72% returned to full duty, whereas 28% were only slightly limited in their vocational capacities. Only seven patients (13%) were unable to return to work. Visual analog scale (VAS) for back pain improved from an average preoperative measurement of 7.4 to 1.3, whereas leg pain improved from 6.7 to 1.9. Oswestry low back disability index improved from a preoperative score of 56 to 14 postoperatively. These changes were both statistically and clinically significant. There were no significant differences between single-level and multilevel outcomes.

Bertagnoli's Criteria

Indications	Disk height	Facets	Adjacent level	Posterior elements	Single	Double	Triple
						Levels	
Prime	> 4 mm	No OA	No degeneration	Intact	✔		
Good	> 4 mm	No primary OA	Minimum degeneration	Minimum posterior segment instability (post-laminectomy)	✔	✔	
Borderline	< 4 mm	Primary OA	Minimum degeneration	Adjacent fusion	✔	✔	✔
Poor	< 4 mm	Secondary OA	Gross degeneration	Instability	✔	✔	✔

Figure 23–7   Bertagnoli's indication criteria for disk reconstruction utilizing the ProDisc.

Radiographic data were very similar to that shown by Bertagnoli. There was an average range of motion at L5–S1 of 8 degrees (2–12 degrees) and 10 degrees (8-18 degrees) at L4–L5. There were no ossifications or implant failure. No degenerative changes were seen at the levels adjacent to disk replacement or at the facet joints.

There was a 9% complication rate. One patient with unrecognized osteoporosis suffered a vertebral body fracture. The device was malpositioned in two patients. Two patients had persistent radicular pain despite the absence of neurological compression on imaging studies. Both patients improved after 3 and 5 months. There was a 6% reoperation rate—one case was a 52-year-old with unrecognized osteopenia who suffered an end plate fracture that was revised to a fusion. There were two patients who required reoperation for laterally malpositioned implants.

◆ U.S. Experience

Based on the optimistic results of the European experience, the U.S. FDA opened an IDE trial that began October 2001. This can be considered level one evidence.[15] The study is a randomized, prospective, multicenter (19 centers) design comparing the ProDisc II implant with a 360 degree fusion in a 2 to 1 fashion. The control fusion group was treated with an anterior femoral ring allograft and a posterior instrumented pedicle screw fusion with iliac crest autograft. At the time of the study design, this was considered the surgical standard of care for disabling degenerative disk disease. Patients were blinded to the randomization selection until immediately postop.

The inclusion criteria were patients 18 to 60 years of age with predominant back pain, although patients could have coexistent leg pain. Patients were required to have failed at least 6 months of conservative care. One or two painful disks at L3–L4, L4–L5, or L5–S1 were included in the study (**Fig. 23–8**). Minimum Oswestry low back pain disability index was 40/100. Patients were excluded if they had undergone a previous lumbar fusion or had compromised vertebral bodies, severe facet degeneration, or metal allergies **Table 23–1**.

Outcome measurements were based on the VAS and the Oswestry measured at 6 weeks, 3 months, 6 months, 1 year, 18 months, and 2 years. The subjective question, "Would you have it done again?" was answered. Neutral anteroposterior/lateral and dynamic films were obtained at each follow-up interval. Radiographic data were collected measuring flexion, extension, and lateral bending.

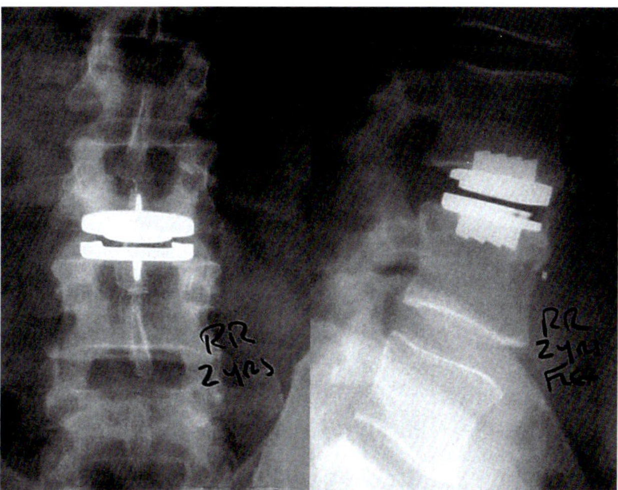

Figure 23–8   Postoperative anteroposterior and lateral radiograph of a ProDisc reconstruction at L3–L4. The U.S. Food and Drug Administration Investigational Device Exemption ProDisc trial included single- or two-level disk space reconstruction at L3–L4, L4–L5, or L5–S1.

Table 23–9   Inclusion and exclusion criteria for the U.S. Food and Drug Administration Investigational Device Exemption study

Inclusion criteria
1. Age between 18 and 60 y
2. At least 6 mo of failed nonoperative therapy
3. DDD at one or two adjacent vertebral levels between L3 and S1, where a diagnosis of DDD requires
   a. Primarily back and/or radicular pain
   b. Radiographic confirmation of any one of the following by CT, MRI, diskography, plain film, myelography, and/or flexion/extension films
      i. Lack of instability (defined at > 3 mm of translation of > 5° of angulation)
      ii. Decreased disk height > 2 mm
      iii. Scarring/thickening of annulus fibrosus
      iv. Herniated nucleus pulposus, or
      v. Vacuum phenomenon
4. Oswestry Low Back Pain Disability Questionnaire score of at least 20/50 (40%)
5. Psychosocially, mentally, or physically able to fully comply with this protocol, including adhering to follow-up schedule and requirements and filling out of form

Exclusion criteria
1. > 2 degenerative levels
2. Endplate dimensions < 34.5 mm in coronal plane and/or < 27 mm in sagittal plane
3. Known allergy to titanium, polyethylene, cobalt, chromium, or molybdenum
4. Prior lumbar fusion
5. Posttraumatic vertebral body compromise/deformity
6. Facet joint degeneration
7. Lytic spondylolisthesis or spinal stenosis
8. Degenerative spondylolisthesis of grade > 1
9. Back or leg pain of unknown etiology
10. Osteoporosis
11. Metabolic bone disease (excluding osteoporosis, eg, Paget disease)
12. Morbid obesity (BMI > 40 or weight > 100 lb over ideal body weight)
13. Pregnant or interested in becoming pregnant in next 3 y
14. Active systematic/local infection
15. Medications or drugs known to potentially interfere with bone/soft tissue healing, excluding smoking (eg, steroids)
16. Rheumatoid arthritis or other autoimmune spondylarthopathies.
17. Systematic disease including but not limited to AIDS, HIV, hepatitis
18. Active malignancy: patient with history of any invasive malignancy (except nonmelanoma skin cancer), unless he/she has been treated with curative intent and there have been no clinical signs or symptoms or malignancy for at least 5 y.

DDD, degenerative disc disease; CT, computed tomography; MRI, magnetic resonance imaging; BMI, body mass index; AIDS, acquired immune deficiency syndrome; HIV, human immunodeficiency virus.
(With permission from Zigler JE, Burd TA, Vialle EN, Sachs BL, Rashbaum RF, Ohnmeiss DD. Lumbar spine arthroplasty: results using the ProDisc II: a prospective randomized trial of arthroplasty versus fusion. J Spinal Disord Tech 2003;16:352–361. Table 1.)

At the time of this writing, the randomized portion of the study has been concluded and data have been submitted to the FDA. Final pooled results have yet to be made public. However, two of the largest ProDisc IDE sites have published interim results—Rick Delamarter's group from Saint John's Health Center in Santa Monica, California, and Jack Zigler's group from the Texas Back Institute in Plano, Texas.

In 2003, Delamarter et al published the results of their first 53 patients enrolled in the study, 35 of which received the ProDisc.[4] Of the 27 patients who had single-level reconstructions, 19 had a ProDisc arthroplasty. Of the 26 patients who had two-level procedures, 16 ProDiscs were placed. In terms of patient-assessed outcome scores, improvements were seen in both scores for each group at each assessment interval. As compared with the control group, the ProDisc group showed significantly greater improvement in the VAS score at both 6-week and 3-month intervals. In relation to disability, the ProDisc group significantly outperformed the fusions Oswestry score improvement at the 3-month assessment.

The radiographic analysis indicates that at the 6-month assessment, there was a significant increase in the sagittal motion as measured on flexion-extension views for the L4–L5 disk replacements. At L5–S1 there was an improvement in sagittal motion but this was not significant in comparison with the fusion cohort, which remained at 4 degrees both

pre- and postoperatively. No significant difference existed between the untreated L3–L4 segment ranges of motion in both the arthroplasty and fusion groups. Importantly, there were no radiographic signs of implant migration, breakage, or mechanical failure. There were no revisions.

Zigler and colleagues published interim results in 2003[16] and more recent results were published in 2004.[12] The most recent data were collected on the first 78 patients enrolled at their site. Fifty-five patients received the ProDisc. The largest differences in this study were the times to recovery. The ProDisc group had no limitation in ambulation in 61% of patients at 3-month follow-up. In contrast, the fusion group had only 45% of patients with unlimited ambulation. Furthermore, 68% patients were performing some type of recreational physical activity at 6 weeks in the arthroplasty group. At 6 months, 25% of patients were improved to the point that they were engaged in noncontact sports. In the fusion group, only 18% of patients were involved in any physical activities at 6 months. Return to work averaged 8 weeks in the ProDisc group as opposed to 16 weeks in the fusion group. The difference might have been even larger had not all four of the workers' compensation patients been randomized to the arthroplasty cohort.

An improvement in VAS was seen in both groups. A trend toward greater improvements was recorded in the ProDisc group, but this was not a statistically significant change. Oswestry scores improved throughout the study period. The difference between arthroplasty and fusion groups was significant at the 3 month assessment. In this study, although most survey questions showed only slight superiority of the ProDisc over the control group, the subjective "Would you do it again?" showed a larger difference. In the ProDisc group 98% of patients answered "definitely" and the other 2% were undecided. In the fusion group, 20% of patients answered "definitely not."

Radiographic measurements showed significantly better range of motion with forward bending, left lateral bending, and right lateral bending at 3 months and 6 months postoperatively as compared with their preoperative measurements. There was also a greater range of motion in the arthroplasty group than that obtained in the fusion cohort.

In terms of technical outcomes, the ProDisc showed a significant advantage. Operative times were shorter in the ProDisc group (75.4 minutes vs 218.2 minutes). Hospital stay was significantly shorter (2.1 days vs 3.5 days). Blood loss was less (68.9 mL versus 175 mL).

Complications in the fusion group included one incidence of bilateral leg pain, one posterior infection that required irrigation and debridement, four patients who experienced graft site pain at 6 weeks, and two patients who continued to experience graft site pain at 6 months.

The ProDisc group had one patient with polyethylene extrusion. This was early in the learning curve and was believed to be from improper seating of the polyethylene. The patient was returned to the operating room within 24 hours and a new polyethylene was placed uneventfully. There was one iliac vein tear that was successfully repaired intraoperatively. Two patients had right-leg pain postoperatively that showed improvement with Neurontin (Pfizer Inc., New York, NY) and epidural steroid injections. One patient had sacroiliac pain that was initially improved with chiropractic care and epidural steroid injections; however, it was reexacerbated in a motor vehicle accident. One patient had a pelvic venous thrombosis treated with anticoagulants and was found to have an underlying genetic coagulopathy.

Overall, the U.S. experience has shown that there are significant advantages to the ProDisc over a circumferential fusion during the first few months. This is most evident during the time frame that the bone graft is in the process of solidifying as a fusion mass. The ProDisc in essence gives patients a several-month "head start" over the fusion group. In terms of surgical technique, the ProDisc requires attention to detail in performing a thorough diskectomy and "soft-tissue balancing," but once this is mastered there is an overall shorter operative time with decreased blood loss and shorter hospital stay. The biggest question has yet to be answered not only for the ProDisc but for all of the disk replacements: Will range of motion help to diminish adjacent segment degeneration? This FDA study cohort will serve as a tremendous source of information as they are followed over the next several decades.

References

1. Marnay T. Lumbar disc replacement: 7–10-year results with ProDisc. Eur Spine J 2002;11:S19

2. Hallab N, Link HD, McAfee PC. Biomaterial optimization in total disc arthroplasty. Spine 2003;28:S139–S152

3. Tropiano P, Huang RC, Girardi FP, Marnay T. Lumbar disc replacement: preliminary results with ProDisc II after a minimum follow-up period of 1 year. J Spinal Disord Tech 2003;16:362–368

4. Delamarter RB, Fribourg DM, Kanim LE, Bae H. ProDisc artificial total lumbar disc replacement: introduction and early results from the United States clinical trial. Spine 2003;28:S167–S175

5. Pearcy MJ, Bogduk N. Instantaneous axes of rotation of the lumbar intervertebral joints. Spine 1988;13:1033–1041

6. Rousseau M, et al. Total disc replacement alters L5/S1 kinematics while partially unloading the facet joints. In: NASS. Chicago: Elsevier; 2004

7. Huang RC, Girardi FP, Cammisa FP Jr, Tropiano P, Marnay T. Long-term flexion-extension range of motion of the ProDisc total disc replacement. J Spinal Disord Tech 2003;16:435–440

8. Hayes MA, Howard TC, Gruel CR, Kopta JA. Roentgenographic evaluation of lumbar spine flexion-extension in asymptomatic individuals. Spine 1989;14:327–331

9. Huang RC, et al. Range of motion and adjacent level degeneration after lumbar total disc replacement. In NASS. Chicago: Elsevier; 2004

10. Tropiano P, Marnay T, Pierunek M, et al. Spinal balance after total disc replacement: preliminary results. In: Global Symposium on Intervertebral Disc Replacement and Non-Fusion Technology, Spine Arthroplasty Society Meeting; 2002; Montpellier, France

11. LeHuec JC, Kiaer T, Friesem T, Mathews H, Liu M, Eisermann L. Shock absorption in lumbar disc prosthesis: a preliminary mechanical study. J Spinal Disord Tech 2003;16:346–351

12. Zigler JE. Lumbar spine arthroplasty using the ProDisc II. Spine J 2004;4(Suppl 6):260S–267S

13. Zigler JE. Clinical results with ProDisc: European experience and U.S. investigation device exemption study. Spine 2003;28:S163–S166

14. Bertagnoli R, Kumar S. Indications for full prosthetic disc arthroplasty: a correlation of clinical outcome against a variety of indications. Eur Spine J 2002;11(Suppl 2):S131–S136

15. Evidence-Based Medicine Working Group. Guyett, GR, Drummond. Users' Guide to the Medical Literature: A Manual for Evidence-Based Clinical Practice. Chicago: AMA Press; 2002

16. Zigler JE, Burd TA, Vialle EN, Sachs BL, Rashbaum RF, Ohnmeiss DD. Lumbar spine arthroplasty: early results using the ProDisc II: a prospective randomized trial of arthroplasty versus fusion. J Spinal Disord Tech 2003;16:352–361

24

MAVERICK Total Disc Replacement

Matthew F. Gornet

◆ **Male End Plate (Inferior Component)**

◆ **Female End Plate (Superior Component)**

◆ **Design Rationale of the Maverick**
 Posterior Center of Rotation
 Metal-on-Metal Design
 Hydroxyapatite Coating Fixation
 Streamlined Surgical Technique

◆ **Patient Selection**

◆ **Surgical Technique**

◆ **Clinical Outcomes**
 Surgical Data
 Oswestry Disability Questionnaire Scores
 Neurological Status
 Back and Leg Pain
 Work Status
 Patient Satisfaction

◆ **Conclusion**

The current standard of care for the treatment of lumbar degenerative disk disease is spinal fusion. Spinal fusion is designed to increase stability of a diseased motion segment, while necessarily limiting motion. This static stabilization, however, is coming under increased scrutiny as a potential contributor to adjacent level degenerative changes, even as improved materials and surgical techniques drive very high rates of successful fusion.[1–3] Clinical outcomes following fusion may likewise be problematic in that painful loading across the disk space may still occur.[4,5] In response to these apparent shortcomings, it has been proposed that motion stabilization via disk arthroplasty, rather than disk arthrodesis, may be a preferred treatment.[6–9] The two most clinically notable designs in use in the world today, the SB Charité III (DePuy Spine, Raynham, MA) and the ProDisc (Synthes, Inc., West Chester, PA), are both based on articulating cobalt-chromium-molybdenum (CoCrMo) on ultra high molecular weight polyethylene (UHMWPE). The earliest versions of the SB Charité have been in use since ~1984, with the current model III design in use since ~1987. Both Charité[10–13] and ProDisc[14] have been used with some reported clinical success.

Maverick Total Disc Replacement (TDR) (Medtronic Sofamor Danek, Inc., Memphis, TN) is among the next generation of arthroplasty implants and is intended for use in the lumbar spine to treat degenerative disk disease.[8,15] The Maverick TDR was certified for implantation in Europe in 2001 and was first applied clinically in the United States in April 2003. Maverick TDR has already undergone an extensive evaluation of material and design strength, durability, wear, and surgical implantation techniques.[8,15–17]

The unique design characteristics of the Maverick prosthesis allow for improved function with superior wear via a metal-on-metal (MOM) articulation in a ball and socket joint (**Fig. 24–1**). Similar to the experience in total hip prostheses, it is expected that using CoCrMo alloy for both articulating surfaces will provide excellent wear characteristics.[18–21] The Maverick TDR consists of male and female, MOM end plates (**Fig. 24–2**).

◆ Male End Plate (Inferior Component)

The male end plate is intended for positioning on the superior end plate of the inferior vertebra at the treated spinal level. The device is manufactured from cobalt-chromium-molybdenum (CoCrMo). The bone-abutting surface is chemically textured to provide a roughened surface geometry and is subsequently coated with hydroxyapatite (HA) by a thermal plasma-spray deposition process. Protruding from the bone-abutting surface is a keel, which provides for device stability by press-fitting into a prepared channel in the vertebral body. The articulating surface has a male (convex) dome, which mates with the female end plate. The male end plate is available in only one height.

◆ Female End Plate (Superior Component)

The female end plate is identical to the male end plate except that, instead of a convex male dome, it has the mating concave female receiving surface and is offered in several heights. The mated device allows for 16 degrees of motion off the neutral position in all bending directions. Both male and female end plates may be preangled either 3 degrees or 6 degrees. Both end plates are offered in small, medium, and large sizes. All

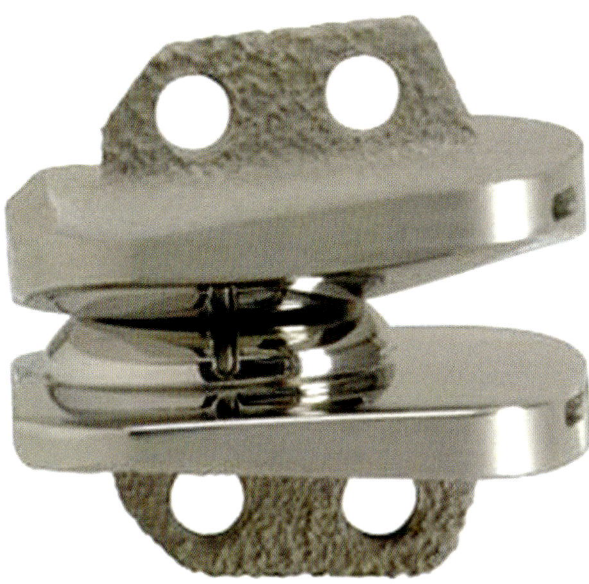

Figure 24–1   MAVERICK Total Disc Replacement two-piece ball and joint prosthesis.

joints are designed to be interchangeable. Therefore, the surgeon is able to interchange components to build a wide configuration of constructs. Some examples include 6 degrees, 9 degrees, or 12 degrees of prelordosis as well as posterior heights of 10 to 14 mm, and may even include a combination of different footprint sizes (**Fig. 24–3**). For example, a small female end plate could be mated with a medium male end plate.

◆ Design Rationale of the Maverick

A thorough analysis and understanding of the biomechanical properties of spinal segments is a critical prerequisite in the design of prosthetics for disk arthroplasty.[4,7–9,16,17,22] Consideration must be given as well to the intended patient population, for whom longevity may be a significant requirement of the motion-preservation device. The Maverick TDR is designed as a permanent implant, intended to maintain segmental motion at the affected level. Testing involved material and design issues such as shear and compressive strength, long-term durability, wear performance, and shock absorption. Furthermore, strategic surgical considerations such as implantation technique[8,16,17,22] were optimized. Several key elements were ultimately incorporated in this design in pursuit of optimal motion stabilization:

Posterior Center of Rotation

The Maverick prosthesis possesses a fixed center of rotation (COR) in the posterior third of the device. Accurate placement of any TDR prosthesis is critical to preserve normal motion and reduce facet loads. Extreme posterior placement of any prosthesis is often difficult. In a ball and cup design, facet loads are sensitive to COR location. Placement of a prosthesis too far anterior is felt to magnify facet loading over 2.5 times normal,[8] which may lead to early degeneration and continued pain. By having the COR posterior within the device itself, Maverick allows "forgiveness" of any surgical placement that is less than optimal (**Fig. 24–4**). In addition, this design provides up to 3 mm of controlled translation while mimicking the normal kinematics of the spine.

Metal-on-Metal Design

Among the benefits of MOM design is longer survivorship.[23] The track record of UHMWPE wear in large joint replacement is well reported.[24,25] Given the fact that any anterior revision of a TDR could be life threatening, the optimal prosthesis should be able to last the patient's lifetime. Wear debris from polyethylene can be associated with osteolysis and foreign body reaction. For that reason, the use of MOM for reduced

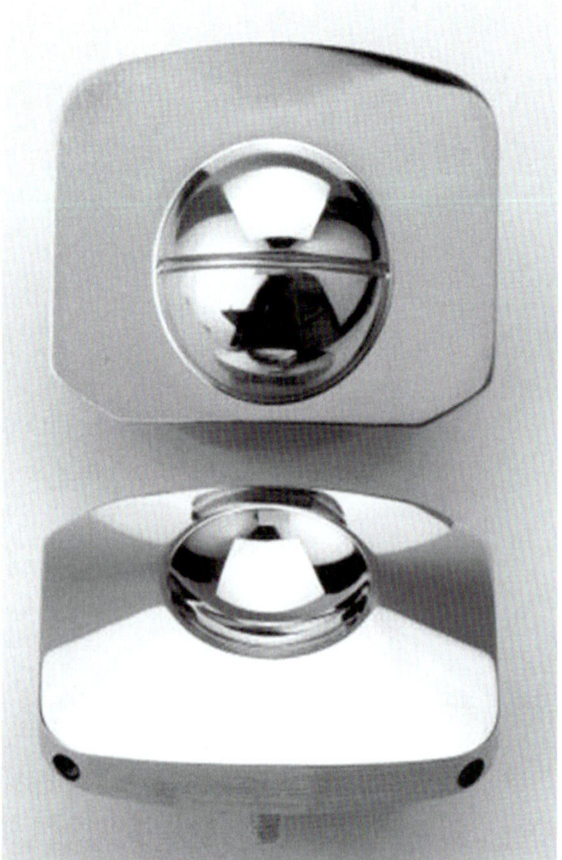

Figure 24–2 Maverick metal-on-metal end plates (cobalt-chromium-molybdenum alloy).

Wear testing of Maverick demonstrated low wear of ~14 mm³ during the 10 million cycle (MC) duration of the test. Assuming that there are 125,000 significant bends in 1 year in situ, this equates to 14 mm³ of wear over ~31.5 years of use or 0.35 mm³/year. Compared with in vitro simulator wear tests of MOM hip implants, which exhibit wear rates of ~0.38 mm³/MC,[18-20] or 0.38 mm³/year with the assumption that the average hip arthroplasty patient takes 1 million steps per year, the wear of Maverick is well within that reported for MOM hips in current clinical use. It is interesting to note that the annualized wear rate of Maverick is further reduced to 0.14 mm³/year with the assumption of 125,000 bends per year as used by Dooris et al.[28] Finally, because all in vitro testing must be validated through comparisons with explanted devices, it is noteworthy that the Maverick was the subject of such a comparison in only the published studies comparing simulator-tested and retrieved implants of the same type.[29,30] These studies compared in vitro–tested Maverick implants to an explanted Maverick device and found marked differences between the surface morphology of the articulating surfaces. In general, the simulator-tested implants showed highly visible wear scars, whereas the surface of the explanted device was highly polished with minimal scratching. This strongly suggests that the in vitro simulator test conditions are harsher than what occurs physiologically. Therefore, the wear rates generated in simulator testing may overestimate the actual in situ wear of the implants.

The main perceived objection to MOM designs is the increased systemic exposure to metal ions due to metal wear debris. In a study where CoCrMo particles were administered to the spine in a rabbit model,[31] CoCrMo wear debris particles were calculated for dosage levels equivalent to 10-year, 30-year, and 60-year exposure after CoCrMo-on-CoCrMo TDR. Intervertebral injection sites at L5 or L6, local lymph nodes adjacent to the implantation site, and distant lymph nodes were evaluated microscopically in both investigational and control animals. In addition, liver, kidneys, spleen, and thymus of all animals were assessed microscopically. The results of this study simulating up to 60 years of clinical use of a CoCrMo-on-CoCrMo device indicated no significant histological changes when comparing treated and control animals. Human studies are now ongoing to look at the production of ions associated with MOM designs.

wear in spinal applications was one of the critical Maverick design considerations. CoCrMo alloy, currently used in large-joint total arthroplasty, may provide the opportunity for long-lasting utilization without the complications of conventional polyethylene wear debris.[23-26] In hip replacement, MOM produces up to two orders of magnitude less wear than metal-on-conventional UHMWPE hip prostheses.[27] Use of a MOM prosthesis in the spine appears to be more advantageous than in the hip due to the different forces generated from this anatomical location.[8]

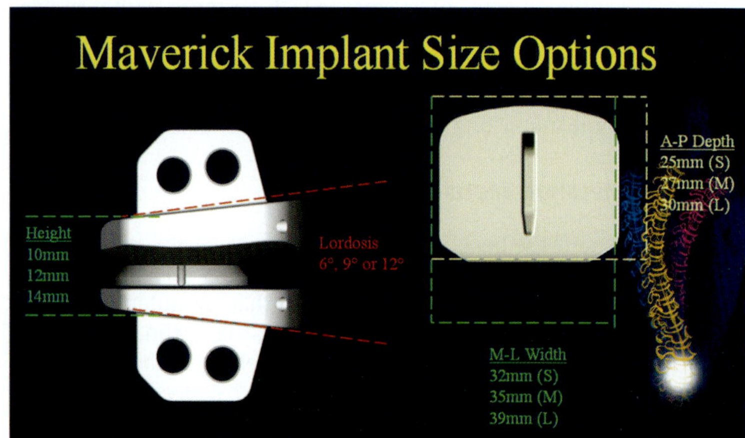

Figure 24–3 Maverick Total Disc Replacement interchangeable components provide flexibility to build a wide range of constructs.

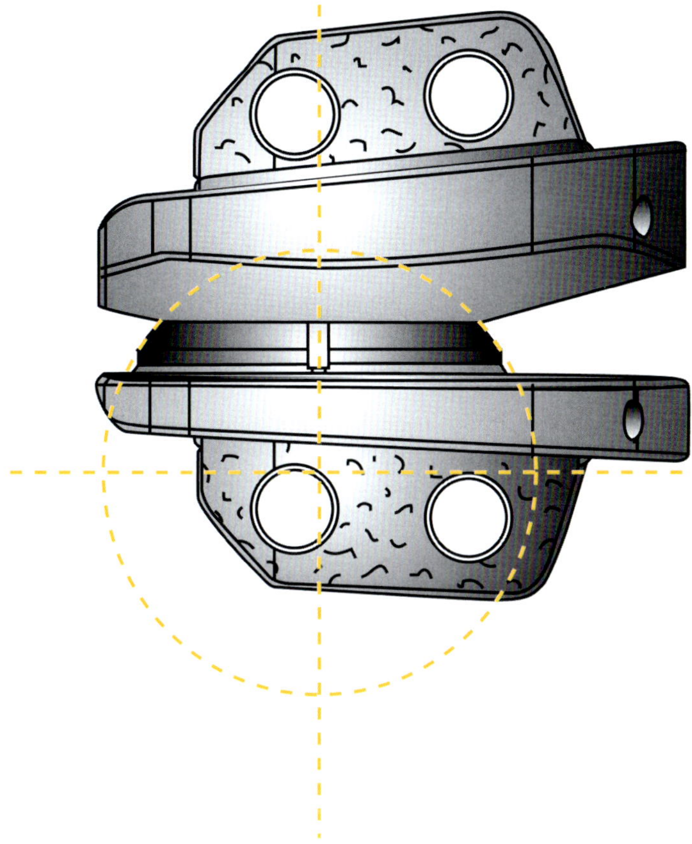

Figure 24–4   Posterior center of rotation corresponds more closely to patient anatomy.

Hydroxyapatite Coating Fixation

Used in arthroplasty for 30 years, this osseoconductive synthetic-bone material is highly crystalline, providing an excellent bone-device fixation surface. In addition, the roughened Chemtex surface (**Fig. 24–5**) provides increased friction for a press fit.

Streamlined Surgical Technique

This final element of the design rationale provides the surgeon with a complete tray for en bloc diskectomy, with the All-in-1 guide (provided in the Maverick kit) (**Fig. 24–6A–C**) for accuracy and reproducibility. The All-in-1 guide maintains lordosis, measures anteroposterior depth, measures height distraction, and guides chiseling. In conjunction with

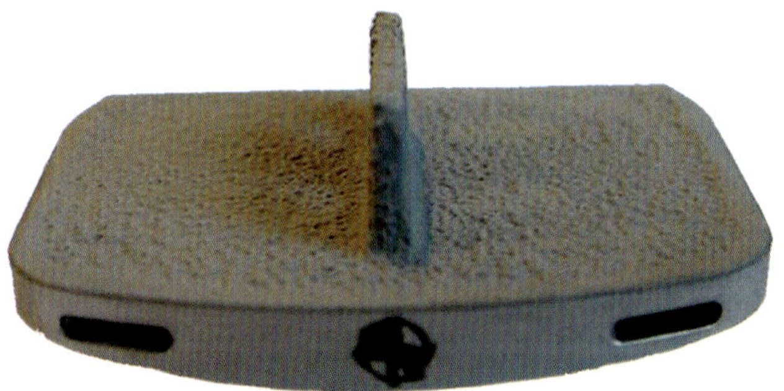

Figure 24–5   Hydroxyapatite and roughened Chemtex provide a surface conducive to bony ongrowth with increased friction for a press-fit.

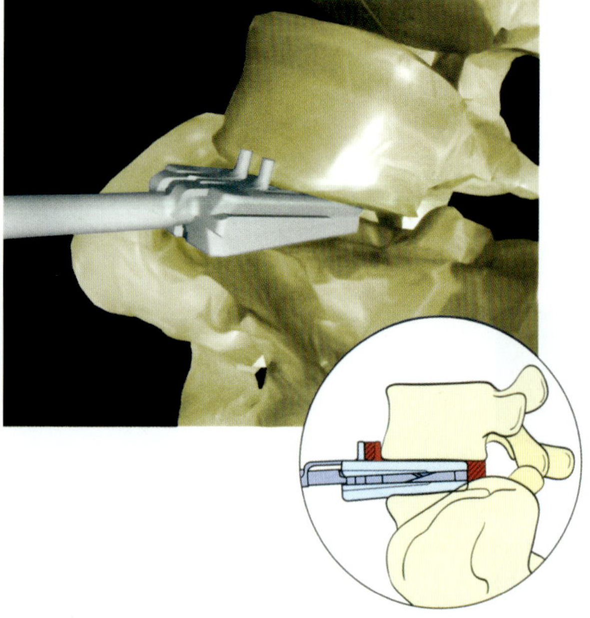

A

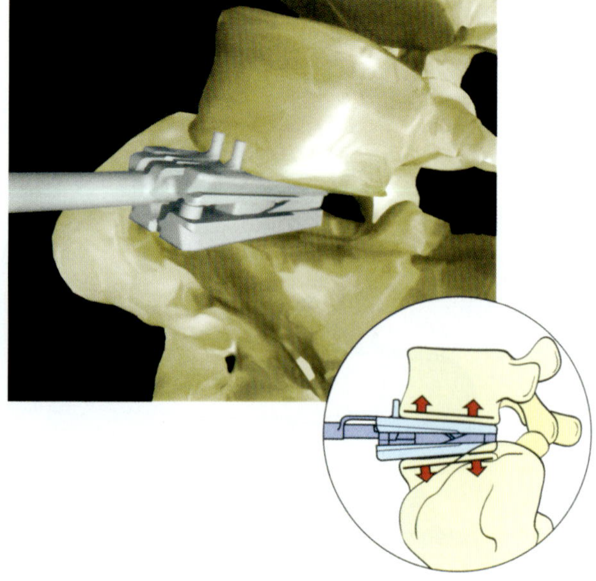

B

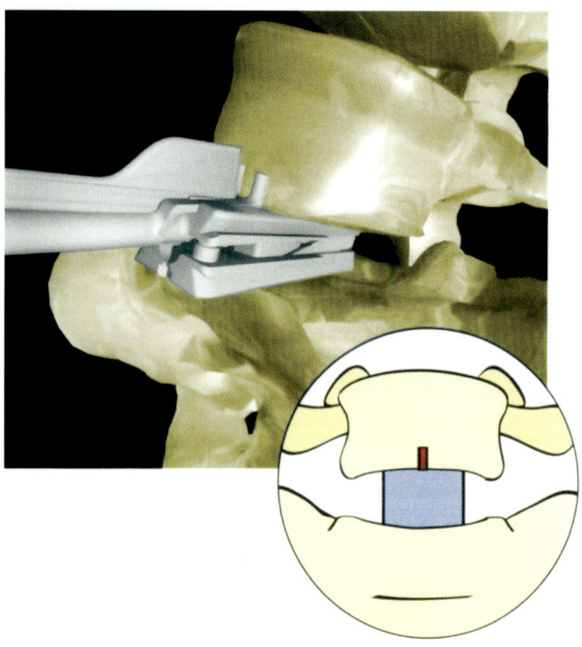

C

Figure 24–6   (A) Templating with the All-in-1 instrument to establish midline and proper depth. **(B)** Parallel distraction with the All-in-1 instrument, establishing in situ parallel tension on the segment. **(C)** Keel cutting with the All-in-1 instrument for ideal midline keel placement.

proper sizing, this guide promotes surgical efficiency and device effectiveness for optimal results.

To summarize, the following were key considerations in the Maverick design:

◆ Posterior COR to optimize unloading of facet joints
◆ Fixed COR to resist shear loading
◆ Two-piece design unit requiring only a single insertion
◆ MOM for excellent wear performance
◆ HA coating and keel design for optimal fixation
◆ Shock transmission of MOM identical to MO-UHMWPE
◆ Restoration of functional motion

◆ Patient Selection

Successful clinical outcomes with the Maverick TDR, as with any intervertebral prosthesis, depend above all on proper patient selection. Patients accepted for the U.S. Food and Drug Administration (FDA)-approved clinical study of the Maverick device beginning in 2003 all had single-level degenerative disk disease (at L4–L5 or L5–S1) as noted by back pain of diskogenic origin, with or without leg pain. Degeneration of the disk was confirmed by patient history, neurological examination, and radiographic testing. Imaging generally revealed Modic changes, zones of high intensity in the annulus, loss of disk height, and decreased disk hydration in patients who were potential candidates for the procedure (**Fig. 24–7**). This

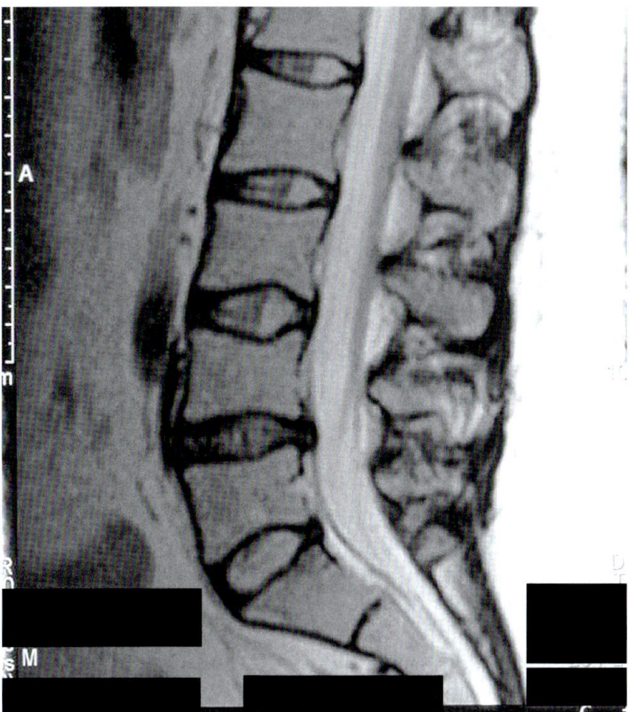

Figure 24–7   A 32-year-old female: magnetic resonance imaging reveals a central annular tear at L4–L5 with a central disk protrusion.

documented annular pathology, in conjunction with intact facet joints suggesting back pain from loading of the disk, and significant elevated Oswestry and visual analog back and leg pain scores, indicate likely candidates for this implantation. For the Investigational Device Exemption (IDE) study, patients with single-level disease between 18 and 70 years of age who had not responded to nonoperative treatment (e.g., bed rest, physical therapy, medications, Transcutaneous Electrical Nerve Stimulation (TENS) manipulation, and/or spinal injections) for a period of 6 months were included.

Equally important in the selection of patients with the highest probability of a successful outcome are the clinical contraindications. Patients with a spinal disorder other than degenerative disk disease at the involved level, those who had a previous posterior lumbar spinal fusion or any anterior lumbar spinal surgery at the involved level, and patients who require either or both spinal fusion and arthroplasty at more than one lumbar level would be excluded in the U.S. IDE study. Posterior element insufficiency (e.g., facet resection, spondylolysis, or pars fracture), severe pathology of the facet joints of the involved vertebral bodies, spondylolisthesis, spinal canal stenosis, and segmental scoliosis are also considered contraindications for the Maverick TDR.

◆ Surgical Technique

As previously discussed, the patient is selected who is considered an appropriate candidate for disk replacement. Particular care should be taken to eliminate patients with significant bone abnormalities that may produce subsidence in the prosthesis, as well as patients with severe facet disease. Once the appropriate patient is selected, the surgical team

should attempt to match the largest disk replacement footprint possible to the anatomy. In my experience, this can be accomplished by using the axial images of a magnetic resonance imaging (MRI) or computed tomographic (CT) scan prior to surgery. Templates are available for preoperative planning; once the surgeon gains adequate experience utilizing the Maverick prosthesis, however, templating can be eliminated and sizing can be determined intraoperatively.

Proper position is achieved by placing the patient supine on the operative table. We use a radiolucent Orthopedic Systems, Inc. (OSI) table, which allows adequate utilization of the image intensifier for prosthetic positioning during surgery. A bump or bolster can be used under the patient's pelvis to facilitate exposure; this will often allow greater access to the disk space by opening the anterior margin.

The lumbar spine is then approached anteriorly. This can either be transperitoneal or retroperitoneal. The vessels are retracted to gain exposure at the diseased segment. At the L4–L5 level, special care should be taken to identify any iliolumbar vessels that may limit the immobilization of the left common iliac. Once we feel we have adequate exposure at the diseased segment, markers are placed directly anteriorly at what we feel visually is the midline of the vertebral body. A centering pin is provided as part of the Maverick disk replacement instrumentation. This pin allows the surgeon to mark the center of the disk space and bring the imaging intensifier into the AP position, allowing the vessels to safely retract directly over the center pin. The AP image will aid in the confirmation at the midline and allow the surgeon to access any rotation of the vertebral body that may be present. Once the midline position is confirmed by fluoroscopy, I mark the vertebral body with a Bovie to permanently preserve the midpoint. With the midline identified and appropriately checked and marked, we bring the fluoroscopy machine into the lateral position. This also confirms our operative level from a lateral viewpoint. The fluoroscopy machine is then maneuvered up toward the patient's head and out of the way of the operating surgeon.

A block diskectomy is then performed (**Fig. 24–8**). Care is taken to limit the size of the block diskectomy and to not remove too much of the lateral annulus. The lateral annular fibers are considered to be an important stabilizing structure in disk replacement surgery. We remove all disk material

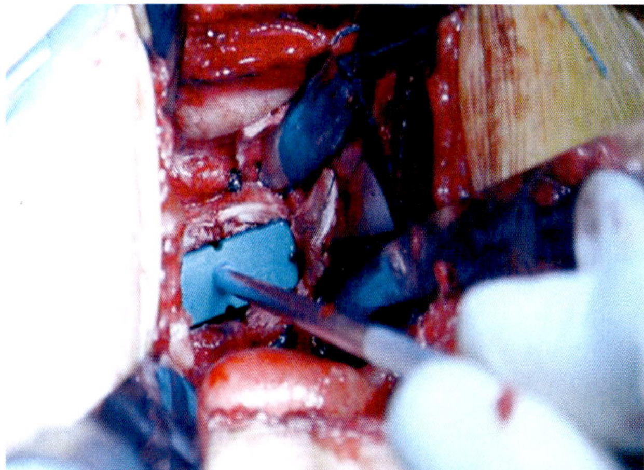

Figure 24–8   Diskectomy should clear the disk space all the way to the posterior ligament.

down to the cartilaginous end plate. The operating surgeon is cautioned not to violate the bone itself because this may allow destabilization of the end plate and create the potential for subsidence of the disk prosthesis. Once a complete diskectomy is performed, the surgeon may need to mobilize the disk space. Osteophytes that may inhibit placement of the prosthesis can also be removed at this time.

In my experience, mobilization of the disk space can be performed using a series of central dilators. The dilators are standard instruments for performing an anterior lumbar fusion. By progressively dilating the space, the surgeon can feel quickly whether the segment is mobile. With a collapsed disk space, the segment will often mobilize anteriorly but tether at the posterior annulus. In essence, the disk space moves like a bellows, with only one side mobile. If this finding occurs intraoperatively, the posterior aspect of the annulus remains tethered. This is easily rectified by additional posterior dilation or by using a curette to release the annulus itself. Once the tether is removed, symmetric dilation of the motion segment can occur. The surgeon can confirm symmetric dilation by obtaining a lateral fluoroscopic image.

After the space has been determined to be freely mobile, trials can be utilized to determine the appropriate disk height. I tend to select a disk height that is 1 to 2 mm less than the snug dilator I would use for an anterior lumbar interbody fusion (ALIF). The disk trial should fit in snugly but be more easily removed than the standard distractors for an anterior lumbar fusion. Selecting a disk height size that is too large will cause overtensioning of the lateral annulus and the facet joints, and may contribute to decreased motion of the prosthesis while increasing the incidence of subsidence.

Trialing to estimate the correct lordosis is much more difficult. The positioning on the table affects the perceived lordosis intraoperatively. The surgeon must remember that, unlike an ALIF, a disk prosthesis is freely mobile, and the position templated and eventually achieved intraoperatively will not necessarily mimic the position of the prosthesis when the patient is standing. For this reason, we attempt to estimate the maximum lordosis of the interspace using the trials provided. The trial should parallel the superior and inferior end plates. This will allow us to better determine the midrange of motion between flexion and extension. Once maximum lordosis is determined, we decrease the degree measured a minimum of 3 degrees to allow mobility of the segment. For example, if the maximum lordosis was determined to be 12 degrees, we would ask for a 9 degree or even a 6 degree prosthesis.

After the disk height is estimated and the preferred lordotic angle is noted, the All-in-1 device provided in the Maverick kit is used to establish all remaining size parameters (**Fig. 24–6A**). One can double check the actual disk height by distracting the segment using the All-in-1 guide while performing lateral fluoroscopy. I have found that the All-in-1 guide gives me less feel for the actual disk height than the interspace dilators, and therefore I tend to use dilators.

Once the All-in-1 guide is in position and is centered on the AP mark on the vertebral body, we perform keel osteotomy cuts (**Fig. 24–6C**). Before making the osteotomy cuts, the surgeon should always check that the All-in-1 guide is positioned as far posteriorly as possible. Place the tip of the device as close as possible to the posterior vertebral body line. This will allow the prosthesis to be seated as far

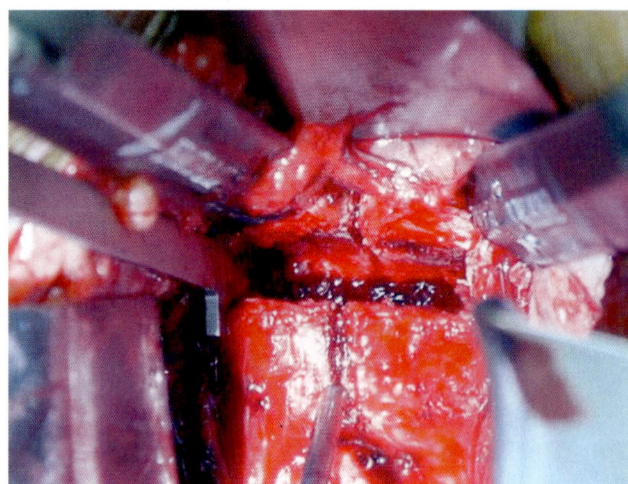

Figure 24–9   Final view of the prepared disk space.

posteriorly as possible and will maximize unloading of the facet joints (**Fig. 24–6B**). Placing the All-in-1 guide at the posterior vertebral body line will not create a risk of the chisel going completely through the vertebral body. The chisel will stop ~10 mm proximal to the posterior tip of the All-in-1 guide. The guide allows for both keel cuts to be made at one time. Usually there is brisk bleeding from the keel cuts once the chisels are removed. This bleeding can often be limited by using Flowseal and Surgicel in the disk space for ~30 seconds.

The surgeon now has a feel for disk height, lordosis, and the footprint of the implant (**Fig. 24–9**). The surgeon should try to place the largest footprint that the anatomy allows. In this author's experience, Maverick is not prone to subsidence. With our previous patients, the most commonly used prosthesis has been a small 10 mm height with 6 degrees of lordosis. The larger prosthesis will allow slightly greater medial to lateral surface area as well as anterior posterior footprint. It is rare that one would require a large prosthesis with greater than 12 mm of height.

The prosthesis the surgeon requests is offered in 3 degree lordotic increments. Both the superior and inferior components of the prosthesis contribute to the lordosis achieved. For example, a request for 9 degrees of lordosis could be achieved from combining one 3 degree and one 6 degree prosthetic component, regardless of end plate position. There is no advantage from placing the smaller lordotic component on either the inferior or superior end plate because this does not seem to alter the clinical outcome.

Depending on end plate morphology, corner cuts can be made to allow the prosthesis to sit in a more uniform position. The author's experience is that this phenomenon is quite rare, and usually the additional corner chisel cuts are not required.

The prosthesis is now ready to be inserted. It is assembled on the driver and tamped home. The depth of insertion is verified under x-ray control using the image intensifier. The final position of the prosthesis should be as far posterior as possible and should correlate with the previous chisel cuts made. Because the prosthesis assembles and enters the disk space similarly to a wedged dilator, as the prosthesis is tamped home, it tends to dilate this space quite easily. This is in direct comparison with other prostheses that require distraction once the implant is in position to place a polyethylene core. Overdistraction often leads to the creation of stress risers within the end plate and to eventual subsidence. Care should be taken not to overtamp the prosthesis posteriorly because pulling the prosthesis back anterior is often difficult. Should this occur, there are special guides that allow extraction of the prosthesis itself. Tamping the prosthesis too far posteriorly could lead to potential foramen encroachment by the lateral margins of the prosthesis. The image intensifier is used to confirm the final position in both lateral and AP planes. At this point, the incision is closed in the standard fashion.

◆ Clinical Outcomes

The early clinical and radiographic results for patients receiving the Maverick TDR system have been encouraging. In a prospective study of the influence of TDR on sagittal balance, there was no significant change versus preoperative status in any of the studied variables including sacral tilt, pelvic tilt, or overall lordosis after placement of the Maverick prosthesis.[32] Separately, Le Huec et al report on 2-year follow-up in a prospective study of 64 patients receiving the Maverick at one European site.[15] With Oswestry, back pain, and leg pain scores all significantly improved versus preoperative scores at 6, 12, and 24 months, the Maverick results in this study compare favorably with the best ALIF series.[33]

Although data for the complete U.S. IDE study are not available as of this writing, a review of 12-month data for 151 investigational patients from five participating centers shows promise for the Maverick TDR system. In this group, the average age of patients was 40 years, with 46% male and 54% female patients. Of these patients, 37% were smokers. The percentage of patients with pending litigation was 22%, and 25% were seeking workers' compensation.

Patient assessments were completed preoperatively, during hospitalization, and postoperatively at 6 weeks and at 3, 6, and 12 months. Clinical outcomes were assessed using the Oswestry Low Back Pain Disability Questionnaire, neurological status, short form (SF)-36 Health Survey, and back and leg pain questionnaires.

Surgical Data

The level L4–L5 was treated in 26% of patients, with 74% receiving treatment at L5–S1. The mean operative time for the Maverick TDR procedure was 1.7 hours; average blood loss was 243.9 mL. On average, patients were hospitalized for 2.2 days. Discharge from the hospital was based on the treating surgeon's standard criteria for discharge, with no objective discharge parameters used in the study. There was one severe (grade 3) implant/surgical procedure–associated adverse event in this investigational group at the time of the annual report to the FDA in May 2005.

Oswestry Disability Questionnaire Scores

The Oswestry Low Back Pain Disability Questionnaire measures pain associated with patient activities. The Oswestry questionnaire was administered preoperatively and at each postoperative visit. At 12 months, the mean Oswestry score was 20.6, an improvement of 33.4 ($p < .001$) versus preoperative scores. Oswestry scores showed statistically significant improvement versus baseline at all measured postoperative intervals. In addition, patient results demonstrated sequentially better outcomes at all measured time intervals starting at 6 weeks (**Table 24–1**).

Table 24–1 Clinical Results Compared with Preoperative Benchmark at Follow-Up Intervals

Period	Variable	Oswestry	Low Back Pain	Leg Pain	SF-36 PCS
Preoperative	n	151	151	151	151
	Mean	54.6	72.3	54.0	27.1
6 weeks	n	145	145	145	144
Improvement from	Mean	35.0	23.4	27.6	34.8
preoperative	n	145	145	145	144
	Mean	−19.6	−48.6	−26.3	7.6
	p value*	<.001	<.001	<.001	<.001
3 months	n	144	144	144	144
Improvement from	Mean	26.3	20.1	23.9	39.7
preoperative	n	144	144	144	144
	Mean	−28.2	−51.9	−31.5	12.5
	p value	<.001	<.001	<.001	<.001
6 months	n	142	142	142	142
Improvement from	Mean	22.6	19.8	20.0	41.8
preoperative	n	142	142	142	142
	Mean	−32.0	−52.3	−24.7	14.5
	p value	<.001	<.001	<.001	<.001
12 months	n	118	118	118	118
Improvement from	Mean	20.6	17.9	17.5	42.9
preoperative	n	118	118	118	118
	Mean	−33.4	−53.3	−36.6	15.8
	p value	<.001	<.001	<.001	<.001

p values for change from preoperative are from paired t-test.

Neurological Status

To determine neurological status of the patients, four neurological measurements were evaluated: motor function, sensory function, deep tendon reflexes, and sciatic tension signs. The values for each of these measurements were totaled and reported as a percentage of the maximum possible score, which was then compared with the preoperative score for each patient. Success was defined as maintenance of or improvement in all four measurements. At 12 months, the overall neurological success rate was 94.1% for Maverick patients.

Back and Leg Pain

The assessment of back pain intensity and duration is accomplished with the use of a 20-point numeric rating scale. A composite score is calculated by multiplying the numeric rating scores for back pain intensity and back pain duration. The mean back pain scores at all postoperative periods were significantly improved versus the preoperative mean value, with sequential improvement at each postoperative interval (**Table 24–1**).

In the same fashion, leg pain is assessed using a numeric rating scale for both intensity and duration of pain. Mean leg pain scores improved significantly versus the preoperative baseline at all postoperative periods, and there was sequential improvement at each follow-up interval (**Table 24–1**).

Work Status

Work status is another variable that may be assessed in an effort to evaluate a patient's overall success following spinal surgery. There are numerous factors that affect the work status of these patients, including the nature of their work, the ability and willingness of the workplace to accommodate work restrictions, and the patients' personal circumstances. In this investigational group, 49% of patients were working prior to surgery. The number of patients working after receiving the Maverick TDR increased at each postoperative interval.

Patient Satisfaction

At 12 months, 82.2% of the Maverick TDR patients reported that they were satisfied with the results of the surgery, and 78.0% reported that they were helped by their surgery as much as they expected. Of 92 patients responding, only 6.7% indicated that, all things considered, they would not elect to have the surgery again for the same condition.

◆ Conclusion

The Maverick TDR system shows considerable promise as a therapeutic technique (**Fig. 24–10**). Unique design characteristics, including a metal-on-metal ball and joint construct and a posterior COR with controlled translation, attempt to address key biomechanical and longevity requirements. Although years of follow-up study are needed to ultimately determine the Maverick's place in the evolution of treatment for single-level lumbar degenerative disk disease, patient outcomes equivalent to the current gold standard of treatment for this disease are an important first step in the validation of this new approach to improved patient outcomes.

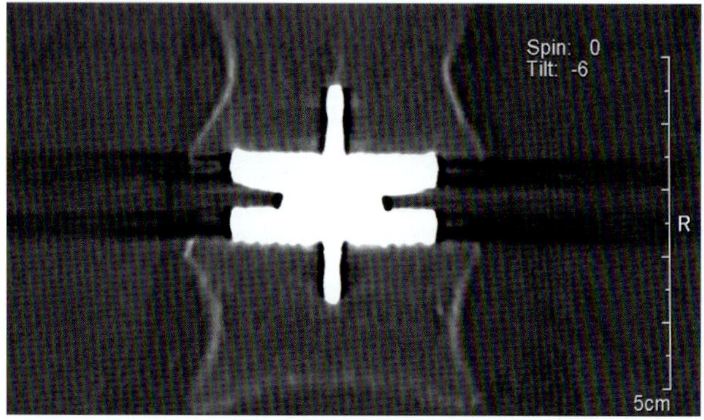

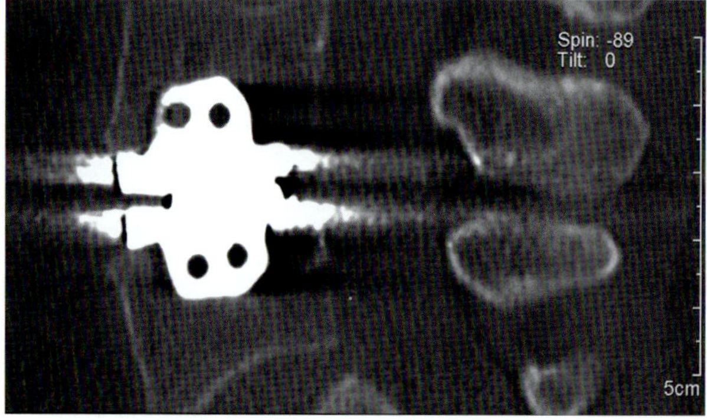

Figure 24–10 **(A)** Coronal and **(B)** sagittal reformatted images from a computed tomographic (CT) scan show excellent position at the L4–L5 intervertebral disk space in a 32-year-old woman. (With permission from Williams AL, Gornet MF, Burkus JK. CT evaluation of lumbar interbody fusion: current concepts. AJNR Am J Neuroradiol 2005; 26:2057–2066.)

References

1. Eck JC, Humphreys SC, Hodges SD. Adjacent-segment degeneration after lumbar fusion: a review of clinical, biomechanical, and radiologic studies. Am J Orthop 1999;28:336–340
2. Lee CK. Accelerated degeneration of the segment adjacent to a lumbar fusion. Spine 1988;13:375–377
3. Chou WY, Hsu CJ, Chang WN, Wong CY. Adjacent segment degeneration after lumbar spinal posterolateral fusion with instrumentation in elderly patients. Arch Orthop Trauma Surg 2002;122:39–43
4. Mulholland RC, Sengupta DK. Rationale, principles and experimental evaluation of the concept of soft stabilization. Eur Spine J 2002; 11(Suppl 2):S198–S205
5. West JL III, Bradford DS, Ogilvie JW. Results of spinal arthrodesis with pedicle-screw fixation. J Bone Joint Surg Am 1991;73A: 1179–1184
6. Errico TJ. Lumbar disc arthroplasty. Clin Orthop Relat Res 2005;435: 106–117

7. Gamradt SC, Wang JC. Lumbar disc arthroplasty. Spine J 2005;5: 95–103

8. Mathews H, LeHuec JC, Friesem T, Zdeblick T, Eisermann BS. Design rationale and biomechanics of Maverick Total Disc arthroplasty with early clinical results. Spine J 2004;4(Suppl 6):268S–275S

9. Dooris AP, Goel VK, Grosland NM, Gilbertson LG, Wilder DG. Load-sharing between anterior and posterior elements in a lumbar motion segment implanted with an artificial disc. Spine 2001;26:E122–E129

10. McAfee PC, Fedder IL, Saiedy S, Shucosky EM, Cunningham BW. Experimental design of total disc replacement: experience with a prospective randomized study of the SB Charité. Spine 2003;28:S153–S162

11. Geisler FH, Blumenthal SL, Guyer RD, et al. Neurological complications of lumbar artificial disc replacement and comparison of clinical results with those related to lumbar arthrodesis in the literature: results of a multicenter, prospective, randomized investigational device exemption study of Charité intervertebral disc. J Neurosurg Spine 2004;1:143–154

12. Blumenthal S, McAfee PC, Guyer RD, et al. A prospective, randomized, multicenter Food and Drug Administration investigational device exemptions study of lumbar total disc replacement with the Charité artificial disc versus lumbar fusion, I: Evaluation of clinical outcomes. Spine 2005;30:1565–1575

13. McAfee PC, Cunningham B, Holsapple G, et al. A prospective, randomized, multicenter Food and Drug Administration investigational device exemption study of lumbar total disc replacement with the Charité artificial disc versus lumbar fusion, II: Evaluation of radiographic outcomes and correlation of surgical technique accuracy with clinical outcomes. Spine 2005;30:1576–1583

14. Delamarter RB, Bae HW, Pradhan BB. Clinical results of Pro Disc-II lumbar total disc replacement: report from the United States clinical trial. Orthop Clin North Am 2005;36:301–313

15. Le Huec JC, Mathews H, Basso Y, et al. Clinical results of Maverick Total Disc Replacement: two year prospective follow-up. Orthop Clin North Am 2005;36:315–322

16. LeHuec JC, Kiaer T, Friesem T, Mathews H, Liu M, Eisermann L. Shock absorption in lumbar disc prosthesis: a preliminary mechanical study. J Spinal Disord Tech 2003;16:346–351

17. Hitchon PW, Eichholz K, Barry C, et al. Biomechanical studies of an artificial disc implant in the human cadaveric spine. J Neurosurg Spine 2005; 2:339–343

18. Chan FW, Bobyn JD, Medley JB, Krygier JJ, Yue S, Tanzer M. Engineering issues and wear performance of metal on metal hip implants. Clin Orthop Relat Res 1996;333:96–107

19. Goldsmith AA, Dowson D, Isaac GH, Lancaster JG. A comparative joint simulator study of the wear of metal-on-metal and alternative material combinations in hip replacements. Proc Inst Mech Eng [H] 2000; 214:39–47

20. Fisher J, Hu XQ, Tipper JL, et al. An in vitro study of the reduction in wear of metal-on-metal hip prostheses using surface-engineered femoral heads. Proc Inst Mech Eng [H] 2002;216:219–230

21. Firkins PJ, Tipper JL, Saadatzadeh MR, et al. Quantitative analysis of the wear and wear debris from metal-on-metal hip prostheses tested in a physiological hip joint simulator. Biomed Mater Eng 2001;11: 143–157

22. Bao QB, McCullen GM, Higham PA, Dumbleton JH, Yuan HA. The artificial disc: theory design and materials. Biomaterials 1996;17:1157–1167

23. Schmalzried TP, Peters PC, Maurer BT, Bragdon CR, Harris WH. Long-duration metal-on-metal total hip arthroplasties with low wear of the articulating surfaces. J Arthroplasty 1996;11:322–331

24. Goodman S. Wear particulate and osteolysis. Orthop Clin North Am 2005;36:41–48

25. Jacobs JJ, Shanbhag A, Glant TT, Black J, Galante JO. Wear debris in total joint replacements. J Am Acad Orthop Surg 1994;2:212–220

26. Jacobs JJ, Skipor AK, Doorn PF, et al. Cobalt and chromium concentrations in patients with metal-on-metal total hip replacements. Clin Orthop Relat Res 1996;329(Suppl):S256–S263

27. Chan FW, Bobyn JD, Medley JB, Krygier JJ, Yue S, Tanzer M. Engineering issues and wear performance of metal on metal hip implants. Clin Orthop Relat Res 1996;333:96–107

28. Dooris AP, Ares PJ, Gabriel SM, Serhan HA. Wear characterization of an artificial disc using ASTM guidelines. Transactions of the Orthopaedic Research Society, 51st Annual Meeting, Orthopaedic Research Society; 2005; Poster 1335

29. Chan F, Pare P, Buchholz P, Kurtz S, McCombe P. Is unidirectional motion clinically relevant for wear testing of artificial disc implants? International Meeting on Advanced Spine Technology; 2005

30. Pare PE, Chan FW, Buchholz P, Kurtz SM, McCombe P. Is unidirectional wear testing clinically relevant for artificial disc implants? Submitted to the ASTM Journal of Testing and Evaluation; September 2005

31. Mathews H, High W, McLay C, et al. Evaluation of wear debris in the rabbit spine. Study presented at: Spinal Arthroplasty Society (SAS) 3, "The Journey of the Spine: Global Symposium on Intervertebral Disc Replacement and Non-Fusion Technology"; May 3, 2003; Scottsdale, AZ

32. Le Huec J, Basso Y, Mathews H, et al. The effect of single-level, total disc arthroplasty on sagittal balance parameters: a prospective study. Eur Spine J 2005;14:480–486

33. Burkus JK, Gornet MF, Dickman CA, Zdeblick TA. Anterior lumbar interbody fusion using rhBMP-2 with tapered interbody cages. J Spinal Disord Tech 2002;15:337–349

25

The Mobidisc Prosthesis

Jean-Paul Steib, J. Beaurain, J. Delecrin, and the Mobidisc group
(J. Allain, M. Ameil, H. Chataigner, M. Gau, J. Huppert, M. Onimus, and W. Zeegers)

◆ **Biomechanics of the Spine and of the Intervertebral Space (Junghanns)**

◆ **The Mobidisc Prosthesis**

Principles

Design

Biomechanical Tests

Centers of Rotation

◆ **Operative Technique: Anterior Approach**

◆ **Clinical Results**

◆ **Conclusion**

Spine surgery is in relative infancy within the scope of orthopedics. As with the hip and the knee, spine surgery started with arthrodeses and osteotomies, which were immobilized by plasters and then by osteosyntheses. Today, hip and knee prostheses, or other articulations, achieve considerable excellence and the functional results speak for themselves. But while there are only two hips and two knees, there are multiple vertebral levels. Each level is triple with two posterior articulations and one anterior articulation: the disk. Spinal mobility is concentrated on the lordotic segments (cervical and lumbar). Working segments—crucial to quality of life—worsen with time with the loss of the anatomical ratios, lordosis, and movement. The replacement of the disk is logical from the point of view of reconstructive surgery.

The first disk prostheses appeared in the 1950s and '60s. They were made of cement or steel balls placed inside the disk.[1,2] Today we find nucleus prostheses, such as the PDN (prosthetic disk nucleus; Raymedica, Inc., Minneapolis, MN), serpentine of Husson, hydrogel injection,[3,4] and total disk prostheses (TDPs).[5] The TDPs are semiconstrained or nonconstrained depending on whether their center of rotation is fixed or mobile. They adopt the same principles: superior and inferior metal plates with or without an intermediate polyethylene element. Since 1987, the date of the first implantation of the Charité prosthesis (DePuy Spine, Raynham, MA),[6] more than 14,000 total disk prostheses have been implanted. The prosthesis Mobidisc (LDR Spine, Austin, TX) is a nonconstrained total disk prosthesis with a mobile polyethylene core.

◆ Biomechanics of the Spine and of the Intervertebral Space (Junghanns)

There are three axes and 6 degrees of freedom in a spinal mobile segment[7]: flexion-extension (horizontal frontal axis), lateral bending (horizontal sagittal axis), and rotation (vertical axis). These movements are controlled by "guides" (articular facets) and "brakes" (ligaments, capsules, and muscles).[8] Nearly 80% of the load supported by the spine[9] is on the anterior part of the disk which, due to its elastic distortion/deformation, adapts itself to the movement. The "wear-and-tear" effect will degrade the disk, which will be at the very origin of lumbago, even of lumbago-sciatica.

Spinal movements are characterized by the center of rotation. The centers of rotation of the movement in flexion-extension are determined by geometrical construction based upon the shape and spatial position of the posterior articular processes.[10,11] This center of rotation is located one third posterior to the intervertebral space and underneath the surface of the superior plate of the inferior vertebra, a location that was confirmed by models in finite element analysis[12] and through the use of software applied to radiographs in flexion and extension (**Fig. 25–1**). It is, in fact, a median center of rotation. This median center of rotation is resultant of the instantaneous centers of rotation (ICR). These ICR are defined as being, at a given moment T, the distribution of speeds of the points of a mobile plan compared with a fixed plane. The ICR is the I point where speeds are canceled. The ICR and their spatial evolution make it possible to know and to measure the mechanical solicitations at a precise spot of the studied solid or two solids, one compared with the other. The center of rotation of the flexion-extension movement is thus not single and moves within a physiological area. The ICR in lateral flexion and torsion are still different. Pure rotation around the axis of the vertebral body is impossible because of the anatomical shape of the posterior articular facets. This rotation is thus a torsion[12] resulting from a frontal translation on a circle, the center of which is at the level of the spinal processes and of a slight rotation on the axis of the vertebral body (**Fig. 25–2**). This physiological movement

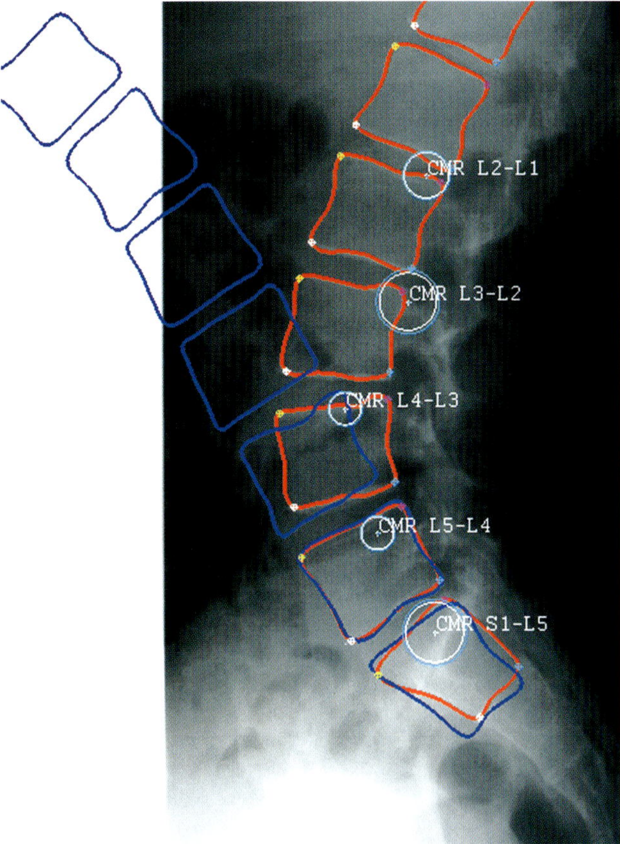

Figure 25–1   Spine view: flexion-extension.

varies from 3 to 6 degrees depending on the age and the morphotype.[8] The majority of the physiological movements are combined movements and the ICR are very variable. At the time of growth, one can think that there is harmony between the development of the disk and posterior articular

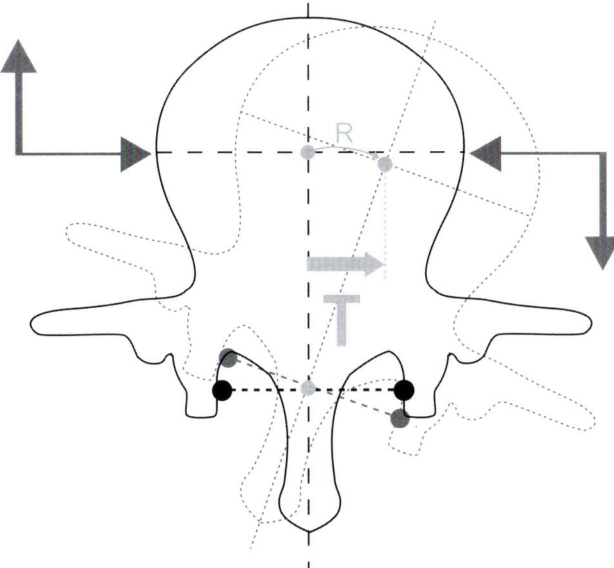

Figure 25–2   Rotation of the intervertebral segment.

facets with adapted ICR. With the aging process and the degeneration of facets and disk, instability moves the ICR away from the physiological areas. The articular facets especially will undergo abnormal strain in torsion.[8] Under the influence of the proprioceptive nervous system, the evolution proceeds toward the progressive expulsion of the degenerated disk and the transfer of the loads behind on the articular facets by loss of height and by putting lordosis on the intervertebral space (evolution in the three stages of Kirkaldy-Willis and Farfan).[13,14] The evolution of the ICR is thus closely related to the function and dysfunction of the intervertebral mobile segment.

A total disk prosthesis must restore the intervertebral height and standard mobility with adapted ICR. The current semiconstrained prostheses have an average posterior and inferior center of rotation corresponding to the Median Center of Rotation (MCR) in flexion-extension. The absence of lateral movement does not favor a physiological rotation of the intervertebral segment. Nonconstrained prostheses respect displacements of the ICR, particularly in rotation. The combined movements are favored and the wear of the posterior articulations and of the prosthesis is reduced.[5]

◆ The Mobidisc Prosthesis

Principles

The Mobidisc prosthesis has a posterior and inferior center of rotation associated with a 2.5 mm translation in all directions of the horizontal plane allowing 6 degrees of freedom. The mobile core moves back and forward in flexion-extension ($\pm$12 degrees), authorizing lateral bending ($\pm$10 degrees), and rotation ($\pm$7 degrees). The intervertebral rotation (torsion) is facilitated by the translation but is limited by its own inherent limitation (2.5 mm of translation Æ 7 degrees of torsion). The mobility of the central core allows the adaptation of the superior plate to the curvature. This core allows automatic centering and can follow the displacement imposed by the anatomy of the articular facets. The prosthesis is thus "personalized" and adapted to each individual. It also allows implantation that is not strictly median and posterior, the mobile inlay reducing a surgical approximation. If the variation of the ICR reproduces Mother Nature as nearly as possible, it spares the posterior articulations moving with a minimal constraint and an amplitude of physiological movement. The constraints between the prosthetic elements are low if the ICR of the prosthesis is the closest to the ICR of the operated mobile segment.

Design

The Mobidisc prosthesis consists of two vertebral plates, one superior and one inferior, and a polyethylene core (**Fig. 25–3**). The plates (three sizes: 29/24, 34/27, 39/29) have a truncated elliptical form and are manufactured from cobalt-chromium. The surface in contact with the bone has a coating of plasma-sprayed porous titanium to facilitate osseous integration. A directional keel allows a primary fixation. Its orientation allows a strict or oblique anteroposterior (AP) implantation.

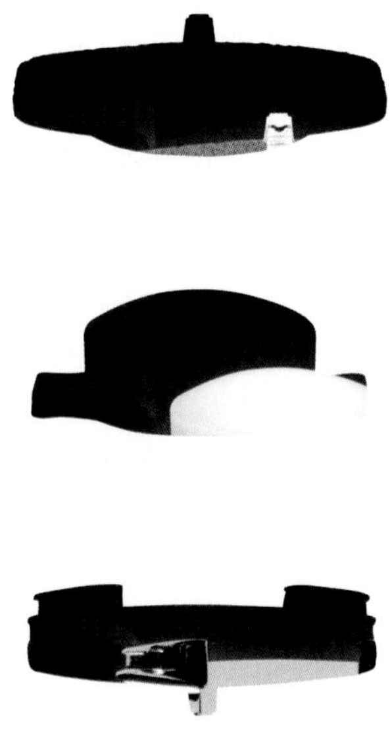

Figure 25–3   Mobidisc design.

The superior plate has a concave inferior surface that adapts to the convexity of the polyethylene inlay. The superior side of the inferior plate is flat and has four stops capturing the polyethylene inlay and limiting its mobility. The inferior plate exists in three versions with 0, 5, and 10 degrees of lordosis. The polyethylene inlay, which is made of ultra high molecular weight polyethylene (UHMWPE), has a flat base and a dome shape with a 15 mm diameter. This dome can be median or lateralized posteriorly so the MCR may be pushed further backward. Two lateral wings on the core slot between the stops of the inferior plate. Any luxation of the inlay is impossible. Its dimension adapts in width to the size of the prosthesis chosen and in height to the intersomatic space. The plate-polyethylene core unit allows all the physiological movements of a normal intervertebral disk.

Biomechanical Tests

Various biomechanical tests were performed before the prosthesis became available for clinical use. These tests were performed at the Centre Régional d'Innovation et de Transfert de Technologie (CRIT) laboratory in Charleville Mézières and at the Laboratoire de Biomécanique of the Ecole Nationale Supérieure d'Arts et Métiers (ENSAM) in Paris. First of all, repeated sliding movements of the polyethylene core on the inferior plate with the wings were performed, hitting the stops of the inferior plate: 5,000,000 cycles with a load ranging from 25 to 450 daN and a frequency of 2 Hz. Neither fracture nor wear were noted. The prosthesis was tested to more than 15,000,000 cycles under a load ranging from 30 to 200 daN at a frequency of 1.1 Hz in a physiological environment of bovine serum at a temperature of 37.5°C ± 0.5°C. The lubricant was changed every half million cycles and was filtered with 1 m m mesh before each test period. The movements successively tested were the flexion-extension (10/−5 degrees, F = 1 Hz), lateral bending (5/−5 degrees, F = 0.95 Hz) and axial rotation (3/−3 degrees, F = 1.05 Hz). Few or no modifications were noticed (**Fig. 25–4**). The studies on anatomical specimens were undertaken on seven lumbar segments

	Before test	500 000	1 000 000
Diameter	-	-1,8%	0%
Height	-	-2,2%	-1%
Ra (mm) (Superior part)	0,44	0,04	0,02
Rt (mm) (Superior part)	2,7	0,29	0,14
Ra (mm) (Inferior part)	1,22	0,08	0,13
Rt (mm) (Inferior part)	7,56	0,65	1,29
Anteroposterior mobility (+10°/-5°) (m)	610	708	868
Lateral mobility (+5°/-5°) (m)	1 125	988	1 083

Figure 25–4   Biomechanical tests.

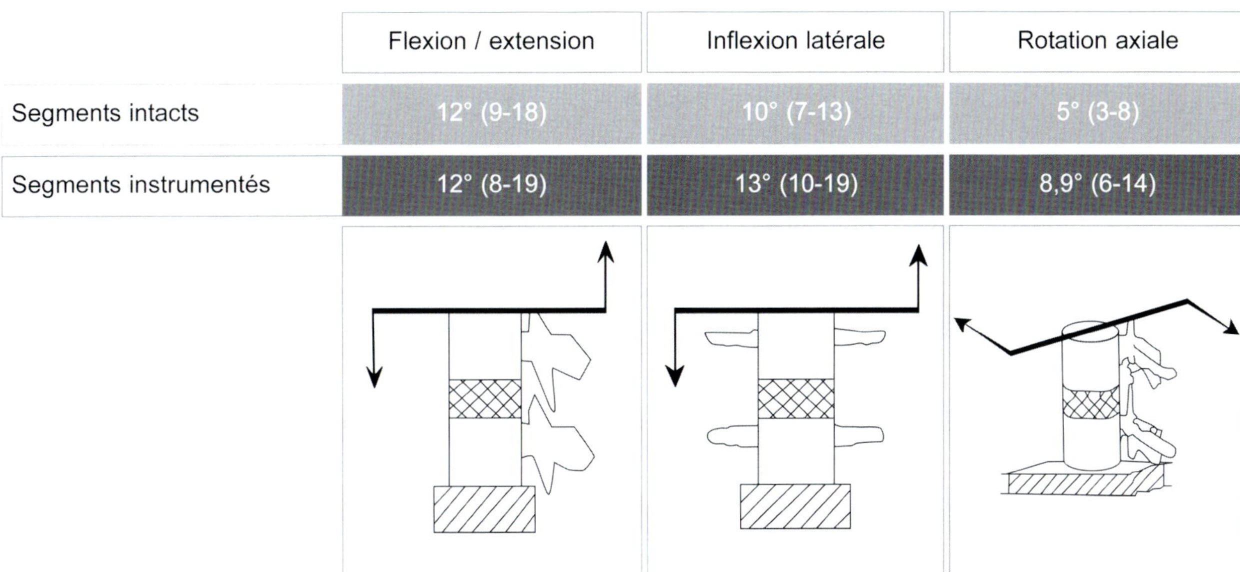

	Flexion / extension	Inflexion latérale	Rotation axiale
Segments intacts	12° (9-18)	10° (7-13)	5° (3-8)
Segments instrumentés	12° (8-19)	13° (10-19)	8,9° (6-14)

Figure 25–5   Biomechanical tests.

[L3–L5: 5 M, 2 F; 62 years (50–67), conservation at −20°C] instrumented by prosthesis in L4–L5. L5 was immobilized and the loads applied in L3 by stages of 1 Nm (**Fig. 25–5**). The parts were tested in flexion-extension, lateral bending, and axial rotation before and after implantation. There were no important variations in flexion-extension but an increase of the main rotations in lateral bending (3 degrees) and in axial rotation (3.9 degrees). Axial rotation was studied in the coupled movements: coupled rotations (flexion-extension, lateral bending), coupled translations (transverse, posteroanterior, and vertical). There were no important variations for coupled rotations but an increase of the lateral translation coupled with axial rotation (4 mm).

Centers of Rotation

We mapped the intervertebral rotation centers of the lumbar spine before and after the implantation of the Mobidisc. The goal of the study was to investigate the concept that disk arthroplasty might restore physiological motion of the operative disk and not modify the center of rotation of the adjacent levels.

Lateral flexion-extension radiographs were obtained in a sitting position with a stabilized pelvis from 32 patients before and after the implantation of the lumbar disk prosthesis. Specific software using digitized radiographs allowed automatic recording of the vertebral body contours on films and numerical calculation of the "mean" center of rotation. The minimum rate of motion was 5 degrees to allow the analysis because of the error sensitivity in determining the center of rotation.

Preoperatively, few centers of rotation were determined because of the absence of mobility. In two cases they appeared as disturbed. Postoperatively, they were located in 13 cases in the posterior half of the disk space or in the posterior half of the inferior vertebral body close to the inferior end plate (**Fig. 25–6**). In 14 cases, they were not determined because the intervertebral segmental motions were

±0.5 degrees. In three cases, the thickness of the implant appeared oversized and the tendency of the center of rotation was to move upward compared with normal states. In two cases, the center of rotation appeared too anterior with a prosthesis implanted too anterior. No disturbance of the centers of rotation at the adjacent levels was observed.

In conclusion, the determination of a preoperative abnormal center of rotation may be an indicator of presumed instability. Disk arthroplasty could restore physiological centers of rotation at some operative levels. But the position and the thickness of the implant could influence their locations. The restoration of normal mapping of segmental motion at the operative level and preservation of adjacent level motion support the concept that arthroplasty may reduce the incidence of adjacent segment degeneration compared with arthrodesis.

◆ Operative Technique: Anterior Approach

The patient is placed in the supine position with the patient's frontal plane parallel with the plane of the table. The anteroposterior (AP) axis of the patient must correspond with the vertical plumb line. The spine and the disk are exposed via the anterior retroperitoneal approach. Extra care should be given to the blood vessels, which should be gently retracted. At the L4–L5 level, ligature of the ascending lumbar vessels gives improved access. When the disk is largely exposed, the median aspect of the spine is located by x-ray. A radiopaque centering pin is placed at the inferior edge of the superior plate or the upper edge of the inferior plate of the vertebrae of the operated level. It will be used as a reference mark throughout the surgery to ensure accurate centering of the prosthesis. At the end of surgery, one mustn't forget to withdraw this pin. The instrumentation for the prosthesis is designed to direct every operative step from this pin. At this stage, one can choose the size of the prosthesis using a width gauge centered on the centering pin. At this moment, verify

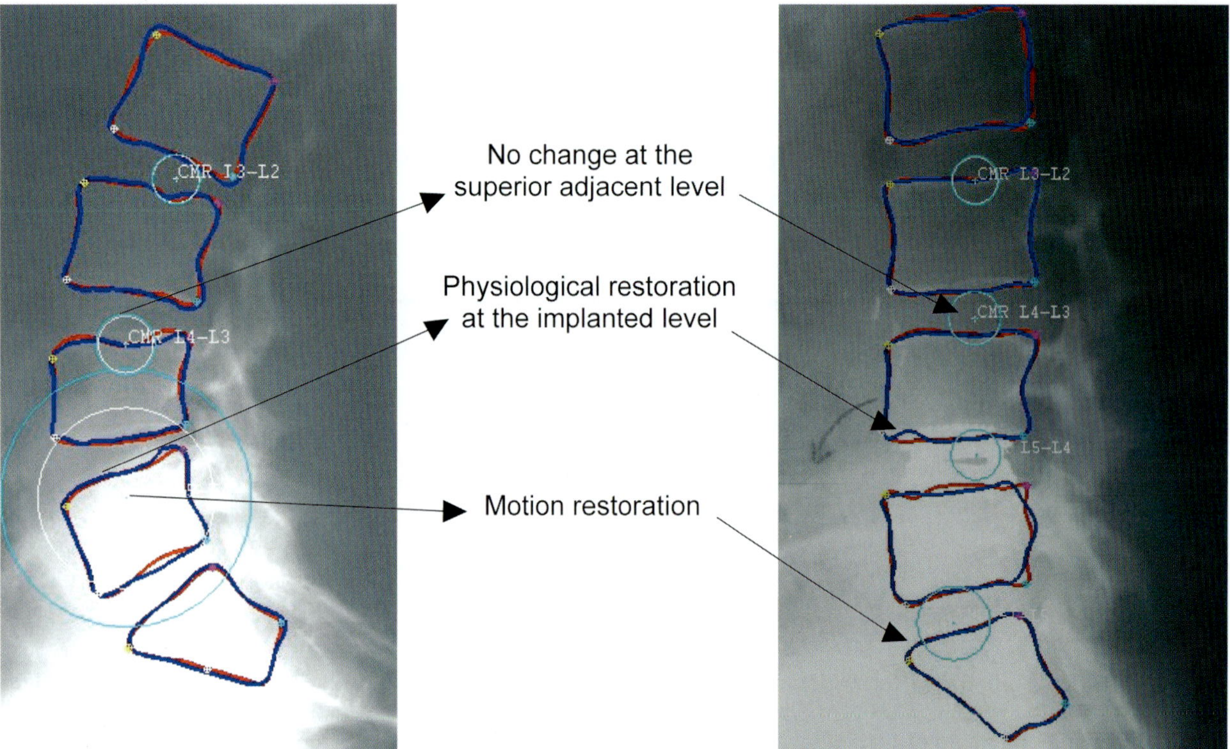

Figure 25–6   Centers of rotation before and after prosthesis.

that the left and right exposures are sufficient. A further exposure can be made if necessary. The disk is then opened with or without a flap. The anterior two-thirds of the disk is removed, and the vertebral plates are cleaned (detachment with the rongeur). It is necessary to check for and remove any anterior osteophytes and the hypertrophic margins of the disk on the anterior side of the vertebrae. The unilateral distractor is introduced into the intervertebral space. It is possible to clean the back of the disk with posterior release: detachment of the posterior intervertebral ligament is recommended. The vertebral end plates are cleaned with the curette or chisels to remove the osteophytes and to make the flattest surface possible. The aim is to be able to push the prosthesis to the posterior limit of the disk space. This distractor will be placed on the right and on the left to release the left and the right side, respectively.

Once the disk is perfectly cleaned and freed the prosthesis can be chosen. The depth gauge gives the AP length in mm of the vertebral end plate. This measurement, thanks to the charts included in the Mobidisc kit (**Fig. 25–7**) will make it possible to calibrate the chisel and the prosthesis impactor to place the implant at the posterior edge of the vertebra. The bilateral distractor will open the intervertebral space. This space, particularly posterior, will be helped by the placement of a spacer between the side jaws to keep the end plates parallel. Once the desired space is obtained, the selected spacer will be placed between the right and left jaws of the distractor. Thus is obtained Lume height of the future prosthesis (10, 12, or 14 mm). The distractor is then withdrawn, leaving the spacer in place, maintaining the gap.

One will be able to introduce the guide that corresponds with the size and height of the prosthesis with the spacer

still in place. This guide will be centered on the pin (a groove in the guide corresponds to the pin). This introduction is sometimes difficult and may require some widening of the lateral disk resection. One must be careful with the vessels and protect them with gentle retraction. The spacer and guide holder are withdrawn, making sure that the guide is strictly in the AP plane (check the vertical position of the guide holder with an AP x-ray). It is also necessary to be certain that the guide is retained in the axis and parallel to the vertebral end plates (lateral x-ray). This guide must be inserted to the maximum depth because its position will dictate the correct placement on the prosthesis, particularly in depth. The chisel corresponding to the height of the prosthesis, adjusted to the given depth (using the charts), will be placed in the rails of the guide. It will be inserted with a hammer until the safety stop and will be withdrawn with a slap hammer. The preparation stage is complete.

The prosthetic plates are installed with their keels. The polyethylene core is clipped into the inferior plate. The assembled prosthesis is grasped with the prosthesis holder. One should ensure that the superior plate is in the uppermost position, and the inferior plate and the polyethylene core should have the anterior part facing the surgeon. The prosthesis is introduced and released into the guide. It is then punched home with the impactor, which was adjusted the same way as the chisel, using the charts provided. The guide is withdrawn as well as the pin. An x-ray control confirms the satisfactory position of the prosthesis. It is possible, if needed, to push it further in with the impactor. The prosthesis is in place (**Fig. 25–8**). Closure can be made by normal methods. The patient should be out of bed the following day in the absence of any other clinical problems.

Instruments adjustments for the Mobidisc® implantation

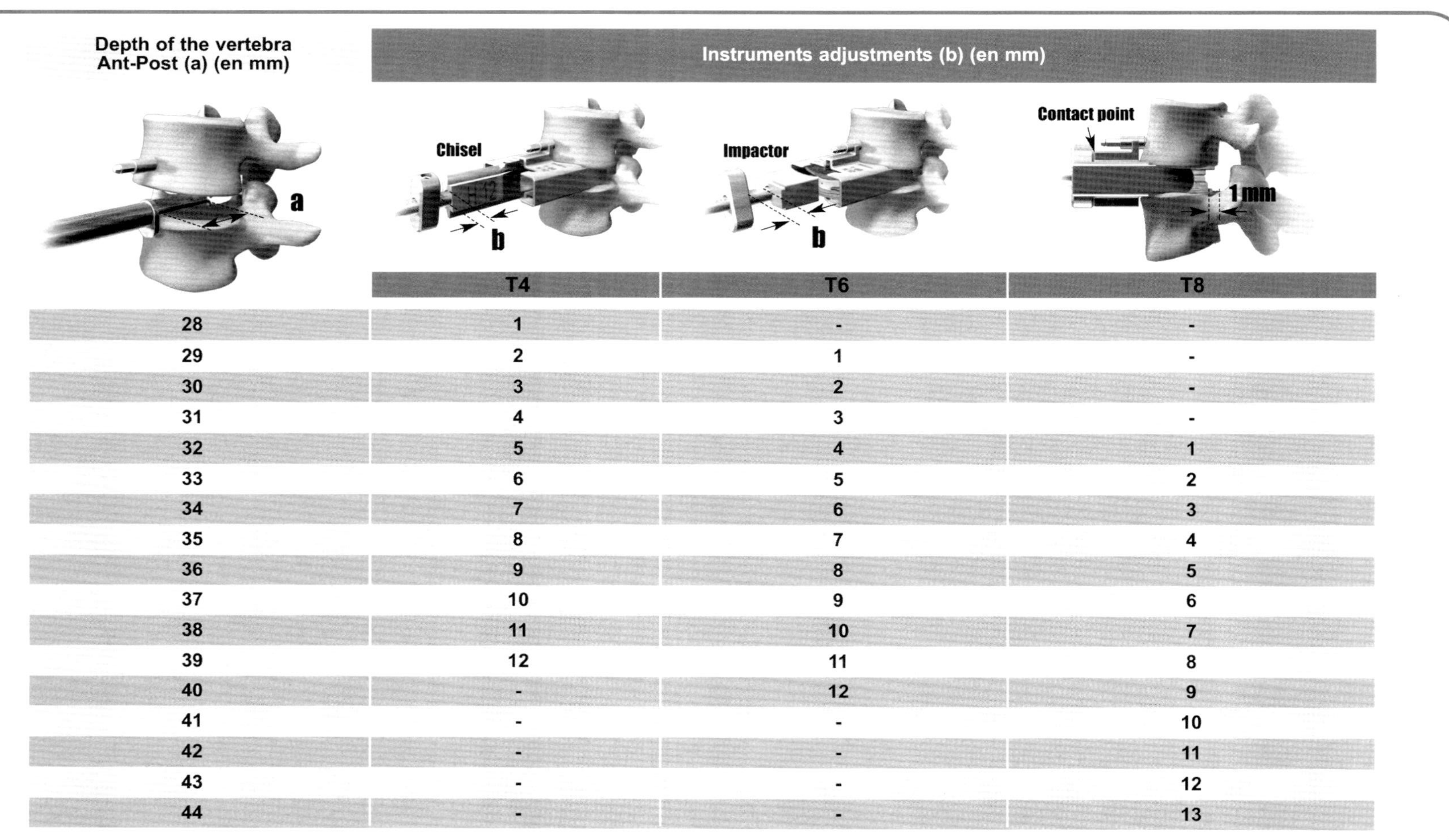

Depth of the vertebra Ant-Post (a) (en mm)	T4	T6	T8
28	1	-	-
29	2	1	-
30	3	2	-
31	4	3	-
32	5	4	1
33	6	5	2
34	7	6	3
35	8	7	4
36	9	8	5
37	10	9	6
38	11	10	7
39	12	11	8
40	-	12	9
41	-	-	10
42	-	-	11
43	-	-	12
44	-	-	13

Figure 25–7   Charts included in the Mobidisc kit.

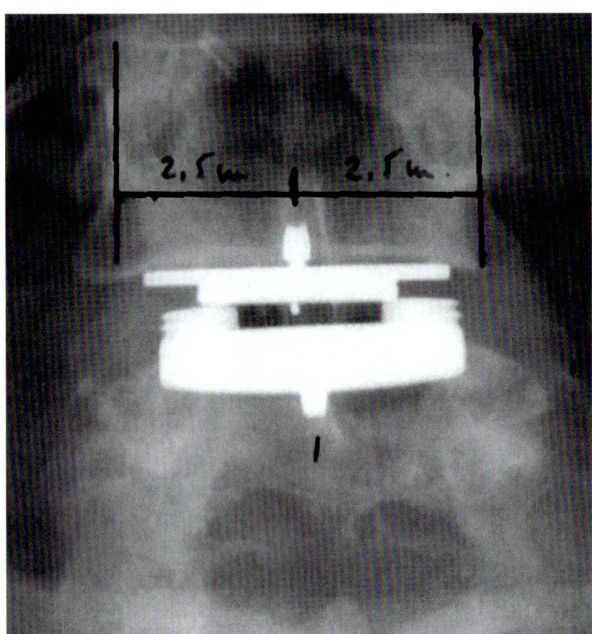

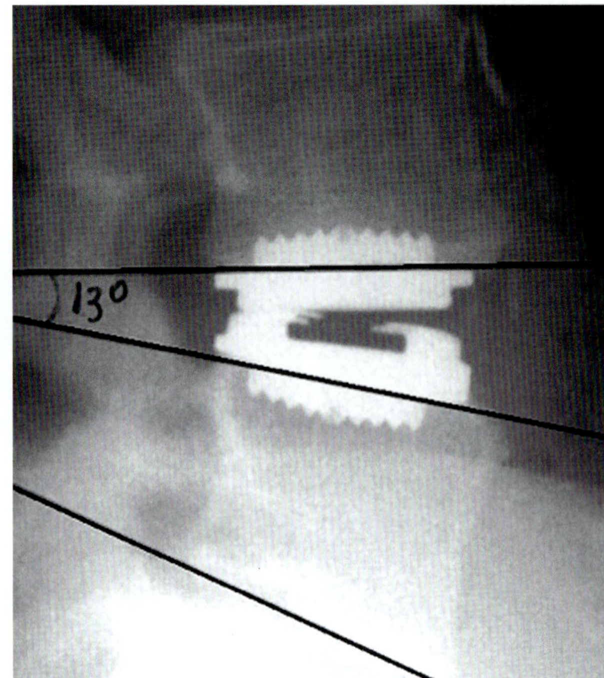

Figure 25–8   Prosthesis L4–L5.

◆ Clinical Results

The first Mobidisc prosthesis was implanted in November 2003. More than 150 prostheses were implanted within the first year. These prostheses have been regularly reviewed, clinically and radiologically. Radiological assessments include a lateral big standing radiograph (30 × 90 cm) and AP and lateral lumbar radiographs with lateral views in flexion and extension. Preoperatively, all examinations necessary to the diagnosis and the indication were performed, including scanner, magnetic resonance imaging (MRI, Modic), and diskography (memory pain). The clinical assessment included a clinical examination and the completion of questionnaires, including the visual analog scale (VAS), Oswestry Disability Index, short form (SF)-36 Health Survey, and sexual function and satisfaction index.

A series of 40 patients (nine males, 31 females) with consistent baseline characteristics (primary and secondary degenerative disk disease) were operated on in 2004 by five surgeons in France (**Fig. 25–9**). The average age of the patients was 41 years (range, 19-54 years) and the average follow-up was 9 months (with 6-month minimal follow-up). All the patients suffered from back pain and radicular pain with failure of medical treatment and intensive physiotherapy for more than 6 months. Twenty-seven percent of the patients had undergone one or more previous surgical operations.

The back pain VAS was decreased by 71% (7.46 to 2.18). The leg pain score was decreased by 72% (5.7 to 1.6).

The Oswestry score (**Fig. 25–10**) was improved by 25% in 90.6% of patients, with 84.3% improving by over 30% and 68.7% improving by over 50%.

The pain intensity score was decreased by 72%. The mean improvement at final follow-up was also more than 75% regarding personal care, walking, sleeping, sexual function, and social life. Almost 90% of patients were satisfied (51.7%) and very satisfied (37.9%) concerning the decrease in lumbar pain.

There was no implant breakage, migration, or loss of disk height except for one case of subsidence at 2 months in a 45-year-old man. No osteolysis was noted in response to the presence of the implant. There was no heterotopic ossification. The mean range of motion found at the final follow-up was 8 degrees for L4–L5 and 7 degrees for L5–S1. There was one implant revision due to persistent leg pain related to a prosthesis misplacement (laterality and contact with the root). This technical error was corrected by the replacement of the prosthesis in good position, with an excellent clinical result.

Number Of Patient	Gender		Number of prosthesis	Level of prosthesis				# of disc/Pt	
	Male	Female		L2-L3	L3-L4	L4-L5	L5-S1	1	2
40	9	31	45	1	3	14	27	35	5

Figure 25–9   Operated levels.

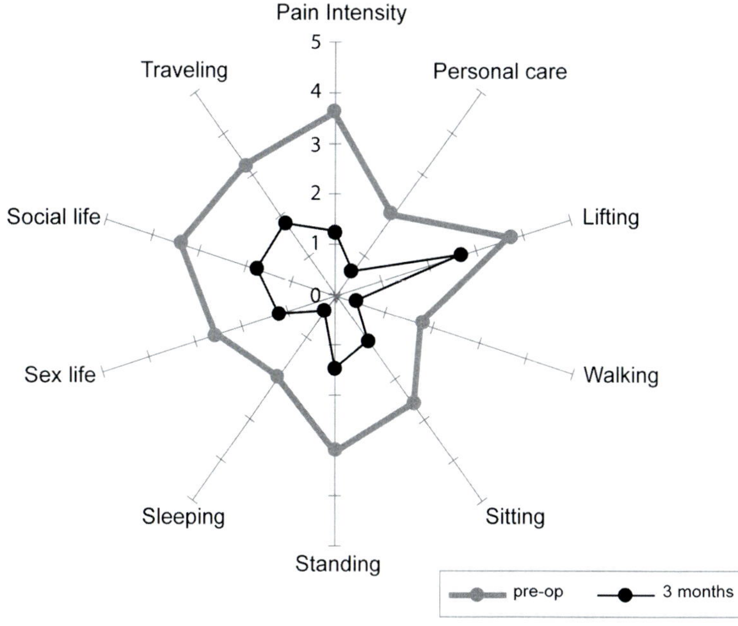

Figure 25–10 Oswestry score.

◆ Conclusion

The concept of the total disk prosthesis seems validated with a follow-up of more than 15 years. Mobidisc is a new, original prosthesis thanks to its mobile inlay. With this mobile inlay, the movements of the instrumented segment follow the articular guide and resemble the movements of the healthy segment. The ICR protect the elements of the mobile segment and the prosthesis from early wear. This prosthesis is "tailor-made" because it adapts itself to the mechanics of the operated segment. The surgical operative procedure is made possible via an operative technique and specific instrumentation. An oblique implantation using an antero-lateral approach avoiding the vessels should soon be possible. The current clinical results are good and the follow-up continues. The future results should confirm the advantages of this new implant. The same principle was recently applied to the cervical spine (Mobi-C).

References

1. Cleveland DA. The use of methylacrylic for spinal stabilization after disc operations. Marquet Med Rev 1955;20:62

2. Fernström U. Arthroplasty with intercorporal endoprosthesis in herniated disc and in painful disc. Acta Chir Scand Suppl 1966;357:154–159

3. Szpalski M, Gunzburg R, Mayer M. Spine arthroplasty: a historical review. Eur Spine J 2002;11(Suppl 2):S65–S84

4. Sagi HC, Bao QB, Yuan HA. Nuclear replacement strategies. Orthop Clin North Am 2003;34:263–267

5. Anderson PA, Rouleau JP. Intervertebral disc arthroplasty. Spine 2004;29:2779–2786

6. Buttner-Janz K. The Development of the Artificial Disc SB Charité. Ann Arbor, MI: Hundley & Associates; 1992

7. Kapandji IA. The Physiology of the Joints. Vol 3: The Trunk and the Vertebral Column. New York: Churchill Livingstone; 1974

8. Louis R. Chirurgie du rachis: Anatomie chirurgicale et voies d'abord. 2nd ed., rev. and enl. New York: Springer-Verlag; 1993

9. Goel VK, Kim YE, Lim TH, Weinstein JN. An analytical investigation of the mechanics of spinal instrumentation. Spine 1988;13: 1003–1011

10. Fick R. Handbuch der Anatomie und Mechanik der Gelenke unter Berücksichtigung der bewegenden Muskeln. Jena, Germany: Fischer; 1904–11

11. Lysell E. Motion in the cervical spine: an experimental study on autopsy specimens. Acta Orthop Scand 1969;(Suppl 123):1

12. Templier A, Skalli W, Lemaire J-Ph. Three-dimensional finite-element modeling and improvement of a bispherical disc prosthesis. Eur J Orthop Surg Traumato 1999;9:51–58

13. Kirkaldy-Willis WH, Farfan HF. Instability of the lumbar spine. Clin Orthop Relat Res 1982;165:110–123

14. Farfan HF, Cossette JW, Wells RV, Robertson GH, Kraus GH. The effect of torsion of the lumbar intervertebral joints. J Bone Joint Surg Am 1970;52:468–497

26

Activ-L Lumbar (Aesculap) Total Disk Arthroplasty

James J. Yue and Rolando Garcia

- ◆ **Indications**
- ◆ **Description of System Components**
- ◆ **Operative Technique**
  - **Preparation and Positioning**
  - **Disk Space Preparation**
  - **Trialing and Chiseling**

  Anterior-Posterior Implant Insertion
  Oblique Implant Insertion
- ◆ **Tips and Pearls**
- ◆ **Complications**
- ◆ **Conclusion**

Several innovative and promising nonfusion spinal implant devices and accompanying techniques have recently been proposed for the treatment of debilitating axial diskogenic low back pain.[1–14] Over the past $2\frac{1}{2}$ decades, the early focus has been in the utilization of total disk arthroplasty. Biomechanically, there are presently three main types of artificial disk replacements (ADR): unconstrained, semiconstrained without translation, and, the next generation, semiconstrained with translation. This last type of motion we term mobilization. A more recent design, the Activ-L (Aesculap, Inc., Tuttlingen, Germany) (**Fig. 26–1**), allows for mobilization as well as implant stability and variability, uncomplicated prosthetic implantation, and revision instrumentation.

Design improvements for the next generation of prostheses include those as outlined in **Table 26–1**. Material and biomechanical properties should be optimized to minimize wear debris, prosthetic designs should allow for ease of insertion via multiple angles, and surgical revision instrumentation should be available. In addition, the implant should provide maximal end plate coverage with minimal or no end plate recontouring, and the implant height should be minimized to protect neurological structures while concurrently allowing ease of implant delivery at single or multiple levels. The Activ-L prosthesis was designed to satisfy all of the foregoing next-generation requirements for lumbar ADR. We emphasize the concept that both implant design and insertional technique should be harmonious and considered as equally vital and important when comparing one implant with another.

◆ Indications

The indications for Activ-L intervertebral lumbar disk arthroplasty include severe lumbar diskogenic back pain as a result of lumbar spondylosis with or without radiculopathy. Clinical findings should be closely correlated with radiological imaging findings, including magnetic resonance imaging, standing plane x-rays, diskography, and computed tomography (CT) to assess the integrity of facet joints and the pars interarticularis. Other sources of back pain such as facet disease, myofascial syndromes, inflammatory arthritic conditions, and others should be excluded. The patient should have had at least 6 months of conservative measures prior to pursuing lumbar intervertebral total disk arthroplasty.

Contraindications to this procedure include chronic infections such as periodontal sources of infection, urinary sources of infection, and chronic skin ulcerations. Patients with a body mass index greater than ~34 should be counseled extensively in an attempt to achieve a body mass index of less than or equal to 30 before proceeding with any intervertebral disk arthroplasty procedure. Patients

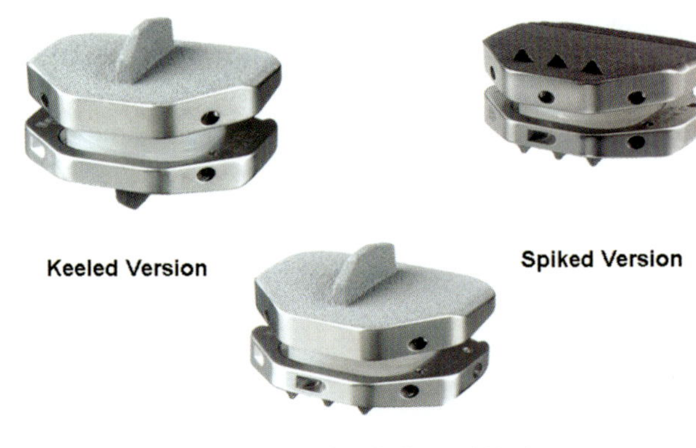

Figure 26–1 Activ-L lumbar disk replacement.

Table 26–1 Implant Design Characteristics

Artificial Disk Replacement	, 9 mm Height	Variable Fixation	Revision Instruments	Controlled Mobilization	Variable Surgical Approach
Activ-L (Aesculap)	+	+	+	+	+
ProDisc (Synthes)	–	–	–	–	+
Charité (DePuy Spine)	–	–	–	–	–
Kineflex (SpinalMotion)	–	–	–	±	–
Maverick (Medtronic Sofamor Danek)	–	–	–	–	+
Mobidisc (LDR Spine)	–	–	–	+	+

should be appropriately screened and tested for osteoporosis prior to ADR surgery.

◆ Description of System Components

The Activ-L implant consists of three primary components (**Fig. 26–2A,B**). The superior and inferior components are composed of a three-metal alloy (cobalt, chromium, and molybdenum). The superior component is composed of a solid one-piece design with a central keel or three anterior spikes and is available in two lordotic angles—6 and 11 degrees. The superior component has a concave polished surface that articulates with the second component, an ultra high molecular weight polyethylene inlay (available in 8.5,10,12, and 14 mm). This inlay rests in the third (i.e., inferior) component, which is composed of a solid one-piece design with a central keel or three anterior spikes. The inferior component also has a highly polished surface that permits translation in the anteroposterior (AP) direction only during flexion and extension (**Fig. 26–3**). The S size permits for 1.5 mm of polyethylene inlay translation in the AP direction. The M, L, and XL sizes permit 2 mm of AP translation. None of the implants permit medial-lateral translation of the inlay.

Four implant sizes are available: S, M, L, and XL (**Fig. 26–4**). The anteroposterior dimension of the S size is 26 mm. The medial-lateral dimension is 31 mm. The XL size is 33 mm in the AP dimension and 40 mm in the medial-lateral dimension. In terms of anatomical sizing, the AP dimension of each vertebral end plate must be at least 26 mm to permit the use of the Activ-L implant. The medial-lateral dimensions of the end plate must be at least 31 mm also, to allow for successful implantation. These measurements can be best evaluated on axial CT scan images, which are parallel to the intervertebral disk space in question. Both the superior and inferior components are plasma sprayed with a pure titanium coating as well as a thin layer (20 m m) of dicalcium phosphate dehydrate (m -CaP) to enhance bony ingrowth.

Instrumentation for the Activ-L surgical procedure includes a set of disk space mobilization/distraction instruments (curettes, distractors, and disk space bullet distractors). Trial implant end plates for end plate sizing are available

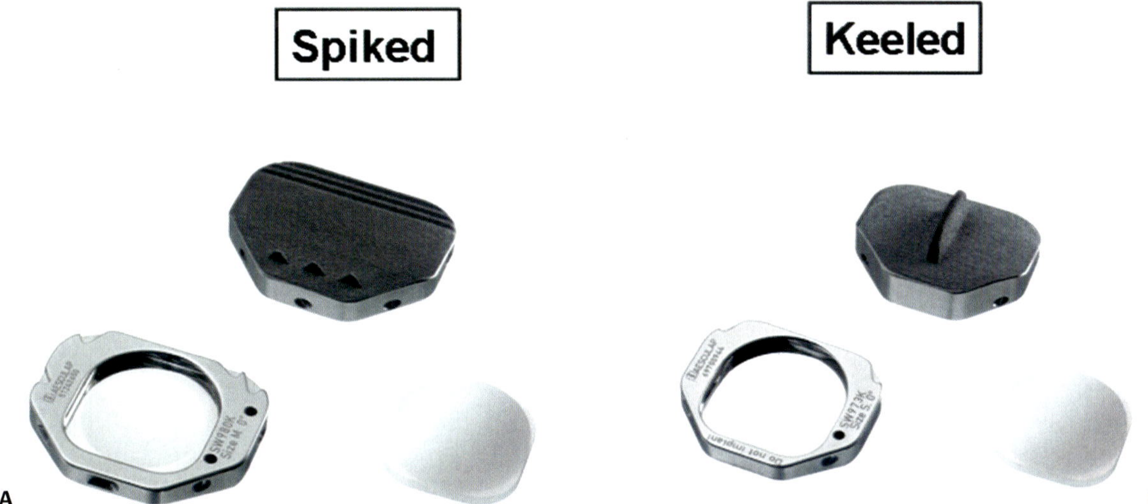

A

B

Figure 26–2A,B   Components of Activ-L disk replacement.

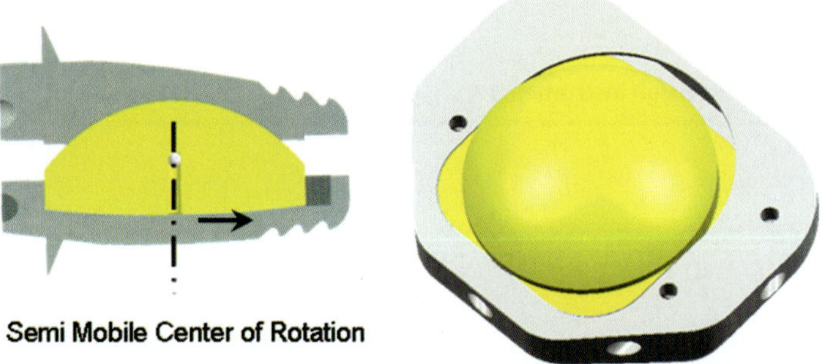

Figure 26–3   Polyethylene (PE) inlay translates 2 mm in anteroposterior direction producing more physiological motion of vertebral segment.

and can be placed directly on a mechanical distractor and intervertebral space sizer (**Fig. 26–5**). A midline pin marker can be placed to assist in midline accuracy. When an oblique insertion is desired, a radiolucent marker with radiopaque midpoint alignment markers is available to assist in midline marking in the AP and lateral projections (**Fig. 26–6**).

The end plates of the Activ-L implant are available in either keeled or spiked versions. These end plates can be mixed (superior keeled with inferior spiked or vice versa). When a keeled implant technique is desired, a protected chisel is available to cut the keel groove. The chisel is available in a double- or single-chisel design.

Revision instruments are included that permit for translation of the implant in an anterior direction if so desired. This same set of instruments allows for complete removal of the implant. A separate revision instrument allows for removal and replacement of the polyethylene insert.

◆ Operative Technique

Preparation and Positioning

The preparation for surgery begins 24 hours prior to the surgical procedure. Patients are permitted only a clear liquid

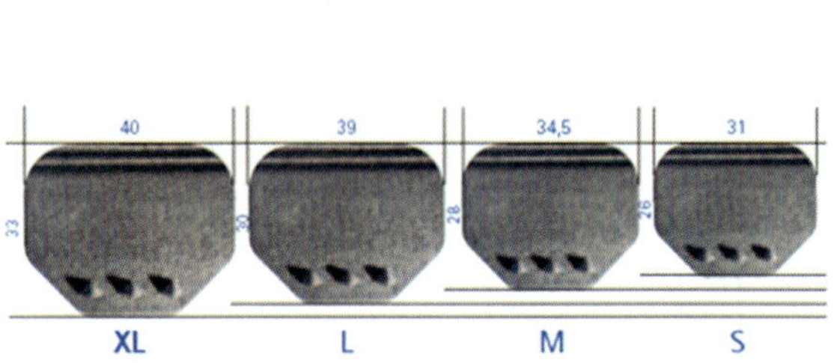

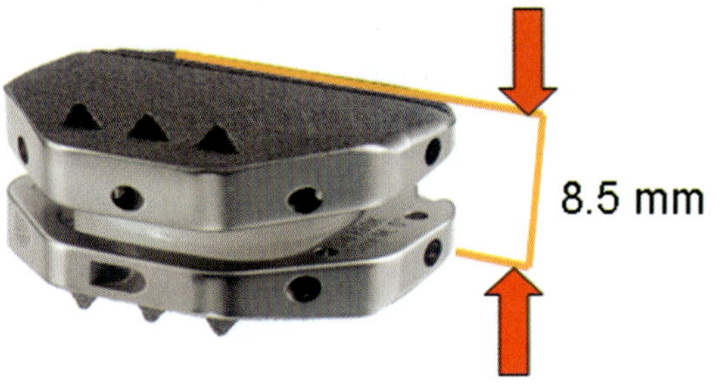

Implants	Description		Sizes			
			S (26x 31)	M (28x 34.5)	L (30x 39)	XL (33x 40)
Superior Plate	Angle	6°	SW97 1K	SW98 1K	SW99 1K	SW89 1K
		11°	SW97 2K	SW98 2K	SW99 2K	SW89 2K
Superior Plate with Keel	Angle	6°	SW97 4K	SW98 4K	SW99 4K	SW89 4K
		11°	SW97 5K	SW98 5K	SW99 5K	SW89 5K
Inlay	Height	8,5 mm	SW965			
		10 mm	SW966			
		12 mm	SW967			
		14 mm	SW968			
Inferior Plate		0°	SW970K	SW 980 K	SW99 0K	SW89 0K
Inferior Plate with Keel		0°	SW973K	SW 983 K	SW99 3K	SW89 3K

Figure 26–4   Available component dimensions of Activ-L prosthesis (mm).

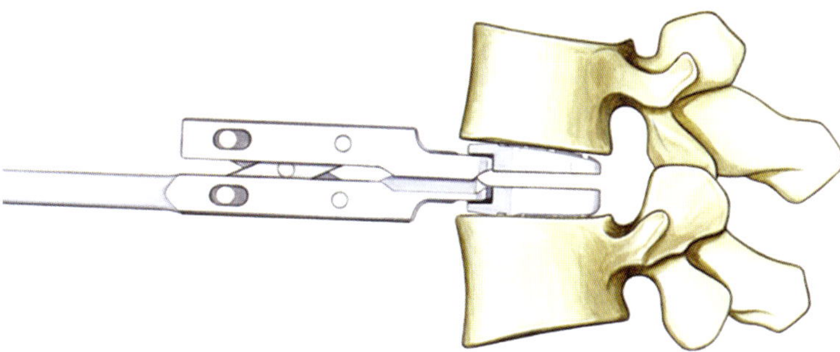

Figure 26–5   Trial/distractor instrument.

diet beginning 24 hours prior to surgery and are NPO beginning 8 hours before surgery. Patients are placed on a fluoroscopic imaging table, which allows for abduction of both legs so that the patients can be positioned with both arms and legs abducted. This allows the surgeon to work between the patient's legs. The patient's hips are slightly extended to allow for greater access potential to the lumbosacral junction. If such a fluoroscopic imaging table is not obtainable, patients can be positioned on a flat fluoroscopic imaging table with their legs in the neutral position.

Disk Space Preparation

Once the patient has been properly positioned, fluoroscopy is then brought into the field and appropriate skin markings are made prior to sterile technique. The fluoroscopic image viewer should be at the patient's head level. To aid in the minimally invasive approach to the spine, exposure of the disk space is enhanced with an appropriate self-retaining retractor. Standard retroperitoneal or transperitoneal approaches to the spine are then performed.

Once the anterior disk has been exposed and the appropriate level of dissection reverified, the midpoint of the disk space is marked under fluoroscopic imaging in the AP plane. It is critical that the distance between the spinous process and both pedicles be equal to ensure a perfect AP projection for midline marking and implant insertion. The midline pin marker is then placed. The annulus is then incised and two halves of the annulus are retracted laterally with a stay suture secured to the surrounding circular frame, thereby providing further protection of the lateral vascular structures.

A complete diskectomy and distraction of the disk interspace using the handheld distractors and bullets are mandatory. A small curved curette should always be placed along the posterior ridge of both vertebral bodies. This palpation will aid in the release of the posterior longitudinal ligament and removal of extruded disk fragments and posterior inflammatory granulation tissue when indicated. The bony end plate must be preserved. The disk space must be distracted and mobilized to allow for easy distraction. It is not mandatory to remove the entire posterior longitudinal ligament unless extruded disk material needs to be removed or greater intervertebral disk space distraction is necessary.

Trialing and Chiseling

After end plate preparation and disk space mobilization are completed, implant trialing is performed. Both disk space height and intervertebral lordotic angles should be reestablished. Close attention is needed when one is determining the largest possible end plate coverage using the end plate trials.

Depending on the type of end plate configuration (**Fig. 26–7**) as well as surgeon's preference, the decision for a keeled or spiked implant is then made. The distractor/sizer instrument is then placed into the disk space and the disk space is simultaneously distracted and measured by turning the handle of this instrument. If a keeled implant is chosen, the appropriate chisel trial is placed carefully in the midline of the disk space, and chiseling is performed. Correct positioning of this trial implant is imperative. A keeled implant cannot be used for oblique insertion. Chiseling is performed under fluoroscopic imaging control. A safety block can be adjusted to allow for

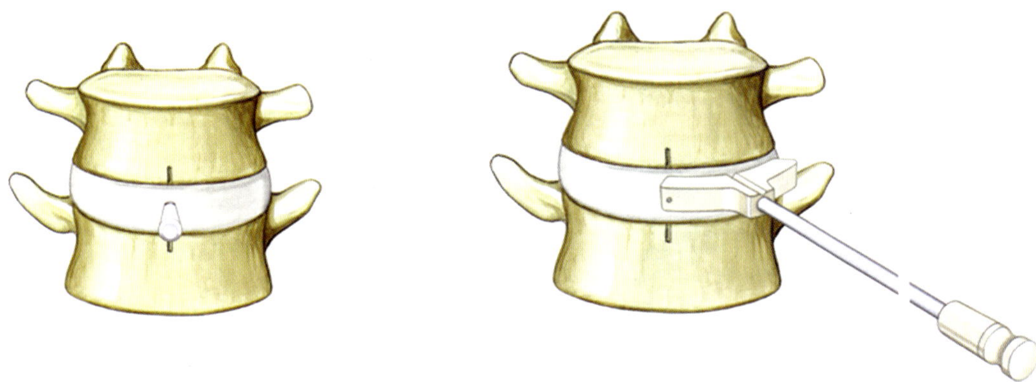

Figure 26–6   Midline marker for anterior and lateral approaches.

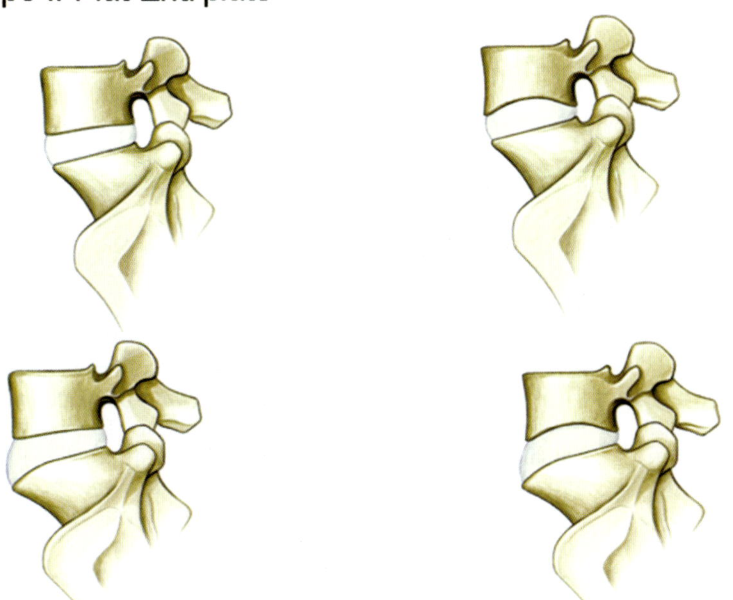

Figure 26–7   End plate morphologies: Yue-Bertagnoli classification.

appropriate chiseling depths. After chiseling is performed, the disk space should be thoroughly inspected for any loose pieces of bone, which may have been produced as a result of the chiseling and trial impaction. If any loose pieces of bony material are evident or soft tissue materials are present, these should be removed immediately prior to final implantation of the final implant components. It is not necessary to perform chiseling if a spiked implant is chosen.

Anterior-Posterior Implant Insertion

Once disk size, height, and lordotic angle have been determined, and chiseling has been performed (in cases of a keeled implant only), an appropriately sized implant (two end plates and polyethylene insert) is chosen and placed onto the inserter instrument (**Fig. 26–8**). From a disk height perspective, undersizing is preferred. Undersizing of the implant will allow for more anatomical range of motion following implantation. The implant is then placed using fluoroscopic assistance in the AP and lateral planes.

Once all three components of the implant have been inserted, the insertion device should be removed. Final visual inspection of the implant should be performed both fluoroscopically and visually (**Fig. 26–9A–C**).

Oblique Implant Insertion

If during anterior exposure it has been determined that an oblique insertion is desired, three insertional steps are required. (1) Although an oblique insertion is to be performed,

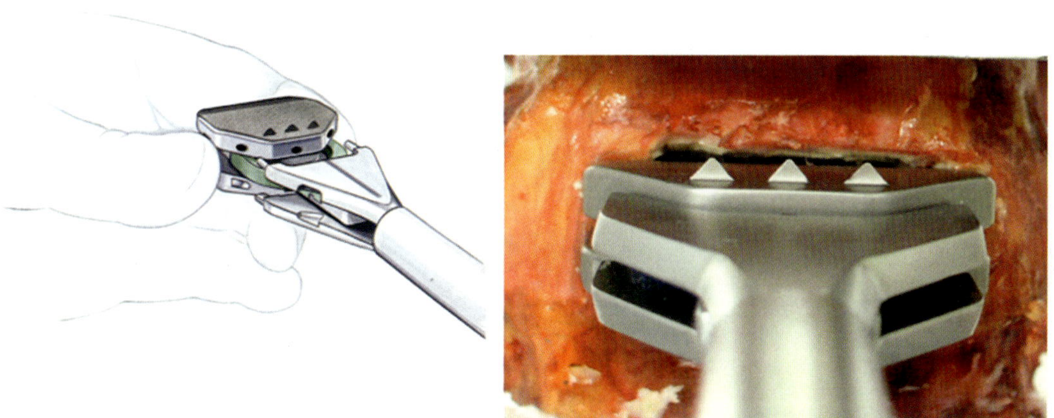

Figure 26–8   Assembly of prosthesis into insertor and en bloc insertion.

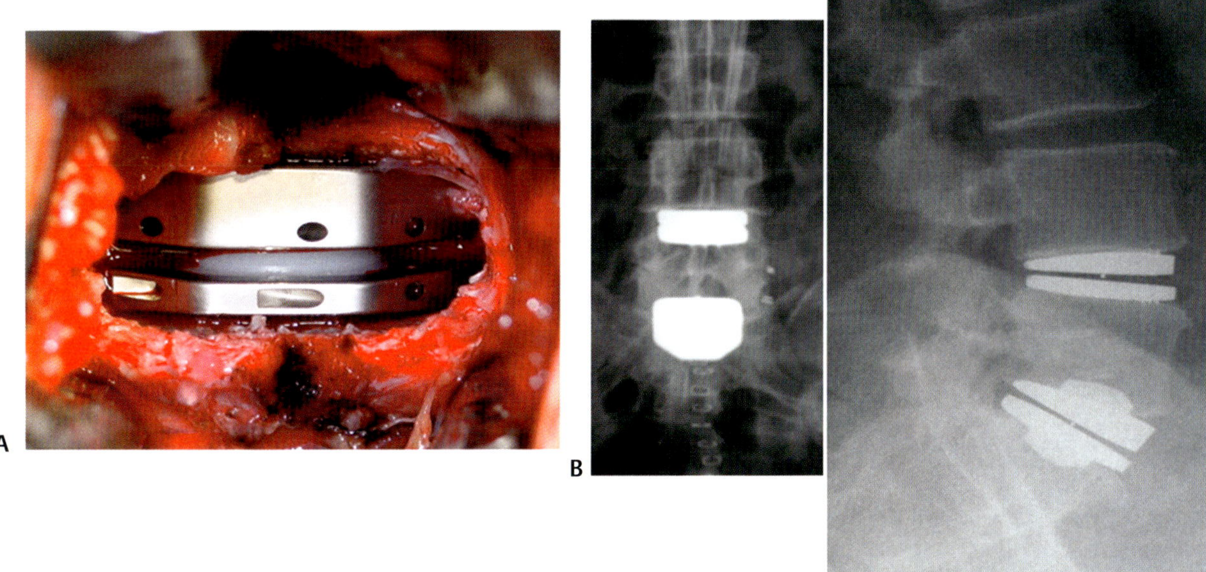

Figure 26–9 In vivo and radiographic final positioning of prosthesis. (Provided by Dr. S. Sola.) **(A)** Anterior view of implanted prothesis. **(B)** An x-ray of bisegmented case. **(C)** Lateral view of bisegmented case.

vascular mobilization ~2 cm past the midline of the vertebral interspace is recommended. (2) Once the vascular structures have been mobilized, the radiolucent trial is placed on the disk space prior to diskectomy and a small notch is made on the superior vertebra thereby defining the insertional angle for the final prosthesis. The next steps for disk preparation and implant selection are similar to the AP insertion. If at all possible, complete release of the anterior annulus should be performed to allow for proper balancing of the spine to avoid causing iatrogenic scoliosis. (3) Using fluoroscopy in the AP plane, the implant should first be positioned in the final medial-lateral position. Once the implant has been positioned in the anatomical center of the interspace in the AP plane, the implant is then positioned posteriorly using fluoroscopy in the lateral plane. If possible, biplanar simultaneous fluoroscopy is useful in oblique positioning of the implant.

◆ Tips and Pearls

1. Although implant selection allows for 8.5 mm ADR implantation, it is highly recommended that disk distraction and mobilization be performed meticulously and thoroughly using handheld spreader/distractors and, if necessary, release of the posterior longitudinal ligament (PLL).

2. End plate coverage should be maximized.

3. Preoperative and intraoperative evaluation of end plate contour should be considered when choosing between spiked versus keeled implant configurations.

4. Slight implant undersizing is preferred over implant oversizing.

5. During oblique insertion, the final implant should be positioned in the medial-lateral plane first and then the lateral AP plane second.

◆ Complications

Careful preoperative planning and intraoperative attention to detail will decrease complications when performing an Activ-L lumbar disk arthroplasty. Preoperatively, patients should be advised to achieve a body mass index of 30 or less, thereby allowing for easier visualization fluoroscopically and also surgically. Careful end plate evaluation should be performed. CT scans should be obtained in all patients to evaluate for facet arthrosis and for pars interarticularis defects. Flexion-extension films should be utilized in all cases to assess for spondylolisthesis and intervertebral disk height. Patients with severe disk height loss and marginal osteophyte formation must be warned that mobilization of the intervertebral disk height will be intensive, and then if appropriate distraction cannot be performed, other procedures such as a fusion surgery may be necessary.

Intraoperatively, great care should be taken to avoid vascular injury. Extensive retraction of vessels should be avoided and should be limited to 45 minutes at one particular time. Pulse oximetry should be utilized intraoperatively in higher-risk individuals such as smokers or revision cases. Postoperatively, these patients should also be evaluated very carefully for delayed vascular compromise. Patients with prior abdominopelvic surgery should be considered for ureteral stents.

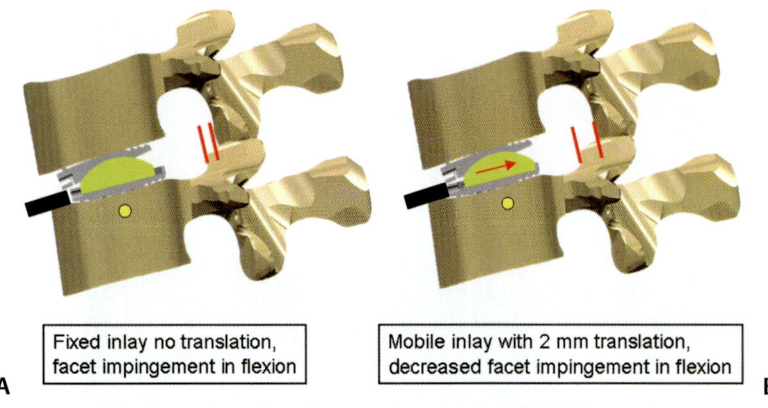

Figure 26–10A,B   Combined translation and rotation equals mobilization.

Postoperatively, patients are permitted to ambulate as soon as possible. They are permitted to drive and walk as tolerated. Clerical and light duty work is also permitted immediately. Lifting is limited to 15 pounds primarily to protect the abdominal wall repair. After 10 weeks and after appropriate confirmation of implant stability on dynamic radiographs, patients are allowed to participate in all non-contact recreational activities. Avoidance of high-impact activities should be a lifelong restriction as well as other forms of aggressive contact activities.

◆ Conclusion

The technique of lumbar total disk arthroplasty is gaining more widespread acceptance as implant designs exploit both mechanical and biological technological advances in arthroplasty design.[15–26] The Activ-L implant achieves an effective and safe balance between intervertebral motion and implant stability. The Activ-L implant allows for semi-constrained flexion-extension, rotation, and translation. This combined motion we term *mobilization* (**Fig. 26–10A,B**). Mobilization allows for more anatomical motion as well as smaller disk heights in the restoration of diseased intervertebral disk space. Immediate primary stability is achieved through the keel and/or spiked design of the implant, and secondary stability is achieved through the osseous integration of the titanium and dicalcium phosphate dehydrate (m -CaP) coating. Meticulous surgical exposure is mandatory to avoid injury to soft tissue structures. Before attempting to perform intervertebral disk arthroplasty, surgeons should familiarize themselves with surrounding anatomical structures and also have extensive experience in mobilizing intervertebral disk spaces.

References

1. de Kleuver M, Oner FC, Jacobs WC. Total disc replacement for chronic low back pain: background and a systematic review of the literature. Eur Spine J 2003;12:108–116

2. Zeegers WS, Bohnen LM, Laaper M, Verhaegen MJ. Artificial disc replacement with the modular type SB Charité III: 2-year results in 50 prospectively studied patients. Eur Spine J 1999;8:210–217

3. Zigler J. Clinical results with ProDisc: European experience and U.S. investigation device exemption study. Spine 2003;28:S163–S166

4. Bertagnoli R, Karg A, Voigt S. Lumbar partial disc replacement. Orthop Clin North Am 2005;36:341–347

5. Blumenthal S, McAfee PC, Guyer RD, et al. A prospective, randomized, multicenter Food and Drug Administration investigational device exemptions study of lumbar total disc replacement with the Charité artificial disc versus lumbar fusion, I: Evaluation of clinical outcomes. Spine 2005;30:1565–1575 discussion E387–391

6. Delamarter RB, Bae HW, Pradhan BB. Clinical results of ProDisc-II lumbar total disc replacement: report from the United States clinical trial. Orthop Clin North Am 2005;36:301–313

7. Errico TJ. Lumbar disc arthroplasty. Clin Orthop Relat Res 2005;435: 106–117

8. Frelinghuysen P, Huang RC, Girardi FP, et al. Lumbar total disc replacement, I: Rationale, biomechanics, and implant types. Orthop Clin North Am 2005;36:293–299

9. Gamradt SC, Wang JC. Lumbar disc arthroplasty. Spine J 2005;5: 95–103

10. Le Huec JC, Mathews H, Basso Y, et al. Clinical results of Maverick lumbar total disc replacement: two-year prospective follow-up. Orthop Clin North Am 2005;36:315–322

11. Mayer HM. Total lumbar disc replacement. J Bone Joint Surg Br 2005; 87:1029–1037

12. McAfee PC, Cunningham B, Holsapple G, et al. A prospective, randomized, multicenter Food and Drug Administration investigational device exemption study of lumbar total disc replacement with the Charité artificial disc versus lumbar fusion, II: Evaluation of radiographic outcomes and correlation of surgical technique accuracy with clinical outcomes. Spine 2005;30:1576–1583 discussion E388–390

13. Shuff C, An HS. Artificial disc replacement: the new solution for discogenic low back pain? Am J Orthop 2005;34:8–12

14. Tropiano P, Huang RC, Girardi FP, et al. Lumbar total disc replacement: seven- to eleven-year follow-up. J Bone Joint Surg Am 2005;87:490–496

15. Joshi A, Mehta S, Vresilovic E, et al. Nucleus implant parameters significantly change the compressive stiffness of the human lumbar intervertebral disc. J Biomech Eng 2005;127:536–540

16. Bertagnoli R, Zigler J, Karg A, et al. Complications and strategies for revision surgery in total disc replacement. Orthop Clin North Am 2005;36:389–395

17. Huang RC, Wright TM, Panjabi MM, et al. Biomechanics of nonfusion implants. Orthop Clin North Am 2005;36:271–280

18. Taksali S, Grauer JN, Vaccaro AR. Material considerations for intervertebral disc replacement implants. Spine J 2004;4:231S–238S

19. Hopf C, Heeckt H, Beske C. Indication, biomechanics and early results of artificial disc replacement [in German]. Z Orthop Ihre Grenzgeb 2004;142:153–158

20. LeHuec JC, Kiaer T, Friesem T, et al. Shock absorption in lumbar disc prosthesis: a preliminary mechanical study. J Spinal Disord Tech 2003;16:346–351

21. Huang RC, Girardi FP, Cammisa FP Jr, et al. The implications of constraint in lumbar total disc replacement. J Spinal Disord Tech 2003;16:412–417

22. McAfee PC, Fedder IL, Saiedy S, et al. Experimental design of total disc replacement-experience with a prospective randomized study of the SB Charité. Spine 2003;28:S153–S162

23. Takahata M, Kotani Y, Abumi K, et al. Bone ingrowth fixation of artificial intervertebral disc consisting of bioceramic-coated three-dimensional fabric. Spine 2003;28:637–644 discussion 44

24. Hallab N, Link HD, McAfee PC. Biomaterial optimization in total disc arthroplasty. Spine 2003;28:S139–S152

25. McAfee PC, Cunnigham BW, Orbegoso CM, et al. Analysis of porous ingrowth in intervertebral disc prosthesis: a nonhuman primate model. Spine 2003;28:332–340

26. Eijkelkamp MF, Hayen J, Veldhuizen AG, et al. Improving the fixation of an artificial intervertebral disc. Int J Artif Organs 2002;25:327–333

27

The FlexiCore Disk

Alok D. Sharan and Thomas Errico

◆ **FlexiCore Disk Design**

◆ **Indications**

◆ **Contraindications**

◆ **Description of System Components**
   Distraction Spacers
   Static Distractors
   Static Distractor Handle
   Dynamic Distractor
   Inserter/Impactor
   Repositioners/Extractors
   Leveling Tool
   Wedge-Ramp Distractor
   Parallel Insertion Distractor
   FlexiCore Intervertebral Disk

◆ **Operative Techniques**
   Preparation and Surgical Approach
   Diskectomy and End Plate Preparation
   Distraction (Disk Height Restoration)
   Establishing Proper Implant Size
   Inserting the FlexiCore
   Repositioning (or Extracting) the FlexiCore
   Seating the FlexiCore
   Closure and Postoperative Care

◆ **Complications**

◆ **Conclusion**

◆ **Caution**

Degenerative disk disease (DDD) represents a significant morbidity in our health care system. Back pain, the clinical manifestation of DDD, results in major disability, time lost from work, and a significant effect on quality of life for the patient. It is estimated that a significant episode of back pain will affect 80% of the U.S. population at least once in their lifetime.[1] More than $50 billion in annual health care expenditures for both direct and indirect costs will be spent in the treatment of back pain. This unfortunately makes back pain a significant problem for society.

Treatment strategies for back pain initially begin with an exhaustive course of nonoperative therapy. Most back pain can be treated with rest, medication, and physical therapy. When this has failed, surgical treatment is indicated. Spine surgeons generally agree that surgical treatment for DDD typically involves some type of fusion of the lumbar spine. The rationale for fusion is that immobilizing the degenerated segment can eliminate painful motion of that joint while also eliminating the disk as a pain generator. Historically, posterolateral fusion was the most common technique used to fuse the lumbar spine, but as our clinical skills and technology have improved, newer techniques have been developed. Today DDD can be treated with lumbar interbody fusion, posterior spinal fusion, or a combination of the two procedures. As newer techniques have been developed our success at achieving radiological fusion has increased.

Unfortunately our improvement in clinical results has not equaled the radiological results.[2,3]

Mobility of the spine is a result of interconnected motion between each intervertebral level. Fusing one segment of the spine results in increased load across other levels. This leads to adjacent level degeneration, which can result in further morbidity. In addition there could be an alteration in sagittal balance due to graft collapse, and stress shielding/disuse osteoporosis.[3–6] For this reason spine surgeons have begun to investigate and use newer techniques to treat DDD while still restoring motion across the segment.

The total disk replacement (TDR) represents a new generation of devices that can preserve motion in the spine while removing the painful degenerative disk. Currently there are four TDRs that are undergoing investigational trials in the United States. The FlexiCore Lumbar Intervertebral Disc Replacement (Stryker Spine, Allendale, NJ) represents a metal-on-metal device.

◆ FlexiCore Disk Design

The FlexiCore disk is a cobalt-chromium-molybdenum highly polished ball and socket metal-on-metal prosthesis. The device is designed as a tension-bearing device that prevents separation and potential dislocation of the superior and inferior baseplates. There is also a rotational stop in the device that prevents the facets from being overloaded. A unique design feature of the FlexiCore disk is the central dome shape of the baseplate. This shape enables the prosthesis to match the normal end plate concavity of the vertebral body. This helps both to facilitate bony fixation and to optimally locate the device's center of rotation slightly posterior to the spinal midline. The domes are flanked by short spikes to establish initial fixation and are coated with a titanium plasma spray to encourage long-term fixation.

The two baseplates are joined by a central ball and socket joint that establishes the device's center of rotation. This provides a range of motion that does not limit the natural range of motion of the intervertebral segment. In addition, it prevents any translation of the baseplates that would mimic subluxation. The device provides 15 degrees of flexion-extension and lateral bending. This exceeds the natural range of motion of an intervertebral segment but does not lead to the baseplates sliding anteriorly-posteriorly, or later-ally, relative to one another. There is an internal rotational stop that is designed to minimize pathological facet loading by preventing axial rotation beyond 5 degrees, which is just outside the natural range of motion. The bearing surfaces of the ball and socket components are highly polished cobalt-chromium. This has been shown in the joint replacement literature to have a lower coefficient of friction and generates a decreased amount of wear debris compared with bearing surfaces that include polyethylene. Further, metal-on-metal bearing surfaces are not subject to the "creep" seen in metal-on-polyethylene interfaces.[7,8]

The ball of the joint is captured in the socket during the manufacturing process before delivery to the surgeon. This prevents the device from separating under tension loads and permits it to be held, manipulated, and inserted into the disk space as a single unit. This, combined with the implantation instrumentation, not only permits the device to be inserted from multiple anterior angles but also minimizes the implantation misalignments and other errors associated with multipiece assembly and implantation. Some repositioning is also possible even after the device is seated in the disk space.

◆ Indications

The FlexiCore intervertebral disk is currently under investigation in the United States. It is indicated for implantation in patients with DDD who are between ages 18 and 60. Other indications include:

- Back pain of diskogenic origin with degeneration of a single disk (L1–S1)
- Axial back pain greater than leg/radicular pain
- Radiographic evidence of decreased disk height by 2 mm compared with adjacent (cranial) disk height and/or[1]: Translational instability ($\geq$ 3 mm translation)[2]; angular instability ($\geq$ 5 degrees)
- A preoperative visual analog scale (VAS) score for back pain of at least 40/100
- A preoperative Oswestry score of at least 40/100
- Failed conservative treatment for back pain for a minimum of 6 months

◆ Contraindications

The FlexiCore intervertebral disk is contraindicated for study in patients having:

- DDD at more than one level
- Previous lumbar fusion or bilateral open decompressive procedures
- Compromised vertebral body structure
- Degenerative spondylolisthesis/retrolisthesis > 25%
- Spondylolysis with or without spondylolisthesis
- Lumbar scoliosis > 15 degrees
- Facet joint disease or degeneration
- Poor bone quality
- Medications that interfere with bone/tissue healing
- Infection, hepatitis, rheumatoid arthritis, autoimmune diseases, or malignancy
- Obesity, pregnancy, or allergy to implant materials

◆ Description of System Components

The components of the FlexiCore intervertebral disk implantation system include:

- Distraction spacers (**Fig. 27–1**)
- Static distractors (**Fig. 27–2**)

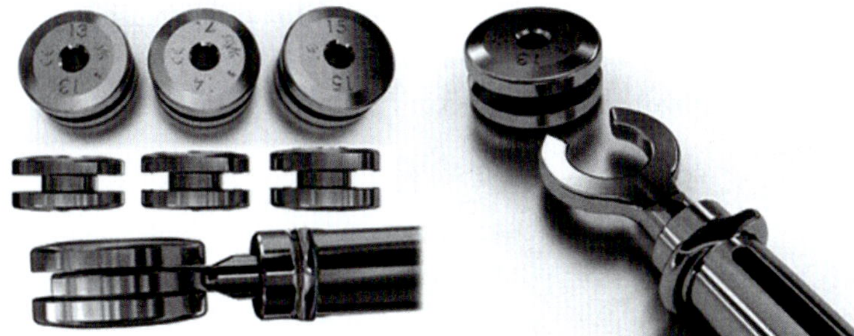

Figure 27–1   Distraction spacers.

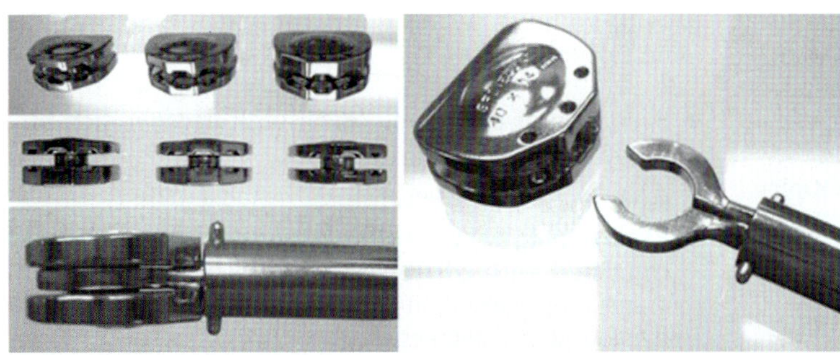

Figure 27–2   Static distractors.

- Static distractor handle (**Fig. 27–3**)
- Dynamic distractor (**Fig. 27–4**)
- Inserter/impactor (**Fig. 27–5A–C**)
- Repositioner/extractor (**Fig. 27–6A,B**)
- Leveling tool (**Fig. 27–7**)
- Wedge-ramp distractor (**Fig. 27–8**)
- Parallel insertion distractor (**Fig. 27–9**)
- FlexiCore intervertebral disk (**Fig. 27–10A–C**)

A brief description of each component follows.

Distraction Spacers

- Cylindrical spacers with heights ranging from 8 to 18 mm in 1 mm increments
- Cylindrical core for engagement by static distractor handle (**Fig. 27–3**)
- Parallel upper and lower surfaces with beveled perimetrical edges for insertion
- Effect distraction by sequential insertion and removal with increasing heights

Static Distractors

- D-shaped spacers with two footprints, 28×35 mm and 30×40 mm
- Heights ranging from 12 to 18 mm in 1 mm increments
- Baseplates in fixed lordosis at 5 degrees
- Beveled posterior edge for inserting between vertebral end plates

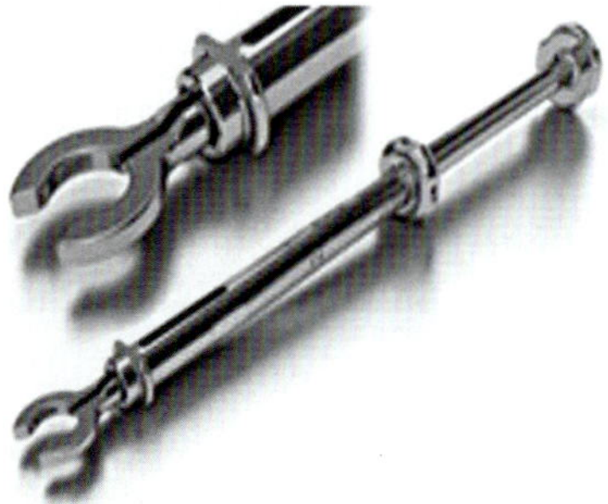

Figure 27–3   Static distractor handle.

- Cylindrical core for engagement by static distractor handle (**Fig. 27–3**)
- Designed for initial implant sizing and distraction by sequential insertion and removal with increasing heights

Static Distractor Handle

- Distal enclosure snaps on and off cylindrical cores of distraction spacers and static distractors to facilitate their sequential use.
- Central knob rotates to lock distal enclosure for rugged manipulation of distraction spacers and static distractors.

Dynamic Distractor

- Distal baseplates with a 28×35 mm footprint can be inserted into intervertebral space and separated from 13 mm to 20 mm by analog adjustment for gradual distraction.
- Forward movement of central bar separates baseplates; rotation of central knob provides mechanical advantage as height increases.
- Baseplate domes fit into and prepare vertebral end plate concavities for receipt of domes of implant's baseplates.

Inserter/Impactor

- Movement of central flange extends and retracts a spring-biased J-hook from the tool's distal head to grip holes in implant baseplates to hold and manipulate implant.
- Angled surfaces of distal head prevent axial rotation of implant baseplates and hold them in 5 degrees of lordosis.
- Configuration of distal head, in cooperation with holes and angled surfaces of implant baseplates, facilitates an anterior and two anterolateral insertion approach angles.

Repositioners/Extractors

- Distal end provides pins for engagement of pairs of holes in implant and static distractor baseplates to facilitate intraoperative repositioning or removal.
- Symmetric, right-offset, and left-offset versions provide multiple approach angles in cooperation with three- and four-hole sets on upper and lower baseplates.

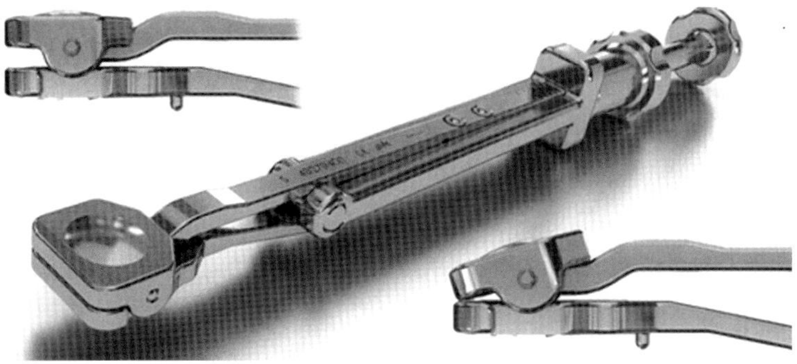

Figure 27–4   Dynamic distractor.

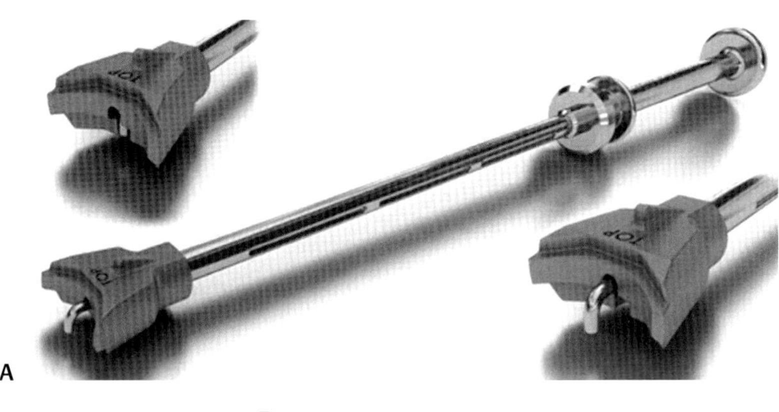

A

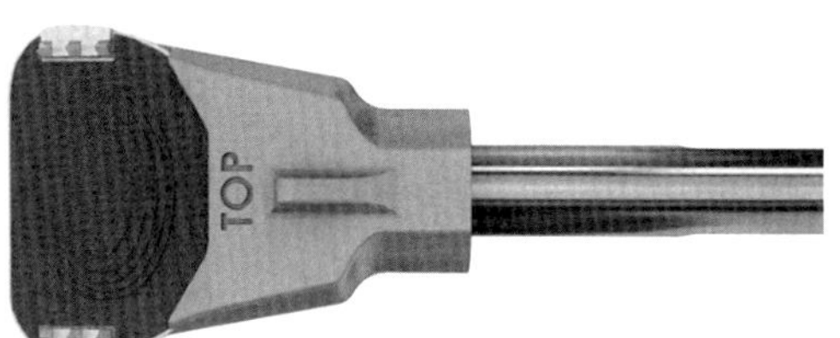

B

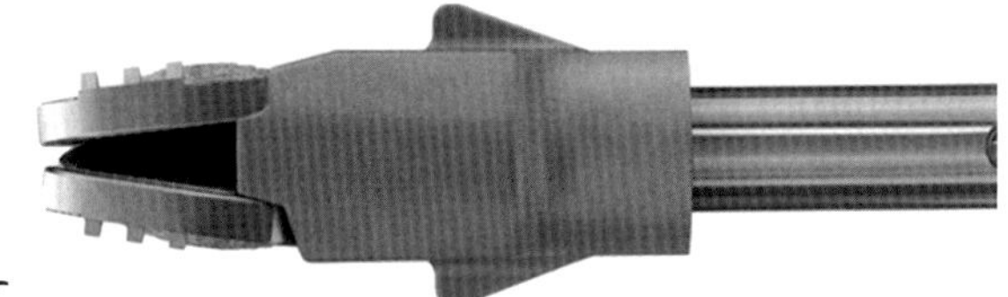

C

Figure 27–5   (A) Inserter/impactor. (B) Inserter/impactor gripping implant (top view). (C) Inserter/impactor gripping implant (lateral view).

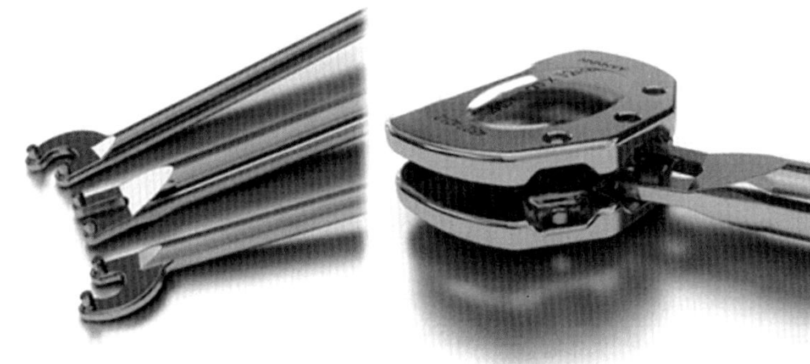

A

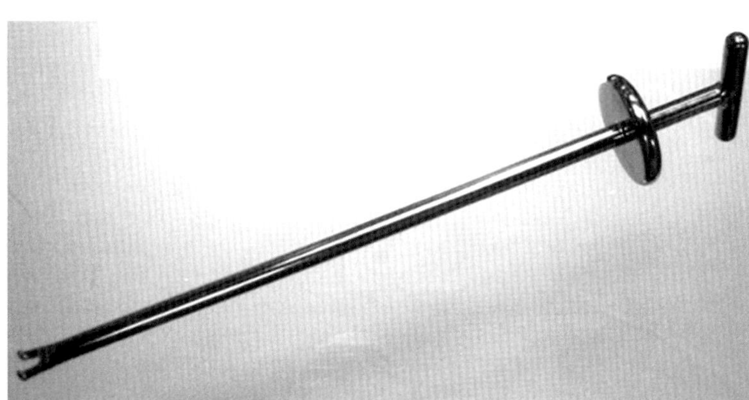

B

Figure 27–6   (A) Repositioners/extractors (distal ends). (B) Symmetric repositioner/extractor.

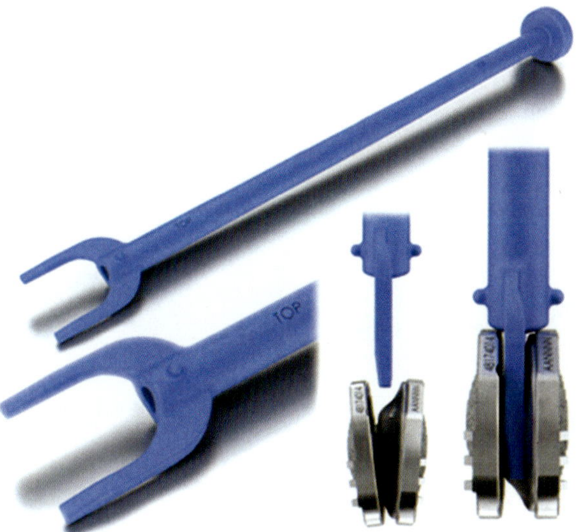

Figure 27–7 Leveling tool.

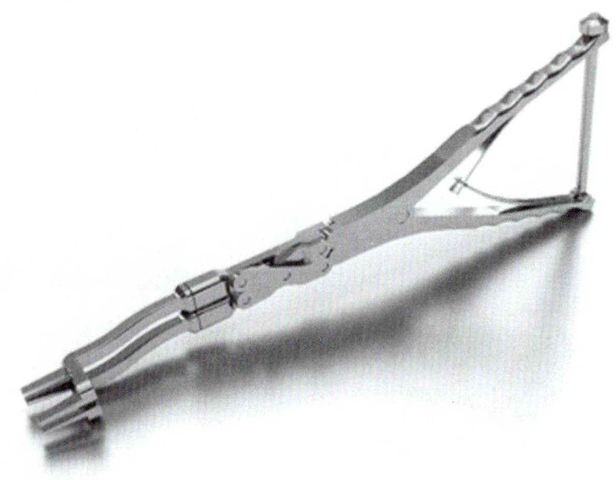

Figure 27–9 Parallel insertion distractor.

Leveling Tool

◆ Double prongs at distal end are inserted between implant baseplates around the ball and socket joint to force baseplate spikes into the vertebral end plates.

Wedge-Ramp Distractor

◆ Effects distraction simultaneous with insertion
◆ Ramps are double-hinged at proximal ends by a C-clip connector.
◆ Implant's baseplate spikes ride in ramp tracks for insertion.

Parallel Insertion Distractor

◆ Holds intervertebral space in distraction during insertion
◆ Distal tongs can be opened by closing scissor handle and held in open position by set screw on scissor handle.
◆ Features behind tongs guide insertion of implant into intervertebral space

FlexiCore Intervertebral Disk

◆ TDR device with tension-bearing structure for single-unit manipulation and insertion

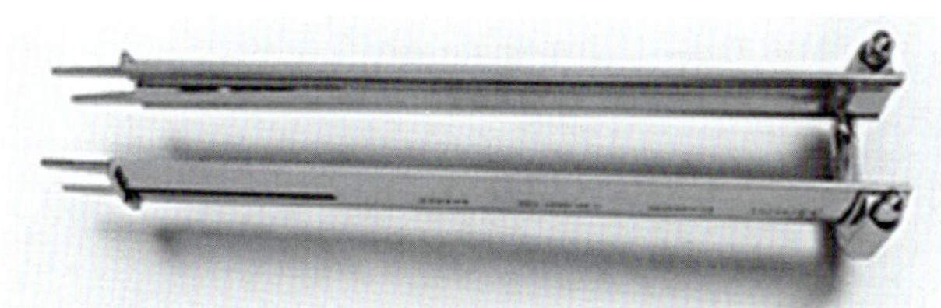

Figure 27–8 Wedge-ramp distractor.

◆ All-metal construction with cobalt chromium baseplates joined by a central 13 mm ball and socket joint with highly polished cobalt-chromium bearing surfaces
◆ Each baseplate has a central dome that seats in an adjacent vertebral end plate concavity and is flanked by short spikes and a porous titanium plasma spray layer.
◆ Central ball and socket joint, in conjunction with baseplate domes, establishes a stationary center of rotation centrally between the baseplate and slightly posterior to the spinal midline.
◆ Each baseplate is featured for engagement by instrumentation from an anterior and two anterolateral surgical approach angles: three angled perimetrical surfaces, three- and four-hole sets on the inferior and superior baseplates.
◆ Flexion-extension and lateral bending range is ± 15 degrees; internal stop limits axial rotation beyond ± 5 degrees.
◆ Available in seven disk heights (12–18 mm in 1 mm increments) and two baseplate footprint sizes (28 × 35 mm and 30 × 40 mm)

◆ Operative Techniques

Preparation and Surgical Approach

The FlexiCore Lumbar Intervertebral Disc Replacement implantation procedure is performed with the patient under general anesthesia in the supine decubitus position for an anterior or anterolateral approach to the lumbar spine. A Pfannenstiel minilaparotomy transverse incision (usually 5–8 cm long) may be used for a single-level disk replacement from L3–S1. A midline longitudinal incision may be used if a previous midline scar is present. At the L4–L5 level, the bifurcation of the aorta into the common iliac vessels should occur to allow for easier exposure of the bare L5–S1 disk space. The middle sacral artery or vein or both should be identified and ligated at the L5–S1 interspace.

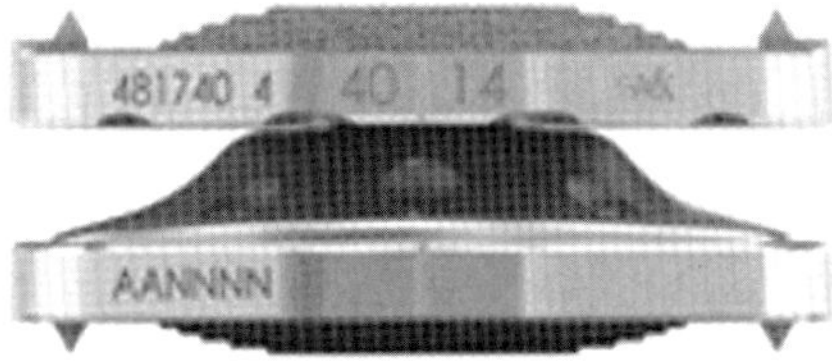

A

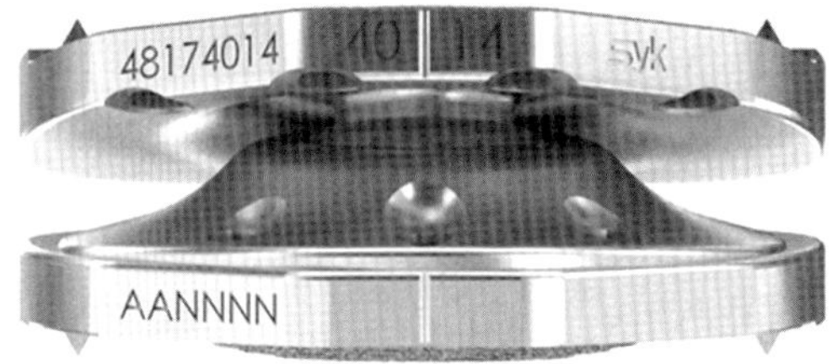

B

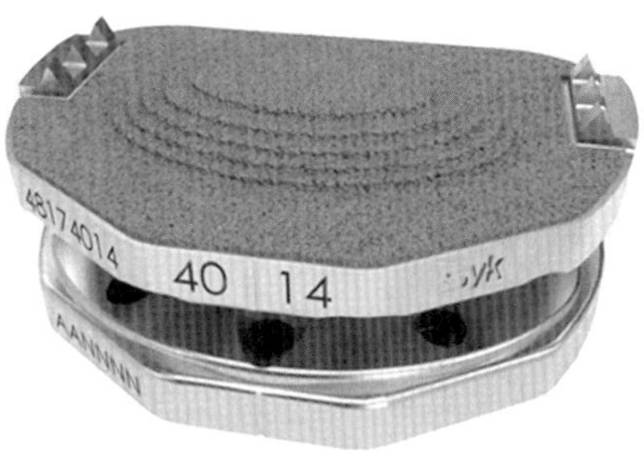

C

Figure 27–10 **(A)** FlexiCore Lumbar Intervertebral Disc Replacement (anterior view). **(B)** FlexiCore Lumbar Intervertebral Disc Replacement (anterior view lordosed). **(C)** FlexiCore Lumbar Intervertebral Disc Replacement (perspective view).

For exposure of the L4–L5 disk space, the iliolumbar vein must be exposed and ligated to allow for the remaining artery and vein to be swept medially. The entire disk must be exposed from each lateral margin to allow for proper centralized placement of the prosthesis. The midline of the disk space should also be intraoperatively determined and marked prior to starting the diskectomy. The midline of the disk space can be determined by placing a metal marker and comparing its location to the spinous processes on an anteroposterior (AP) fluoroscopic view.

Diskectomy and End Plate Preparation

After a localizing radiograph has been taken to identify the proper disk space, the annulus–end plate interface is incised to dissect an anterior hole in the annulus that approximates the width of the implant. The disk and the end plate cartilage are removed to expose the subchondral bone until punctate bleeding is produced. The posterior margin of the disk space should be cleared of any osteophytes or soft tissue material that may inhibit the full distraction of the posterior portion of the disk space. It is not required that the posterior longitudinal ligament or the remaining portion of the annulus be sacrificed.

Distraction (Disk Height Restoration)

Once the end plates have been prepared properly, the disk space is serially distracted. Restoring the disk height begins by gently twisting large, thin periosteal elevators. When enough height is available to insert an 8 mm distraction spacer (**Fig. 27–1**), the spacer is gently inserted into the disk space, rocked back and forth to loosen the surrounding ligaments, and removed. Distraction continues with the sequential insertion and removal of progressively larger distraction spacers in 1 mm increments, until the 13 mm spacer can be inserted easily.

Establishing Proper Implant Size

The static distractors (**Fig. 27–2**) are used to further distract the disk space and to determine the proper implant size. The height of the first static distractor used should be 1 mm less than the height of the last distraction spacer used for distraction. When inserted, each static distractor should be centered laterally and positioned 2 to 3 mm within the anterior margin and 1 to 2 mm within the posterior margin. The domes of the baseplates should be seated within the concavities of the vertebral end plates. Sequential insertion of the static distractors in 1 mm increments continues until the posterior soft tissue elements are loosened but not stretched.

The dynamic distractor (**Fig. 27–4**) is used to confirm the final implant size and ensure that the intervertebral space is wide enough to accommodate the spikes of the implant's baseplates. The baseplates of the dynamic distractor are inserted between the vertebral bodies and separated to the height of the last static distractor used by moving the central flange of the instrument forward, using the central knob if necessary. The dynamic distractor provides tactile feedback regarding whether the surrounding ligaments are suitably loosened but not overly tightened, to help determine or confirm the optimal height of the implant. Once the optimal height is determined, the dynamic distractor is used to further distract the disk space by an additional 2 mm to permit easy passage of the implant's baseplate spikes. Under the compressive forces of this additional distraction, the central domes on the instrument's baseplates prepare the natural vertebral end plate concavities to receive the domes of the implant's baseplates.

Inserting the FlexiCore

Intervertebral Disk

After the intervertebral space is prepared and distracted and the optimal implant size is determined, an appropriately sized FlexiCore intervertebral disk (**Fig. 27–10A–C**) is secured to the inserter/impactor (**Fig. 27–5A**) by extending the instrument's J-hook and engaging it with one of the three holes in the implant's baseplate (**Fig. 27–5B,C**). The central hole is used for a directly anterior surgical approach, and the offset holes are used for anterolateral approaches. When released, the spring-biased J-hook will retract to hold the angled perimeters of the baseplates against the angled surfaces of the inserter/impactor head, which prevents them from axially rotating during the insertion. The central wedge of the inserter/impactor head seats between the baseplates to hold them in 5 degrees of lordosis to allow for easier insertion into the intervertebral space.

The inserter/impactor can be used alone to insert the implant into the intervertebral space, similar to the manner in which a femoral ring is inserted during an anterior lumbar interbody fusion (ALIF) procedure. The posterior edges of the baseplates are positioned between the vertebral end plates' edges, and the implant is advanced into the space. The implant should be centered laterally and positioned 2 to 3 mm within the anterior margin and 1 to 2 mm within the posterior margin of the intervertebral space. The domes of the baseplates should be seated within the vertebral end plate concavities.

Two alternative insertion instruments are provided to accommodate surgeon preferences. The first instrument is the wedge-ramp distractor (**Fig. 27–8**), which is used to distract the intervertebral space as the implant is inserted. It includes a pair of ramps that are double-hinged to one another at their proximal ends with a C-clip connector. The ramps converge toward one another such that their proximal ends are separated to receive the implant (previously loaded on the inserter/impactor) between them, and their distal ends converge toward one another to meet at the intervertebral space. The distal ends are inserted between the vertebral end plates, and the implant is slid between the ramps toward the intervertebral space. As the implant is being advanced, the height of the implant forces the distal ends of the ramps apart, which distracts the restervertebral space to the necessary height as the implant is positioned in the space. After the insertion, the ramps are removed one at a time.

The second instrument is the parallel insertion distractor (**Fig. 27–9**), which is used to hold the intervertebral space open as the implant is inserted. It includes a scissor handle that when closed separates distal upper and lower tongs of the instrument. The closed tongs are inserted between the vertebral end plates and then separated (by closing the scissor handle) to hold the intervertebral space open to receive the implant. The tongs are held in separation by advancing a screw at the proximal end of the instrument to hold the scissor handle in the closed position. The implant (previously loaded on the inserter/impactor) is inserted between the tongs and into the intervertebral space. After the insertion, the scissor handle is released and the tongs are slid out from between the implant and the vertebral end plates.

Repositioning (or Extracting) the FlexiCore

Intervertebral Disk

If the lateral or AP images indicate that the implant is not in the optimal position, the implant can be repositioned using the repositioners/extractors (**Fig. 27–6A,B**). Symmetric, right offset, and left offset instruments are provided, each with a pair of pins on its distal end that can be inserted into any pair of holes in the upper or lower baseplates of the implant, to provide multiple surgical approach angles. Once the pins are engaged with a hole pair, the baseplates can be moved in the lateral and AP planes and axially rotated. The baseplate can be engaged for individual or simultaneous adjustment (by using two repositioners/extractors, one on each baseplate). The repositioners/extractors can also be used to extract the implant by engaging the pins into any pair of holes on the implant baseplates and pulling on the handle's flange.

Seating the FlexiCore

Intervertebral Disk

Once the implant is optimally positioned in the intervertebral space, the radiolucent leveling tool (**Fig. 27–7**) is used to force the spikes of the baseplates into the vertebral end plates to facilitate initial and long-term fixation. The distal prongs of the instrument are inserted and advanced between the baseplates, straddling the ball and socket joint, until the baseplates become parallel to one another. Using fluoroscopy, the final intraoperative position of the implant can be verified to determine proper posterior seating against the posterior annulus, parallel alignment of the device's baseplates with the adjacent end plates, and a centralized position in relation to the vertebral bodies (**Fig. 27–11A,B**).

Closure and Postoperative Care

Standard closure procedures for anterior or anterolateral spine surgery are followed. The patient is extubated immediately after the operation and taken to the recovery room. The patient is kept NPO until there are signs of bowel activity. By the first postoperative day, the patient is encouraged to ambulate with the assistance of a physical therapist. By the second or third postoperative day, the patient should be tolerating a regular diet and ambulating hallways with the assistance of a physical therapist. The patient can usually

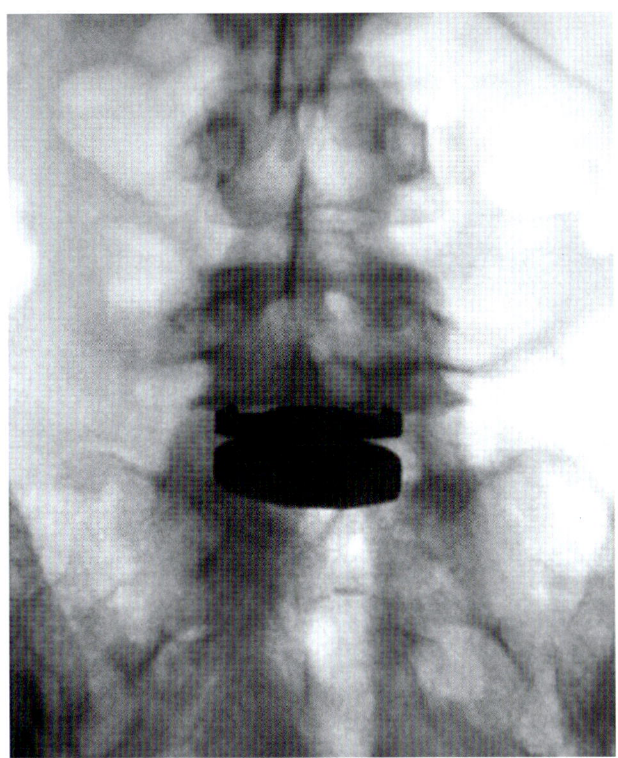
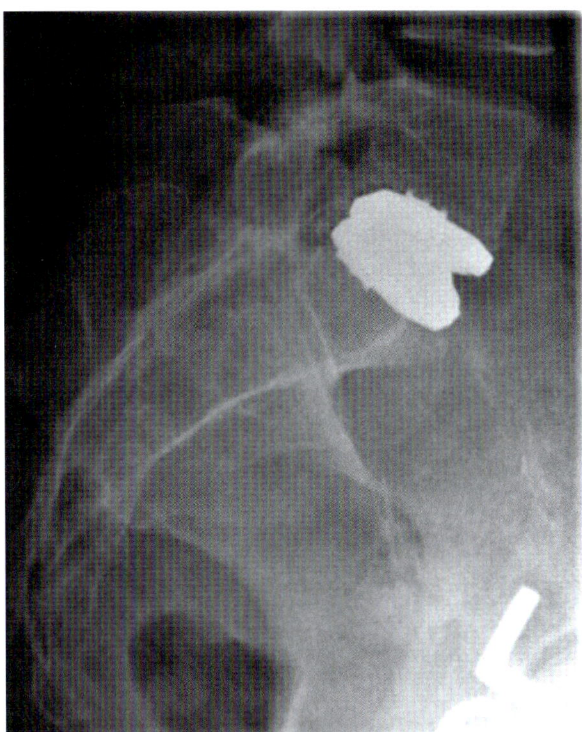

Figure 27–11 **(A)** Anteroposterior fluoroscopy view of final position. **(B)** Lateral fluoroscopy view of final position.

be discharged home between the second and fourth postoperative days. Whether the patient should be allowed to return to work is determined by the individual's specific job-related activities. Heavy lifting should be restricted until the patient is fully rehabilitated, which typically occurs after 8 to 12 weeks.

◆ Complications

Complications associated with the insertion of the FlexiCore disk can be due to the surgical technique/approach or to the implant itself. The lack of pain relief can occur if there was an inappropriate selection of the surgical candidate. It is important to do a proper workup of the patient to determine if the back pain is truly diskogenic. During this workup, it is important that the correct level contributing to the back pain be chosen for disk replacement. Patients may have multiple levels of symptomatic disk degeneration contributing to their disease. In addition, patients may often have an unrecognized instability contributing to their pain that would not be amenable to a disk replacement.

During surgery, technical errors during the approach may result that could lead to morbidities for the patient. Inadvertent violation of the peritoneum may occur, which requires immediate repair. During the exposure and placement of the retractors, it is critical to be aware of the vessels in this region. Injury may occur to the common iliac vessels, aorta, iliolumbar vein, or the inferior vena cava, which also requires immediate repair. In males, the use of electrocautery should be limited because this may lead to injury to the superior hypogastric plexus, which could result in retrograde ejaculation.

With regard to the implant, it is important to check the implant on fluoroscopy via AP and lateral views. If the implant is placed too anterior, some remaining posterior disk material or posterior osteophytes may need to be removed. If the implant is too posterior it can signify excessive resection or rupture of the posterior longitudinal ligament.

Postoperative complications can develop that could be a direct result of the surgical exposure or related to the implant itself. Often these patients will develop an ileus due to the transabdominal or even retroperitoneal approach. A prolonged ileus may require the insertion of a nasogastric tube. During closure, it is important that the fascia be closed properly, otherwise an incisional hernia can develop. Manipulation of the great vessels can sometimes lead to deep vein thrombosis, which requires anticoagulation. As with other joint replacements, it is important to maintain good sterile technique to avoid infection.

With regard to the implant, undersizing or oversizing the prosthesis can result in excessive or insufficient motion. Sometimes the implant can subside or change positions if the end plate preparations were too excessive. And, finally, there have been cases reported with other disk replacements of spontaneous fusion developing if inadequate motion is not restored.

◆ Conclusion

The FlexiCore disk represents a unique design for a total disk replacement that offers many benefits. The baseplate dome and central ball and socket joint are designed to establish a stationary center of rotation that is located centrally between the end plates and slightly posterior to the midline.

This position closely matches the center of rotation of a normal intervertebral disk. The metal-on-metal bearing surfaces are anticipated to maintain their shape over the lifetime of the device with minimal wear debris. The internal stop that limits axial rotation beyond a point just outside the natural range of motion prevents over-rotation and pathological facet loading. The design of the baseplates as well as the titanium plasma sprayed bone ongrowth allows the implant to fit flush within the concavities of the end plates. This will assist in early and late bony fixation without compromising the structure of the vertebral body. The tension-bearing structure is expected to prevent separation and dislocation of the bearing surfaces. The FlexiCore intervertebral disk is manipulated and implanted as a single unit, which is expected to assist in the proper alignment, reduce implantation errors, and minimize inventory. Finally, the implant can be inserted and manipulated via multiple angles, which can accommodate individual patient anatomy.

◆ CAUTION

The devices depicted in Figs. 27–1 through 27–10 are investigational. Limited by United States law to investigational use.

References

1. Frymoyer J, Cats-Baril W. An overview of the incidence and costs of lower back pain. Orthop Clin North Am 1991;22:263–270
2. Barrick WT, Schofferman JA, Reynolds JB, et al. Anterior lumbar fusion improves discogenic pain at levels of prior posterolateral fusion. Spine 2000;25:853–857
3. Buttermann GR, Garvey TA, Hunt AF, et al. Lumbar fusion results related to Diagnosis. Spine 1998;23:116–127
4. Kumar MN, Jacquot F, Hall H. Long-term follow-up of functional outcomes and radiographic changes at adjacent levels following lumbar spine fusion for degenerative disc diseases. Eur Spine J 2001;10:309–313
5. Lehmann TR, Spratt KF, Tozzi JE, et al. Long-term follow-up of lower lumbar fusion patients. Spine 1987;12:97–104
6. Shono Y, Kaneda K, Abumi K, McAfee PC, Cunningham BW. Stability of posterior spinal instrumentation and its effects on adjacent motion segments in the lumbosacral spine. Spine 1998;23:1550–1558
7. Chan FW, Bobyn JD, Medley JB, Krygier JJ, Tanzer M. Wear and lubrication of metal-on-metal hip implants. Clin Orthop Relat Res 1999;369:10–24
8. Dorr LD, Wan Z, Longjohn DB, Dubois B, Murken R. Total hip arthroplasty with the use of the Metasul metal-on-metal articulation: four- to seven-year results. J Bone Joint Surg Am 2000;82:789–798

28

Management of Vascular and Surgical Approach–Related Complications for Lumbar Total Disk Replacement

Sang-Ho Lee and Sang-Hyeop Jeon

◆ **Preoperative Evaluation and Planning**

◆ **Management of Vascular Complications**
  Venous Tear and Bleeding
  Arterial Obstruction
  Deep Venous Thrombosis

◆ **Other Approach-Related Complications**
  Visceral Complications
  Urogenital Complications
  Peripheral Nerve Complications
  Miscellaneous Wound Problems

◆ **Conclusion**

Wide exposure of the ventral disk space is necessary for good implant position and safety of instrumentation in relation to heavy and complex artificial disk instruments. Therefore, extensive vascular mobilization is inevitable, resulting in the fact that surgeons are confronted with the risk of vascular injury. However, most approach-related complications are avoidable when surgeons are more experienced. The surgical planes of properly selected patients are more easily separable due to less degenerative inflammatory change, as well the patients' being relatively young and less obese compared with fusion patient cases.[1]

The authors' collaborative professional surgical team, composed of vascular and general surgeons, has a great amount of surgical experience with the anterior retroperitoneal approach for spine surgery, with more than 1000 cases per year.[2] We present our clinical experiences with complication-reducing techniques and the skill developed in the management of vascular and surgical-related complications, with a review of the literature.

◆ Preoperative Evaluation and Planning

It is important to obtain information about the prevertebral vascular structure and its status. Preoperative computed tomographic (CT) scans and magnetic resonance (MR) axial images should contain not only spine pathology but the prevertebral vascular anatomy as well. Digitalized image-viewing systems are especially useful in understanding the three-dimensional relationship between the vascular structure and the ventral vertebral surface. Louis has described six primary variants of the aortocaval anatomy based on the level of the aortic split and vena cava bifurcation.[3] In our experience, many unclassified vascular variations exist, including dual infrarenal inferior vena cava (IVC) and situs inversus (**Fig. 28–1**).

Additionally, combinations of lumbar spine segment variants, lumbarization, or sacralization make it more complex. Such exact recognition of the vasculature at the targeted disk level helps to determine an apt approach plan (e.g., entrance between aortocaval bifurcation is better even at the L4–L5 level in some cases) and avoid encountering surprises, such as aortic aneurysm or the rare variations already mentioned.

In cases of calcified atherosclerotic plaques, as noticed on CT scan, duplex Doppler ultrasound for lower extremity arterial blood flow can provide more meaningful information. If, due to atherosclerosis, any stenotic portion is noted on a lower-extremity duplex scan, an anterior retroperitoneal approach for total disk replacement (TDR) is contraindicated.

Preoperative abdominal ultrasound checks are routinely performed to rule out urogenital, visceral anomaly, or an unexpected pathology, such as a congenital single kidney, ureter duplication, hidden abdominal solid organ malignancy, gynecological abnormalities, or abdominal aortic aneurysms.

All these efforts may lead to decreases in vascular and other approach-related complications.

◆ Management of Vascular Complications

Venous Tear and Bleeding

In our clinical experience of TDR in 620 patients, the incidence of venous bleeding was 1.3% (eight cases), with tearing of the left common iliac vein being the most common during L4–L5 disk space exposure. Six cases sustained minor pinpoint bleeding caused by either an avulsion of small radicular branches hidden beneath perivascular soft tissue, containing lymphatics, or losing sight of a tethered perforating vein to the L5 body. Although it was possible to control such occurrences

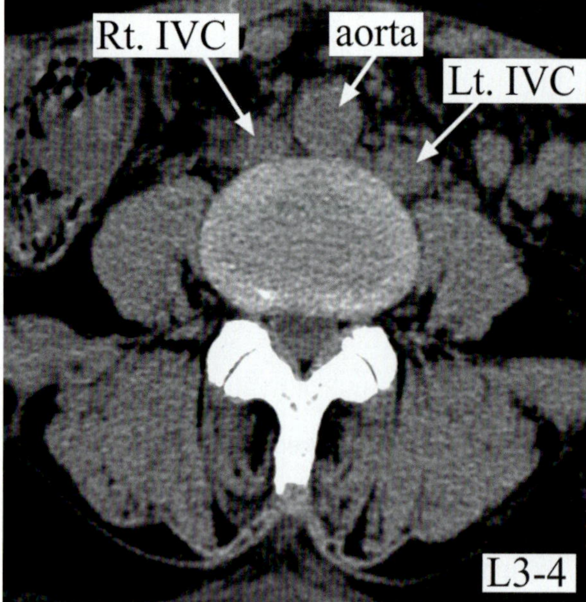

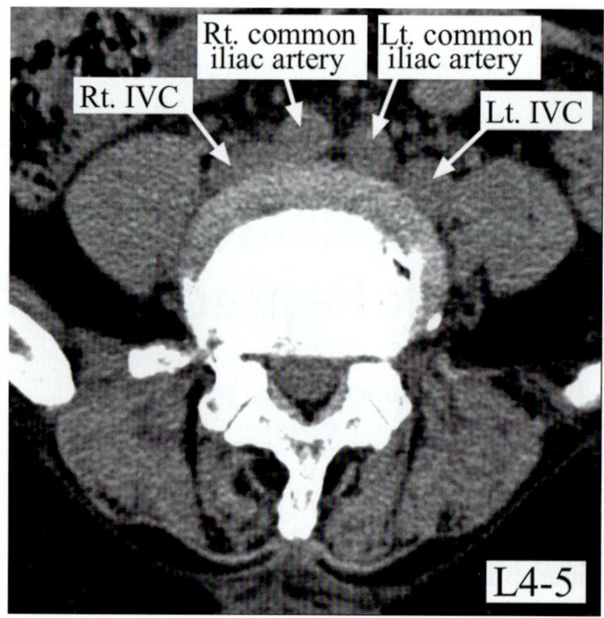

Figure 28–1 Unusual left infrarenal dual inferior vena cava (IVC). **(A)** Axial computed tomography (CT) scan showing the left-sided infrarenal dual inferior vena cava (IVC) at the L3–L4 level. **(B)** Axial CT scan showing the left-sided infrarenal dual IVC at the L4–L5 level.

by compression with coagulants, we performed a simple suture with 5–0 Prolene to complete further vessel mobilization. At times, venous injury of the main trunk with large amounts of bleeding can occur due to the laceration of a misread collapsed vein under retraction of underlying soft tissue when the surgeon is less experienced. Therefore, the surgeon should dissect perivascular soft tissue with careful attention to the lateral margin of the venous trunk, especially under conditions of perivascular scarring and adherence caused by reactive inflammation at an osteophytic spur, degenerative changes of the spine, or prior abdominal surgery. Two cases of major venous injury occurred during artificial disk implantation (**Table 28–1**). One was caused by anesthetic complications; the abdominal pressure suddenly increased with ventilator fighting at the midterm of the ProDisc (Synthes, Inc., West Chester, PA) implantation at the L4–L5 level. The left iliac vein injury occurred during the temporary removal of the retractor system and artificial disk instruments. The other venous injury was caused by the SB Charité instruments (DePuy Spine, Raynham, MA); we had failed at secure retraction transiently because the patient had a heavy abdominal musculature and bulky psoas

muscle. Therefore, some of my anesthesiologist colleagues prefer to implement continuous infusion of muscle relaxants during anterior retroperitoneal spine surgery.

The iliolumbar vein can often be extremely troublesome for most surgeons. Special attention should be paid to this precarious structure early during its exposure. For wide exposure, enough for TDR, ligation of the ascending iliolumbar vein is necessary to prevent avulsion from the mother vessel. If iliolumbar vein injury occurs, it is impossible to control using direct compression alone or with direct suturing due to the large amount of bleeding and the narrow surgical field. In such situations, tentative clipping and cutting of the remnant vein followed by an elective suture and tie are more effective than blind cauterization or a direct suture (**Fig. 28–2**).

Table 28–1 Approach-Related Complications of Total Disk Replacement in 620 Consecutive Patients

Complications	Numbers*
Major venous injury	2
Arterial embolism	1
Deep vein thrombosis	0
Visceral complication	0
Retrograde ejaculation	0
Sympathetic nerve damage	0
Anterior rectus facia defect	2

*Results of the clinical review involved four vascular surgeons at the Wooridul Spine Hospital, Seoul, Korea.

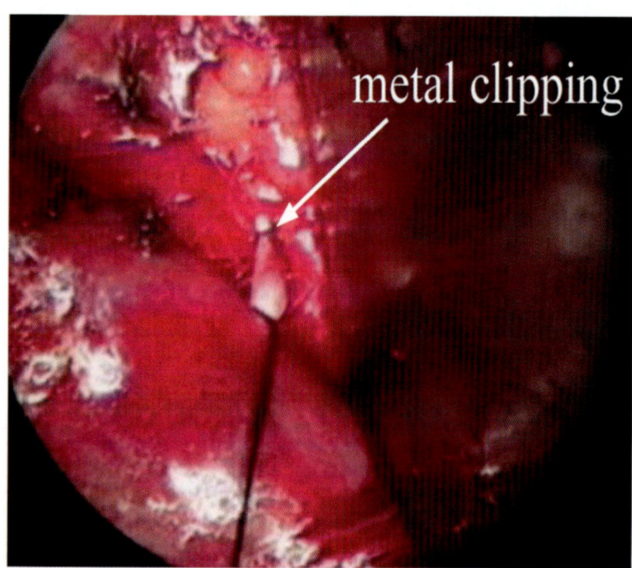

Figure 28–2 Similar normal situation of ligation of the ascending iliolumbar vein: metal clipping of the distal end, with proximal stump ligation.

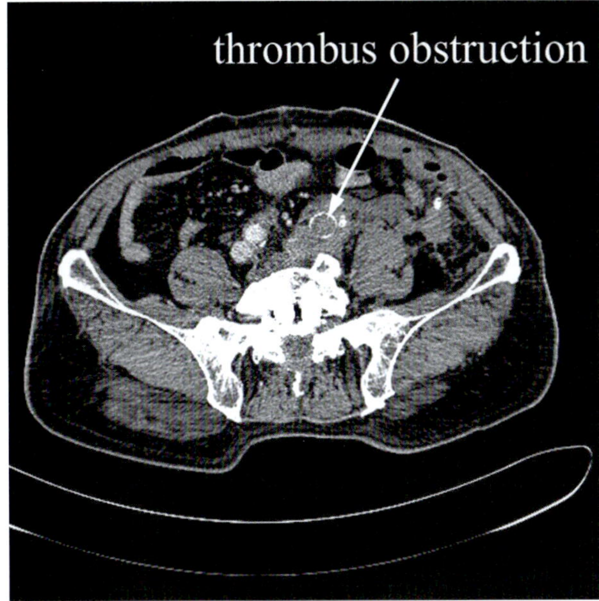

A

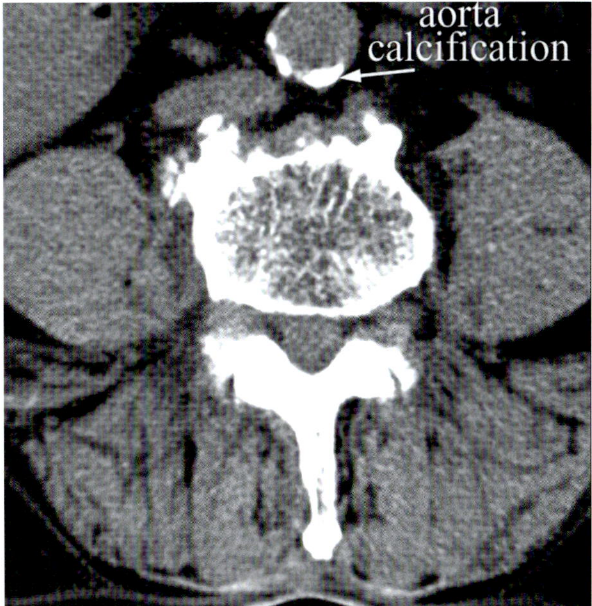

B

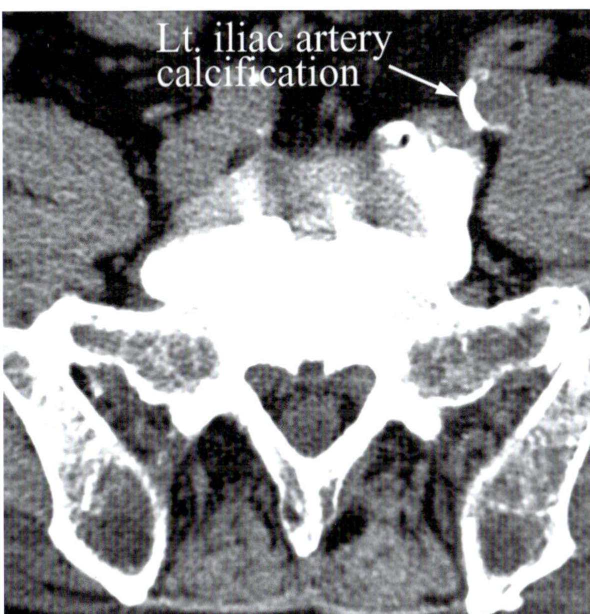

C

Figure 28–3 **(A)** Immediate postoperative angiographic computed tomography (CT) showing left common iliac artery obstruction. **(B)** Preoperative CT scans of the same patient showing aortic and **(C)** left common iliac artery calcification.

Arterial Obstruction

In our series of 620 TDR cases, only one arterial thromboembolism occurred. Although this is a rare complication of TDR, the result can be catastrophic if it occurs, with prompt diagnosis being the key to fixing the problem (**Fig. 28–3**). Intermittent intraoperative palpation of the iliac arterial pulse may be helpful, but it is not definite evidence of patent peripheral arterial blood flow. Intraoperative application of a pulse oximeter at the foot could prove effective.[4] Postoperative palpation of the dorsalis pedis artery pulse should be included in the routine checkup. In our thromboembolism case, the patient complained of severe leg pain, with a cyanotic cold sign of the left lower extremity an hour after the operation. A left iliac artery thromboembolism was diagnosed from the CT angiography, and an aortofemoral bypass graft was then performed, followed by an emergent thrombectomy within the "golden hour." A sensory deficit may be the only early sign of a progressive thrombotic arterial occlusion.[5]

The method of management is different according to the angiographic findings and the time interval for diagnosis. A simple thrombectomy with a Fogarty catheter through the femoral artery at the inguinal region, or an artificial bypass graft, can be considered. As with any complication, the best treatment is prevention. Various efforts to reduce arterial intimal damage are required. For example, gentle manual retraction is safer than early application of a retractor, with broad-based mobilization to prevent acute angled torsion or stretching of the iliac artery. The use of a self-retaining retractor system for periods longer than an hour should be avoided, but intermittent release of retraction is mandatory.[4,6]

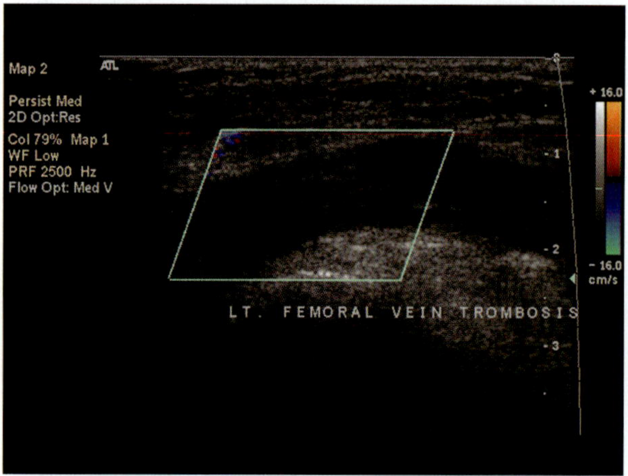

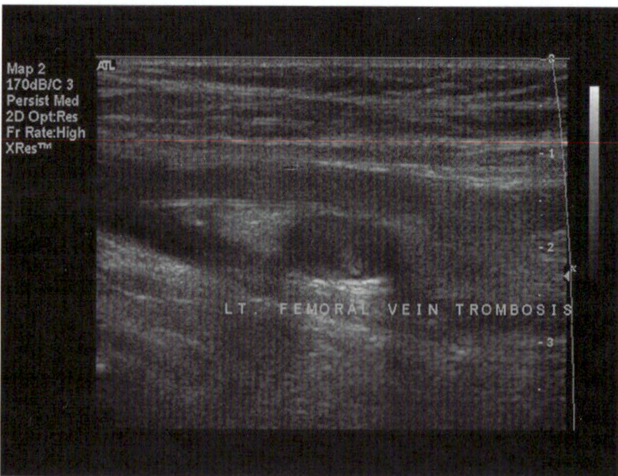

A   B

Figure 28–4   (A,B) Deep vein thrombosis after retroperitoneal approach.

Deep Venous Thrombosis

Prolonged retraction of large veins and venous injury have been considered risk factors for venous thrombosis. In the study by Baker et al,[7] however, a 15.6% incidence of venous injury translated into only a 0.9% incidence of deep venous thrombosis, and with no cases of pulmonary embolus in anterior lumbar surgery. Rajaraman et al[8] reported a 1.6% incidence of deep venous thrombosis, but no cases of pulmonary embolus in their 60 consecutive patients who underwent anterior lumbar interbody fusion (ALIF) using the transabdominal retroperitoneal approach performed by general surgeons.

Compression ultrasonography is the preferred initial diagnostic test when symptoms and signs suggest acute deep venous thrombosis, and a positive test confirms the diagnosis (**Fig. 28–4**). However, a negative compression ultrasound examination requires additional testing because a calf vein thrombosis can be overlooked. Venography or MR imaging could be helpful if serial compression ultrasonography cannot be performed or if iliac vein thrombi are suspected.

A minor embolism, when detected early, can be treated with combined heparin and warfarin anticoagulation therapy.[9] However, some patients need an IVC filter to prevent the development of a pulmonary embolism. Perioperative application of a compression elastic stocking, a preoperative low molecular heparin injection in selected patients with high risk factors, intermittent release of retractor, and minimal contusion and stretching techniques are all effective for prevention.[10]

In our large series of TDR, there were no cases of deep venous thrombosis or pulmonary embolism. We consider early ambulation after dynamic stabilization and active prophylaxis efforts beneficial.

◆ Other Approach-Related Complications

Visceral Complications

With retroperitoneal approaches, delicate handling of the peritoneum itself will ensure safety of containing the visceral contents; hence, visceral injury is extremely rare. During exposure, the peritoneum may accidentally open and should be repaired securely to prevent further visceral injury, such as a small bowel injury or postoperative bowel strangulation.

Although a benign and transient condition, postoperative paralytic ileus is the most frequently encountered problem, considered almost inevitable and a usual response to surgery. However, early mobilization and postoperative feeding, the use of prokinetic drugs, and balancing the use of opioid analgesics and nasogastric intubation in some severe patients are useful to reduce postoperative ileus.

Urogenital Complications

The ureter may be damaged during retroperitoneal exposure due to forceful sustained retraction or electrocautery. If the diagnosis is made during surgery, the injury can be sutured over a catheter by a urologist. However, if delayed, a large amount of retroperitoneal serous fluid collection is detected postoperatively. A concealed ureteral injury should be considered in such cases, although in most cases, lymphatic fluid collection should be suspected. For the differential diagnosis, an aspirated fluid analysis, including the creatine level, and a ureterogram, is needed in some rare cases. In our clinical experience of more than 5000 anterior retroperitoneal approaches, ureteral injury has not been encountered, with only two cases of delayed hydronephrosis (**Fig. 28–5**). These were managed with transient percutaneous nephrostomy drainage by the urologist. Delayed hydronephrosis can be caused by retroperitoneal fibrosis and stricture.[11] We suspect that a past history of either or both renal and ureteral stone is an underlying risk factor.

Retrograde ejaculation is a most frequent urogenital complication. In 1965, Sacks[12] originally described retrograde ejaculation as a consequence of anterior lumbar surgery. Since that report, the true incidence of these complications has been debated. A recent worldwide survey, conducted by Flynn and Price[13] of 20 surgeons who performed ~4500 anterior approaches to the spine revealed a remarkably low (0.42%) incidence of retrograde ejaculation and infertility. The incidence of retrograde ejaculation may be different

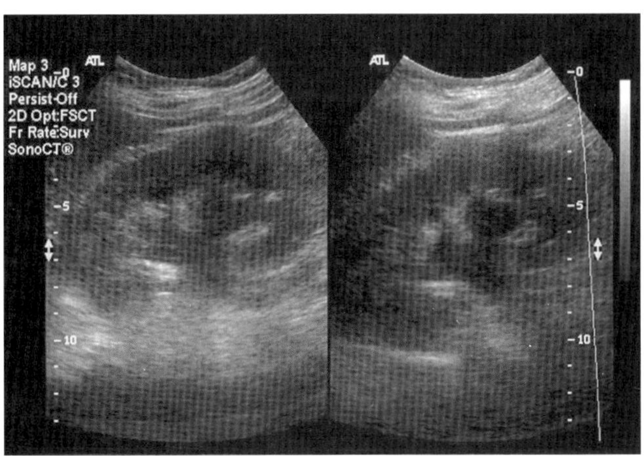

Figure 28–5   Left delayed hydronephrosis after retroperitoneal approach.

according to the proficiency of the surgical technique, with anatomical comprehension of hypogastric sympathetic plexus variants, direction of approach (left retroperitoneal, right retroperitoneal, or transperitoneal), level of operation (above L4–L5 or L5–S1), and method of study (retrospective or prospective).[14–17]

The principles of avoiding midline dissection, performing clip ligation of the middle sacral artery and vein, using blunt dissection when possible, and avoiding a second approach to the L5–S1 disk space are, however, uniformly emphasized.[13,18–21] The use of electrocautery should also be avoided in this area.[15]

No cases of retrograde ejaculation were seen in our series of TDR. We did not use a transperitoneal approach, but preferred a right retroperitoneal approach at the L5–S1 level, considering the possibility of a left retroperitoneal approach at the upper junctional level at a later stage. However, above the L4–L5 level, the anterior surface of the aortoiliac artery is not exposed more than lateral one third of its area to prevent injury of the prevascular hypogastric sympathetic plexus. At the L5–S1 level, we never violate the anterior prevertebral and prevascular soft tissue transversely or mobilize the whole structure to the contralateral side, with the exception of a vasculature at the approach side.

Peripheral Nerve Complications

The lumbar sympathetic chain lies along the medial margin of the psoas muscle attachment. Most commonly, patients who have unilateral sympathetic nerve injury complain that their contralateral foot is cold. In actual fact, it is the ipsilateral foot that is warm as the result of unopposed vasodilation of the parasympathetic fibers.[22] Although quite disconcerting, it is a clinically benign condition, and, typically, reassurance of the patient is all that is needed. However, routine evaluation of the distal pulses in the cold extremity is warranted to exclude the rare case of a vascular complication.[20] Partial sympathectomy at any level is not associated with erectile dysfunction or impotence in the majority of normal men. However, up to 50%

of patients with advanced peripheral vascular disease can develop erectile impotence after undergoing an extensive sympathectomy.[23] It is thought that the adverse effect of the peripheral blood flow is the underlying cause of this phenomenon.[5,14]

In our experience, the dissection plane of periaortic soft tissue is essential following blunt swap-out of the peritoneal content to the aorta and left common iliac artery lateral margin; sharp and blunt dissection is started just beside the aorta and periaortic lymphatic fat tissue, including sympathetic chain leaves to the left side under the retractor. In our opinion, the preservation of the lymphatic pathway and sympathetic nerve may prevent postoperative incomprehensible leg edema. Also, avoidance of monopolar cauterization is crucial in preventing iatrogenic sympathetic chain damage.

Additionally, the genitofemoral nerve, which lies on the anterior surface of the psoas muscle, can be damaged during retroperitoneal dissection. This can result in anterior medial thigh and inguinal pain or paresis postoperatively. Based on our clinical experience, we believe that gentle and careful dissection, retaining some retroperitoneal fat over the abdominal wall and psoas muscle, may prevent iatrogenic genitofemoral nerve damage and also decrease the degree of retroperitoneal fibrosis postoperatively.

Miscellaneous Wound Problems

Although immediate postoperative wound bulging, with sanguineous drainage, occurs in some cases, it can be detected early. The differential diagnoses include incisional hernia, hematoma under the rectus muscle, and retroperitoneal delayed fluid collection. Ultrasonography is useful, and is often enough for diagnosis, but an abdominal CT scan may be needed in some cases. Factors associated with the formation of an anterior rectus fascia defect include wound infection, morbid obesity, and previous operations. However, most immediate postoperative wound problems result from an inadequate suture technique. In addition to careful bleeding control, cautious closure and reapproximation of each individual layer with slowly absorbing sutures are crucial in preventing incisional hernias. An incisional hernia detected during the early postoperative period can be managed with primary repair, but in patients suffering from hernia with a large defect for an extended period after surgery, prosthetic polyethylene meshes might be required (**Fig. 28–6**). A hematoma under the abdominal muscle could have been caused by inferior hypogastric vessel bleeding or drain insertion site bleeding (**Fig. 28–7**).[24] The management plan varies according to the amount of bleeding and postoperative interval. Simple aspiration or reopening may be a chosen technique, but meticulous bleeding control should be made before wound closure. There are several potential incision methods with an anterior retroperitoneal approach, but we prefer a midline muscle-sparing incision, which is much less traumatic to the abdominal wall structure. This also provides good surgical vision, with low retractor tension, which may reduce visceral and vascular complications.

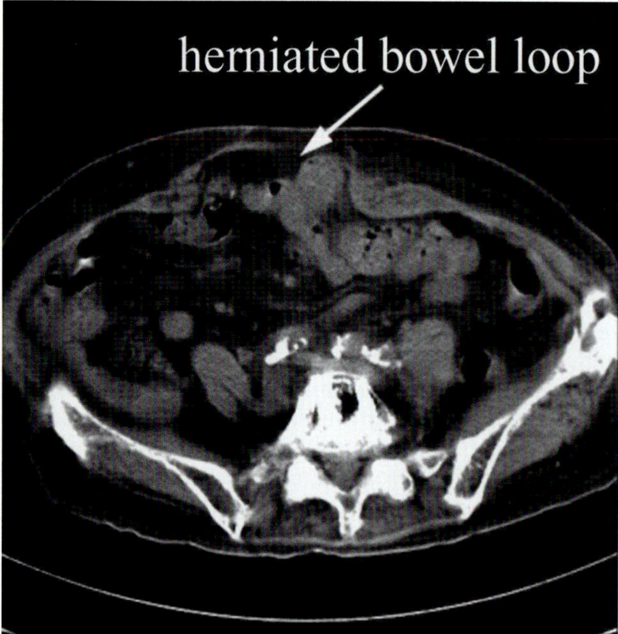

Figure 28–6 Anterior rectus fascia defect after retroperitoneal approach.

Figure 28–7 Hematoma under the abdominal muscle due to drain insertion site bleeding after retroperitoneal approach.

◆ Conclusion

Although collaborative surgery with a vascular surgeon is convenient, an anterior retroperitoneal approach for TDR is a safe procedure in the hands of an experienced spine surgeon. If one is not available, the emergency on-call system with multiple specialists such as vascular surgeons, general surgeons, and urologists can be activated for the management of vascular and surgical approach–related complications. To prevent and minimize approach-related complications, sufficient knowledge of anatomy and pathophysiology is essential.

References

1. Kleuver M, Oner FC, Jacobs WCH. Total disc replacement for chronic low back pain: background and a systemic review of the literature. Eur Spine J 2003;12:108–116

2. Lee SH. Minimally invasive spinal surgery: evolution and actual practice in Korea. Paper presented at: International Society for Minimal Intervention in Spinal Surgery; January 29, 2004; Zurich, Switzerland

3. Louis R. Chirurgie du rachis: anatomie chirurgicale et voies d'abord. New York: Springer-Verlag; 1982

4. Brau SA, Delamarter RB, Schiffman ML, Williams LA, Watkins RG. Vascular injury during anterior lumbar surgery. Spine J 2004;4:409–412

5. Khazim R, Boos N, Webb JK. Progressive thrombotic occlusion of the left common iliac artery after anterior lumbar interbody fusion. Eur Spine J 1998;7:239–241

6. Kulkarni SS, Lowery GL, Ross RE, Ravi Sankar K, Lykomitros V. Arterial complications following anterior lumbar interbody fusion: report of eight cases. Eur Spine J 2003;12:48–54

7. Baker JK, Reardon PR, Reardon MJ, Heggeness MH. Vascular injury in anterior lumbar surgery. Spine 1993;18:2227–2230

8. Rajaraman V, Vingan R, Roth P, Heary RF, Conklin L, Jacobs GB. Visceral and vascular complications resulting from anterior lumbar interbody fusion. J Neurosurg 1999;91(Suppl 1):60–64

9. Heit JA. Current management of acute symptomatic deep vein thrombosis. Am J Cardiovasc Drugs 2001;1:45–50

10. Rokito SE, Schwartz MC, Neuwirth MG. Deep vein thrombosis after major reconstructive spinal surgery. Spine 1996;21:853–859

11. Cleveland RH, Gilsanz V, Lebowitz RL, Wilkinson RH. Hydronephrosis from retroperitoneal fibrosis and anterior spinal fusion: a case report. J Bone Joint Surg Am 1978;60:996–997

12. Sacks S. Anterior interbody fusion of the lumbar spine. J Bone Joint Surg Br 1965;47:211–223

13. Flynn JC, Price CT. Sexual complications of anterior fusion of the lumbar spine. Spine 1984;9:489–492

14. Johnson RM, McGuire EJ. Urogenital complications of anterior approaches to the lumbar spine. Clin Orthop Relat Res 1981;154:114–118

15. Mirbaha MM. Anterior approach to the thoraco-lumbar junction of the spine by a retroperitoneal-extrapleural technique. Clin Orthop Relat Res 1973;91:41–47

16. Tropiano P, Huang RC, Girardi FP, Marnay T. Lumbar disc replacement: preliminary results with ProDisc II after a minimum follow-up period of 1 year. J Spinal Disord Tech 2003;4:362–368

17. Frymoyer JW. Indications for consideration of the artificial disc. In: Weinstein JN, ed. Clinical Efficacy and Outcome in the Diagnosis and Treatment of Low Back Pain. New York: Raven; 1992:227–236

18. McCormack B, Maher D, Fessler RG. Anterior approaches to the lumbar spine. In: Menezes AH, Sonntag VKH eds. Principles of Spinal Surgery. New York: McGraw-Hill; 1995:1293–1306

19. Sturgill M, Fessler RG, Woodward EJ. The lumbar and sacral spine. In: Benzel EC, ed. Spine Surgery: Techniques, Complication Avoidance, and Management. New York: Churchill Livingstone; 1999:169–191

20. Watkins R. Anterior lumbar interbody fusion surgical complications. Clin Orthop Relat Res 1992;284:47–53

21. Watkins R. Cervical, thoracic, and lumbar complications: anterior approach. In: Grafin SR, ed. Complications of Spine Surgery. Baltimore: Williams & Wilkins; 1989:211–247

22. Bell GR. Complications of lumbar spine surgery. In: Wiesel SW, and the Editorial Committee of the International Society for the Study of the Lumbar Spine, eds. The Lumbar Spine. Philadelphia: WB Saunders; 1996:945–969

23. Whitelaw GP, Smithwick RH. Some secondary effects of sympathectomy with particular reference to disturbance of sexual function. N Engl J Med 1951;245:121–122

24. Zeegers WS. Artificial disc replacement with the modular type SB Charite III: 2-year results in 50 prospectively studied patients. Eur Spine J 1999;8:210–217

29

Complications of Lumbar Disk Arthroplasty

Sang-Ho Lee and Chan Shik Shim

◆ **Early Complications**
    Subsidence
    Migration of Polyethylene Core
    Device Migration, Dislocation, or Subluxation
    Fracture of the Vertebral Body
    Postoperative Radiculopathy
    Persistent Back Pain
    Cerebrospinal Fluid Leakage and Root Injury
    Infection

◆ **Late Complications**
    Facet Arthrosis
    Polyethylene Wear and Osteolysis
    Heterotopic Ossification

◆ **Conclusion**

Recent successful clinical results of lumbar disk arthroplasty have provoked widespread enthusiasm. The early- and intermediate-term clinical results of total disk replacement (TDR) were promising.[1–15] Early results of prospective randomized studies comparing TDR with spinal arthrodesis have shown that TDR is doing as well or better than fusion.[16–20] But the complications of TDR reported so far are neither rare nor minor in their potential severity. The incidence of complications even with experienced surgeons are not negligible and it is expected that the incidence will increase if TDR is widespread and done by less experienced surgeons.[21] Furthermore, some of the reported complications are significantly dangerous and difficult to deal with.[22] Therefore, it is worth appreciating all of the reported complications in this early period of enthusiasm to be aware of the real advantages and disadvantages of lumbar TDR and to avoid complications, if possible, when it is adopted in one's own practice.

This chapter discusses the complications of lumbar disk arthroplasty that are not related to surgical approach.

◆ Early Complications

Subsidence

Subsidence of the prosthesis is one of the common complications of TDR. It is generally regarded as a late complication of disk arthroplasty and Cinotti et al[4] stated that subsidence occurred in patients who had an undersized prosthesis. In our series, however, subsidence occurred in the early postoperative period in relation to a fracture of the vertebral body (**Fig. 29–1**) or in patients with osteoporosis (**Fig. 29–2**).

Marked subsidence and the resultant change in the configuration of the prosthesis could make the polyethylene core extrude. Because the extruded core may damage the great vessels that lie in front of the vertebral column, the prosthesis should be removed when the subsidence is identified in the immediate postoperative period or the configuration of the prosthesis is distorted significantly. However, in cases where the subsidence is not significant, reinforcement of the vertebral body with polymethyl methacrylate (PMMA) can prevent further sinking of the prosthesis (**Fig. 29–2C**).

Technical error may be one cause of the subsidence. End plate preparation should be carefully done to make the plates of the prosthesis parallel because obliquity in the coronal plane may cause subsidence (**Fig. 29–2A**). The prosthesis should be positioned in the center of the coronal plane of the disk space to maintain the coronal balance of the spinal motion segment. Advanced segmental scoliosis preoperatively should be regarded as a relative contraindication of TDR because it is difficult to restore the scoliotic segment with an artificial disk. A patient with significant osteoporosis also should be excluded from TDR. In patients who have osteoporosis and refuse to accept fusion, augmentation of the vertebral body with PMMA may be a possible solution. There has been a successful report of concomitant augmentation of the vertebral body with PMMA in a patient with osteoporosis who underwent TDR,[23] but long-term data are needed to prove its long-term efficacy.

Delayed subsidence several years after the successful implantation of the prosthesis is another concern. When the vertebral body becomes osteoporotic as the patient ages, because of the discrepancy of the strength between bone and prosthesis, the prosthesis could subside. Although some investigators presumed that the porous-coated end plates (titanium and hydroxyapatite) would improve biological fixation of the metal plates to the vertebral bodies,[24] it is uncertain that it could prevent late subsidence of the prosthesis.

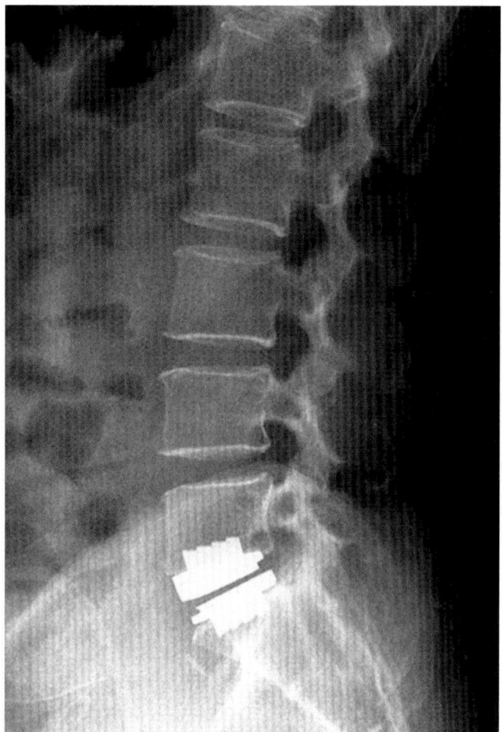
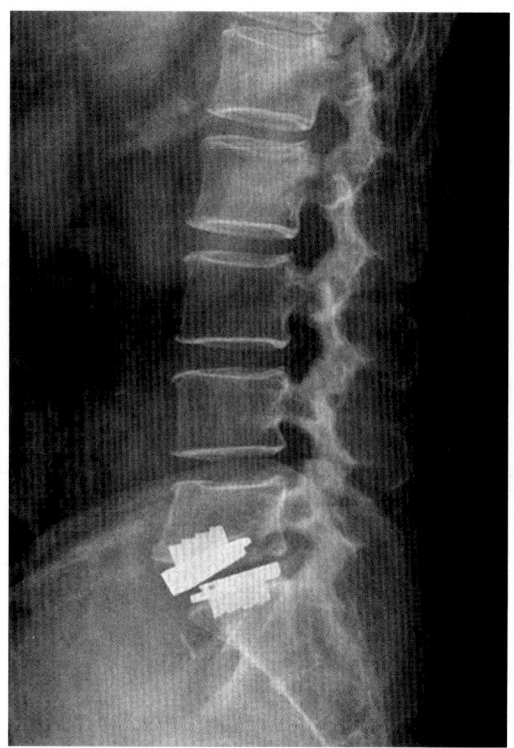

A

B

Figure 29–1   (A) Fifty-eight-year-old female. Lateral radiograph taken postoperative day 1 showed proper positioning of the implant. **(B)** On postoperative day 6, she felt severe back pain and radiography revealed subsidence of the implant with a transverse fracture of the L5 vertebral body. The prosthesis was removed and anterior lumbar interbody fusion was done. (Courtesy of Dr. Byung-Joon Kong.)

Migration of Polyethylene Core

There was a case of migration of the polyethylene core reported in the ProDisc series and it was attributed to technical fault.[19] With the SB Charité (DePuy Spine, Raynham, MA) it occurred at the L5–S1 level where there was a large lumbosacral angle and hyperlordosis with a large distance between the two vertebral end plates anteriorly and a narrow posterior disk space. In such a case, David[24] proposed to use the prosthesis with a more acute angle and place it more posteriorly. In our experience of 620 TDR cases, we have encountered one case of extrusion of the polyethylene core with resultant subluxation of the upper plate of the ProDisc (Synthes, Inc., West Chester, PA). In our opinion, the extrusion of the core is closely related to surgical technique. It is important to see that the core is securely positioned after the insertion. With the ProDisc, it is easy to see if the core is properly placed because the anterior margin of the core is at the same level of the device plates and it should not protrude over the edges of the plates of the prosthesis. With the SB Charité, it is better to confirm the position of the core with fluoroscopy because there is a metallic marker around the polyethylene core.

Device Migration, Dislocation, or Subluxation

Device migration or dislocations were reported in the study of previous models of the SB Charité (Charité I and Charité II)[7,25] but with the SB Charité III, the incidence of migration or subluxation has decreased.[4,5] With the ProDisc, though, there is no reported device migration or subluxation in the literature.[8,11,12] We experienced a case of device subluxation in our ProDisc series. One reason that the ProDisc showed no incidence of device migration or subluxation may be that it has a high keel on the plates that gives more solid fixation in the immediate postoperative period than does the SB Charité.

Fracture of the Vertebral Body

Fracture of the posterior corner of the vertebral body is a well-known complication of the SB Charité replacement (**Fig. 29–3**). The SB Charité has spikes on the anterior and posterior margin of the plates and these spikes can cause fracture of the posterior lips of the vertebral body during insertion of the prosthesis. It is better to prepare the posterior portion of the vertebral end plates adequately for smooth insertion of the prosthesis with a high-speed drill or a curette. It was also recommended that once the polyethylene core has been inserted, the prosthesis should not be hammered to be placed posteriorly.[24] If the fracture of the posterior lip of the vertebral end plate is identified immediately after the surgery and the patient has symptoms of neural compression, the bony fragment should be removed by either an anterior or a posterior approach. We prefer the posterior approach because it can allow removal of the bony fragment compressing the thecal sac and root without the need to manipulate the prosthesis.

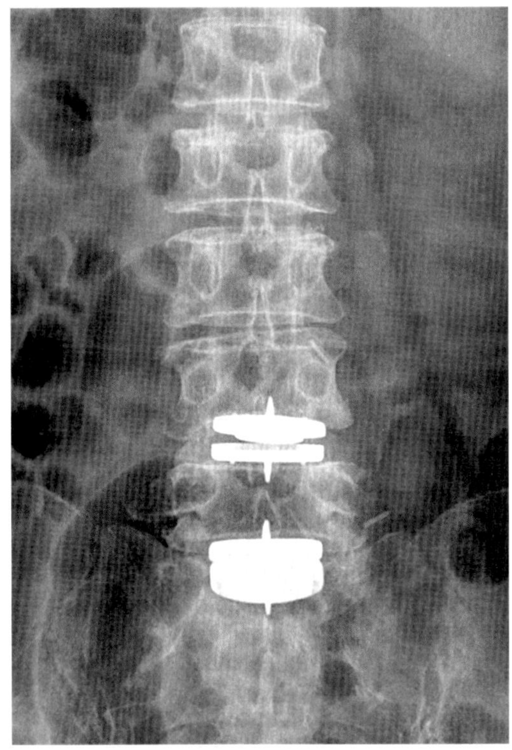
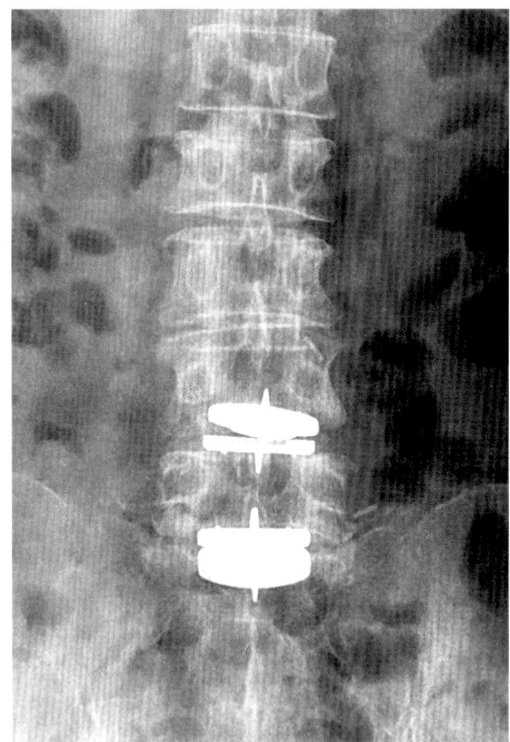
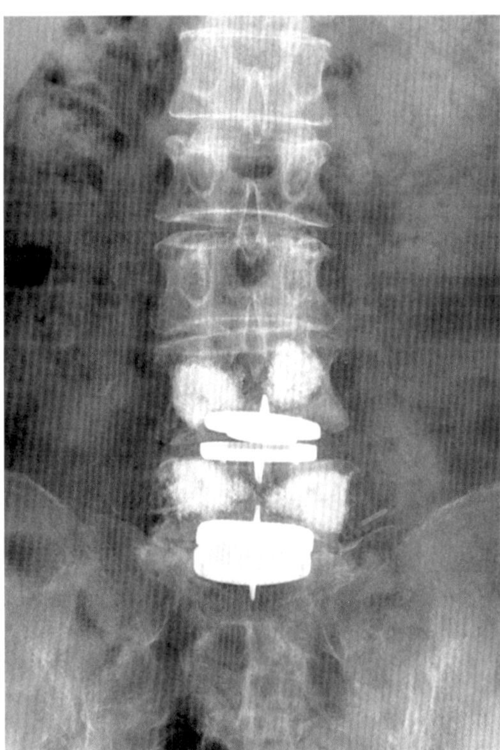

Figure 29–2 **(A)** Sixty-two-year-old female. The immediate postoperative anteroposterior plain radiograph showed unparallel plates of L4–L5 prosthesis. **(B)** The radiograph taken on postoperative day 4 showed the subsidence of the upper plate of the L4–L5 prosthesis into the L4 vertebral body. **(C)** Reinforcement of the vertebral body with polymethyl methacrylate was done to prevent further sinking of the prosthesis. (Courtesy of Dr. Won-Cheol Choi.)

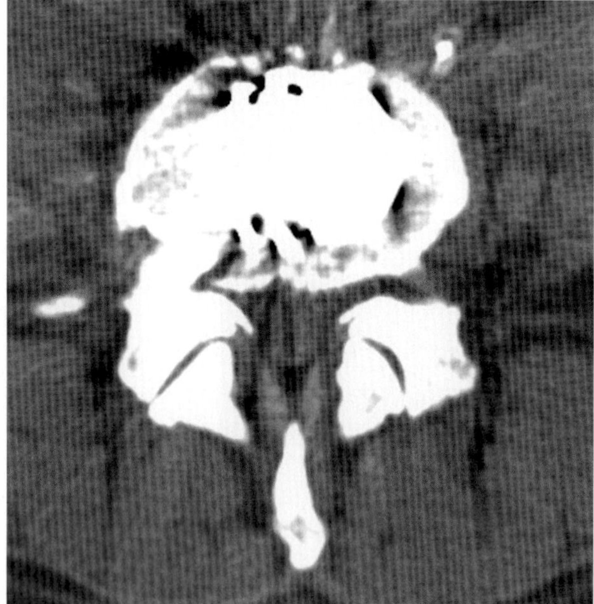

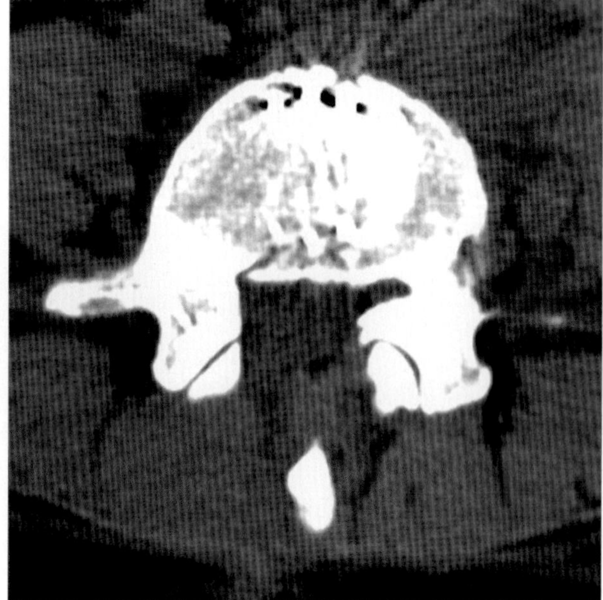

A   B

Figure 29–3   Thirty-two-year-old female. **(A)** Postoperative computed tomographic (CT) scan showed posterior lip of L5 upper end plate fracture. The patient had weakness of right big toe in dorsiflexion. The fractured fragment compressing the neural tissue was removed via a posterior approach. **(B)** CT scan taken after revision surgery showed removal of offending bony fragment. (Courtesy of Dr. Gun Choi.)

Vertical split fracture of the vertebral body after arthroplasty with the ProDisc has been reported (**Fig. 29–4**).[26] Because the ProDisc has a large keel on the plates, chiseling is needed to make grooves on the vertebral bodies for the insertion of the prosthesis. This step of the procedure can cause a vertical split fracture of the vertebral body. Therefore, care should be exercised during the chiseling of the bodies and insertion of the ProDisc, especially when it is implanted in a patient with small dimensions of the vertebral body, or when replacement is planned at multiple levels.

There were two cases of facet fracture after artificial disk replacement in patients who underwent previous laminectomy for disk herniation.[27] It was recommended that in a patient with a history of laminectomy, the extent of laminectomy and amount of facet remaining should be checked before the artificial disk replacement is planned.

Postoperative Radiculopathy

Some patients experience postoperative radicular pain that was not present before the surgery. In most cases, the cause

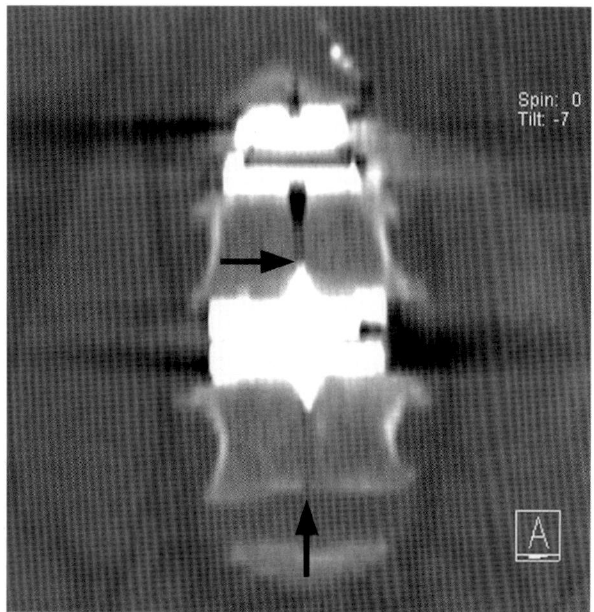

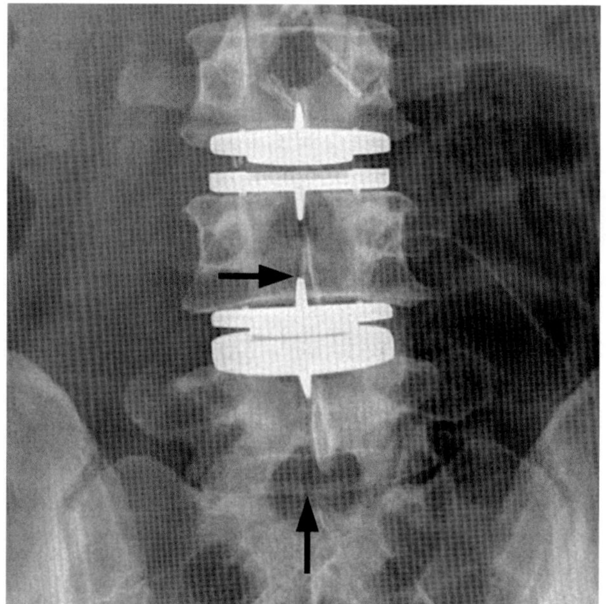

A   B

Figure 29–4   **(A)** Vertical split fracture of the vertebral body after ProDisc replacement. Plain radiograph showed vertical split fracture lines (arrows) at L4 and L5 vertebral bodies. **(B)** Coronal reformation of computed tomographic image showed the fracture lines (arrows).

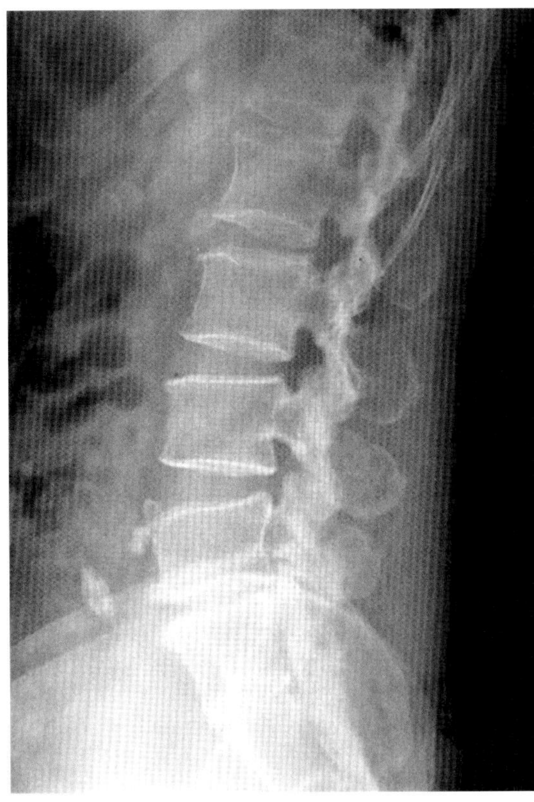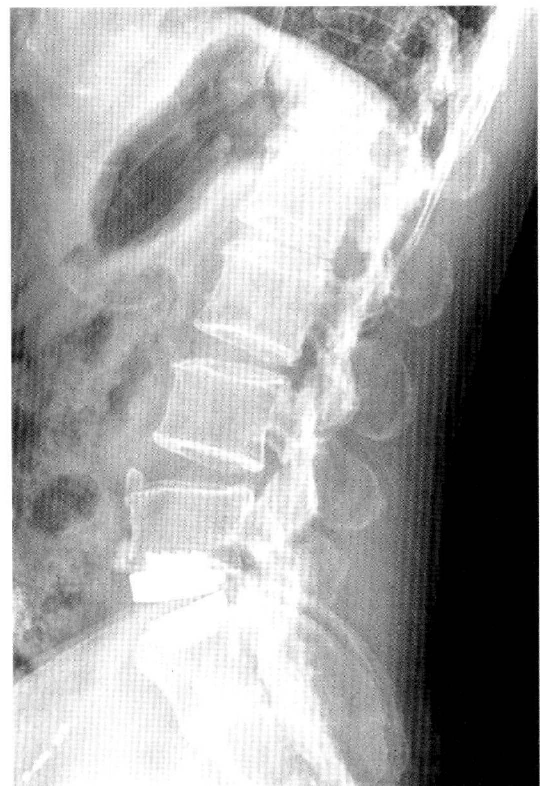

A   B

Figure 29–5   **(A)** Preoperative and **(B)** postoperative plain lateral radiographs of 44-year-old female. Note the marked postoperative increment of disk height of the operated level. The patient complained of severe postoperative back and right leg pain.

is unknown.[24] We consider the cause to be traction of the nerve root due to the overdistraction of the disk space in patients who already have decreased disk height due to degenerative disk disease for a prolonged period of time. The majority of the radiculopathy has been transitory, resolving within 3 months. But in cases with severe radicular pain, the device should be removed and replaced with a device of smaller height or a conversion to anterior lumbar interbody fusion.

Persistent Back Pain

Some patients complain of severe back pain in the immediate postoperative period, most of which is caused by the overdistraction of the disk space (**Fig. 29–5**). We encountered one patient with severe intolerable back pain in the recovery room. The patient was revised immediately, replacing the polyethylene core with a smaller one. If the postoperative back pain is significant immediately after surgery, the prosthesis should be removed or changed to a smaller one. But, because most of the patients who have had a disk replaced with an artificial disk prosthesis experience some kind of transitory, vague, and dull back pain in the immediate postoperative period, the revision surgery should be decided based on the severity of the pain and the patient's disability.

In the case of overdistraction there is no quantitative method with which to measure the distraction of the disk space. The proper size of the prosthesis is determined empirically by the surgeon according to the extent of

distraction of the disk space when it is distracted. The manuals of the surgical technique for both prostheses recommend choosing a device as big as possible to prevent the problems of device migration or extrusion of the polyethylene core. Therefore, there is a tendency to choose a prosthesis with maximal distraction of the disk space. We feel this tendency causes the problems of postoperative radicular pain or back pain caused by traction of the nerve root or distraction of the facet joints. Another problem is that devices currently available are too big for certain patients who are short in stature and have small vertebral body dimensions. It is inevitable that disk arthroplasty in those patients would cause overdistraction of the disk space.

Another type of persistent postoperative back pain is one caused by poor patient selection. TDR is not appropriate in a patient who already has significant facet arthropathy, and in fact may cause facet pain by distraction and mobilization of the already degenerated, hypertrophied, and immobile joint. In that case, disk arthroplasty should be withheld and spinal arthrodesis should be considered.

Cerebrospinal Fluid Leakage and Root Injury

Cerebrospinal fluid (CSF) leakage due to a dural tear can occur in patients who have undergone previous posterior surgery.[24] The tear of the dura in such a circumstance is difficult to repair. Usually, it can be managed with hemostatic sponges and fibrin glue. Root injury can occur when aggressive decompression of the neural foramen is attempted. We experienced a case of a partial avulsion injury of the L5 root during the removal of a concomitant foraminal disk herniation in a patient with degenerative disk disease, resulting in footdrop after the surgery. The patient eventually recovered from the footdrop, but the experience was painful. Care should be exercised not to damage an exiting nerve root when the neural foraminal area is decompressed from an anterior approach.

Infection

Infection after TDR is rare. There were no reported case of infection after TDR in the literature, and there was only one case of infection in our series. The patient underwent a hybrid type of disk replacement at L5–S1 in combination with posterior fusion at the above levels. The dorsal wound became infected and later the infection was disseminated into the L5–S1 space making the prosthesis loosen and subside. The revision was done via a transperitoneal route, removing the prosthesis and grafting an iliac bone strut after careful debridement.

If infection around the prosthesis occurs, conservative care with antibiotics is generally not recommended because the bulk of the implant hinders the antibiotics' ability to eradicate the infection.[28] Surgical treatment is indicated, but a concern arises about this revision surgery because removal of the implant can be life-threatening given the extensive scarring around the great vessels. As Santos et al[29] pointed out, although infection after disk arthroplasty per se has not been reported in the literature, a protocol to handle it needs to be put in place.

Another issue is prophylactic use of antibiotics in a medical procedure that can cause bacteremia after disk arthroplasty. After joint arthroplasty, medical procedures that cause bacteremia, such as dental work, require prophylactic antibiotics.[30] Although it is generally not recommended in spinal fusion, this will need consideration in spinal arthroplasty because once the prosthesis is infected via the hematogenous route the consequence can be disastrous.

◆ Late Complications

Facet Arthrosis

Van Ooij et al[22] reported 11 patients with facet arthrosis after TDR with the SB Charité prosthesis in a series of ~500 patients operated on at a single institution near their hospital. They performed posterior fusion on eight of the patients and found that facet joint hypertrophy reached huge dimensions. They postulated that the cause of the facet arthrosis was abnormal movement patterns of the segment containing the disk prosthesis. In the ProDisc series, there is no report addressing the issue of facet arthrosis. This is because the history of the ProDisc is shorter than that of the SB Charité, and facet arthrosis is a long-term complication. Link[31] described the biomechanics of disk prostheses and differences in impingement and stress on the facet joint in relation to movement of the core of the prosthesis. He theorized that the sliding core of the SB Charité prosthesis was biomechanically superior to the fixed core of the ProDisc in unloading the facet joint in flexion and extension of the lumbar motion

segment. Link's theory may be true in some respects, but long-term evidence is needed to confirm the superiority of the sliding core over the fixed core in preservation of the facet joint because there is also a concern that too much unloading and mobilizing of the facet joint can cause laxity of the facet capsule, which in turn causes hypertrophy of the facet joint. David[24] described bilateral symmetric facet arthritis in a patient whose prosthesis had been placed too far anteriorly. Anteriorly placed prostheses can cause marked movement of the facet joint in flexion and extension because the center of rotation locates much more anteriorly than the instantaneous axis of rotation of the normal motion segment. This case reinforces the concern that too much mobilization of the facet joint can cause late problems in that joint.

Polyethylene Wear and Osteolysis

Polyethylene wear was reported by van Ooij et al[22] in a patient with a prosthesis in situ for more than 13 years. However, there is no other report of polyethylene wear thus far in both the SB Charité and ProDisc series. Although the cobalt-chromium-molybdenum alloy was known to make less polyethylene wear debris,[32,33] the production of wear particles has not been completely prevented and many questions about wear debris from material other than polyethylene remain unanswered. Although there has been no other reported case of osteolysis or polyethylene wear in either the SB Charité or the ProDisc series, long-term results are needed to answer the question of wear debris.

Heterotopic Ossification

Heterotopic ossification in artificial disk replacement has been described by several authors.[4,5,7,24] McAfee et al[34] developed a classification of heterotopic ossification based on the classification of heterotopic ossification of the hip following total hip replacement. Heterotopic ossification after disk arthroplasty did not affect clinical outcome, however. There have been reports of spontaneous fusion after disk arthroplasty.[4] In our series, there are several cases in which the implanted segment showed no movement at all, although spontaneous fusion around the prosthesis has not been observed. Regardless of the clinical outcomes, those cases should be regarded as surgical failures because the preservation of motion is one of the major purposes of disk arthroplasty.

◆ Conclusion

Several complications in lumbar disk arthroplasty exist. Encouraged by the favorable early clinical outcomes and potential advantage of prevention of accelerated degeneration of the adjacent segment, TDR will be widely used in spinal practice. However, it is obvious that TDR will face more frequent complications when it is used widely by less experienced hands. Additionally, there is room for improvement of the device design and instruments. To reduce the complications of TDR in which treatment can sometimes be life threatening, the surgeon should be well informed about detailed surgical techniques and the deficiencies of each prosthesis and should stick to the most important principle for successful surgery—proper patient selection. It should be kept in mind that, with current technology, total disk replacement cannot completely replace spinal arthrodesis like total joint replacement has replaced joint arthrodesis in other fields of joint surgery.

References

1. Anderson PA, Rouleau JP. Intervertebral disc arthroplasty. Spine 2004; 29:2779–2786
2. Bertagnoli R, Kumar S. Indications for full prosthetic disc arthroplasty: a correlation of clinical outcome against a variety of indications. Eur Spine J 2002;11(Suppl):S131–S136
3. Blumenthal SL, Ohnmeiss DD, Guyer RD, Hochschuler SH. Prospective study evaluating total disc replacement: preliminary results. J Spinal Disord Tech 2003;16:450–454
4. Cinotti G, David T, Postacchini F. Results of disc prosthesis after a minimum follow-up period of 2 years. Spine 1996;21:995–1000
5. David T. The surgical and medical perioperative complications of lumbar "Charité" disc prosthesis: a review of 132 procedures. J Bone Joint Surg Br 1997;79:328
6. David TJ. Lumbar disc prosthesis: five-year follow-up study on 66 patients. J Bone Joint Surg Br 1999;81:252
7. Griffith SL, Shelokov AP, Buttner-Janz K, LeMaire JP, Zeegers WS. A multicenter retrospective study of the clinical results of the Link SB Charité intervertebral prosthesis: the initial European experience. Spine 1994;19:1842–1849
8. Guyer RD, Ohnmeiss DD. Intervertebral disc prosthesis. Spine 2003; 28:S15–S23
9. Hochschuler SH, Ohnmeiss DD, Guyer RD, Blumenthal SL. Artificial disc: preliminary results of a prospective study in the United States. Eur Spine J 2002;11(Suppl):S106–S110
10. Lemaire JP, Skalli W, Lavaste F, et al. Intervertebral disc prosthesis: results and prospects for the year 2000. Clin Orthop Relat Res 1997; 337:64–76
11. Marnay T. Lumbar disc replacement: 7- to 11-year results with ProDisc. Spine J 2002;2:94S
12. Mayer HM, Wiechert K, Korge A, Qose I. Minimally invasive total disc replacement: surgical technique and preliminary clinical results. Eur Spine J 2002;11(Suppl):S124–S130
13. Sott AH, Harrison DJ. Increasing age does not affect good outcome after lumbar disc replacement. Int Orthop 2000;24:50–53
14. Tropiano P, Huang RC, Girardi FP, Marnay T. Lumbar disc replacement: preliminary results with ProDisc II after a minimum follow-up period of 1 year. J Spinal Disord Tech 2003;16:362–368
15. Zeegers WS, Bohnen LMLJ, Laaper M, Verhaegen MG. Artificial disc replacement with the modular type SB Charité III: 2-year results in 50 prospectively studied patients. Eur Spine J 1999;8:210–217
16. Delamarter RB, Fribourg DM, Kanim LE, Bae H. ProDisc artificial total lumbar disc replacement: introduction and early clinical results from the United States clinical trial. Spine 2003;28:S167–S175
17. Guyer RD, McAfee PC, Hochschuler SH, et al. Prospective randomized study of the Charité artificial disc: data from two investigational centers. Spine J 2004;4:252S–259S
18. McAfee PC, Fedder IL, Saiedy S, Shucosky EM, Cunningham BW. SB Charité disc replacement: report of 60 prospective randomized cases in a United States center. J Spinal Disord Tech 2003;16:424–433
19. Zigler JE, Burd TA, Vialle EN, Sachs BL, Rashbaum RF, Ohnmeiss DD. Lumbar spine arthroplasty: early result using the ProDisc II: a prospective randomized trial of arthroplasty versus fusion. J Spinal Disord Tech 2003;16:352–361
20. Zigler JE. Lumbar spine arthroplasty using the ProDisc II. Spine J 2004; 4(Suppl 6):260S–267S
21. Polly DW. Adapting innovative motion-preserving technology to spinal surgical practice: what should we expect to happen? Spine 2003;28:S104–S109
22. van Ooij A, Oner FC, Verbout AJ. Complications of artificial disc replacement: a report of 27 patients with the SB Charité disc. J Spinal Disord Tech 2003;16:369–383
23. Kim WJ, Chang SB, Yoo KH, Lim ST, Lee SH. Prevention of artificial disc subsidence with intraoperative polymethylmethacrylate vertebroplasty in osteoporotic patients: 2-year result of a prospective study. Paper presented at: 2nd annual meeting of Korean Spine Arthroplasty Society, April 30, 2005, Seoul, Korea
24. David T. Complications with the SB Charité Artificial Disc. In: Buttner-Janz K, Hochschuler SH, McAfee PC, eds. The Artificial Disc. Berlin: Springer-Verlag; 2003
25. Gamradt SC, Wang JC. Contemporary concepts review: lumbar disc arthroplasty. Spine J 2005;5:95–103
26. Shim CS, Lee S, Maeng DH, Lee SH. Vertical split fracture of the vertebral body following total disc replacement using ProDisc. J Spinal Disord Tech 2005;18:465–469
27. Regan JJ, Bray R, Johnson P, Goldstein T, Anand N. Charité III artificial disc: evaluation of surgical complications in the early postoperative period. Paper presented at: 5th annual meeting of Spine Arthroplasty Society, May 5, 2005, New York, NY
28. Kostuik JP. Complications and surgical revision for failed disc arthroplasty. Spine J 2004;4(Suppl 6):289S–291S
29. Santos EG, Polly DW, Mehobod AA, Saleh KJ. Disc arthroplasty: lessons learned from total joint arthroplasty. Spine J 2004;4(Suppl 6): 182S–189S
30. Deacon JM, Pagliaro AJ, Zelicof SB, Horowitz HW. Prophylactic use of antibiotics for procedure after total joint replacement. J Bone Joint Surg Am 1996;78:1755–1770
31. Link HD. History, design and biomechanics of the LINK SB Charité artificial disc. Eur Spine J 2002;11(Suppl 2):S98–S105
32. Bono CM, Garfin SR. History and evolution of disc replacement. Spine J 2004;4:145S–150S
33. McAfee PC, Cunningham BC, Dmitriev A, et al. Cervical disc replacement: porous coated motion prosthesis: a comparative biomechanical analysis showing the key role of the posterior longitudinal ligament. Spine 2003;28:S176–S185
34. McAfee PC, Cunningham BW, Devine J, Williams E, Yu-Yahiro J. Classification of heterotopic ossification (HO) in artificial disc replacement. J Spinal Disord Tech 2003;16:384–389

Section III

Restoration of Lumbar Motion Segment
C. Dynamic Posterior Stabilization

30

Rationale for Dynamic Stabilization

Donal S. McNally

- **Modes of Action of Dynamic Posterior Stabilization Devices**
- **Modification of Neutral Angle and Disk Space Height**
- **Control of Sagittal Plane Bending**
- **Unloading of the Intervertebral Disk**
- **Modification of Motion of the Treated Segment**
- **Modification of the Distribution of Loads within a Segment**
- **Conclusions**

Dynamic posterior stabilization is now a popular form of surgical intervention employing a highly diverse range of devices. These devices are designed to relieve several different pathological conditions, including spinal stenosis and diskogenic pain, by fulfilling a range of biomechanical functions. The purpose of this chapter is not to describe individual devices in great detail or to evaluate their clinical effectiveness in different applications because this will be covered in subsequent chapters. The proposed biomechanical actions of these devices will be analyzed in generic terms so that the reader develops an understanding of the fundamental principles involved in their usage.

Simplistically, dynamic posterior stabilization devices have the potential for affecting the spine in several ways:

- Control of neutral posture of the segment. Many devices aim to modify the neutral angulation of the affected segment or to distract the disk space or both.
- Control of sagittal plane bending of the treated level. Most devices aim to prevent extremes of either or both flexion and extension without totally preventing such motion.
- "Unloading" of the intervertebral disk of the treated level. There is a hypothesis, discussed further later in this chapter, that diskogenic pain results from an overloading of the disk that can be prevented through surgical intervention. Several devices aim to share a proportion of the compressive load, hence reducing the magnitude of disk loading.
- Modification of the motion of the treated segment. The spinal motion segment is a mechanically complex structure; its response to applied bending moments arises from the sum of the effects of its component parts. Hence, any surgical intervention is going to change its behavior in bending. In particular, the effect of devices on the instantaneous center of rotation (ICR) of the segment will be discussed. More importantly, an insight into the functional/clinical relevance of the ICR will be introduced.
- Modification of the distribution of loads within the segment, and in particular within the intervertebral disk. It should be remembered that for all mechanical systems deformation and load are linked. If a device modifies how the segment deforms; for example, by changing the position of the ICR, this can have dramatic effects on the internal distribution of loads.

The extent to which a given device achieves any or all of the foregoing depends upon its design and mode of action and also on the mechanics of the segment that is treated.

Modes of Action of Dynamic Posterior Stabilization Devices

Posterior stabilization devices fall within two broad categories of design: interspinous process spacers and pedicle screw–based systems. Interspinous spacers have the potential to cause the segment to flex, distract the disk space, block extension, unload the disk, and subtly change loading and motion patterns in extension. Those that have additional tension bands, such as the Wallis Mechanical Normalization System (Abbott Spine, Inc., Austin, TX), also have the potential to limit flexion and modify flexional loading and motion patterns. Pedicle screw based–systems have the potential to modify the full range of segment behavior. The extent to which these potentials can be achieved is discussed in the remainder of this chapter.

◆ Modification of Neutral Angle and Disk Space Height

All posterior stabilization devices have the potential to increase the flexion or extension angle of the unloaded segment. The degree to which they do this, or indeed if they do it at all, depends on the size of the device relative to the separation of the pedicle screws or spinous processes. For example, if the spacer height of a Dynesys Dynamic Stabilization System (Zimmer Spine, Inc., Warsaw, IN) is greater than the separation of the pedicle screws in the neutral position, the segment will be forced into flexion, whereas if they are shorter it will be forced into extension. Tension band–only devices, such as the Graf Ligament System (Neoligaments, Leeds, U.K.), will force the segment into extension, the degree of angulation being dependent upon the tension in the ligament. This ability comes from the fact that the posteriorly positioned device can apply a bending moment to the segment. Motion segments have a highly nonlinear bending moment versus bending angle relationship where, close to the neutral position, small applied bending moments result in large, angular displacements (**Fig. 30–1**). It is therefore relatively easy for a device to apply a bending moment that is sufficient to alter the angulation of the segment.

It should be noted that in more complex devices such as the Dynesys, the relationship between spacer length and flexion-extension angle is complicated by the application of tension through the cord, which results in postimplantation deformation of the spacer. For example, application of the standard tension to the cord of a Dynesys device will result in a 2 mm shortening of the spacer. Such deformation must be taken into account if it is wished to control the flexion-extension angle of the segment using the device.

Study of **Fig. 30–1** indicates why it is very difficult to use a posterior stabilization device to change the neutral position disk height of a segment (i.e., to apply distraction). Clearly it is possible to apply many devices in such a way as

to apply a distractive force either to the spinous processes or the pedicles. Such a force is, however, applied posteriorly to the ICR of the segment and will therefore also apply a bending moment. This bending moment is greater for a given distractive force the more posteriorly the device is mounted. From **Fig. 30–1** we can see that from the neutral position (the origin of the graph) comparatively small moments are required to cause relatively large changes of angulation. However, the intervertebral disk is very stiff (~2 kN/mm) in the axial direction. Very large forces must therefore be applied to achieve small amounts of distraction. Hence, application of distraction forces using posterior stabilization devices will result in flexion rather than distraction.

The only circumstance under which this is not the case is if the stabilization device is itself very stiff to bending. It will then be able to apply an opposing bending moment to the segment that will prevent it from flexing. However, such rigid fixation devices by definition do not stabilize dynamically; they will prevent any form of bending to the segment.

It is possible for a device to prevent loss of disk height, particularly in extension. Consider, for example, the X-STOP Interspinous Process Decompression system (St. Francis Medical Technologies, Inc., Alameda, CA), which provides no rigidity in flexion, but which becomes very stiff in extension when the spinous processes come into contact with the titanium spacer. In this case the ICR will move posteriorly, attracted to the point of maximum stiffness (see later for a detailed explanation). The segment will then rotate about the device (**Fig. 30–2**) maintaining vertebral canal width and distracting the disk. This is an example of a device with low stiffness in some situations (allowing motion) and high stiffness in others (preventing motion).

◆ Control of Sagittal Plane Bending

Control of sagittal plane bending has been the primary design criterion for the majority of dynamic stabilization devices. The degree to which they achieve this, and under what circumstances, is more fully described in the device-specific chapters. The fundamental principles by which they operate is discussed in this chapter.

Control of sagittal plane bending really means that additional bending stiffness is created by the device at some point in flexion-extension of the segment. This additional stiffness comes directly for the device or by modifying the geometry of the segment (particularly the position of the ICR) so that it becomes stiffer in bending. Illustrative examples are given following here.

Consider the case of a Graf ligament in flexion (**Fig. 30–2A,B**). In this case the device resists bending by adding a bending moment through the action of the ligament directly. The tension in the ligament material acts on the motion segment to create a bending moment acting in the extension direction (thereby reducing the overall flexion moment applied to the segment). In common with all posterior devices, such limiting of flexion results in increased compressive

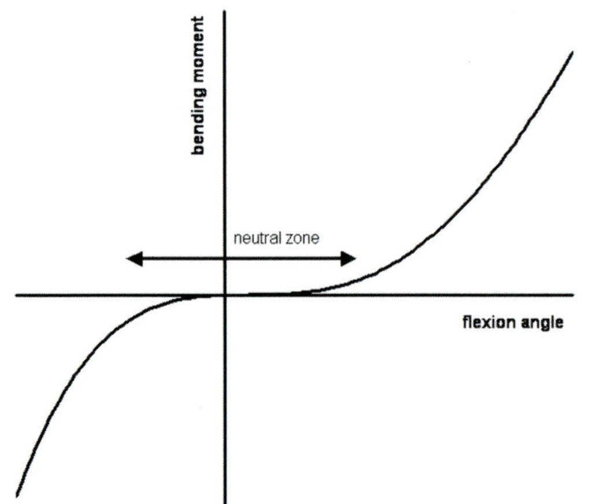

Figure 30–1 A typical bending moment versus flexion angle for a motion segment. Note the neutral zone where small changes in bending moment result in large changes of angle.

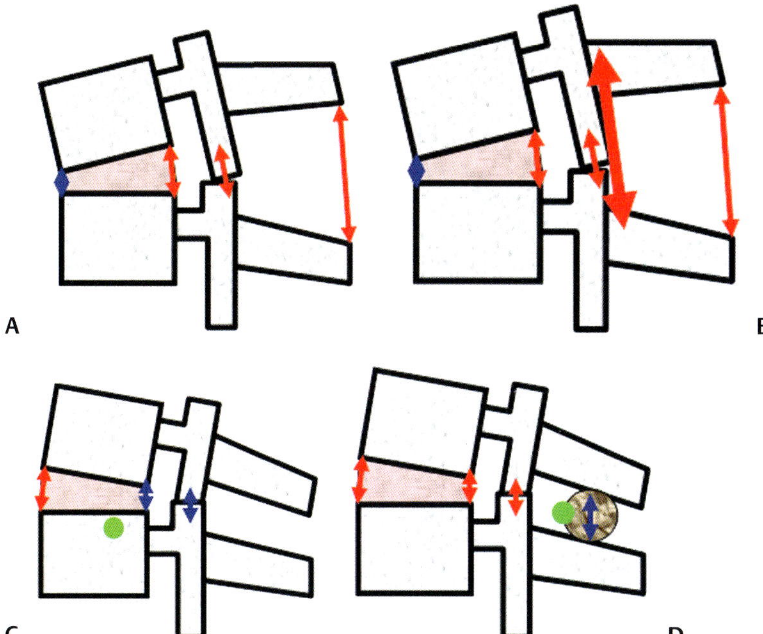

Figure 30–2   The effects of different stabilization devices on distribution of bending moments. Red and blue arrows represent tensile and compressive forces, respectively, and the green dots represent the location of the instantaneous center of rotation (ICR). **(A)** The uninstrumented flexed segment has flexion resisted by compression of the anterior annulus and tension in the posterior annulus, facet capsule, and interspinous ligaments. **(B)** The Graf stabilized segment has an additional moment resisting bending from tension in the ligament. **(C)** The uninstrumented segment has extension resisted by tension in the anterior annulus and compression in the posterior annulus and facet joints. **(D)** The X STOP stabilized segment has its ICR shifted posteriorly toward the device resulting in extension being resisted by tension in the anterior and posterior annulus and facet joints and to a lesser extent compression at the device itself (due to the small distance from the ICR).

loading of the segment as a whole because of the contribution of the tensile force in the ligament.

A slightly different mechanism is employed by the X STOP in extension (**Fig. 30–2D**). In this case, the spinous processes contact the titanium spacer, which is very stiff in compression. This high stiffness results in a posterior shift of the IRC from anterior of the posterior annulus. With the center of rotation in its new location, the anterior and posterior annuli are now in tension (and applying a large moment due to the greater distance from the IRC). The device itself carries a compressive load posterior to the ICR and hence contributes a moment that opposes extension. This moment may be small, however, because, although the force is large, its point of action is close to the center of rotation.

It should be noted that many of these devices, including the Graf ligament and Dynesys, are sensitive to variation in disk space height. Because this can be reduced by compressive loading (and even creep through sustained loading) it is important to evaluate the bending properties of the device under a realistic compressive load. If this is not done, the resistance to the bending of the device might be overestimated.

◆ Unloading of the Intervertebral Disk

An often-cited aim of dynamic posterior stabilization is to unload the intervertebral disk. Such unloading can only take place if the load is transferred to the device itself. Were this to happen there are significant implications for the long-term success of the implant—stand-alone instrumented fusions posterior are know to loosen and fail if solid bony fusion does not take place. However, it is unlikely that the device will carry significant loads for the following reason:

A simplistic model of the motion segment and device is that of two springs in parallel as shown in **Fig. 30–3**. For this

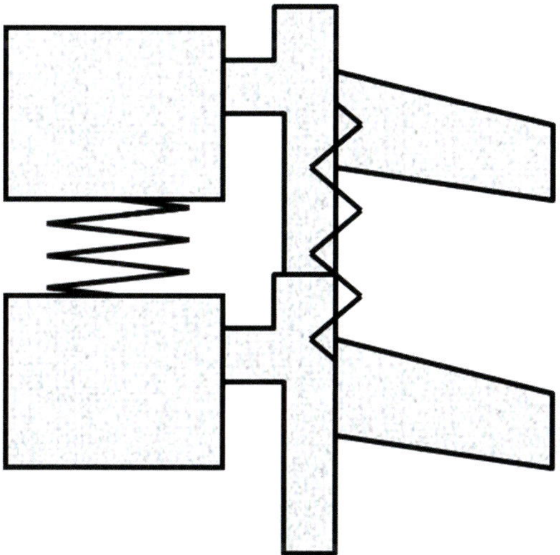

Figure 30–3   The disk and implant can be thought of as springs in parallel.

arrangement of springs it can be shown that the proportion of load, $\frac{F_{disk}}{F_{total}}$ and $\frac{F_{implant}}{F_{total}}$, taken by the disk and implant, respectively, are functions of their respective stiffness, s_{disk} and $s_{implant}$. Stiffness is the load acting on a spring divided by its change in length. The stiffer the spring, the less it deforms. In the case of implant stiffness, this includes not only the deformation of the implant (including any pedicle screws) but also the implant vertebral body interface (including the spinous process and pedicle).

$$\frac{F_{dics}}{F_{total}} = \frac{s_{dics}}{s_{dics} + s_{implant}}$$

$$\frac{F_{implant}}{F_{total}} = \frac{s_{implant}}{s_{dics} + s_{implant}}$$

These proportional loads can be plotted as functions of relative stiffness of the implant (**Fig. 30–4**). It can be seen that even when the implant and the disk have equal stiffness, the load carried by the disk is only reduced by 50%. An implant that has 10% of the stiffness of the disk will carry only 10% of the load.

Intervertebral disks are extremely stiff in compression—most implants are not. This theoretical explanation is backed up by experimental quantification of intervertebral disk and fixator loads in vitro[1] and in vivo[2] where rigid stainless steel posterior fixators have been shown to provide negligible unloading of disks and carry comparatively small axial loads. A biomechanical study has demonstrated the off-loading effects of a posterior stabilization device[3]; however, this used neoprene rubber as a model for the disk that is not as stiff in compression. This is an illustration of the beauty of the "design" of a natural disk, in that it can be very stiff in compression and very compliant in flexion-extension in a way that a block of a single material cannot.

Posterior dynamic stabilization devices should therefore not be considered to have a primary role in unloading the intervertebral disk. However, this is not to say that they

cannot have a profound effect on the loading of particular regions of the disk (see Modification of the Distribution of Loads within a Segment).

◆ Modification of Motion of the Treated Segment

A previous section has described how stabilization devices can modify the overall flexion-extension characteristics of the segment. This section discusses the effect that the device has on local regions of the disk. Unfortunately, the variability of devices, surgical usage, and most importantly the characteristics of intervertebral disks themselves prevents detailed generalized conclusions from being drawn; however, this section explains the important basic principles that can be applied to any device.

An important concept to understand is the ICR. Any structure, no matter how complex, has a point at which if a load is applied no bending will occur. This is the ICR. Similarly, if the load is offset slightly from the ICR a bending rotation will occur that is centered on the ICR. This is important in identifying which structures will be stretched and which compressed when a segment is placed in extension or compression.

For example, **Fig. 30–5A** shows the relative motions of two vertebrae on extension when the ICR is located at the green dot, whereas **Fig. 30–5B** shows the same motions when the ICR is moved posteriorly. Clearly, in this example the posterior annulus changes its loading from compression to tension. Indeed, it is this mechanism that the X STOP employs to reduce spinal stenosis on extension. The location of the ICR is therefore very important in predicting the deformation of particular structures such as the annulus and facet capsules.

Unfortunately, prediction of the position of the ICR in structures that are as complex as vertebral motion segments is not easy. Generally, the position of the ICR in the sagittal plane of a healthy motion segment is posterior of the center of the disk and just below the superior end plate of the inferior vertebra. It does tend to move slightly both in the anterior-posterior and superior-inferior directions during flexion and extension. In disk degeneration and particularly when there are degenerative changes of the facet joints, there is considerable variability in both mean location and motion of the ICR.

There is a simple rule that can be used to predict the effect of a stabilization device on the location of the ICR. Put basically, the ICR will move toward an increase in stiffness. Hence, a rigid interspinous spacer will move the ICR posteriorly (**Fig. 30–5B**) in extension but not in flexion, whereas a tension band ligament will do the same thing on flexion.

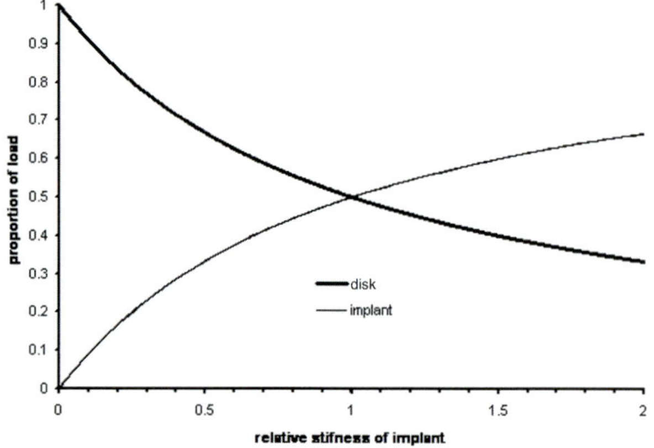

Figure 30–4 The proportion of load taken by the disk and implant as a function of the relative stiffness of the implant.

◆ Modification of the Distribution of Loads within a Segment

Previous sections discussed how, in most cases, it is unlikely that the application of a posterior stabilization will result in a significant overall unloading of the intervertebral disk. It has also been demonstrated that should such a device limit

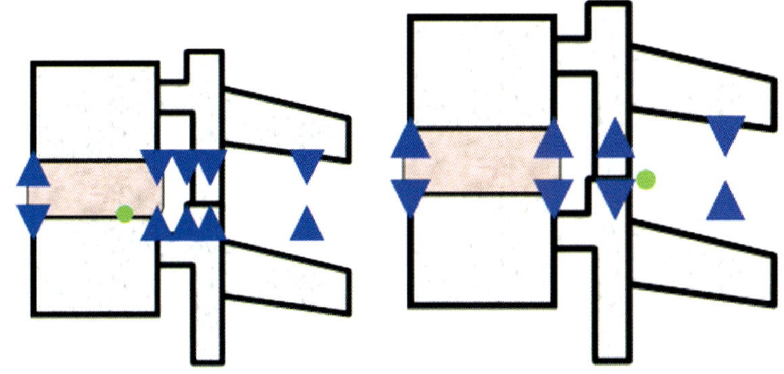

Figure 30–5   **(A,B)** Relative motion of two adjacent vertebrae on extension about different ICRs (green dots).

the amount of flexion of the segment resulting from the application of a particular bending moment, it will increase the overall compressive loading of the segment. However, it has also been shown that changes in the location of the ICR will change the deformation of local areas of tissue such as the posterior annulus and facet capsule. It can therefore be predicted that the distribution of loading within the segment may be modified. The same rule for the effect of such ICR movement as already described can be applied to predict qualitatively the effects of a device on tissue loading. However, experimental investigation (or very complex and well-validated finite element modeling) is the only method by which such changes can be quantified. Unfortunately, there is a paucity of such investigation in the literature.

We performed such an experiment using the standard technique of stress profilometry.[4] A small, needle-mounted pressure transducer[5] was drawn through the disk so that a record of internal stress with position could be made. A posterior dynamic stabilization device (Dynesys) was applied to the segment with different spacer lengths (neutral and ±2 mm). It should be noted that spacer length was taken from the space between the pedicle screws in the neutral posture and that the spacers compressed when the cord was tightened. The true spacer lengths were therefore neutral, 2 mm extension, and 4 mm extension.

We found that the effects of the device varied between disks, and in particular were dependent upon the state of degeneration of the disk.[6] This is not surprising because degeneration will reduce the stiffness of the disk and therefore the contribution of the device will be greater. In general, the device had very little effect on nondegenerate disks (**Fig. 30–6A**), whereas the distribution of load was changed in more degenerate disks (**Fig. 30–6B**). In such cases the device increased the loading in the posterior annulus (recall that the configuration was such to place the segment into extension), did not change the load within the nucleus, and decreased stress peaks in the anterior annulus. It can therefore be seen that, although the overall loading of the disk was not changed significantly, the distribution of that load was shifted posteriorly. This is consistent with both the application of a small amount of flexion and a posterior movement of the ICR toward the device.

Similarly, it has been shown that interspinous spacers, such as the X STOP, have the ability to change the mechanical environment of the facet joints.[7] Again, this is consistent with the device, which is stiff in extension, attracting the

ICR, with the result that the facet joints are opened by extension rather than closed.

◆ Conclusions

Posterior dynamic stabilization devices have a rich potential to modify the mechanical behavior of the treated segment. They can change the neutral posture of the segment, control its range of motion, and change both the loading and the deformation of individual regions of the segment.

In their current forms, they do not have the ability to significantly "off load" the segment because they must be sited away from the center of rotation of the segment and be relatively less stiff. They may, however, lead to additional loading of the segment. Posteriorly mounted devices that limit flexion will impose additional loads during flexion. Tension band–type devices that do not have a spacer component will also load the segment simply through the tension in the band. Stiff, interspinous devices will lead to a reduction of loading in the anterior structure of the segment on extension. However, they will also lead to high compressive loads in the spinous processes.

The question is still open as to whether increased loading of the disk is actually a bad thing. Obviously, when taken to extremes, any structure can be overloaded and will fail. However, intervertebral disks are well designed to function under high compressive loads. For example, compressive overload of a segment will invariably lead to failure of the adjacent vertebra before that of the disk.[8] Similarly, when disk loads have been measured in vivo,[9] the magnitude of the load was unrelated to the results of provocative diskography. It is often cited that low back pain is aggravated by activity that causes high loading of the spine. However, such activities normally involve large muscle forces as well. It could well be that the muscles are the source of pain.

There is a clear application for interspinous devices in the prevention of spinal stenosis on extension. They will prevent such extension movements and will move the ICR posteriorly so that the disk space opens up rather than closes down.

The use of posterior dynamic stabilization as a treatment for diskogenic pain is rather less clear-cut. It is conceivable, if the source of pain is known, to design a stabilization device that will modify the deformation or loading of the pain source. This may well be the mechanism by which a range of such devices achieves favorable outcomes. However, it is the

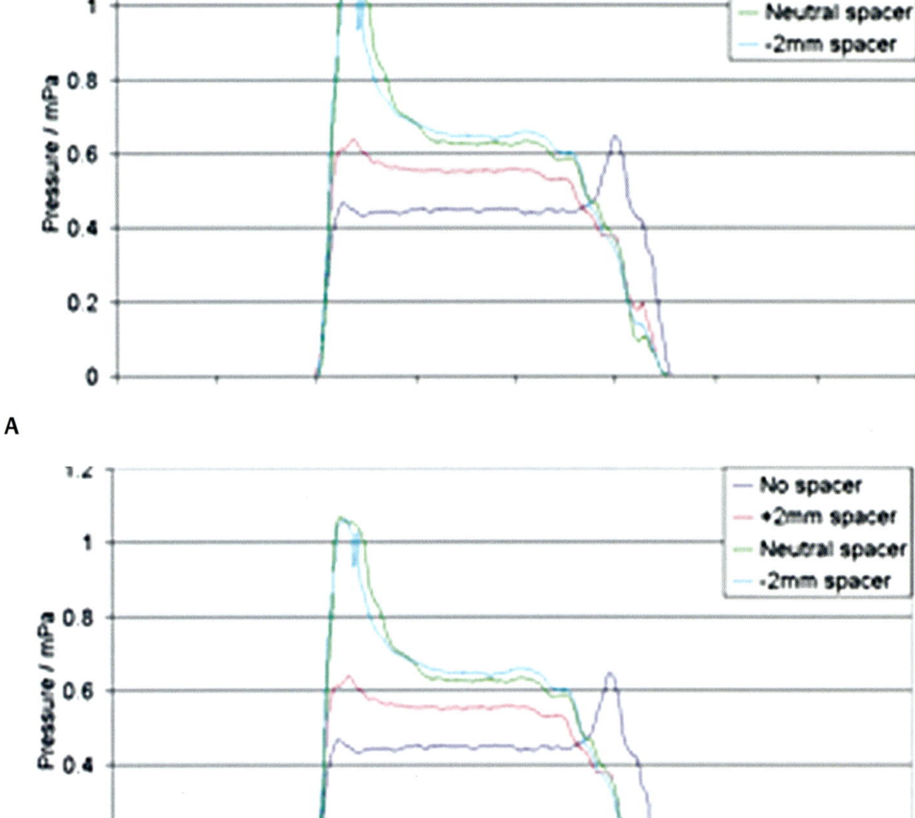

Figure 30–6   Distribution of load within a **(A)** nondegenerate and **(B)** moderately degenerate intervertebral disk and the effects of applying a Dynesys device with different spacer lengths (left = posterior, right = anterior).

author's opinion that present diagnostic techniques are not currently sufficient to identify such regions of tissue, and our understanding of pain etiology is insufficient to predict the most appropriate change. For dynamic stabilization techniques to be truly successful both these deficiencies need to be addressed so that treatment can be tailored to the specific pathology of an individual.

It is possible to illustrate how such treatment might be effective. For example, one possible mechanism for diskogenic pain is inward bulging of the posterior annulus. Some degenerate disks that will reproduce pain on diskography have been shown to have a depressurized nucleus that results in an inward rather than outward bulging of the posterior annulus.[9] This may well be painful in itself because the inner annulus bulges inward while the outer annulus bulges outward. Hence, somewhere in the annulus there will be a point where the deformation is pulling the lamellae apart. Indeed, circumferential lesions are often seen in degenerate disks in precisely this location. It is know that the peripheral annulus is innervated[10,11] as is the vertebral end plate into which the annulus fibers insert. It is therefore quite possible to expect such loading to result in a painful stimulus.

So how could a dynamic stabilization device be used to prevent internal bulging of the posterior annulus? Current devices would be very useful were such bulging a problem only on extension. Interspinous spacers, or rigidly spaced pedicle screw devices, will move the ICR posteriorly outside of the disk resulting in the posterior annulus being placed in tension on extension and therefore will reduce any bulging. If, however, the bulging was a problem in the neutral position, stabilization devices offer fewer possibilities for correction. The best that could be hoped for would be a pedicle screw/rigid spacer device mounted as anteriorly as possible with as long a spacer as possible. In this case the segment may be forced into flexion; however, the posterior annulus would be kept as distracted as possible. There may even be more unloading possible than is typically the case because such inward bulging tends to occur in "depressurized" low-stiffness disks.

It is therefore evident that there is a continuing potential for dynamic stabilization devices to have a role in the treatment of several pathologies. They have a unique ability to be customizable to the requirements of a particular patient. However, results will continue to be disappointing until better diagnostic techniques and understanding of pain production mechanisms are achieved.

References

1. Edwards AG, McNally DS, Mulholland RC, Goodship AE. The effects of posterior fixation on internal intervertebral disc mechanics. J Bone Joint Surg Br 1997;79:154–160

2. Rohlmannt A, Claes LE, Bergmannt G, Graichen F, Neef P, Wilke HJ. Comparison of intradiscal pressures and spinal fixator loads for different body positions and exercises. Ergonomics 2001;44:781–794

3. Sengupta DK, Mulholland RC. Fulcrum assisted soft stabilization system: a new concept in the surgical treatment of degenerative low back pain. Spine 2005;30:1019–1029 discussion 1030

4. McNally DS, Adams MA, Goodship AE. Measurement of stress distribution within intact loaded intervertebral discs. In: Little EG, ed. Experimental Mechanics: Technology Transfer between High Tech Engineering and Biomechanics. Amsterdam: Elsevier Science; 1992: 139–150

5. McNally DS, Adams MA, Goodship AE. Development and validation of a new transducer for intradiscal pressure measurement. J Biomed Eng 1992;14:495–498

6. Aylott CEW, Mckinlay KJ, Freeman BJC, Sheperd J, McNally DS. In-vitro Biomechanical Effects of DYNESYS (Dynamic Neutralisation System for the Spine). Proceedings of SpineWeek 2004 (SSE). Porto, Portugal: 2004:747

7. Wiseman CM, Lindsey DP, Fredrick AD, Yerby SA. The effect of an interspinous process implant on facet loading during extension. Spine 2005;30:903–907

8. Adams MA, McNally DS, Chinn H, Dolan P. Posture and the compressive strength of the lumbar spine. Clinical Biomechanics 1994;9:5–14

9. McNally DS, Shackleford IM, Goodship AE, Mulholland RC. In-vivo stress measurement can predict pain on discography. Spine 1996;21: 2580–2587

10. Jackson H, Winkelman R, Bichel W. Nerve endings in the human lumbar spinal column and related structures. J Bone Joint Surg Am 1966;48:1272–1280

11. Wiberg G. Back pain in relation to the nerve supply of the intervertebral disc. Acta Orthop Scand 1949;19:211–221

31

Rationale for Dynamic Stabilization II—SoftFlex System

Dilip K. Sengupta

◆ **Instability**

◆ **The Requirements of a Dynamic Stabilization System**

◆ **SoftFlex Flexible Rod System**

◆ **Surgical Technique**

◆ **Clinical Results**

◆ **Conclusion**

The concept of nonfusion and motion preservation has generated considerable clinical interest in the surgical treatment of chronic low back pain in recent years. Fusion has been the mainstay of surgical treatment in the last 3 decades, and the common experience is that, although fusion works for many patients with back pain, a successful fusion does not guarantee a successful clinical outcome with pain relief. Even if it works, most surgeons believe that successful fusion may increase the incidence of, or at least accentuate, adjacent segment disease.[1,2] Prosthetic disk or nucleus replacements are attractive alternatives, but these are not applicable in the presence of significant facet arthrosis and instability of the motion segment.[3,4] All these factors have raised the demand for a dynamic stabilization system to restore stability in an unstable, painful motion segment, to protect an adjacent segment from previous or concomitant fusion, or to salvage a failed disk or nucleus prosthesis without losing motion.

◆ Instability

In degenerative lumbar spine disorder, "instability" as a cause of chronic low back pain is not well understood. Degeneration in the lumbar spine often results in decreased range of motion (ROM).[5] Most authors describe spinal instability as an abnormal motion.[6–9] However, it is not an increase in the quantity of abnormal motion but in the abnormal quality of motion that characterizes spinal instability.[6,10–12] Mulholland and Sengupta[13] hypothesized that the mechanism of pain production related to the instability is in fact abnormal load transmission; the abnormal motion leads to an abnormal distribution of load across the vertebral end plate, which is pain sensitive. The aim for motion preservation by dynamic stabilization is therefore to permit normal motion as much as possible but to limit any abnormal motion, and more importantly to unload or to uniformly load the disk and prevent any large spikes of spot loading at any stage throughout the ROM.

◆ The Requirements of a Dynamic Stabilization System

Even such a well-defined goal of dynamic stabilization may not be adequate to understand exactly what is needed from dynamic stabilization unless the abnormal quality of motion is defined or can be determined. The characteristics of quality of motion that can be determined in the laboratory are ROM in each individual direction (like flexion, extension, etc.), neutral zone (NZ) motion, stiffness [load-deformation (L-D) curve], and instantaneous axis of rotation (IAR). The ROM, NZ motion, and L-D curve are easy to determine in the laboratory, whereas IAR is difficult to determine and not easily reproducible. A more practical alternative is to determine a continuous pressure tracing in the center of the disk during motion, measurement of which is more precise and reproducible. Although the pressure profile does not indicate the location of the IAR, it is a sensitive parameter, which may sharply reflect any abnormal load transmission through the disk as a result of an abnormal IAR or quality of motion during the ROM.

The biomechanical requirements of an ideal dynamic stabilization system may be summarized as follows:

1. Preserve motion and prevent any abnormal motion
2. Unload the disk and prevent any abnormal load distribution throughout the ROM

The clinical requirements of an ideal dynamic stabilization device include:

1. Minimally invasive surgical insertion
2. Survive fatigue failure

3. Maintain normal resting posture of the spine—no excessive kyphosis or lordosis

4. Easy salvage (e.g., conversion to fusion in case of failure)

A classification of the various dynamic stabilization systems has been described by the author.[14] All dynamic stabilization devices restrict motion. Some of them restrict motion unevenly (e.g., one may restrict predominantly flexion, whereas others restrict extension permitting a relatively free motion in the opposite direction). Some devices alter the resting posture of the lumbar spine. The Graf ligament (SEM Sarl, Montroge, France) device locks the spine in extension, spinous process distraction devices cause flexion, and the Dynesys Dynamic Stabilization System (DSS) (Zimmer Spine, Inc., Warsaw, IN) produces loss of lordosis or flexion depending on the degree of distraction between the pedicle screws. Very little information is available on the effect of these devices on the IAR or disk load (pressure). The spinous process distraction devices are not rigidly fixed to the spine and therefore are less subjected to fatigue failure with continued movement of the segment. Ligament devices connected rigidly to the spine through pedicle screws may undergo creep over time and become ineffective and thereby avoid fatigue failure. Most devices can be inserted by minimally invasive techniques except the Dynesys, which requires standard posture exposure like fusion. However, flexible metallic devices like the DSS, fixed rigidly to the spine, may not escape fatigue failure by way of becoming ineffective or creep after a certain period. A more detailed description of the DSS system, developed by the author, is provided in chapter 41. In the following section another flexible metallic rod device, SoftFlex (Globus Medical, Inc., Phoenixville, PA) has been described.

◆ SoftFlex Flexible Rod System

The SoftFlex system (**Fig. 31–1**) consists of a 6.5 mm titanium rod, which is the same diameter of solid rod used for rigid fixation for spinal fusion. The rod is made flexible by cutting out a helical pattern. The two ends of the rod are solid and can be attached to regular pedicle screw systems. Because the flexibility is incorporated by creating helical rods in a solid rod, it is possible to make only one end of a solid rod flexible, leaving the rest as solid rod (**Fig. 31–1B**). Such a combination is very convenient to stabilize a segment by fusion and the adjacent segment by dynamic stabilization using the same device (**Fig. 31–1C**). Lordosis can be built into the solid section of the rod (**Fig. 31–1B**). It is important to maintain the lumbar lordosis while instrumenting with the SoftFlex system.

The biomechanical tests with the SoftFlex system on L-D character in the cadaver spine showed that it can restore the normal flexibility of the spine after it has been destabilized by laminectomy and diskectomy. The effect was uniform in all directions of motion. The stiffness of the spine was not significantly increased with SoftFlex compared with the intact spine in any direction of motion (**Fig. 31–2**).

The intradiskal pressure profile from the center of the disk space was tested in flexion-extension motion. There was no change in the resting pressure profile. But the peak pressures at full flexion was reduced by 33% and that at full extension was reduced by 29% (**Fig. 31–3**). This shows that the SoftFlex system unloads the disk symmetrically in both flexion and extension.

Fatigue properties were tested in the laboratory by applying the SoftFlex system between two polyethylene blocks representing vertebral bodies, according to the American Society for Testing and Materials (ASTM) corpectomy model.[15] The test specimens were cyclically loaded with axial compression/tension load of ± 500 N, at 10 Hz, and also in shear load of ± 140 N, at 10 Hz, and they survived 10 million cycles in both (**Fig. 31–4**). It is well known that perfect simulation of in vivo actions of a dynamic stabilization system is never possible in a laboratory setting. The ASTM corpectomy model does not have the disk or the facet joint; the test construct has to take the full load and may show a shorter fatigue life in the laboratory. On the other hand, the implant may be subjected to complex loading, in a combination of axial compression, side bending, and rotation or shear, which may lead to a shorter fatigue life than predicted by in vitro testing. Therefore, it may not be possible to accurately predict the fatigue failure after implantation of the system. Interpretation of the fatigue testing results should be made in the light of such understanding.

◆ Surgical Technique

The surgical rod can be implanted in a minimally invasive, open paraspinal muscle—splitting approach described by Wiltse and Spencer.[16] The patient is positioned prone on rolls under the chest and pelvis or using a Jackson frame. This must allow a physiological lordotic posture of the lumbar spine, which is checked by preoperative fluoroscopy. The knee-chest position or the prone position on a Wilson frame should be avoided because it leads to loss of lordosis of the lumbar spine. The pedicle screws (Protex CT Occipito-Cervico-Thoracic Stabilization System; Globus Medical, Inc., Phoenixville, PA) are inserted percutaneously over guide pins under fluoroscopy. This may be possible through a single 2 to 3 cm skin incision on each side because of the lordosis of the lumbosacral junction. The flexible rods are then inserted into the pedicle screw heads and locked into position. When additional lordosis is desired, the soft rods may be held in a kyphotic position in a rod holder before application to the pedicle screw heads. When the rod holder is released, the rod recoils, producing lordosis of the motion segment. Distraction between the pedicle screw heads may be applied to restore any significant collapse of the disk height. However, an excessive distraction may lead to loss of lordosis, or even a frank kyphosis of the motion segment, and must be avoided (**Fig. 31–5**).

◆ Clinical Results

The SoftFlex system has not yet been used in clinical practice. However, a precursor to the SoftFlex flexible rod is the AccuFlex system (Globus Medical, Inc., Phoenixville, PA), which has been approved by the U.S. Food and Drug Administration (FDA) as a fusion device, to provide less rigid stabilization. AccuRod has been started in clinical applications recently, and

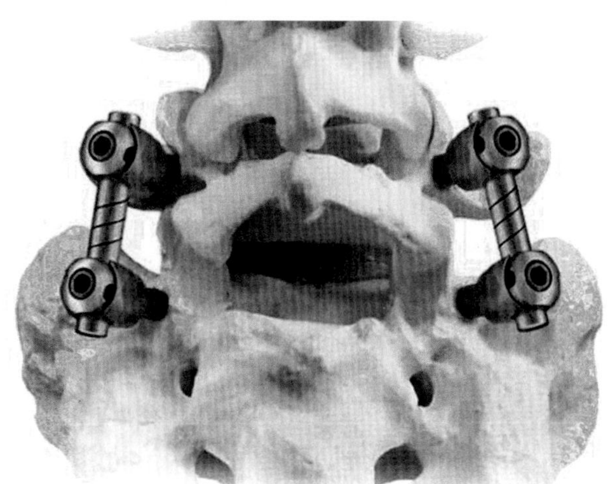

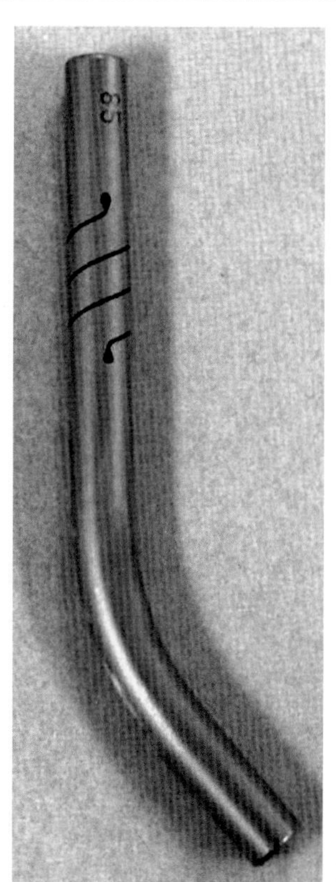

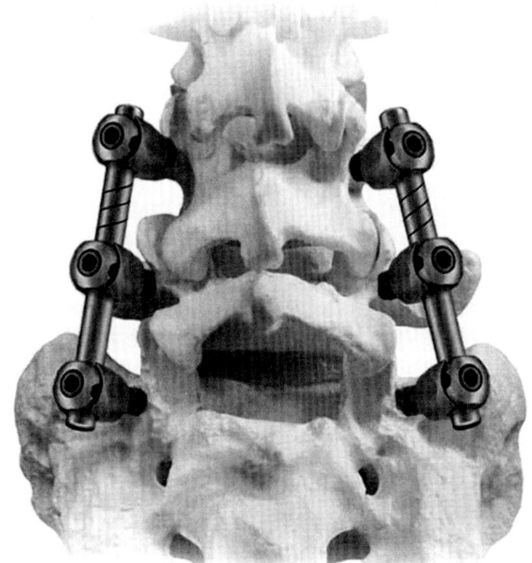

Figure 31–1 **(A)** The SoftFlex system, applied to a plastic vertebral model using the threaded Protex pedicle screw system, which can be inserted percutaneously over guide pins. **(B)** The flexible section may be present in combination with the solid section in the same rod, and lordosis may be built in in the solid section for application of the system for **(C)** fusion as well as adjacent segment stabilization in the same patient.

early clinical experience has been encouraging (**Fig. 31–6**). No catastrophic failure has been observed as yet. All cases have significant relief of symptoms. However, the early clinical cases consist not only of isolated disk degeneration along with back pain but also concomitant surgery like decompressive laminectomy or fusion. A prospective, controlled, clinical trial on isolated degenerative back pain where dynamic stabilization will be performed alone, using a minimally invasive technique, without any other concomitant surgery like decompression or fusion, is needed to evaluate the SoftFlex system. This will contribute to the study of the clinical efficacy of the SoftFlex system in the surgical treatment of chronic low back pain. To the author's knowledge, an FDA Investigational Device Exemption clinical trial of the SoftFlex system is being planned in the United States.

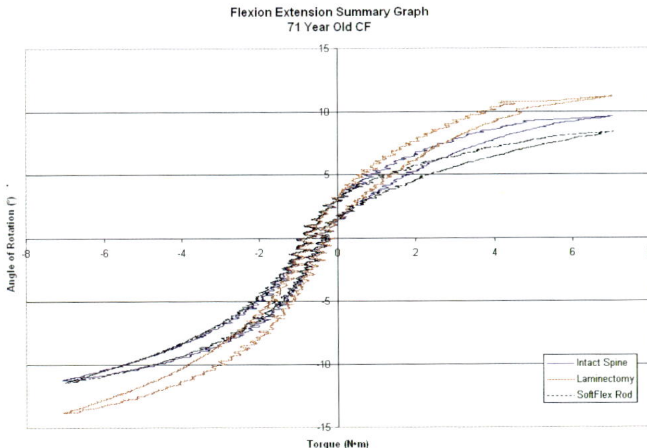

A

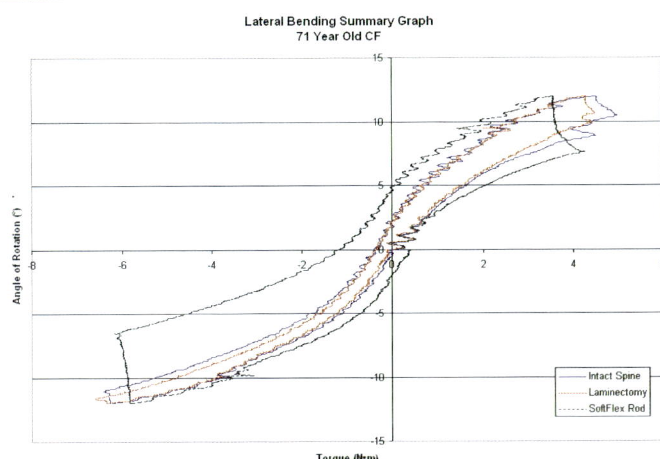

B

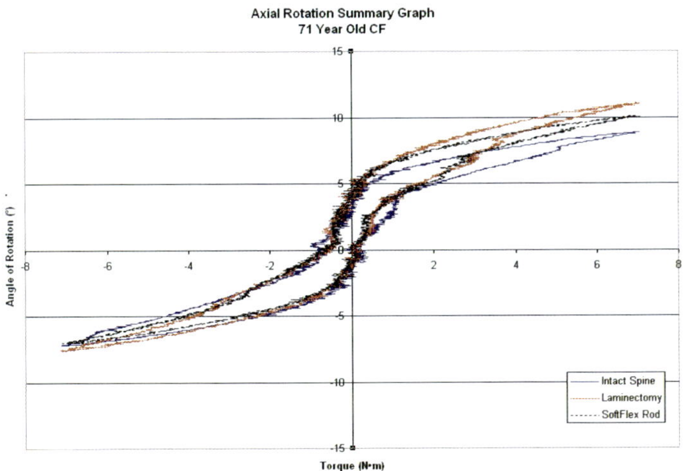

Figure 31–2 Load-deformation curve in an intact spine, after destabilization, and after dynamic stabilization with the SoftFlex system. **(A)** In flexion (right) and extension (left). **(B)** In lateral bending. **(C)** In rotation.

C

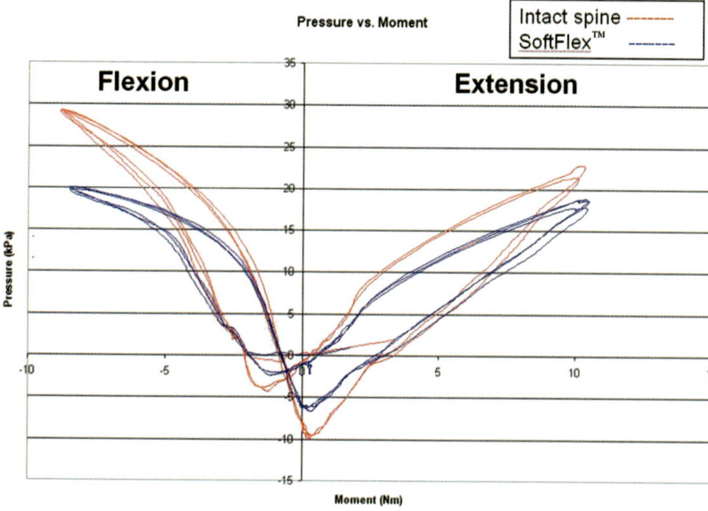

Figure 31–3 The intradiskal pressure tracing from the center of the disk, during flexion-extension motion in the intact spine and after stabilization with the SoftFlex system.

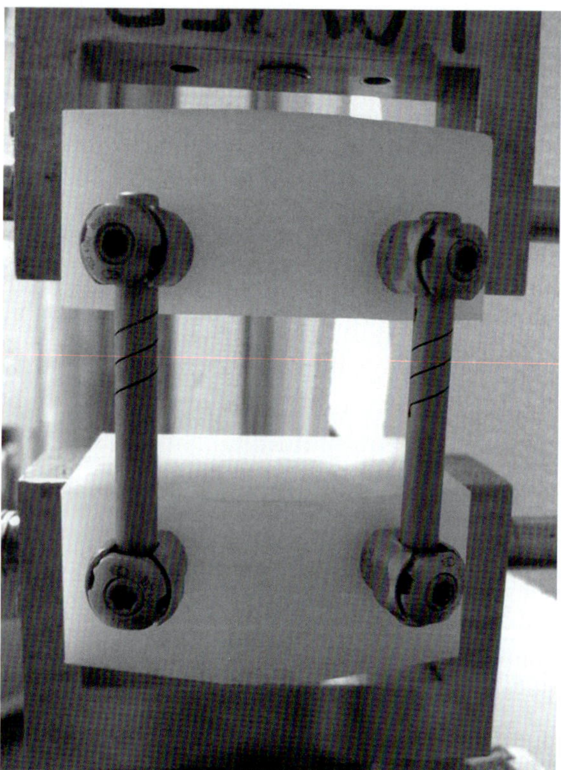
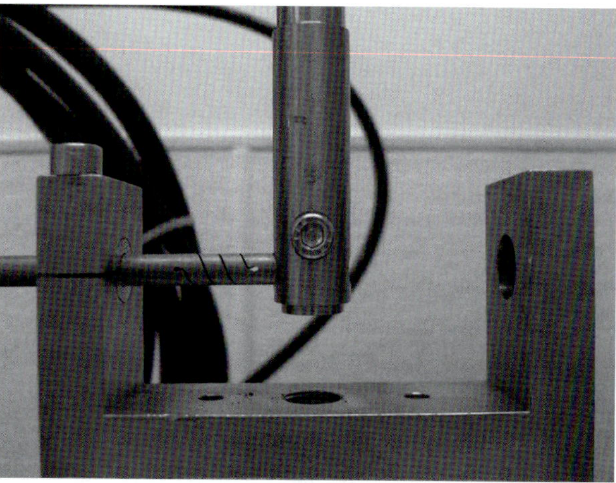

A   B

Figure 31–4 Fatigue testing of the SoftFlex system on an ASTM F1717 vertebrectomy model in **(A)** axial compression/tension loading and **(B)** shear loading.

◆ Conclusion

The bench tests with the SoftFlex system show promise that the device will achieve uniform unloading of the disk throughout the ranges of motion, and it restores the normal flexibility of the spine in all directions. The fatigue test, within the limitation of the laboratory test conditions, shows that it survives 10 million cycles without failure. The clinical advantages of this system include compatibility with a regular pedicle screw, minimally invasive implantation, easy salvage, and combination of a solid section for fusion with a flexible section for dynamic stabilization in the same rod. The early clinical results with a similar device (AccuRod system) are encouraging for the AccuRod as a fusion device, but the system requires prospective, controlled, clinical trials for proper evaluation of its efficacy and survival in vivo as a nonfusion device.

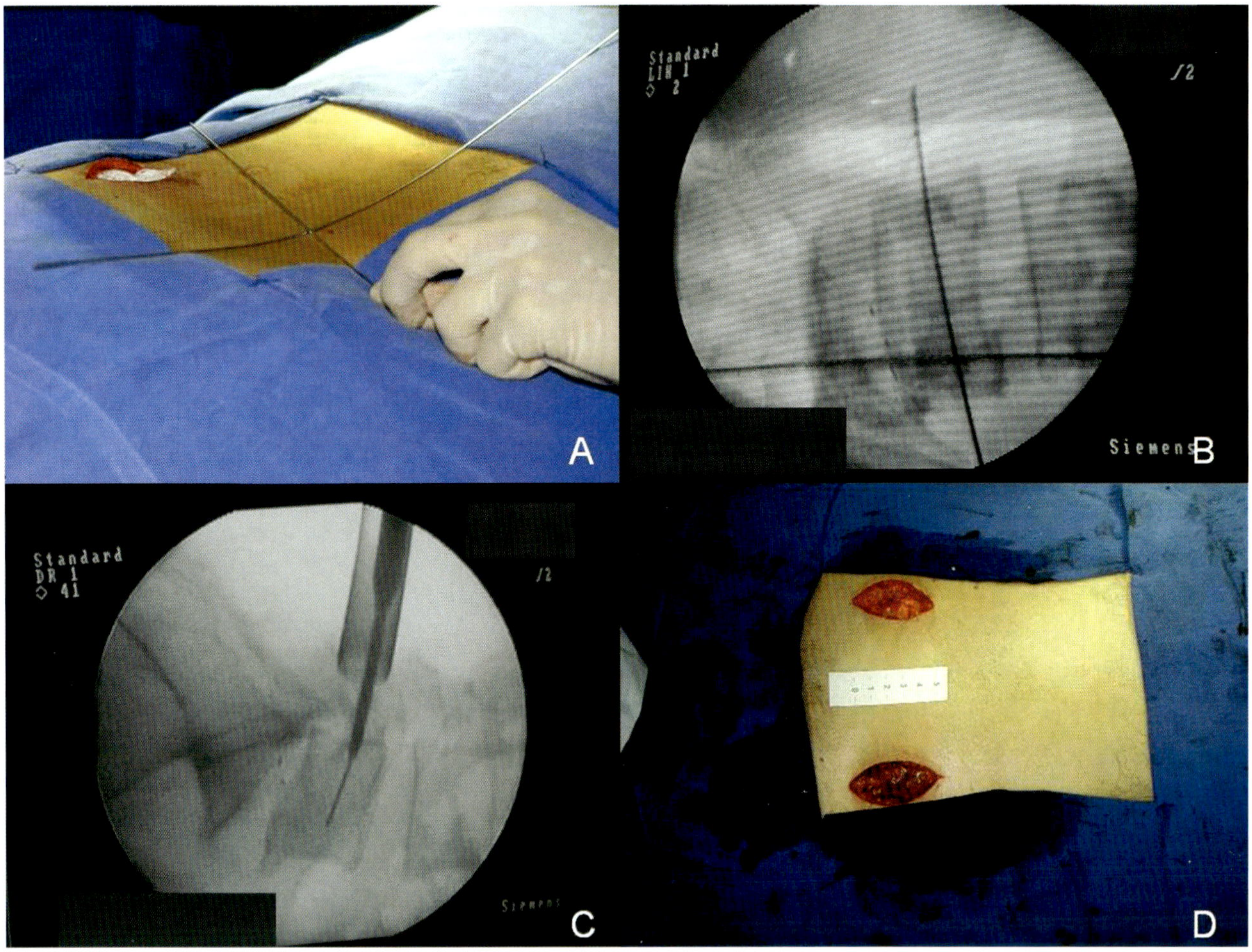

Figure 31–5 Surgical technique of minimally invasive implantation of the flexible rod, over a percutaneous pedicle screw inserted under fluoroscopic guidance. **(A)** The entry point of guide pin for the pedicle is marked by a cross K-wire over the skin and **(B)** checked under fluoroscopy. **(C)** A guide pin is inserted into the pedicle, and a track for insertion of the pedicle screw is created using dilators of progressively increasing sizes over the guide pin. The procedure is repeated for insertion of second pedicle screw in the adjacent vertebra through the same skin incision, and finally the rod is inserted. **(D)** Shows the final skin incisions on either side at the completion of the procedure.

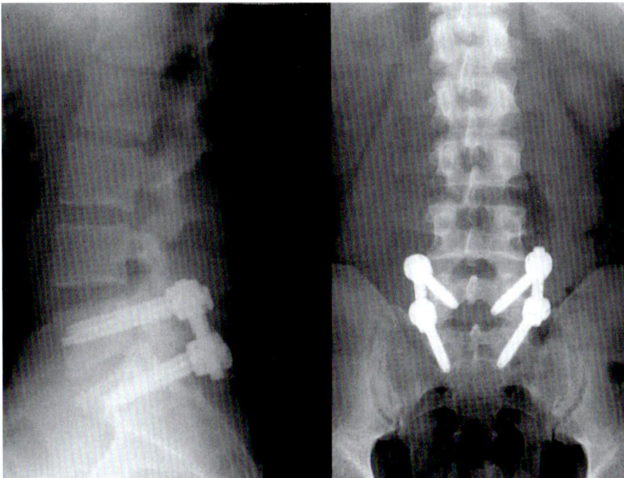

Figure 31–6 Anteroposterior and lateral radiographs following stabilization of the L5–S1 motion segment using the AccuRod system.

References

1. Bono CM, Lee CK. Critical analysis of trends in fusion for degenerative disc disease over the past 20 years: influence of technique on fusion rate and clinical outcome. Spine 2004;29:455–463 discussion Z455

2. Gibson J, Waddell G, Gibson JA. Surgery for degenerative lumbar spondylosis. Cochrane Database Syst Rev 2005;4:CD001352

3. Guyer RD, Ohnmeiss DD. Intervertebral disc prostheses. Spine 2003;28:S15–S23

4. Errico TJ. Lumbar disc arthroplasty. Clin Orthop Relat Res 2005;435:106–117

5. Fujiwara A, Lim TH, An HS, et al. The effect of disc degeneration and facet joint osteoarthritis on the segmental flexibility of the lumbar spine. Spine 2000;25:3036–3044

6. Pope MH, Frymoyer JW, Krag MH. Diagnosing instability. Clin Orthop Relat Res. 1992;279:60–67

7. Frymoyer JW, Selby DK. Segmental instability: rationale for treatment. Spine 1985;10:280–286

8. Graf H. Lumbar instability: surgical treatment without fusion. Rachis 1992;412:123–137

9. Kirkaldy-Willis WH, Farfan HF. Instability of the lumbar spine. Clin Orthop Relat Res 1982;165:110–123

10. Panjabi MM. The stabilizing system of the spine, II: Neutral zone and instability hypothesis. J Spinal Disord 1992;5:390–396 discussion 397

11. Panjabi MM. Clinical spinal instability and low back pain. J Electromyogr Kinesiol 2003;13:371–379

12. Panjabi MM, Lydon C, Vasavada A, Grob D, Crisco JJ III, Dvorak J. On the understanding of clinical instability. Spine 1994;19:2642–2650

13. Mulholland RC, Sengupta DK. Rationale, principles and experimental evaluation of the concept of soft stabilization. Eur Spine J 2002;11(Suppl 2):S198–S205

14. Sengupta DK. Dynamic stabilization devices in the treatment of low back pain. Orthop Clin North Am 2004;35:43–56

15. American Society for Testing and Materials. The Handbook of Standardization: F1717. West Conshohocken, PA: ASTM; 2003

16. Wiltse LL, Spencer CW. New uses and refinements of the paraspinal approach to the lumbar spine. Spine 1988;13:696–706

32

The X STOP Interspinous Process Decompression System for the Treatment of Lumbar Neurogenic Claudication

Richard M. Thunder, Ken Y. Hsu, and James F. Zucherman

◆ Historical Perspective

◆ Current Treatments

◆ X STOP Design Rationale and Preclinical Confirmation

◆ Operative Technique

◆ The X STOP Multicenter Randomized Trial

◆ Study Results

◆ Discussion

◆ Conclusion

Neurogenic intermittent claudication is the most common and characteristic syndrome of lumbar spinal stenosis. Patients typically obtain relief from sitting and positions of flexion, and exacerbate the pain while standing or walking.

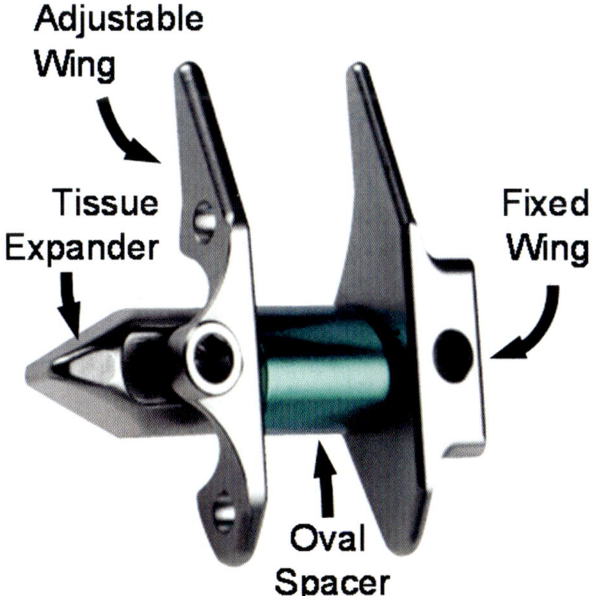

Figure 32–1 An image of the X STOP depicting the adjustable universal wing, tissue expander, fixed wing, and spacer. The tapered tissue expander allows for easier insertion between the spinous processes. The universal and fixed wings limit anterior and lateral migration. The spacer limits extension of the treated spinous processes.

The X STOP Interspinous Process Decompression (IPD) system (St. Francis Medical Technologies, Inc., Alameda, CA) is an interspinous spacer developed to treat patients with neurogenic intermittent claudication (**Fig. 32–1**). The implant limits extension of the stenotic levels of the lumbar spine by means of a spacer placed between the spinous processes. The procedure typically requires no general anesthesia and can be performed in under an hour. The X STOP is an alternative therapy to conservative treatment and decompressive surgery for patients suffering from lumbar spinal stenosis.[1] The X STOP IPD system is indicated in patients whose symptoms are exacerbated in extension and relieved in flexion. Implanted between the spinous processes, the X STOP reduces extension at the symptomatic level and allows motion in flexion, axial rotation, and lateral bending.[2]

◆ Historical Perspective

Although spinal stenosis had been observed in animals[3–5] and found in Egyptian mummies, it was probably first described in 1803, by Portal of France, who observed that narrowed spinal canals were associated with leg pain and atrophy.[6] Our understanding of this condition, however, really starts with Verbiest, who described the anatomical changes of hypertrophic articular processes causing spinal canal stenosis.[7] Subsequently, Kirkaldy-Willis et al wrote about the three-joint complex and the pathological changes found in degenerative spinal stenosis.[8] Degenerative processes may start in one-, two-, or three-joint complexes, including the disk anteriorly and the two facet joints posteriorly. With time, all three joints are involved. The degeneration of the joint also causes abnormal motion, which may produce osteophyte formation. Ultimately, disk protrusion or osteophyte formation, and hypertrophy of the facet joints and ligamentum flavum result in spinal stenosis. Medical literature regarding this condition became more available after the mid-1970s.[9] The significant increase in the diagnosis of spinal stenosis is attributable to the introduction of axial imaging provided by computed tomographic (CT) and magnetic resonance imaging (MRI) scans.

In the United States, lumbar spinal stenosis is the leading preoperative diagnosis for adults older than 65 who undergo spine surgery.[10] In 1996, almost 90,000 surgeries were performed for lumbar spinal stenosis.[10] Symptoms present with upright posture activity and include unilateral or bilateral radicular pain, sensation disturbance, and loss of strength in the lower extremities.[7] Symptoms are typically relieved with flexion of the lumbar spine.

The incidence of degenerative lumbar stenosis ranges from 1.7 to 8%.[11] There does not appear to be gender predominance; however, degenerative spondylolisthesis associated with lumbar spinal stenosis is four times more common among women. Symptoms typically develop in the fifth or sixth decade of life in association with osteoarthritic changes in the lumbar spine. No known relationship exists between incidence of lumbar spinal stenosis and race. Spinal stenosis did not have the socioeconomic significance that we see today until the 1970s. The aging of our population is resulting in an increased incidence of degenerative stenosis. In 1900, the life expectancy was 45 years. People older than 65 constituted less than 4% of the population.[12] The estimated life expectancy in 2026 is 86 years with 20% of the population expected to be older than 65 years of age. The U.S. Census Bureau projections estimate doubling of the population older than age 64 to 64 million by 2040.

◆ Current Treatments

Symptoms of spinal stenosis may respond to nonoperative management. Conservative measures often begin with a period of rest as well as nonsteroidal anti-inflammatory drugs (NSAIDS), physical therapy, and, sometimes, oral steroids. In physical therapy, trunk stabilization and core muscle strengthening are typically the goals. Epidural steroid injection is often used as an adjunct, particularly in patients with unremitting radiculopathy and neurogenic claudication. There is no clear evidence of long-term efficacy of epidural steroids; however, they can give significant short-term relief and allow participation in physical therapy.

Outcomes with nonoperative treatment reported by Hurri et al showed 44% of patients had at least some improvement in neurological symptoms.[13] In other studies, Atlas et al found that 45% percent of patients had improvement in leg pain with nonoperative treatment, whereas Johnsson et al reported 32% of patients treated nonoperatively considered their condition improved.[14,15]

Operative treatment is indicated for patients with worsening pain that is resistant to conservative treatment. Patients with moderate to severe stenosis who do not improve with nonoperative interventions are likely to improve with surgical decompression. Historically, the literature supporting operative treatment has been shown to have methodological flaws with respect to indications for surgery and surgical outcome.[16] However, in the last decade, prospective studies such as the Maine Lumbar Study have shown superior outcomes for operative treatment of symptomatic lumbar stenosis compared with nonoperative treatment.[14]

Surgical decompression, while offering the potential to improve the quality of life for individuals, also has the potential for significant complications, especially when a fusion is performed. Postoperative complications may include infection, epidural hematoma, instability, nonunion, instrumentation failure, and the need for future surgery due to the development of disease at adjacent levels. From a general medical perspective there is also a cardiac and respiratory risk, particularly in elderly patients undergoing procedures with extensive blood loss. The risk for postoperative infection remains significant despite the practice of antibiotic prophylaxis and strict sterile technique. In a study by Yuan et al 2 to 3% of patients undergoing lumbar decompression and arthrodesis with or without internal fixation suffered an infection.[17] In this same study, the risk of nerve root injury from placement of pedicle screws was 0.4%.

In addition to nerve root injury, dural tears are not uncommon during decompressive procedures. In a study by Wang et al, there was a 13.7% incidence of dural tears in 641 patients undergoing lumbar spine surgery, half of which were revisions.[18] A meta-analysis of the literature performed by Turner et al in 1992 showed the following complication rates for neurogenic claudication surgery: perioperative mortality (0.32%), dural tears (5.91%), deep infection (1.08%), superficial infection (2.3%), deep venous thrombosis (2.78%), and any complication (12.64%).[16]

◆ X STOP Design Rationale and Preclinical Confirmation

The X STOP was developed to fill the large void of treatment options between the safer yet less effective conservative care and the riskier but more effective surgical decompression. The X STOP was designed specifically to limit the terminal extension movement at only the individual level(s) that provoke symptoms, while allowing unrestricted movement of the remaining motion axes of the treated level(s). In addition, the implant was designed to be placed using a minimally invasive surgical technique with the patient under local anesthesia. Finally, it was designed to be placed without removing any bony or soft tissues, and removal is very straightforward should revision surgery become necessary.

Several key design features allow for the straightforward implantation of the X STOP. The oval spacer separates the spinous processes and restricts extension at the implanted level (**Fig. 32–2**). The two lateral wings prevent the implant from migrating anteriorly or laterally, and the supraspinous ligament prevents the implant from migrating posteriorly. The tapered tissue expander facilitates lateral insertion while allowing the supraspinous ligament to be preserved.

Biomechanical studies have shown that the X STOP significantly prevents narrowing of the spinal canal and neural foramina, limits extension, and reduces intradiskal pressure and facet loading.[2,19–21] In an MRI cadaver study, Richards et al reported that X STOP placement increases the neural

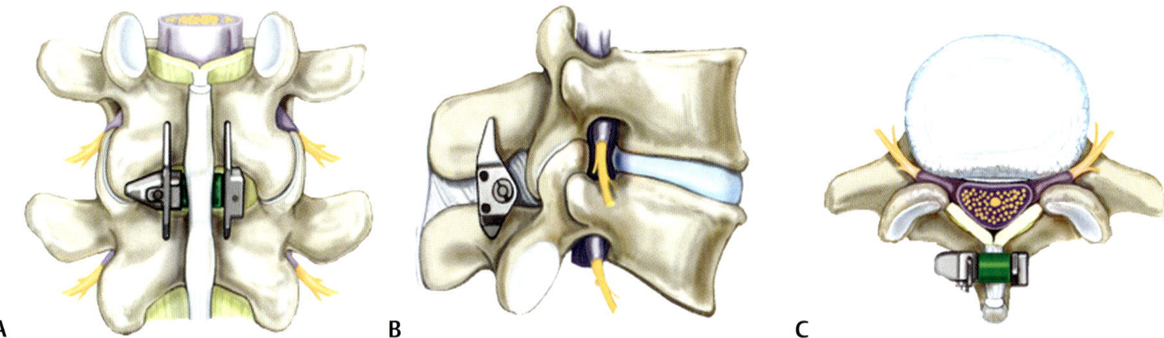

Figure 32–2 **(A)** Posterior, **(B)** lateral, and **(C)** axial views of a lumbar motion segment with an implanted X STOP. The implant is placed posterior to the lamina and away from the nerve roots and spinal cord. The supraspinous ligament is retained to prevent posterior migration. The implant is not fixed to any bony structures.

foramina area by 26% and the spinal canal area by 18% during extension.[19] In addition, the foraminal width was increased by 41% and the subarticular canal diameter by 50% in extension.[19] In a kinematics cadaver study, Lindsey et al reported that terminal extension at the implant level was reduced by 62% following X STOP placement, whereas lateral bending and axial rotation range of motion were unchanged.[2] In a cadaveric disk pressure study, Swanson et al reported that the posterior annulus and nucleus pulposus pressures were reduced by 63% and 41%, respectively, during extension, and by 38% and 20%, respectively, in the neutral, standing position.[20] Finally, Wiseman et al performed a cadaveric facet loading study and reported that the mean facet force during extension decreased by 68% during extension.[21] In each of these studies, the adjacent level measurements were not significantly changed from the intact specimen state. These preclinical studies indicate that the X STOP increases spinal canal and neural foramina space and also produces significant unloading of the disk and facets.

◆ Operative Technique

Patients are placed on a radiolucent table in a right lateral decubitus position (**Fig. 32–3**). The level to be treated is identified by fluoroscopy. After administration of a local

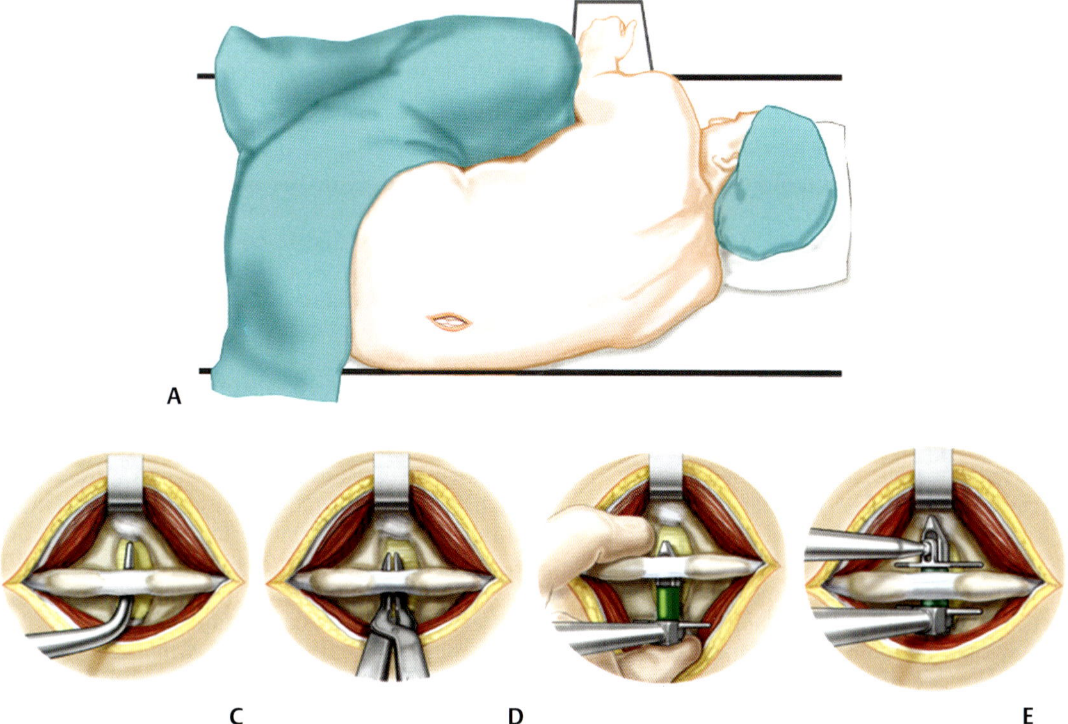

Figure 32–3 Surgical technique. **(A)** Patients are placed in a right lateral decubitus position and a midsagittal incision of ~4 cm is made over the spinous processes of the stenotic level(s). **(B)** The small, curved dilator is inserted at the most anterior margin of the interspinous space. **(C)** The sizing instrument is inserted and dilated. **(D)** The X STOP is inserted between the spinous processes. **(E)** The universal wing is attached to the tissue expander.

anesthetic, a midsagittal incision of ~4 cm is made over the spinous processes of the stenotic level(s). This is carried down to the fascia, which is incised to the right and to the left 2 cm from the midline. The supraspinous ligament is left intact. Paraspinal musculature is then elevated off the spinous processes and medial lamina bilaterally. Occasionally, hypertrophied facets that block entry into the anterior interspinous space are partially trimmed to enable anterior placement of the implant. The small curved dilator is inserted across the interspinous space abutting the posterior facet joints at the most anterior margin of the interspinous space. After the correct level is verified by fluoroscopy, the small dilator is removed and the larger, curved dilator is inserted. After the larger dilator is removed, the sizing distractor is inserted. The interspinous space is distracted until the supraspinous ligament becomes taught. The correct implant size is indicated on the sizing instrument. The appropriately sized X STOP is inserted between the spinous processes to the point where the wing is flush with the right side of the spinous processes. The screw hole for the universal wing on the left side is identified and the universal wing screw is engaged with the main body hole. The two wings are approximated medially and the left-sided universal wing screw is secured with a torque-limiting hex driver. Anteroposterior and lateral fluoroscopy views are taken to verify proper level and position. The incision is then closed. The procedure is typically done within a 24-hour hospitalization.

◆ The X STOP Multicenter Randomized Trial

A multicenter, prospective, randomized, controlled trial was performed comparing the outcomes of mild to moderate neurogenic intermittent claudication patients treated with the X STOP IPD system to those treated nonsurgically.[1] There were 191 patients treated in a prospective, controlled trial at nine centers over a 15-month period. Inclusion criteria included age greater than 50 years; leg, buttock, or groin pain with or without back pain that could be relieved during flexion; ability to sit for 50 minutes without pain; ability to walk 50 feet or more; at least 6 months of prior nonoperative therapy; stenosis confirmed by CT or MRI scan at one or two levels; and ability to comply with scheduled clinical and radiographic follow-up evaluations.

Exclusion criteria included fixed motor deficit, cauda-equina syndrome, significant lumbar instability, previous lumbar surgery, significant peripheral neuropathy or acute denervation secondary to radiculopathy, scoliotic Cobb angle greater than 25 degrees, spondylolisthesis greater than grade 1 (on a scale of 1 to 4) at the affected level(s), sustained pathological fractures or severe osteoporosis of the vertebrae or hips, obesity, active infection or systemic disease, Paget's disease, metastasis to the vertebrae, or steroid use for more than one month within 12 months preceding the study. Patients were also excluded who had anatomy that would prevent implantation of the device, such as an ankylosed segment, or spinal anatomy that would cause the device to be unstable after implantation.

Eligible patients were randomized to either the X STOP group or the control group. Those randomized to the control

Table 32–1   Patient Demographics and Baseline Variables

Variable	X STOP Mean (SD)	Control Mean (SD)	*p*-Value*
Age (years)	70.0 (9.8)	69.1 (9.9)	0.513
Height (cm)	170.9 (9.7)	168.4 (11.2)	0.117
Weight (kg)	80.4 (15.8)	81.8 (18.9)	0.569
Baseline SS	3.14 (0.56)	3.10 (0.51)	0.582
Baseline PF	2.48 (0.48)	2.48 (0.51)	0.938
Spondylolisthesis present	35/100	24/90	0.272

*Student's *t*-test.
SS, symptom severity; PF, physical function.

group received at least one epidural steroid injection and had the option to receive NSAIDs, analgesics, and physical therapy and additional injections as needed. Physical therapy consisted of back school and modalities such as ice packs, heat packs, massage, stabilization exercises, and pool therapy. Those randomized to the X STOP group underwent surgery.

Assessments were made at baseline (prior to initial treatment), and at 6 weeks, 6 months, 1 year, and 2 years following the initial treatment. Assessments were based on data collected using a validated, patient-completed outcomes measure specific to neurogenic claudication, the Zurich Claudication Questionnaire (ZCQ),[22,23] as well as the short form (SF)-36 Health Survey. The ZCQ has three domains focused on symptom severity, physical function, and patient satisfaction.

There were 100 patients randomized to the X STOP group and 91 patients to the control group. There were no significant differences in age, height, or weight between the two groups (**Table 32–1**). Also, there were no significant differences in baseline symptom severity and physical function scores. All 91 patients in the control group received an epidural steroid injection at baseline. An additional 125 injections were administered to control group patients over the course of the study, for a total of 216 injections.

A total of 136 levels were implanted in 100 patients; 64 single levels (**Fig. 32–4**) and 36 double levels (**Fig. 32–5**). One-level procedures took an average of 51 minutes and two-level procedures took an average of 58 minutes. The average blood loss was 40 mL for a one-level procedure and 58 mL for a two-level procedure. The most common level implanted was L4-L5 (89/136) and the second most common level was L3-L4 (43/136). The most common implant size was 12 mm. The procedure was performed under local anesthesia in 97 patients and under general in three patients. The X STOP was typically implanted in an acute care hospital where patients stayed less than 24 hours.

At 2-year follow-up, data from 93 of the 100 X STOP patients and 81 of the 91 control patients were available for analysis. In the X STOP group, seven patients were lost to follow-up; four patients died, two patients failed to complete the ZCQ, and one patient withdrew. In the control group, 10 patients were lost to follow-up; three patients died, one patient could not tolerate the initial epidural steroid injection,

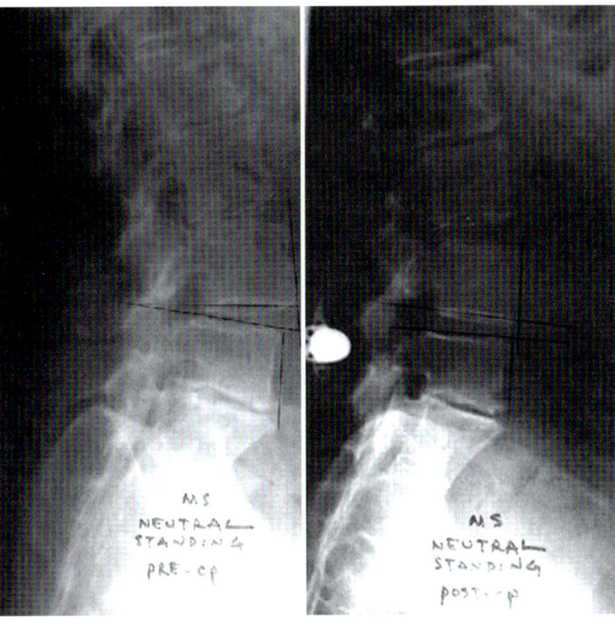

Figure 32–4   Pre- and postoperative lateral radiographs of a patient who received a single-level implantation for symptoms at L4–L5.

which was aborted, and six patients withdrew. During the course of the study, six patients in the X STOP group and 24 patients in the control group underwent decompressive surgery (laminectomy) for relief of their stenosis symptoms during the 2-year follow-up period. Postlaminectomy outcomes were available for 28 of these patients (six X STOP and 22 controls). The mean follow-up time for the laminectomy group was 12.8 months (range, 2.5–26.9 months).

◆ Study Results

The X STOP group had a significantly greater percentage of patients with an improvement in symptom severity than did the control group at each post-treatment visit. At the 24-month evaluation, 56/93 patients (60.2%) reported a

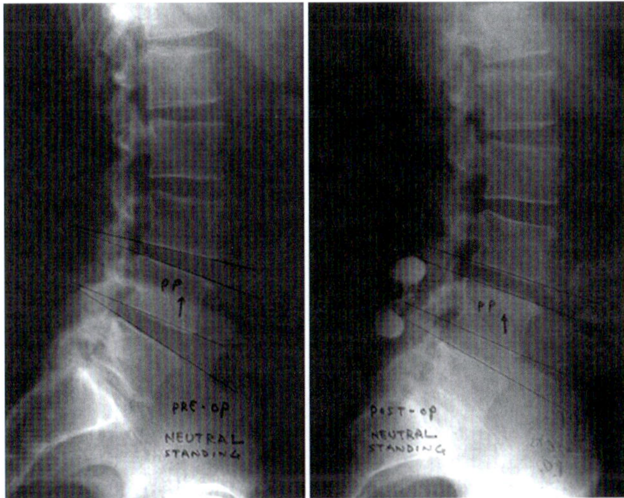

Figure 32–5   Pre- and postoperative lateral radiographs of a patient who received a double-level implantation for symptoms at L3–L4 and L4–L5.

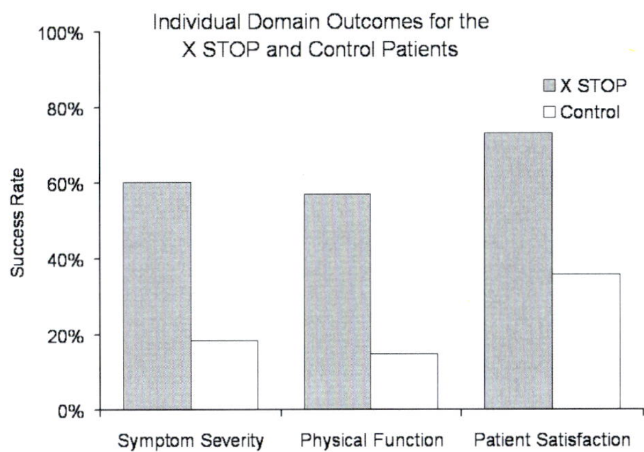

Figure 32–6   A bar chart depicting the percentage of patients in the X STOP and control groups who had significant clinical improvement in the symptom severity and physical function domains and those who were satisfied with the treatment. The X STOP outcomes are significantly greater than those of the control group for each domain.

clinically significant reduction in the severity of symptoms compared with 15/81 patients (18.5%) in the control group (**Fig. 32–6**). The X STOP group also had a significantly greater percentage of patients with an improvement in physical function than did the control group at each post-treatment visit. At the 24-month evaluation, 53/93 patients (57.0%) reported a clinically significant improvement in their physical function compared with 12/81 patients (14.8%) in the control group. The X STOP group had a significantly greater percentage of patients who were at least "somewhat satisfied" in the patient satisfaction domain than did the control group at each post-treatment visit. At the 24-month evaluation, 68/93 patients (73.1%) were at least "somewhat satisfied" compared with only 28/78 patients (35.9%) in the control group. Sixteen of 28 (57.1%) patients undergoing laminectomy had clinically significant improvement in symptom severity, 18/28 (64.3%) had clinically significant improvement in physical function, and 15/28 (53.6%) were satisfied with the outcome of their treatment.

Results of the SF-36 scores show there were no significant differences in the pretreatment enrollment scores between the X STOP and control groups for any SF-36 domain. At all follow-up time points, the X STOP group scored significantly better than the control group in every physical domain. In addition, at each time point, the mean scores in each category for the X STOP group were significantly better than the respective pretreatment scores, whereas in the control group, none of the mean scores was significantly better.

Three complications occurred intraoperatively or within 72 hours following surgery in the X STOP group. There was one episode of respiratory distress and one ischemic coronary episode that resolved without clinical sequelae. One X STOP patient with a history of cardiovascular disease developed pulmonary edema 2 days following device implantation. There were four minor operative site–related complications in the immediate postoperative period: one wound dehiscence, one swollen wound that was aspirated, one hematoma, and one report of incisional pain. There were three device–related complications in the X STOP group. One X STOP patient suffered a fall, which caused the implant to dislodge. The dislodged implant was removed without sequelae. An asymptomatic spinous process fracture was diagnosed in another patient on routine 6-month follow-up radiographs, which required no further medical treatment or surgical intervention. One patient reported worsening pain 382 days following treatment, which was determined to be possibly related to the implant. Finally, one implant was placed posterior enough to be considered malpositioned.

◆ Discussion

The straightforward clinical observation that neurogenic intermittent claudication patients typically get symptom relief from flexion and symptom exacerbation from extension led to the idea that restricting extension at the symptomatic level(s) would likely relieve the patients' symptoms. The concept developed into the X STOP interspinous process implant.

To date no randomized, prospective, multicenter study has been performed for either conservative treatment or a decompressive laminectomy. The ZCQ outcomes measure used in the foregoing study provides a validated instrument to quantify a change in the symptoms, physical function, and patient satisfaction following an intervention for neurogenic intermittent claudication.[22,23]

Approximately 44% of control patients in the present study experienced some improvement in their pain symptoms, and 43% experienced some improvement in their physical function. In addition, 24 of 91 (26%) patients in the control group elected to undergo a laminectomy compared with 6% in the X STOP group. This crossover rate in the control group is consistent with those reported in the literature.[14,24–27]

The outcomes assessed by the ZCQ scores in the present study for patients who underwent a decompressive laminectomy are consistent with the findings from the prospective study reported by Katz et al as well as data reported by others.[28–30] The comparable outcomes for the X STOP group and patients who underwent a laminectomy in the current study provide a basis against which to compare the outcomes of the X STOP group in similar patient populations, using the same outcomes measure and success criteria. The results for X STOP patients and laminectomy patients reported by Katz et al at 2-year follow-up are very similar, as are the mean improvement scores for both symptom severity and physical function (**Fig. 32–7**). In the study by Katz et al, 63% of the patients were significantly improved in symptom severity, 59% were improved in physical function, and 72% were satisfied.[29,30] Comparing these results with results for X STOP patients, 59.8% were improved in symptom severity, 56.5% were improved in physical function, and 72.8% were satisfied. Similar values are present for the 28 patients who went on to a decompressive laminectomy in the foregoing study.

In light of similar outcomes between the X STOP and surgical decompression procedures, there are important differences between the two surgical procedures. The procedural aspects of X STOP implantation compare favorably with those reported in the literature for decompressive surgery. The mean operative time for the X STOP procedure

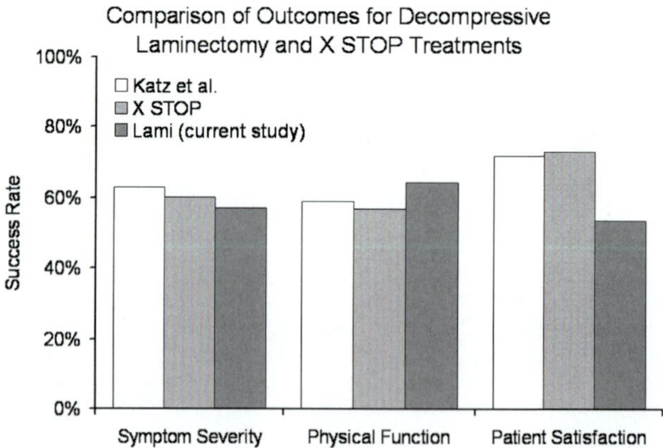

Figure 32–7   A comparison of the Zurich Claudication Questionnaire domain outcomes for the 197 patients reported by Katz et al, the X STOP patients, and six X STOP and 22 control patients who underwent a laminectomy. The outcomes are similar for each group in each domain.

was 51.2 minutes for a single-level procedure and 58.1 minutes for a two-level procedure, which was considerably less than the range of 72 to 278 minutes reported for laminectomy procedures.[31–35] In addition, the mean blood loss of 40.1 mL to 57.9 mL during the X STOP procedure was less than the range of 115 to 1040 mL reported for decompressive surgery.[31–34] Additionally, the ability to perform a majority of the X STOP procedures under local anesthesia significantly reduces the risks associated with the administration of general anesthesia.

Decompressive laminectomy is a relatively invasive surgical procedure and entails significant risks for current nicotine users (NIC) patients with potential complications that include paralysis, myocardial infarction, pulmonary embolism, pneumonia, hematoma, deep venous thrombosis, neurological deficit, deep infection, superficial infection, dural tears, implant failure (when accompanied by a fusion), and pseudarthrosis. Few of these complications were observed during or after the X STOP procedure. Because the X STOP surgical technique is not performed adjacent to the nerve roots or spinal cord, the risk of neurological deficit or paralysis may be considered minimal. No incidence of either complication was reported in this study. Compared with the incidence and severity of complications cited in the laminectomy literature, the X STOP represents a much safer procedure.

Because nonoperative therapy served as a control in the foregoing study, definitive comparisons between the X STOP and decompressive laminectomy cannot be made. In 1992, Turner et al conducted a meta-analysis of 74 stenosis studies in which the authors note that no randomized trials comparing surgery to conservative treatment had been conducted.[16] Few studies were prospective, the follow-up data collection methods were unclear, rarely were the data analyzed by someone other than the physician, and the outcomes were not assessed at consistent time intervals. Subsequent clinical studies have somewhat rectified these shortcomings. Medical therapy was selected as a control, both because it is a common treatment for patients with mild to moderate NIC, and because implantation of the X STOP, like nonoperative care, does not require the patient to undergo a highly invasive procedure.

◆ Conclusion

Implantation of the X STOP is an alternative to laminectomy, with clinical outcomes that are comparable to and consistent with results reported for decompressive surgery. Results of a randomized, prospective trial show that the X STOP improves symptoms and function significantly compared with epidural steroid injections and conservative therapy in patients with mild to moderate symptoms. The absence of any major complications demonstrated that the X STOP is relatively safe.

The X STOP provides an effective treatment option for patients suffering from mild to moderate symptoms of lumbar spinal stenosis.

References

1. Zucherman J, Hsu K, Hartjen C, et al. A multicenter, prospective, randomized trial evaluating the X STOP interspinous process decompression system for the treatment of neurogenic intermittent claudication: two-year follow-up results. Spine 2005;30:1351–1358
2. Lindsey DP, Swanson KE, Fuchs P, Hsu KY, Zucherman JF, Yerby SA. The effects of an interspinous implant on the kinematics of the instrumented and adjacent levels in the lumbar spine. Spine 2003;28:2192–2197
3. Breit S, Kunzel W. Breed specific osteological features of the canine lumbosacral junction. Ann Anat 2001;183:151–157
4. Tarvin G, Prata RG. Lumbosacral stenosis in dogs. J Am Vet Med Assoc 1980;177:154–159
5. Watt P. Degenerative lumbosacral stenosis in 18 dogs. J Small Anim Pract 1991;32:125–134
6. Wiltse LL. History of spinal disorders. In: Frymoyer JW, ed. Adult Spine. New York: Raven, 1991:33–55
7. Verbiest H. A radicular syndrome from developmental narrowing of the lumbar vertebral canal. J Bone Joint Surg Br 1954;36:230–237
8. Kirkaldy-Willis WH, Wedge JH, Yong-Hing K, Reilly J. Pathology and pathogenesis of lumbar spondylosis and stenosis. Spine 1978;3:319–328
9. Verbiest H. Neurogenic intermittent claudication in cases with absolute and relative stenosis of the lumbar vertebral canal (ASLC and RSLC), in cases with narrow lumbar intervertebral foramina, and in cases with both entities. Clin Neurosurg 1973;20:204–214
10. Dartmouth Medical School. Center for the Evaluative Clinical Sciences. The Quality of Medical Care in the United States: A Report on the Medicare Program. The Dartmouth Atlas of Health Care 1999 ed. [Chicago]: AHA Press; 1999
11. Hilibrand AS, Rand N. Degenerative lumbar stenosis: diagnosis and management. J Am Acad Orthop Surg 1999;7:239-249
12. Bakshi S, Miller DK. Assessment of the aging man. Med Clin North Am 1999;83:1131–1149
13. Hurri H, Slatis P, Soini J, et al. Lumbar spinal stenosis: assessment of long-term outcome 12 years after operative and conservative treatment. J Spinal Disord 1998;11:110–115
14. Atlas S, Deyo R, Keller RB, et al. The Maine Lumbar Spine Study, III: 1-year outcomes of surgical and nonsurgical management of lumbar spinal stenosis. Spine 1996;21:1787–1795
15. Johnsson KE, Uden A, Rosen I. The effect of decompression on the natural course of spinal stenosis: a comparison of surgically treated and untreated patients. Spine 1991;16:615–619
16. Turner JA, Ersek M, Herron L, Deyo R. Surgery for lumbar spinal stenosis: attempted meta-analysis of the literature. Spine 1992;17:1–8
17. Yuan HA, Garfin SR, Dickman CA, Mardjetko SM. A historical cohort study of pedicle screw fixation in thoracic, lumbar, and sacral spinal fusions. Spine 1994;19:2279S–2296S
18. Wang JC, Bohlman HH, Riew KD. Dural tears secondary to operations on the lumbar spine: management and results after a two-year-minimum follow-up of eighty-eight patients. J Bone Joint Surg Am 1998;80:1728–1732
19. Richards JC, Majumdar S, Lindsey DP, Beaupre GS, Yerby SA. The treatment mechanism of an interspinous process implant for lumbar neurogenic intermittent claudication. Spine 2005;30:744–749
20. Swanson KE, Lindsey DP, Hsu KY, Zucherman JF, Yerby SA. The effects of an interspinous implant on intervertebral disc pressures. Spine 2003;28:26–32
21. Wiseman CM, Lindsey DP, Fredrick AD, Yerby SA. The effect of an interspinous process implant on facet loading during extension. Spine 2005;30:903–907
22. Stucki G, Daltroy L, Liang MH, Lipson SJ, Fossel AH, Katz JN. Measurement properties of a self-administered outcome measure in lumbar spinal stenosis. Spine 1996;21:796–803
23. Stucki G, Liang MH, Fossel AH, Katz JN. Relative responsiveness of condition-specific and generic health status measures in degenerative lumbar spinal stenosis. J Clin Epidemiol 1995;48:1369–1378
24. Atlas SJ, Keller RB, Robson D, Deyo RA, Singer DE. Surgical and nonsurgical management of lumbar spinal stenosis: four-year outcomes from the Maine Lumbar Spine Study. Spine 2000;25:556–562
25. Cuckler JM, Bernini PA, Wiesel SW, Booth RE Jr, Rothman RH, Pickens GT. The use of epidural steroids in the treatment of lumbar radicular pain. A prospective, randomized, double-blind study. J Bone Joint Surg Am 1985;67:63–66
26. Simotas AC. Nonoperative treatment for lumbar spinal stenosis. Clin Orthop Relat Res 2001;384:153–161
27. Simotas AC, Dorey FJ, Hansraj KK, Cammisa F Jr. Nonoperative treatment for lumbar spinal stenosis: clinical and outcome results and a 3-year survivorship analysis. Spine 2000;25:197–203; discussions 203–204
28. Gunzburg R, Keller TS, Szpalski M, Vandeputte K, Spratt KF. Clinical and psychofunctional measures of conservative decompression surgery for lumbar spinal stenosis: a prospective cohort study. Eur Spine J 2003;12:197–204
29. Katz JN. Spinal Stenosis Data. Boston: Harvard Medical School; 2003:1–33
30. Katz JN, Stucki G, Lipson SJ, Fossel AH, Grobler LJ, Weinstein JN. Predictors of surgical outcome in degenerative lumbar spinal stenosis. Spine 1999;24:2229–2233
31. Benz RJ, Ibrahim ZG, Afshar P, Garfin SR. Predicting complications in elderly patients undergoing lumbar decompression. Clin Orthop Relat Res 2001;384:116–121
32. Iguchi T, Kurihara A, Nakayama J, Sato K, Kurosaka M, Yamasaki K. Minimum 10-year outcome of decompressive laminectomy for degenerative lumbar spinal stenosis. Spine 2000;25:1754–1759
33. Khoo LT, Fessler RG. Microendoscopic decompressive laminotomy for the treatment of lumbar stenosis. Neurosurgery 2002;51(Suppl 5):S146–S154
34. Postacchini F, Cinotti G, Perugia D, Gumina S. The surgical treatment of central lumbar stenosis: multiple laminotomy compared with total laminectomy. J Bone Joint Surg Br 1993;75:386–392
35. Reindl R, Steffen T, Cohen L, Aebi M. Elective lumbar spinal decompression in the elderly: is it a high-risk operation? Can J Surg 2003;46:43–46

33

Dynamic Lumbar Stabilization with the Wallis Interspinous Implant

Jacques Sénégas

◆ **Rationale for Use**

◆ **Basic Concepts**

◆ **The Wallis Implant**
Overall Description
Preclinical Validations
Clinical Validation:
First-Generation Implants

◆ **Clinical Application of the Current Wallis System**
Indications and Contraindications
Surgical Technique
Clinical Results of the Current Wallis Implant

◆ **Discussion**
Technical Aspects
Clinical Aspects

◆ **Conclusion**

◆ Rationale for Use

Dynamic intersegmental stabilization with the Wallis System (Abbott Spine, Inc., Austin, TX) implant lies within the framework of functional articular surgery. This implant, made of an interspinous process spacer that limits extension and two flexion-limiting bands, is intended to improve the stability of the treated intervertebral lumbar segment while preserving its mobility. The implant has an extra-articular design that makes it an easily reversible procedure. Because the operation leaves all the anatomical elements intact except for the interspinous ligament, the entire range of other surgical options remains open, including more invasive surgical solutions such as disk replacement or fusion.

The primary goal of the Wallis System is to relieve or prevent low back pain that accompanies intervertebral segment instability. Furthermore, restoring a more physiological biomechanical environment to the degenerate lumbar segment with a Wallis may foster healing of the disk and facet joint lesions (provided that the disease process has not yet attained an overly advanced stage) and slow the degenerative cascade of adjacent segments.

◆ Basic Concepts

The purpose of this chapter is not to provide a full review of the origin and causes of degenerative disk disease (DDD), but rather to present the rationale and concepts upon which the Wallis System is based. The reader may find more detailed information on DDD elsewhere.[1–4]

Disk degeneration is a multifactorial process, the underlying causes of which remain poorly understood. Nevertheless, in all likelihood, DDD is mediated essentially by biomechanical, environmental, and genetic factors. In healthy intervertebral elements under normal physiological mechanical loads, balance between cellular anabolic and catabolic activity results in optimal remodeling of the nucleus pulposus extracellular matrix. The appropriate balance of disk cell activity results in stable, high proteoglycan concentrations that are necessary for the proper hydration and mechanical properties of the nucleus and annulus. This in turn ensures an adequate nutrient supply and removal of products of metabolism (lactate) as well as a beneficial cellular mechanical environment, further contributing to viable cellular activity and extracellular matrix synthesis and catabolism. Under such conditions, as long as the mechanical demands remain within physiological limits, this process of constant adaptive tissue remodeling maintains the functional anatomical architecture of the intervertebral disk (and of the facet joints as well).

However, the balance between the external gravitational forces and internal forces may change due to either environmental conditions (work-related overloading) or age-related biomechanical changes (trunk deconditioning, insufficient muscular efficacy, or neuromuscular control). These abnormal conditions may disturb the equilibrium between anabolic and catabolic cellular activity (inadequate tissue remodeling) and result in a complex cascade of biological and biomechanical events that can alter the nucleus pulposus structure and ultimately lead to the overall disorganization and degeneration of the disk.

Among other phenomena, this cascade involves either or both cell apoptosis and change in phenotype, which induce an inflammatory response with vascular invasion, macrophage infiltration, and macrophage/chondrocyte interaction. As a result, numerous proinflammatory cytokines, including interleukin (Il)-1a, Il-1b, Il-6, and tumor necrosis factor alpha (TNF-a) are produced in degenerative disks. The presence of these cytokines may further enhance the local inflammation and activate the production of enzymes (notably, matrix mettalo proteinases (MMPs) and aggrecanases) involved in the degradation of the extracellular matrix constituting a detrimental catabolic feedback loop.

This degenerative process begins in the nucleus pulposus with cell loss and extracellular matrix alteration. Progression of the disease causes the outer annulus fibrosus (AF) to lose its normal lamellar arrangement and compromises the mechanical strength of the disk. Tears progressing from the inner AF outward contribute to the loss of mechanical integrity of the spinal segment. These changes increase the mechanical forces transferred to the surrounding vertebral end plates contributing to microfractures and marginal osteophyte formation. This altered mechanical environment could result in further and faster deterioration of the disk itself.

This degeneration, which contributes to excessive mobility and abnormal loading, can transform the fibrocartilaginous architecture of the intervertebral disk into a pseudoarthrodial joint involving cell death in the nucleus pulposus and a cavitation phenomenon in the disk. Cell death rate also increases in the AF as well as in the cartilage of the vertebral end plates and facet joints.

As already stated, susceptibility to this mechanically triggered cascade is widely variable depending on genetic factors, which consequently play a major role in the severity and rate of disk degeneration.

Currently, the only available treatment modalities for disk-related spinal pain focus on alleviating symptoms rather than addressing the underlying cause of degeneration. It is likely that clinical outcomes for patients with painful intervertebral disk degeneration would improve if therapies were more focused on slowing, halting, or even reversing this process. One way of achieving this goal might be to artificially restore the physiological mechanical environment to alter the biomechanical parameters that sustain the catabolic feedback loop and disk destruction process.

As early as 1986, we investigated this concept: rabbit studies performed in our unit showed evidence that disk lesions were reversible by artificially increasing resistance to compression and stretching of the segment using a ligamentoplasty that increased the intervertebral stiffness.[5] These findings prompted us to design an implant that would reduce the range of motion (ROM) and increase the stiffness of a degenerative intervertebral segment.

This approach was recently confirmed by Kroeber et al,[6] who also concluded that degenerative changes could be reversed. Based upon a rabbit model of degenerative disk disease, their results suggested that regeneration of the disk can be induced by unloading of the intervertebral segment by dynamic axial distraction. The decompressed rabbit intervertebral disks showed signs of tissue recovery on biological, cellular, and biomechanical levels after 28 days of distraction.

◆ The Wallis Implant

Overall Description

The implant consists of an interspinous spacer that limits extension and two bands that secure the implant in the interspinous space and limit flexion. It was developed in two phases. In the initial system developed in the 1980s, the interspinous spacer was made of titanium. The spacer was connected to a woven polyester cord, which was looped around the spinous processes and reattached to the spacer by means of a morse taper. An improved Wallis device (Abbott Spine, Inc., Austin, TX) was developed in 2001[7] (**Figs. 33–1 and 33–2**). The former metallic interspinous spacer was replaced by a redesigned spacer made of polyetheretherketone (PEEK). The initial woven polyester cord was replaced by bands made of the same material. Titanium crimping rings are added to prevent fraying of the extremities of the bands after cutting off the excess length. There is one radiodense tantalum marker in each side of the PEEK spacer.

PEEK and polyester were chosen for their excellent biocompatibility, their radiolucency, and their lack of artifacts on magnetic resonance imaging (MRI). In addition, PEEK is highly resistant to degradation in a hydrous environment, and its modulus of elasticity is close to that of cortical bone, thus reducing the contact stresses between the spacer and the spinous processes in extension. The cord of the former device was replaced by flat bands to increase surface contact with the spinous processes, thereby minimizing local concentration of contact stresses on the bone during flexion. The implant also includes small titanium crimping rings and tantalum markers, which are radiodense and biocompatible and do not interfere with MRI.

The PEEK spacer is designed for placement between the spinous processes of two adjacent vertebrae. There are two opposing grooves (proximal and distal) in the device to house the spinous processes. Each of these grooves is inclined 10 degrees with regard to the transverse plane for better adaptation to the anatomy of the spinous processes. The center of the spacer is completely traversed by two identical oval openings, and aligned with the grooves in the sagittal plane. These openings serve to further increase the flexibility of the spacer during compression loading of the intervertebral segment.

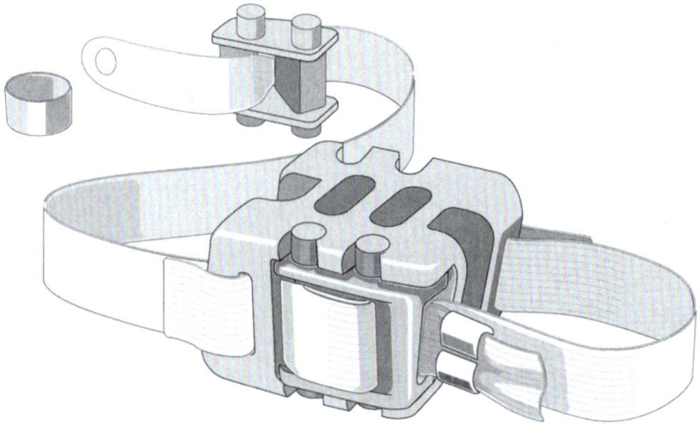

Figure 33–1 The Wallis dynamic stabilization implant.

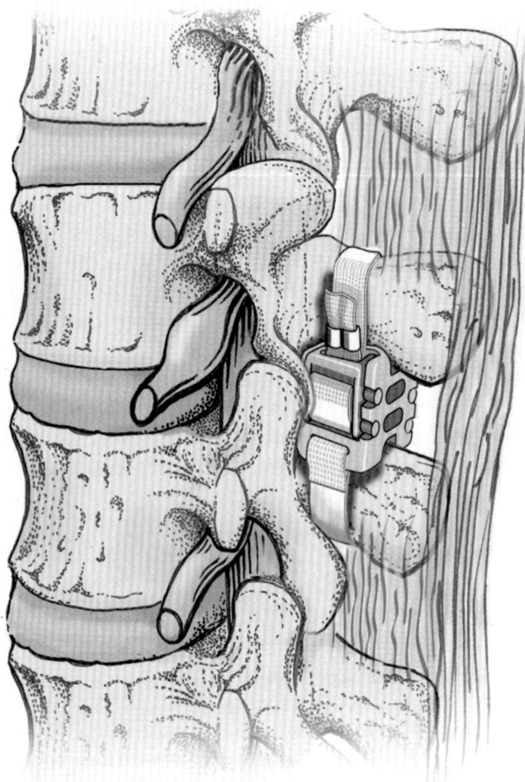

Figure 33–2   A Wallis implant in place.

At one corner of each side of the spacer, there is a tunnel loop around which is sewn one band extremity. After passage around the corresponding spinous process, each band is looped through a PEEK strap fastener, which in turn is snapped on the opposite side of the spacer into four notches located at the edges of a dedicated recess. Small retaining teeth in the floor of this recess prevent back sliding of the band. The implant position can be assessed by means of a radiodense marker (tantalum) in each lateral fastener.

All spacers have the same width. Only the height increases with the size of the spacer. Wallis implants are available with interspinous heights of 8, 10, 12, 14, and 16 mm.

Preclinical Validations

Conventional Biocompatibility Testing

All the materials in the device have a prior history of implant use. The biocompatibility of the PEEK and polyester materials themselves has been extensively tested and confirmed. Biocompatibility testing of the complete Wallis System was established for approval by the U.S. Food and Drug Administration (FDA) Investigational Device Exemption (IDE) study that is under way in the United States. The implant passed a battery of standardized tests, including cytotoxicity, irritation, sensitization, systemic toxicity, genotoxicity (Ames, chromosomal aberration, and mouse lymphoma assay [MLA]), pyrogenicity, and subchronic toxicity (implantation for 28 days, 3 months, and 6 months).

Static Tests

Twelve randomly selected sterilized and packaged size 8 implants were submitted to static testing in saline (0.9%) at 37°C using a stainless steel model of spinous processes. The smallest implant (size 8) was chosen as the worst-case scenario because it has the weakest mechanical properties due to size. The static tension yield load (six implants) was 440 ± 14 N and the static compression yield load (six implants) was 1710 ± 107 N. These values can be put into perspective by comparing them to unpublished cadaver study values of the distractive force shared by the posterior arch during flexion (maximum value at bone failure: 130 N) and to published values of the resistance to compression of the spinous processes (mean value at bone failure, 339 N; 95% CI, 257–447 N).[8]

Dynamic Fatigue Tests

RUN-OUT VALUES IN TENSION AND COMPRESSION

Under identical conditions (5 L of saline at 37°C and the stainless steel model of spinous processes), six sterilized size 8 implants (worst-case scenario) were submitted to 10 million cycles at 5 Hz to test the compressive strength, and six other size 8 implants were submitted to 10 million cycles at 5 Hz to test the tensile strength. The dynamic run-out load was found to be 300 N in tension and 830 N in compression, both findings being more than twice the resistance values of posterior arches and spinous processes cited earlier.

CREEP AFTER 10 MILLION CYCLES

After 10 million cycles of tension at 300 N, the observed creep of the polyester band was 0.16 mm (0.5%). After 10 million cycles of compression at 830 N, the observed creep of the spacer was 0.04 mm (0.5%).

In Vitro Cadaver Testing

Biomechanical evaluation of the effects of the new Wallis on spinal segment mobility and rigidity was performed in cadavers.

Flexion-extension studies performed on intact and damaged disks (nucleotomy) demonstrated that the implant placed on a damaged structure restores the ROM to values similar to those obtained in healthy segments. In the altered segments, the implant also restored the stiffness values in a normal range. The stability of the segment was increased with reduction of the neutral zone and less translation. Although effective in stiffening flexion-extension movements, as intended, this interspinous dynamic system was shown not to affect either lateral bending or axial rotation of the instrumented segments.

Finite Element Analysis

The effects of the new Wallis on the mechanical stresses applied to the disk were also investigated using a finite element model (FEM). The FEM demonstrated similar results in terms of spinal segment mobility when compared with the cadaver study (validating the FEM). Furthermore, the implant did not alter the mechanical behavior of the adjacent segment.

In this FEM, implantation of the interspinous device reduced maximal compressive stresses within the disk, especially on its posterior aspect.

Clinical Validation: First-Generation Implants

A long-term follow-up study is being conducted of first-generation patients operated in my former unit in Bordeaux, France, between 1987 and 1995. Of the 142 patients who could be located for long-term follow-up, 106 (75%) were men. Eighty-two percent were between the age of 30 and 60 at the time of operation. Eighty-eight (62%) had one implant, 27 (19%) were treated at two adjacent levels, 21 (15%) at three consecutive levels, and six (4%) at four consecutive levels. The indications for operation included canal stenosis and disk herniation (20%), isolated canal stenosis (44%), and isolated recurrent herniated disk (24%). Based on this group of 142 patients, the actuarial survival rate of the implant was 84.1% at 10 years with a 95% confidence interval of ±6.1%. There were only three implant-related failures, all of which occurred within 1 year. Moreover, the survival rate of the dynamic construct was independent of the number of implants in the construct (i.e., two-, three-, and four-level procedures had the same success rates as the one-level procedures). Long-term clinical follow-up of these patients is under way.

◆ Clinical Application of the Current Wallis System

Indications and Contraindications

The Wallis posterior stabilization system treats low back pain that accompanies degenerative lesions of grade II, III, and IV according to the MRI classification proposed by Pfirrmann et al[9] in lumbar segments down to L4–L5 in the indications described following here.

The implant is currently the object of an IDE study in the United States in young adults with degenerative disk disease with or without Modic 1 bone changes[10] (not with Modic 2 or 3 changes) at the treated level. Outside of the United States, it is indicated for lumbar canal stenosis in young patients associated with undercutting decompression procedures (*recalibrage* in French) that otherwise destabilize the segment.

Other indications outside of the United States include voluminous herniated disks that can leave behind an instability, and in recurrent herniated disks for the same reason. At L4–L5, a herniated disk associated with an L5 sacralization transitional anomaly can be another source of postoperative lumbar pain if this level is not stabilized. Similarly, it is used for DDD at a segment adjacent to fusion.

Wallis is contraindicated for grade V degenerative lesions in the MRI classification of Pfirrmann, lesions for which no disk tissue is left for healing. Wallis is not suitable for stabilizing spondylolisthesis. Osteoporosis is a contraindication because of the increased risk of spinous process fracture. As already stated, lesions at L5–S1 are contraindicated because of the insufficient size of the spinous process of S1. An implant dedicated to the L5–S1 segment is currently under development. For the same reason, acquired or constitutional spinous process insufficiency is a contraindication. As in other spinal interventions, surgeons should not expect good results in patients with nonspecific low back pain, work-related litigation, or patent psychological disorders.

Surgical Technique

Recommended Preoperative Imaging

Before a Wallis procedure, different imaging studies are recommended. Anteroposterior (AP) films establish the preoperative sagittal alignment of the lumbar spine, and lateral films can be useful later for feedback showing the surgeon that the proper-sized implant was selected to avoid iatrogenic kyphosis. MRI is typically used for the patient selection process, but comparing preoperative and intermediate-term postoperative T2 sagittal sequences can also be used to document changes in the treated segment. Likewise, it is a good idea to obtain preoperative flexion-extension bending films if permitted by the pain status of the patient to monitor the course of the instrumented segment and adjacent segment mobilities.

Potential Complications

Before proposing Wallis to patients, surgeons should inform them of the inherent complications of the decompression that will be associated with the implant placement. As for the dynamic stabilization technique itself, recurrent or primary disk herniation is possible with this implant because of the persistent segment mobility. In such cases, the herniated disk material can be removed, if necessary, without removing the Wallis. If the Wallis is explanted to permit access to the intervertebral disk, it is usually preferable to replace it with a new Wallis instead of resorting to fusion.

Although not specific to the Wallis procedures, surgeons should also provide information on potential complications of anesthesia and spine surgery in general (e.g., allergy to anesthesia, infection, deep venous thrombosis, or pulmonary embolism).

It is also prudent to inform patients of the possibility of persistent low back pain due to concomitant degenerative lesions in other disks or facet joints, unless this possibility has been eliminated by methodical diagnostic procedures performed prior to the operation.[11,12]

Operative Procedure

The operation is performed with the patient under general anesthesia. There are no precautions specific to the use of the Wallis itself.

Depending on the indication, the Wallis implant is placed either after a posterior decompressive procedure or alone through a midline incision. Only the placement technique will be considered here, not the possible accompanying decompression. The patient is placed in the prone position on a frame of foam padding. A neutral position of physiological lumbar lordosis is recommended to choose the proper size of the spacer to avoid local kyphosis at the level treated. Maintaining overall lordosis is important to foster preservation of the adjacent segments. Among the Wallis instruments, there is a novel interlaminar spreader that can be used to transiently obtain local lumbar kyphosis. This spreader facilitates accompanying decompressive procedures without changing the patient to a knee-chest position.

One can never overemphasize the importance of verifying with an image intensifier that the proper segment is being accessed. After incision of the skin, the supraspinous ligament is detached from the two spinous processes of the targeted lumbar level with a conventional scalpel and retracted to one side with the paravertebral muscles. Before proceeding further, a small, sterile surgical drape should be sutured over the wound edge on both sides to preserve the implant from contact with the thin border of skin that may be exposed at the edge of the incision. Although the postoperative infection rate is no higher than in other lumbar interventions, we feel that this added precaution against infection is warranted.

With a gouge, the surgeon removes the interspinous ligament, which is the only anatomical element of the intervertebral segment that is not preserved in this dynamic stabilization technique. In general, if bone trimming is necessary to improve seating of the interspinous spacer, the surgeon should trim the inferior aspect of the upper spinous process rather than the superior aspect of the lower spinous process. Some trimming at the junctions of the laminae with the spinous processes is often advisable, the point being to seat the spacer deeply, not only between the spinous processes but also as much as possible in contact with the laminae. Such trimming is performed along with the accompanying decompressive procedure at this stage if decompression is necessary.

After trying various sizes to determine which spacer to use, the selected implant is placed in the interspinous space (**Fig. 33–3**). To preserve optimal lordosis, when the surgeon

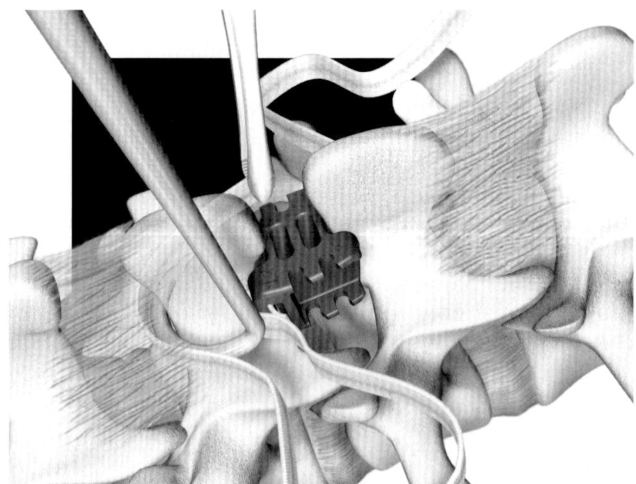

Figure 33–4   Passage of one of the bands around a spinous process.

is uncertain which of two sizes fits better, the smaller one should be used. Given the position of the patient in normal lordosis during the operation, initial strong stability of implant seating is not vital. With a dedicated sharp, curved instrument, the surgeon then pushes the attached polyester band on the rostral end between the overlying interspinous ligament and the rostral edge of the overlying spinous process (**Fig. 33–4**). The band is passed into the clip to secure it to the spacer (**Fig. 33–5**) and to permit final tightening of the band (**Fig. 33–6**). Once the opposing band has been passed around the underlying spinous process and secured to the spacer in an identical manner, and before cutting off the excess band on each side, a small titanium ring is crimped onto each band to stop fraying at the severed end (one must be careful not to damage the functional part of the band that secures the Wallis).

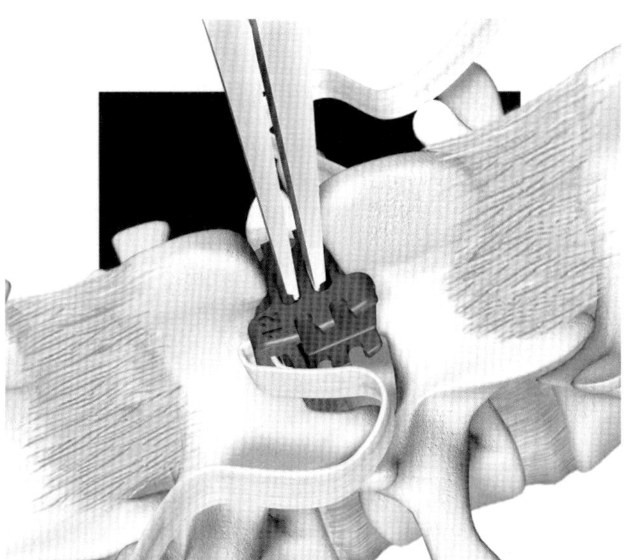

Figure 33–3   Placement of the spacer between the spinous processes.

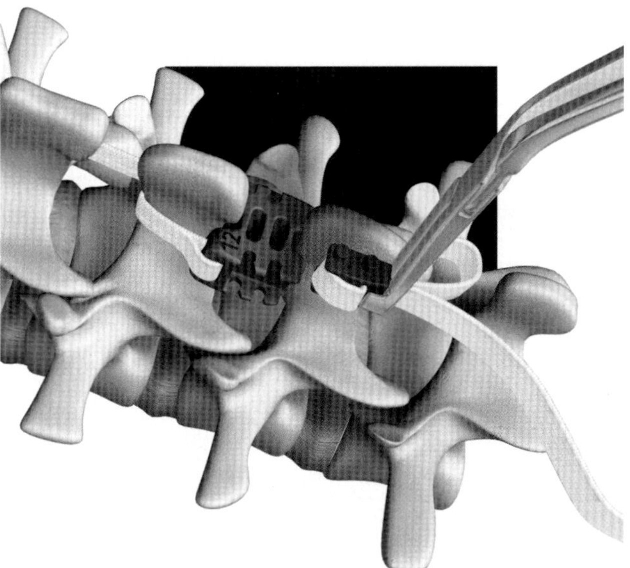

Figure 33–5   Placement of one of the strap fasteners in position to be snapped onto the side of the spacer.

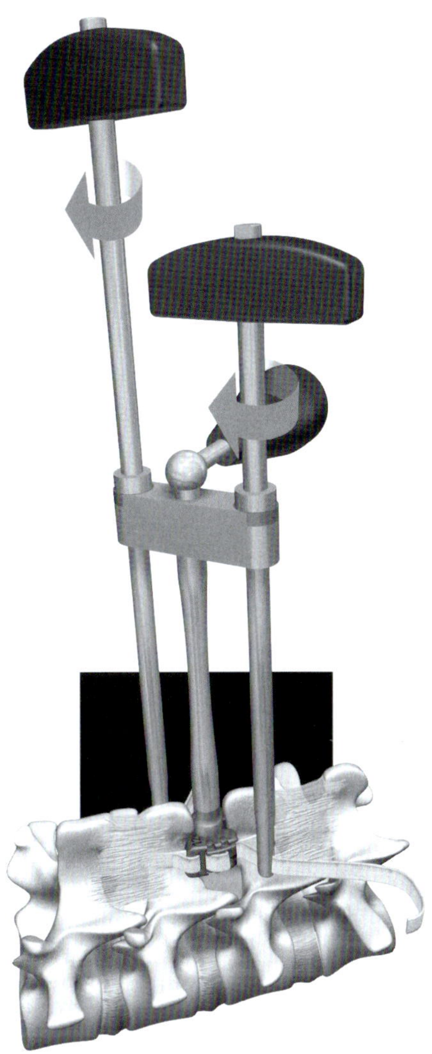

Figure 33–6 Device for final tightening of the bands.

Once the implant is in place, the supraspinous ligament is reinserted onto each spinous process with one suture through a hole made through the tip of the spinous process. To pierce the spinous process, a Backhaus towel clamp works well. The surgeon can make the supraspinous ligament fit more tautly between the spinous processes during its reinsertion.

Finally, the wound is closed over a suction drain (recommended if the Wallis is inserted after a decompressive procedure for proper drainage of possible postoperative epidural bleeding).

The suction drain can be removed the day after surgery in the absence of abnormal discharge. For the first postoperative month, we recommend external lumbar support. Patients should wait for 1 month before starting muscle reinforcement exercises.

Clinical Results of the Current Wallis Implant

A prospective. single-arm, open study of the second-generation implant is under way in eight centers in Europe, South America, and Africa. The results of this study will soon be submitted for publication. Preliminary results on 134 patients at 1-year follow-up are very promising. For example, in terms of the average Japanese Orthopedic Association's scale for evaluating lumbar interventions,[13] the patients improved from 11.9 ± 3.3 (on a scale of 0 to 21) preoperatively to 19.8 ± 1.9 at 1 year. The overall visual analog scale (VAS) for pain reported by patients improved from 7.0 ± 2.1 (on a scale of 0 to 10) preoperatively to 1.1 ± 1.5 at 1 year. According to Odom's criteria, the surgeons reported an excellent or good therapeutic outcome in 88.8% of the patients after 1 year.

The mean operating time for implant placement was low (19 ± 8 minutes) as was the average blood loss (190 ± 135 mL). The majority of patients had a 12 or 10 mm Wallis implant. The most frequently operated level was L4–L5. Among the 262 patients in the study, 11 of the implants have been removed during revision procedures, including three replaced by a second Wallis implant, one after rapid recurrence of herniated disk, one after implant displacement (the initial procedure of the surgeon involved), and the case mentioned earlier involving a band damaged during the operation.

◆ Discussion

Technical Aspects

Safety

The safety of the operation is reflected by the low number of postoperative complications that led to revision procedures in the multicenter study. Among the 262 patients in this study, only 11 of the implants have been removed, including three replaced by another Wallis. This was consistent with the first-generation Wallis retrospective finding that the survival rate of the implant was 84.1% at 10 years. Most certainly contributing to the low complication rate is the fact that the procedure is 100% extra-articular, causing no damage to the disk or the facet joint articular capsules. A particular advantage is the absence of bony purchase such as pedicle screws to secure the implant in place, reducing the potential rate of complications. Pedicle screw placement is a well-documented source of complications in posterior fusion procedures.[14,15] Pedicle screw–based dynamic stabilization systems have high reported rates of loosening attributed to toggling-related osteolysis around the screws.[16]

Other factors to consider in product safety are the implant materials. Both PEEK and woven polyester have established long-term biocompatibility. Among the 142 patients contacted 10 to 15 years after undergoing a first-generation Wallis procedure, none had implant failure related to discomfort or pain. Furthermore, there was no case of spinous process failure related to band debris created by abrasion. This provides additional evidence of the long-term innocuousness of the polyester bands.

Analysis of the first-generation study indicated that the degree of success in terms of implant survival did not depend on the number of implanted levels. This is in stark contrast with the failure rate of lumbar fusion, which is widely reported to increase with the number of fused segments.[17] This improvement over stabilization by fusion would appear to be consistent with both the safety and the efficacy of each segment of these multilevel dynamic constructs.

Reversibility

Among the primary advantages of Wallis is the preservation of all vertebral and intervertebral structures with the exception of the interspinous ligament and slight trimming of the spinous processes. As demonstrated in the international study, when a Wallis had to be removed or replaced by another Wallis, the revision procedure was quite straightforward. The procedure is fully reversible, leaving all subsequent surgical options open, including fusion, disk replacement, and potential future cell therapeutic interventions.[18] Revision of failed arthrodeses or disk replacements are more demanding and are associated with greater risks.[19,20]

Clinical Aspects

Pain Relief

In cadaver studies, Wallis increased stiffness and restored stability to the instrumented level. Clinically, it relieves low back pain induced by instability and is used to prevent low back pain related to postoperative instability that may be created during bony decompression. This is supported by the observed significant improvement in VAS pain scores at 3 months and 1 year postoperatively with respect to the preoperative values.

Among more than 7000 total patients operated in the world, the only documented case of band failure to date inadvertently created a unique crossover therapeutic situation that illustrated the potential of Wallis to relieve degenerative low back pain. In the latter patient, microscopic analysis of the removed implant suggested that the surgeon had partially scored the band with a scalpel, probably when cutting off the excess band at the end of the operation, and this had led to its subsequent failure. The patient in question had been operated primarily for low back pain. After 1 year pain free, the patient began to feel a clicking sensation in the lumbar region, and the low back pain recurred. The surgeon removed the implant and tried physical therapy. After 3 months of unsuccessful conservative treatment, another Wallis was implanted, resulting in immediate relief of this 44-year-old woman's low back pain.

Motion Preservation

While stabilizing the intervertebral level, Wallis still permits motion in the treated segment. In fact, the in vitro studies show that it results in no change in natural lateral bending and rotation of the instrumented segments. This appears to imply that the implant's efficacy can be mediated only by its action on flexion and extension. As can be seen in **Fig. 33–7**, flexion and extension are merely limited by the implant. This 39-year-old man was operated for a median herniated disk

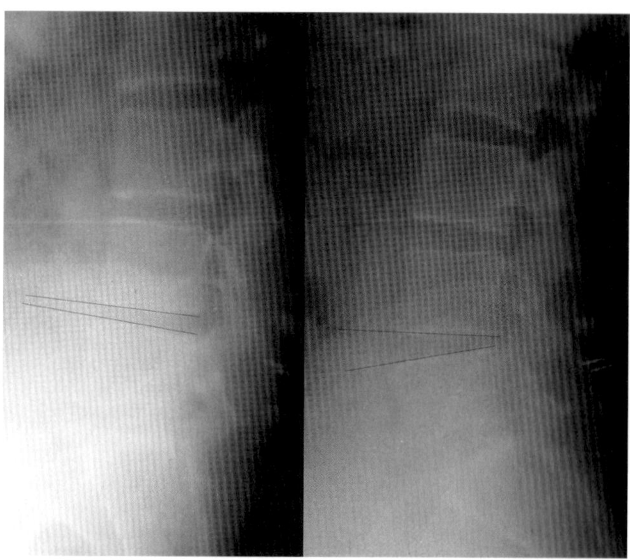

Figure 33–7 Lateral films showing flexion (left), and extension (right). The radiodense markers of the implant are visible as are the clipping rings added to prevent fraying of the bands at each extremity.

at the L4–L5 level with excellent clinical outcome. The bending films in **Fig. 33–7** were made 1 year after the procedure.

Pain relief combined with motion preservation amounts to a functional restoration, especially in patients younger than 60, allowing these individuals to return to their former activities, within reason. For example, contact sports and certain strenuous professions may not be advisable for patients who have a dynamic stabilization system.

Adjacent Segment Preservation

In keeping with one of the initial goals of the concept, according to the finite element model results, Wallis does not change the mechanical loading of the adjacent segments, possibly slowing the progress of degenerative disk disease at those levels compared with the rate of degeneration adjacent to fused segments. Although no study has yet shown the superior outcome of segments adjacent to segments managed by motion preserving techniques with respect to those adjacent to fused segments, the widespread conviction that fusion accelerates the degenerative cascade in adjacent segments is strong enough to fuel the emergence of total disk replacement despite the irreversibility of this solution. For example, in a series of lumbar fusion patients with more than 5 years of follow-up, Gillet[21] observed a 20% rate of revision surgery to extend the arthrodesis to adjacent segments. Similarly, in a survivorship study of 215 patients who had undergone posterior lumbar arthrodesis, Ghiselli et al[22] reported a reoperation rate at adjacent levels of 16.5% at 5 years and 36.1% at 10 years. Interestingly enough, there appeared to be no correlation with the length of fusion or the preoperative arthritic degeneration of the adjacent segment, a finding that may justify the emergence of alternative, motion-preserving techniques.

Stabilization with a Wallis achieves low back pain relief at least as good as that obtained with fusion, while restoring a physiological ROM to the treated segment. Indeed, segments with early degenerative changes and only partially diminished disk height contribute more to lumbar flexion and extension than the healthier segments. This "hinge effect" is thought to constitute a dynamic factor that can worsen the symptoms of canal stenosis.[23] I believe that prevention of both the "hinge effect" and the development of stenosis at adjacent levels by adding Wallis after decompression of canal stenosis should be studied.

Disk replacement has been shown to be at least as effective against low back pain as fusion but is often preferred in view of its putative protective action against adjacent level degeneration. In selected young patients, surgeons may consider to begin by trying a Wallis instead of disk replacement provided that at least 50% of the disk height is preserved, because long-term risks of disk replacements are uncertain.[24] As stated earlier, long-term follow-up of the Wallis system is reassuring. Moreover, Wallis also preserves motion and is easily reversible. Disk replacement would still be possible if the Wallis fails to relieve pain, regardless of whether the low back pain persists postoperatively or develops many years later. Also to be considered are growing concerns that some disk designs may contribute to facet joint changes.[25] In contrast, in view of the unloading effect Wallis has on the facet joints by the placement of an interspinous spacer reported by Minns and Walsh,[26] many users have began applying the Wallis implant to patients with facet joint syndrome with good clinical results.

Potential Disk Restoration

The same study by Minns and Walsh confirms the previously mentioned FEM finding that interspinous process spacers also decrease the compressive forces passing through the disk. They reported load sharing that reached 50% for interspinous process spacer heights of 12 mm. This load sharing is intrinsically related to the stiffness restored to the degenerate disk by a Wallis implant. The hypothesis is that the conjunction of both provides the mechanical conditions that mediate slowing or arrest of the degenerative process. New evidence is emerging to indicate that reversal of degenerative disk changes may even be possible. Although it is not always observed, in several patients, comparison of preoperative and postoperative MRI shows grade IV (in terms of the classification proposed by Pfirrmann et al[9]) treated levels recovering to grade III or even grade II. In other words, on T2-weighted images we are seeing many black disks recovering white, rehydrated signal. Preoperative grade IIIs also appear to be improving to grade II, but this change would probably be more difficult to document than changes involving grade IV disks.

The T2-weighted sequence in **Fig. 33–8** is consistent with rehydration of the L3–L4 disk 6 months after placement of a Wallis above a prior L4–S1 fusion in a 50-year-old stone mason operated for a herniated disk. A 5-year study of the course of degenerate disks in asymptomatic patients[27] has strongly suggested that spontaneous regression of disk degeneration in terms of the Pfirrmann MRI classification never occurs. This suggests that the favorable mechanical environment provided by the implant may replenish or reactivate nucleus cells with subsequent return to a

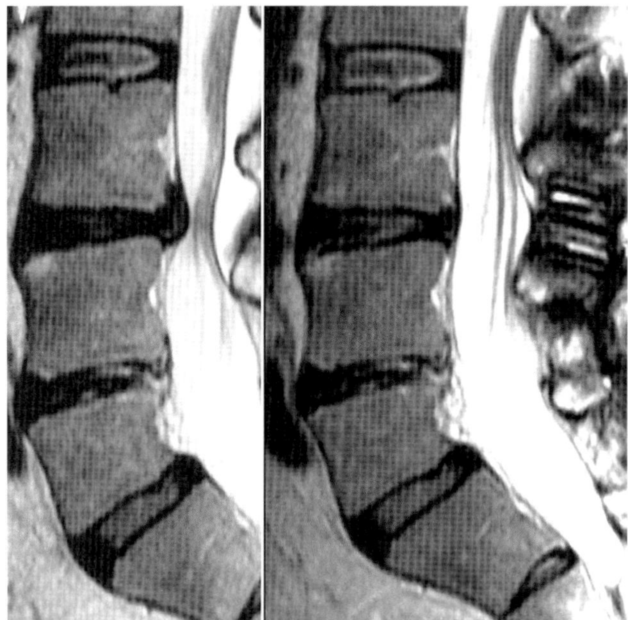

Figure 33–8   Patient with magnetic resonance imaging evidence of disk rehydration at follow-up.

favorable balance of catabolic and anabolic processes affecting the quality of the extracellular matrix (proteoglycan synthesis). On T2-weighted sequences, black disks are black because the water content is diminished, which in turn is due to a reduced concentration in proteoglycan to which the water molecules are bound. Although the half-life of proteoglycans and proteoglycan degradation products in intact disks has been reported to reach 15 years,[28] black disks are often herniated disks, in which case massive proteoglycan loss from the nucleus may have occurred.

Here, once again, an intriguing case from the first-generation series warrants mention. Because of a neck problem, one patient was referred to me 15 years after an enlargement procedure at L3–L4 and L4–L5 stabilized by two first-generation Wallis implants. A follow-up MRI showed white signal in the two treated levels, whereas all of the untreated levels except L5–S1 had become black, presumably with aging (**Fig. 33–9**). The absence of stenosis above the implants is noteworthy as well. Typically within less than 5 years of a lumbar canal enlargement stabilized by fusion, MRI shows narrowing of one or more levels above the treated segments, which remain free of stenosis. This one case is proof of neither disk preservation nor protection of adjacent disks, but it may justify retrospective long-term MRI follow-up of other first-generation patients.

Duration of Effects

The implant includes a posterior tension-band system with no bony fixation because of the theoretical incompatibility of bone screw fixation with a dynamic stabilization device intended to function for years in young patients with early degenerative changes. For an arthrodesis, rod–screw fixation systems must remain securely fastened to the bone for only a few months until bony fusion is obtained. In dynamic

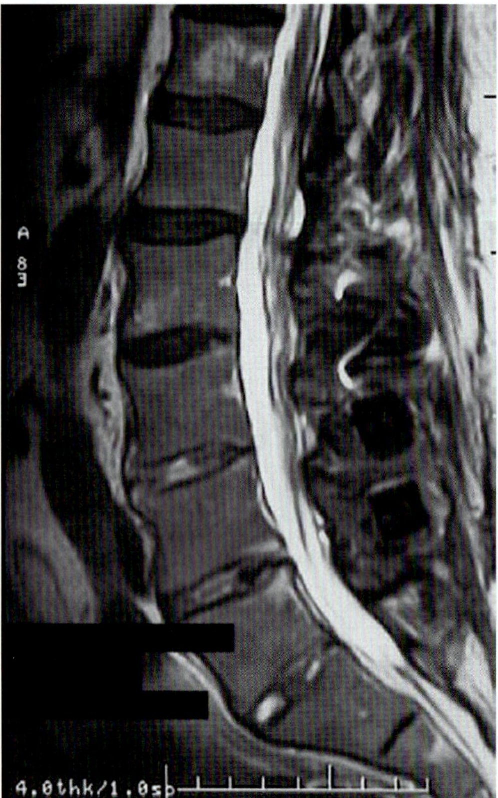

Figure 33–9 Patient with first-generation Wallis implants at L3–L4 and L4–L5 added for dynamic stabilization at the end of an undercutting operation for canal stenosis. Note that this T2-weighted sequence shows greater hydration of the sacralized L5–S1 segment and the two segments treated by Wallis than at the other levels, where the dark signal probably corresponds to normal age-related loss of hydration. Also noteworthy are the preservation of overall lumbar lordosis and the absence of secondary stenosis developing rostral to the treated segments 15 years after the procedure.

stabilization systems, screws may loosen over time under the constant toggling forces. The excellent results of the retrospective long-term survey would seem to indicate that the Wallis system continues to function up to 15 years at least. One may argue that the same results may be possible even if the implant had loosened over time and were no longer mechanically active. Although the anecdote involving white disks in the lone segments stabilized by Wallis for 15 years appears to support its continued mechanical action, this also remains to be determined by future studies, which should concomitantly attempt to distinguish the relative importance of disk off-loading and segmental stiffness in putative disk healing.

◆ Conclusion

The present system has many substantial advantages. Its implementation is straightforward, 100% extra-articular, with a short learning curve and almost no implant-related perioperative or postoperative morbidity. Lesions are avoided by the median approach and patients are generally walking the day after surgery. Although years of follow-up will be necessary to establish whether dynamic stabilization indeed has a protective effect against accelerated changes held to occur in adjacent disks after fusion, Wallis may be as effective in achieving this goal as disk replacements, provided that lumbar lordosis is properly preserved. Furthermore, a surprising number of patients are showing disk rehydration on follow-up MRIs, providing indirect evidence supporting the hypothesis that favorable mechanical conditions should foster healing or scarring of disk tissue.

More importantly than these imaging improvements, very good clinical results are being found using dynamic lumbar stabilization. To date, follow-up shows that the efficacy of the new implant is at least as good as that of fusion.

Wallis fills a therapeutic void that formerly existed between conservative treatment and fusion or disk replacements, both of which may be radical solutions for many young patients with early degenerative changes. Spinal surgery rarely affords definitive solutions. The threshold of Wallis surgery is low and because it leaves other options open, a step-by-step strategy to treat low back pain without compromising future solutions is now possible.

Patients are becoming more sophisticated, many learning of novel biological methods of treating degenerative disks with their own stem cells or fibroblasts.[29] Sports physicians have already begun using stem cell therapy for tendon and ligament lesions. When these techniques extend to include intervertebral disks, patients who have fusion or disk replacements might regret having chosen these options because the possibilities for disk restoration in such patients will be highly compromised, at best. Although Wallis does not restore the disk in all patients, for years it almost always preserves the disk height that was present before the operation. Furthermore, when stem cell therapy does become a reality in the intervertebral disk, the modified cells will probably need favorable mechanical conditions to flourish. Wallis is already being anticipated as a possible adjuvant technique for the new biological solutions in degenerative disk disease.

References

1. Walker MH, Anderson DG. Molecular basis of intervertebral disc degeneration. Spine J 2004;4:158S–166S
2. Battie MC, Videman T, Parent E. Lumbar disc degeneration: epidemiology and genetic influences. Spine 2004;29:2679–2690
3. Silver FH, Siperko LM. Mechanosensing and mechanochemical transduction: how is mechanical energy sensed and converted into chemical energy in an extracellular matrix? Crit Rev Biomed Eng 2003;31:255–331
4. Urban JP, Smith S, Fairbank JC. Nutrition of the intervertebral disc. Spine 2004;29:2700–2709
5. Sénégas J, Vital JM, Guérin J, et al. Stabilisation lombaire souple. In: M'Barek M, Loreiro M, Bouvet R, eds. GIEDA: Instabilités vertébrales lombaires. Paris: Expansion Scientifique Française; 1995: 122–132
6. Kroeber M, Unglaub F, Guegring T, et al. Effects of controlled dynamic disc distraction on degenerated intervertebral discs: an in vivo study on the rabbit lumbar spine model. Spine 2005;30:181–187
7. Sénégas J. Mechanical supplementation by non-rigid fixation in degenerative intervertebral lumbar segments: the Wallis system. Eur Spine J 2002;11(Suppl 2):S164–S169

8. Shepherd DE, Leahy JC, Mathias KJ, Wilkinson SJ, Hukins DW. Spinous process strength. Spine 2000;25:319–323

9. Pfirrmann CW, Metzdorf A, Zanetti M, Hodler J, Boos N. Magnetic resonance classification of lumbar intervertebral disc degeneration. Spine 2001;26:1873–1878

10. Modic MT, Steinberg PM, Ross JS, Masaryk TJ, Carter JR. Degenerative disk disease: assessment of changes in vertebral body marrow with MR imaging. Radiology 1988;166(1 Pt 1):193–199

11. Schwarzer AC, Wang SC, O'Driscoll D, Harrington T, Bogduk N, Laurent R. The ability of computed tomography to identify a painful zy-gapophysial joint in patients with chronic low back pain. Spine 1995;20:907–912

12. Pang WW, Mok MS, Lin ML, Chang DP, Hwang MH. Application of spinal pain mapping in the diagnosis of low back pain-analysis of 104 cases. Acta Anaesthesiol Sin 1998;36:71–74

13. Yorimitsu E, Chiba K, Toyama Y, Hirabayashi K. Long-term outcomes of standard discectomy for lumbar disc herniation: a follow-up study of more than 10 years. Spine 2001;26:652–657

14. Katonis P, Christoforakis J, Kontakis G, et al. Complications and problems related to pedicle screw fixation of the spine. Clin Orthop Relat Res 2003;411:86–94

15. Lonstein JE, Denis F, Perra JH, Pinto MR, Smith MD, Winter RB. Complications associated with pedicle screws. J Bone Joint Surg Am 1999;81:1519–1528

16. Nockels RP. Dynamic stabilization in the surgical management of painful lumbar spinal disorders. Spine 2005;30(Suppl 16):S68–S72

17. Pihlajamaki H, Myllynen P, Bostman O. Complications of transpedicular lumbosacral fixation for non-traumatic disorders. J Bone Joint Surg Br 1997;79:183–189

18. Ganey TM, Meisel HJ. A potential role for cell-based therapeutics in the treatment of intervertebral disc herniation. Eur Spine J 2002;11(Suppl 2):S206–S214

19. Etminan M, Girardi FP, Khan SN, Cammisa FP Jr. Revision strategies for lumbar pseudarthrosis. Orthop Clin North Am 2002;33:381–392

20. Kostuik JP. Complications and surgical revision for failed disc arthroplasty. Spine J 2004;4(Suppl 6):289S–291S

21. Gillet P. The fate of the adjacent motion segments after lumbar fusion. J Spinal Disord Tech 2003;16:338–345

22. Ghiselli G, Wang JC, Bhatia NN, Hsu WK, Dawson EG. The fate of the adjacent motion segments after lumbar fusion. J Bone Joint Surg Am 2004;86-A:1497–1503

23. Vitzthum HE, Konig A, Seifert V. Dynamic examination of the lumbar spine by using vertical, open magnetic resonance imaging. J Neurosurg 2000;93(Suppl 1):58–64

24. van Ooij A, Oner FC, Verbout AJ. Complications of artificial disc replacement: a report of 27 patients with the SB Charité disc. J Spinal Disord Tech 2003;16:369–383

25. Dooris AP, Goel VK, Grosland NM, Gilbertson LG, Wilder DG. Load-sharing between anterior and posterior elements in a lumbar motion segment implanted with an artificial disc. Spine 2001;26:E122–E129

26. Minns RJ, Walsh WK. Preliminary design and experimental studies of a novel soft implant for correcting sagittal plane instability in the lumbar spine. Spine 1997;22:1819–1825

27. Elfering A, Semmer N, Birkhofer D, Zanetti M, Hodler J, Boos N. Risk factors for lumbar disc degeneration: a 5-year prospective MRI study in asymptomatic individuals. Spine 2002;27:125–134

28. Roughley PJ, Melching L, Mort JS, Pearce RH, Sivan S, Maroudas A. The structure, degradation and lifespan of aggrecan in the human intervertebral disc. Eur Cell Mater 2005;10(Suppl 3):17

29. Hildebrand KA, Jia F, Woo SL. Response of donor and recipient cells after transplantation of cells to the ligament and tendon. Microsc Res Tech 2002;58:34–38

34

Coflex

Eun-Sang Kim and Doo-Sik Kong

◆ **Product Design**

◆ **Indications/Contraindications**

  Spinal Stenosis with or without Segmental Instability

  Intraoperative Instability

  Adjacent Level to Rigid Fixation

  Elderly Patients and Osteoporotic Patients with Segmental Instability

◆ **Operative Technique**

◆ **Preliminary Results**

  Clinical Results

◆ **Radiological Outcome**

◆ **Complications**

◆ **Discussion**

◆ **Conclusion**

Since neurogenic claudication secondary to spinal stenosis was first described by Verbiest,[1] decompressive surgery has been required in patients who failed to respond to conservative therapy. However, decompressive surgery sometimes leads to secondary instability. In cases where secondary instability is expected to develop following decompression of the posterior column as well as in cases with instability, additional posterior fusion has been indicated. Although its importance in surgery for spinal stenosis cannot be neglected, posterior fusion is not an ideal treatment modality. Studies have shown that this procedure can result in the adjacent segmental syndrome.[2–4] If surgeons perform fusion surgery with a concern for postoperative potential instability, too many fusions may be done unnecessarily. In addition, rigid fixation may fail to fuse in elderly, osteoporotic patients.

Interspinous implants have been invented to treat lumbar neurogenic claudication secondary to spinal stenosis.[5,6] The indication of Coflex—interspinous implantation—includes minor segmental instability in patients requiring surgery for either or both disk herniation and central spinal canal stenosis. It is implanted in the interspinous space, originally after removal of the interspinous ligaments and resection of their bony attachment. By preventing extension, it relieves the symptoms of lumbar spinal stenosis. However, it cannot be used as a substitute for a rigid fusion in cases of marked instability.[5]

◆ Product Design

French orthopedic surgeon, Jacques Samani, invented the Interspinous "U" in 1994.[7] The Interspinous "U" was renamed the Coflex, which is designed to be inserted between two adjacent lumbar spinous processes (**Fig. 34–1**). Coflex Interspinous Implant (Paradigm Spine, LLC, New York, NY) is a titanium device with a U-shaped body and two wings on each side. The device provides flexible support of the posterior column. Coflex is designed to permit flexion of the lumbar spine, although it restricts mobility in extension and rotation. Coflex can be applied from L1 to L5 (sometimes S1) because it needs the support of the spinous process. Coflex is available in five heights 8, 10, 12, 14, and 16 mm (**Fig. 34–1B**).

◆ Indications/Contraindications

The main controversy about the interspinous implant is its clinical efficacy. Because it is designed to prevent hyperextension, theoretically it can be utilized in any case in which extension aggravates the neurogenic pain. Degenerative spinal stenosis can be an ideal indication, whereas simple disk herniation or spinal stenosis with severe instability is not an indication of this implant. Overuse of this implant may lead to increased medical cost and prolonged operation time.

Until now, the indications for restabilization by interspinous implant documented by many reports are as follows:

1. Spinal stenosis with or without segmental instability

2. Intraoperative instability

3. Adjacent level to rigid fixation

4. Elderly patients or osteoporotic patients with segmental instability

Spinal Stenosis with or without Segmental Instability

We define the mild segmental instability on the standing x-ray lateral film as (1) degenerative spondylolisthesis, grade I ($<$ 4 mm in the sagittal plane), or (2) angular instability [intervertebral range of motion (ROM) $>$ 10 degrees or intervertebral angle (flexion) $<$ 0 degrees], or (3) mild retrolisthesis.

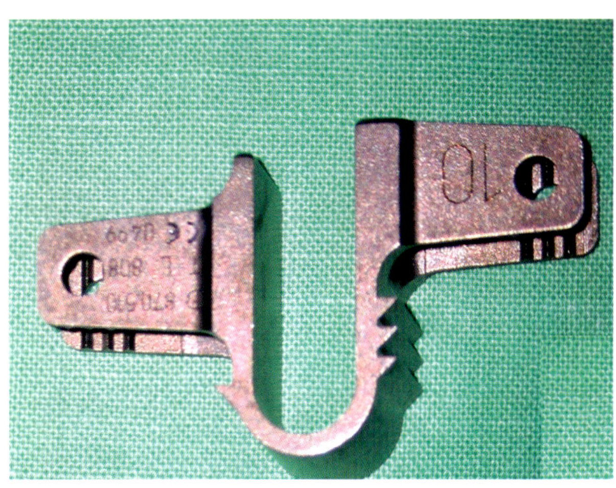 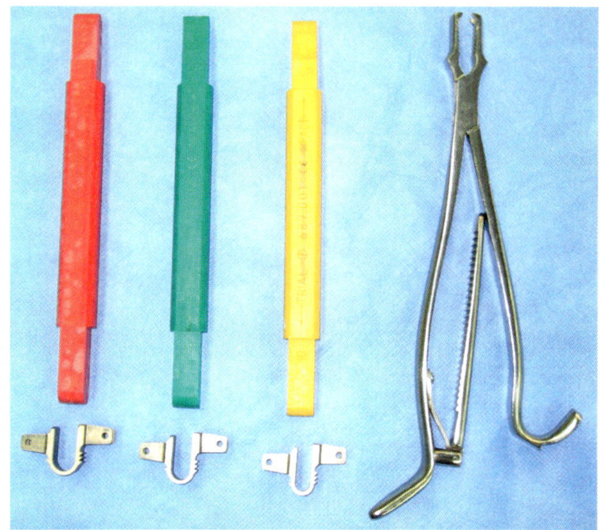

Figure 34–1 (A) The sagittal view of Coflex. This device is designed to be placed between two adjacent spinous processes. Implant migration is prevented by the clamping of the lateral wings. **(B)** Sizes of Coflex and its template.

In addition, this includes conditions that aggravate low back pain and develop referred pain by motion, even if there is no radiological instability.

Intraoperative Instability

Although preoperative evaluation reveals no instability clinically and radiologically, one may encounter segmental instability during surgery. This can be assessed objectively by placing active traction on the spinous processes utilizing clamps during surgery; a significant degree of motion induced by mild traction means decreased stability.[5]

Adjacent Level to Rigid Fixation

Coflex is designed as a cushioning mechanism adjacent to fusion as well as a stand-alone distractor for spinal instability.[7] It is not accurately known whether Coflex adjacent to long, rigid fusion may be effective or not, but this can be used as an adjunctive therapy for stabilizing levels above or below a fusion (topping off) to minimize adjacent level degeneration.

Elderly Patients and Osteoporotic Patients with Segmental Instability

Elderly and osteoporotic patients show lower fusion rates by rigid fixation. These patients tend to have more chances of complication such as loosening of screw fixation and failure of fusion. Therefore, Coflex can be an alternative of rigid fixation in these patients.

Meanwhile, contraindications of Coflex include severe segmental instability, progressive degenerative spondylolisthesis (grade 2 or higher), kyphosis, severe scoliosis, and isthmic spondylolisthesis. Although Coflex was applied previously in some instances, complications such as slippage of the device and progression of spondylolisthesis occurred.

◆ Operative Technique

The procedure for interspinous implantation of Coflex follows. The patient should be placed in the prone position with slight lumbar flexion on the Wilson frame. It requires a midline skin incision of ~4 to 6 cm. Paraspinal muscles are stripped off the lamina and interspinous ligaments and their bony attachments are removed with a rongeur (the supraspinous ligament may be resected depending on the surgeon's preference) (**Fig. 34–2A**). Foraminal decompression with partial laminotomy (microfenestration) can be performed if the surgeon so chooses. In some cases, herniated disk materials can be removed. Following relieving all points of neural compression, a trial is inserted to determine the appropriate implant size (**Fig. 34–2B**). Thereafter, an interspinous implant is introduced tightly with gentle hammering utilizing a mallet (**Fig. 34–2C,D**). Excessive distraction of the interspinous space by the implant may result in postoperative pain from a kyphotic posture. After confirming the purchase of the implant between the spinal processes, the wing clamps of the Coflex against both edges of the spinal process should be tightened (**Fig. 34–2E**). Finally, the proper depth is determined if a nerve hook can be passed freely leaving 3 to 4 mm separation from the thecal sac (**Fig. 34–2F**).

◆ Preliminary Results

Clinical Results

Samani reported that the Interspinous U (now called Coflex) was implanted in 106 patients who underwent surgery from 1994 to 1999.[7] In the follow-up of the 80 patients implanted as a stand-alone, 74% reported good or excellent results, 16% reported average results. Lim et al studied the clinical usefulness of Coflex in 50 patients with lumbar spinal stenosis.[8] They performed the procedure in patients

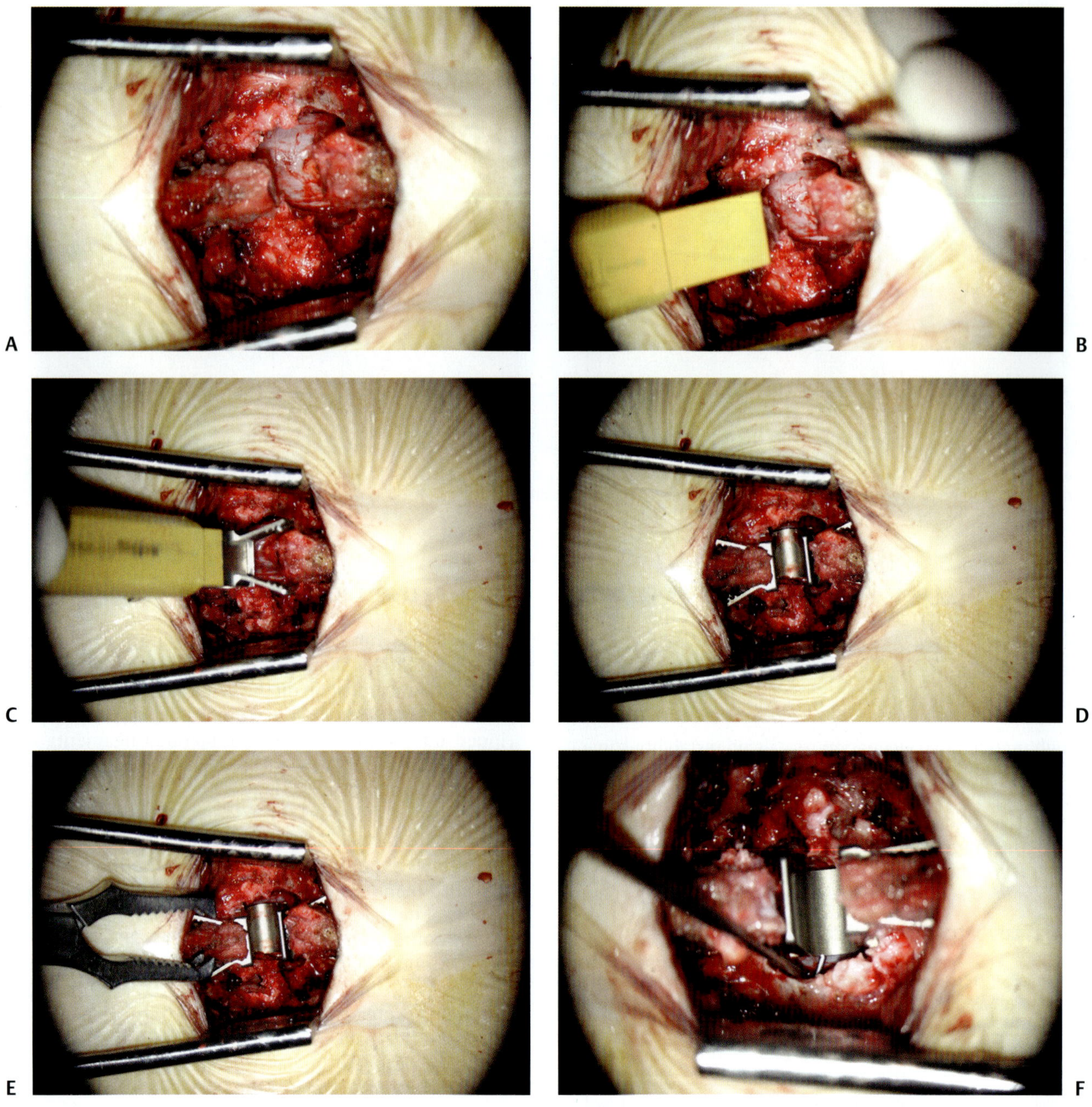

Figure 34–2 Surgical technique. **(A)** The interspinous ligament, its bony attachment, and ligamentum flavum should be removed. If needed, microsurgical penetration including partial laminectomy and foraminotomy can be performed. **(B)** A trial is inserted to determine the appropriate implant size. **(C,D)** The Coflex is introduced tightly with gentle hammering utilizing a mallet. **(E)** The surgeon should tighten the wing clamps of the Coflex against both edges of the spinal process. **(F)** Proper depth is determined if a nerve hook can be passed freely leaving 3 mm separation from the thecal sac.

with spinal stenosis with one or two levels (36), spondylolisthesis (11), and adjacent segment (3). They reported a good or excellent outcome in 88% of patients. Other authors showed similar results.[5,9]

We experienced a total of 42 cases of Coflex (**Table 34–1**). Most of these patients had spinal stenosis with mild segmental instability or were elderly patients who needed posterior fixation. Clinical outcomes were quantified using the visual analog scale (VAS) score for low back pain and leg pain and the Oswestry Disability Index (ODI). Follow-up at the outpatient clinic was after 1, 3, 6, and 12 months postop. In the follow-up

of 1 year, there was a significant improvement in the VAS scores for lower leg pain and low back pain in the interspinous implanted group ($p < .05$) (**Fig. 34–3**).

◆ Radiological Outcome

In our series, preoperative radiological data and their changes after surgery are shown in **Table 34–2**. The postop ROM at the instrumented level decreased significantly compared with the preop ROM (**Fig. 34–4**). Moreover, the posterior disk

Table 34–1 Demographic Data Obtained in Patients Who Underwent Coflex Implantation

	Coflex Group
No. of patients	42
Mean age (yrs)	60.5 (range, 40–71)
Gender Male/female	6/36
Mean follow-up period (months)	16 (range, 11–23)
Diagnosis	22
Degenerative SS	12
SS with minor instability Degenerative SDL, grade I	8

SDL, spondylolisthesis; SS, spinal stenosis.

Table 34–2 Preoperative, Postoperative Range of Motion, and Posterior Disk Height at the Instrumented and Adjacent Segments

ROM (degree)	L3–L4	L4–L5	L5–S1	PDH (mm)
Preop state mean (SD)	6.1 (3.8)	11.4 (4.1)	6.6 (4.8)	7.8 (1.8)
Postop state mean (SD)	5.7 (3.7) $p > .05$	6.4* (5.8) $p < .05$	5.5 (7.7) $p > .05$	9.1* (2.2) $p < .05$

*Significant statistically between preop and postop. ROM, range of motion; PDH, posterior disk height at L4–L5.

of severe back pain, some patients underwent further treatment such as rigid fixation due to aggravation of spondylolisthesis.[9]

height on standing radiographs increased significantly from preop 7.8 mm to postop 9.1 mm ($p < .05$). This result corresponds to other authors' reports.[8,9]

◆ Complications

Some complications, although rare, have occurred. However, slippage of the Coflex was the most common complication. Kaech and Jinkins and Samani reported cases of dislodgment at the L5–S1 levels due to the failure of the device to hold on to the sacral spinous processes.[5,7] Lim et al reported device loosening in seven of 50 cases.[8] In the period of 1 year, among a total of 42 cases in our series, there were two occurrences of slippage of the interspinous implant (**Fig. 34–5B**), one fracture of the spinous process (**Fig. 34–5A**), and three progressions of anterolisthesis. Inadequate removal of the ligamentum flavum and soft tissue was supposedly a cause of the slippage. Additionally, a forced trial of this device into already progressed spondylolisthesis can develop this complication. Although patients who experienced slippage of the device complained

◆ Discussion

Many cases of spinal stenosis are accompanied with degenerative spondylolisthesis, angular instability, and retrolisthesis. In these cases, a detailed microfenestration technique is required for effective decompression, which prevents progressed instability. If wider decompression is inevitable, surgeons should consider spinal fusion as well as decompression. Posterolateral or posterior interbody fusion is the current gold standard in surgical management of lumbar spinal instability.[10,11] However, restabilization of the spine is not without risks. Cunningham et al[12] reported a significant increase in intervertebral disk pressures after destabilization of the lumbar spine followed by stabilization with instrumentation. The motion segment is entirely immobilized following spinal fusion, and the adjacent segments are forced to flex and extend further to compensate for the lack of mobility at the instrumented level. In addition, pedicle fixation with screws often involves the posterior facet joint and may lead to damage in the motion of the upper segment. Several authors have observed that the interval to adjacent segment failure has been considerably shortened in patients who have undergone segmental fusion procedures in which instrumentation is used.[4,13,14] It was notably reported that a total of 18 out of 125 patients developed symptomatic adjacent segment degeneration at a previously asymptomatic level.[2] This risk appeared to be especially high in postmenopausal women. With regard to the potential damage to adjacent segments, some authors advocated nonfusion techniques, such as Graf ligamentoplasty or dynamic instrumentation, showing clinical and radiological outcomes similar to those for posterior lumbar interbody fusion (PLIF).[3,15]

The interspinous implantation is less invasive, and the preliminary clinical results appeared very satisfactory in those whose symptoms were deteriorated by extension.[5,6,16] In a prospective and randomized multicenter study, Zucherman et al[6] showed a success rate of 59% at 1 year postop with an interspinous implant. This result was much better than that of 12% in the control group in which only a conservative treatment was delivered.

In our series, ROM at the instrumented level was significantly decreased postoperatively. This means that the

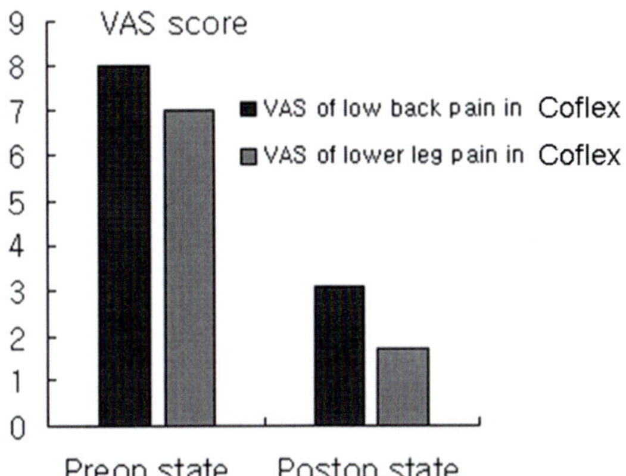

Figure 34–3 Bar graph showing the improvement of symptoms in the Coflex group after surgery ($p < .05$). A: Visual analog scale score, B: Oswestry Disability Index.

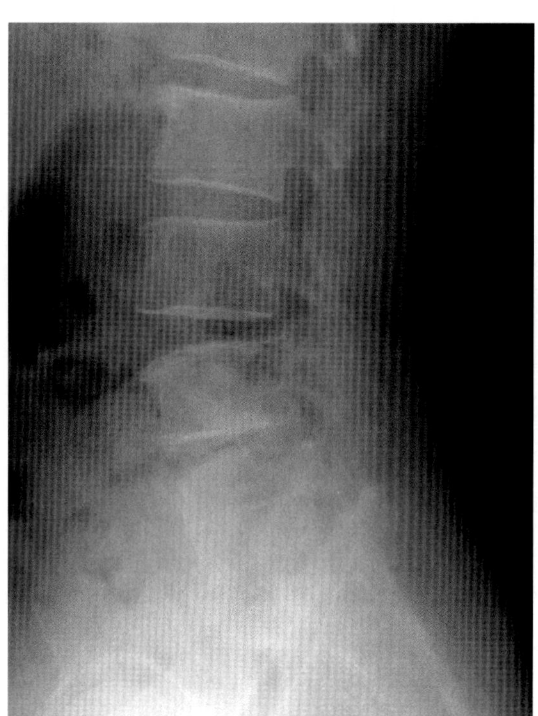

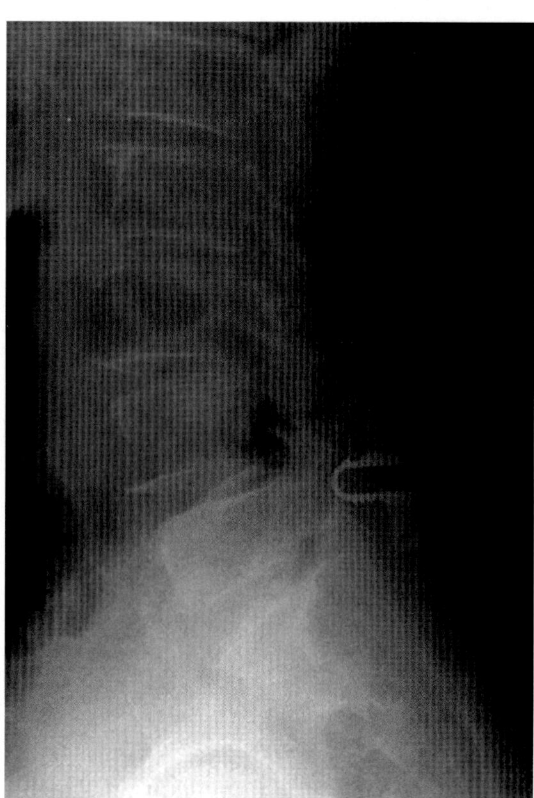

Figure 34–4   Radiographs showing the changes in range of motion after surgery in the Coflex-inserted patient. **(A)** Preoperative lateral x-ray films show the spondylolisthetic instability at the L4–L5 level.

(B) Postoperative flexion and extension images after Coflex insertion reveal improvement of the spondylolisthesis at L4–L5.

Coflex interspinous implant had some ability to restabilize an unstable segment. Remarkably, postoperative radiographs showed less change in ROM at the upper adjacent segment. We assume that interbody fusion renders a more stressful effect to the adjacent segment, which will consequently induce hypermobility and degeneration at the same segment. From this view, the interspinous implant may affect the adjacent segment less than the PLIF. Another biomechanical study showed an unloading of the disk at

the instrumented level with no effect at the adjacent levels with the interspinous distractor device.[17,18] Considering these advantages, the interspinous implantation can be more appropriate than PLIF in treating spinal stenosis with mild segmental instability. If a longer-term follow-up study yields a similar clinical outcome, this technique, which can preserve much of the normal anatomy and biomechanical function of the lumbar spine, will be highly indicated under selective circumstances. Furthermore, this minimally

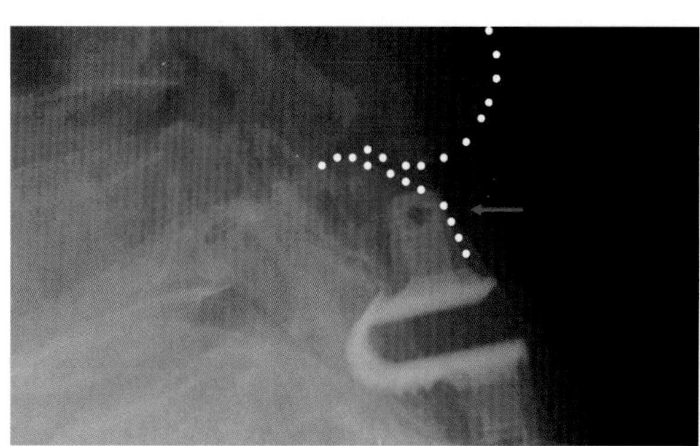

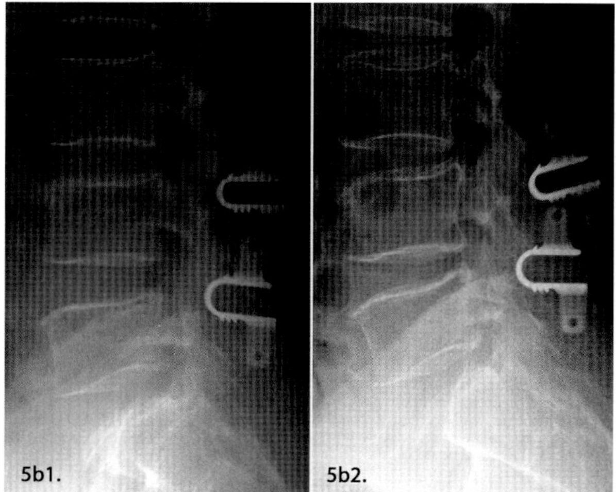

Figure 34–5   Complications of Coflex. **(A)** Radiograph demonstrating spinous process fracture following Coflex implantation. Dotted line represents the line of the spinous process fracture. **(B)** Radiographs showing dislodgment of the Coflex at **(B1)** 2 days postop and **(B2)** 7 days postop.

invasive surgery will benefit elderly patients with osteoporosis or other poor general conditions.

◆ Conclusion

Coflex appears to be a minimally invasive restabilization device appropriate for patients with spinal stenosis accompanying minor instability. In addition, it may be a substitute for elderly or osteoporotic patients who need decompressive surgery and posterior fusion. This procedure can be an alternative or superior treatment for degenerative lumbar stenosis with instability under selected conditions. However, longer-term follow-ups should be performed to prove the clinical benefit and cost effectiveness of this implant.

References

1. Verbiest H. A radicular syndrome from developmental narrowing of the lumbar vertebral canal. J Bone Joint Surg Br 1954;36:230–237
2. Etebar S, Cahill DW. Risk factors for adjacent-segment failure following lumbar fixation with rigid instrumentation for degenerative instability. J Neurosurg 1999;90:163–169
3. Kanayama M, Hashimoto T, Shigenobu K, et al. Adjacent-segment morbidity after Graf ligamentoplasty compared with posterolateral lumbar fusion. J Neurosurg 2001;95:5–10
4. Lee CK. Accelerated degeneration of the segment adjacent to a lumbar fusion. Spine 1988;13:375–377
5. Kaech DL, Jinkins JR. The Interspinous "U": a new restabilization device for the lumbar spine. In: Kaech DL, ed. Spinal Restabilization Procedures. New York: Elsevier Science B.V.; 2002:355–362
6. Zucherman JF, Hsu KY, Hartjen CA, et al. A prospective randomized multi-center study for the treatment of lumbar spinal stenosis with the X STOP interspinous implant: 1-year results. Eur Spine J 2004;13:22–31
7. Samani J. Study of a semi-rigid Interspinous "U" fixation system: 106 patients over 6 years. CD-Rom, Fixano, France, 2000, www.fixano.com
8. Lim DH, Kim DH, Park CK. Preliminary report about clinical usefulness of interspinous stabilization with Interspinous-U in lumbar spinal degenerative diseases. Kor J Spine 2004;1:450–455
9. Lim HJ, Roh SW, Jeon SR, Rhim SC. Early experience with Interspinous U in the management of the degenerative lumbar disease. Kor J Spine 2004;1:456–462
10. Bridwell KH, Sedgewick TA, O'Brien MF, Lenke LG, Baldus C. The role of fusion and instrumentation in the treatment of degenerative spondylolisthesis with spinal stenosis. J Spinal Disord 1993;6:461–472
11. West JL III, Bradford DS, Ogilvie JW. Results of spinal arthrodesis with pedicle screw-plate fixation. J Bone Joint Surg Am 1991;73:1179–1184
12. Cunningham BW, Kotani Y, McNulty PS, Cappuccino A, McAfee PC. The effect of spinal destabilization and instrumentation on lumbar intradiscal pressure: an in vitro biomechanical analysis. Spine 1997;22:2655–2663
13. Penta M, Sandhu A, Fraser RD. Magnetic resonance imaging assessment of disc degeneration 10 years after anterior lumbar interbody fusion. Spine 1995;20:743–747
14. Schlegel JD, Smith JA, Schleusener RL. Lumbar motion segment pathology adjacent to thoracolumbar, lumbar, and lumbosacral fusions. Spine 1996;21:970–981
15. Korovessis P, Papazisis Z, Koureas G, Lambiris E. Rigid, semirigid versus dynamic instrumentation for degenerative lumbar spinal stenosis: a correlative radiological and clinical analysis of short-term results. Spine 2004;29:735–742
16. Lee J, Hida K, Seki T, Iwasaki Y, Minoru A. An interspinous process distractor (X STOP) for lumbar spinal stenosis in elderly patients: preliminary experiences in 10 consecutive cases. J Spinal Disord Tech 2004;17:72–77 discussion 78
17. Lindsey DP, Swanson KE, Fuchs P, Hsu KY, Zucherman JF, Yerby SA. The effects of an interspinous implant on the kinematics of the instrumented and adjacent levels in the lumbar spine. Spine 2003;28:2192–2197
18. Swanson KE, Lindsey DP, Hsu KY, Zucherman JF, Yerby SA. The effects of an interspinous implant on intervertebral disc pressures. Spine 2003;28:26–32

35

DIAM (Device for Intervertebral Assisted Motion) Spinal Stabilization System

Kern Singh and Frank M. Phillips

- ◆ **Biomechanics**
- ◆ **DIAM**
  - **Mechanism**
  - **Indications**
- ◆ **Contraindications**
  - **Precautions**
  - **Contraindications**
- ◆ **Surgical Considerations**
  - **Surgical Technique**
- ◆ **Discussion**
- ◆ **Conclusion**

Spinal arthrodesis is frequently used to treat syndromes related to degenerative pathologies of the lumbar spine.[1–6] Inconsistent clinical results as well as substantial morbidities and complications have been reported following lumbar arthrodesis.[7–10] Biomechanical studies have suggested that the restriction of segmental motion resulting from spinal fusion causes abnormal kinematics at adjacent mobile segments, potentially leading to instability and accelerated degeneration at these levels.[11–13] In an attempt to eliminate problems innate to fusion surgery, the concept of dynamically stabilizing a diseased lumbar motion segment has been proposed. Theoretically, dynamic stabilization preserves lumbar motion while reducing abnormal painful movement.[13,14]

Total disk arthroplasty has been advocated as a *motion-restoring* treatment for pain arising from the intervertebral disk. Alternatively, posteriorly implanted, *motion-limiting* devices that reduce but do not eliminate motion have been widely investigated in Europe for the treatment of mechanical back pain and spinal stenosis.[15–18] Posteriorly-based, dynamic devices include (1) pedicle systems with tethers between the intrapedicular anchors and (2) interspinous process devices.

The first-generation interspinous process implant for nonrigid, lumbar stabilization was developed in 1986.[18] Over the past 20 years, several designs of interspinous process devices have been developed; however, the clinical indications for their use remain poorly defined. The clinical results with these devices have been reported only in anecdotal case reports, with varied indications and incomplete patient follow-up making meaningful interpretation difficult.

The Device for Intervertebral Assisted Motion (DIAM; Medtronic Sofamor Danek, Memphis, TN) is a silicone interspinous process "bumper" designed to provide facet distraction, decrease intradiskal pressure, and reduce abnormal segmental motion and alignment. The rationale for an interspinous spacer dynamic stabilizing device should be based on lumbar biomechanics and anatomy.

◆ Biomechanics

In the healthy spine, the majority of the compressive load is transferred through the anterior column, whereas only 18% is supported posteriorly by the facet joints.[19,20] Anterior compressive forces are distributed uniformly in simple and eccentric loading.[21–25] As the disk degenerates, however, nonuniform stress distributions can develop in eccentric loading, and the disk exhibits properties more characteristic of a solid.[19,26] Stress concentrations are directed toward the outer annulus and away from the nucleus. Advancing degeneration shifts load to the posterior elements of the spine.[27–29] Yang and King indirectly measured facet forces and demonstrated a significant increase in facet load for segments with degenerated disks.[30] The increase in facet load was greater as the eccentricity of the posteriorly applied compressive load increased.

The facet joints have an absorbing and stabilizing role,[31] with the axis of motion centered along the junction of the spinous process and lamina.[11,12] As disk degeneration progresses and anterior column support is lost, the facet joints bear more weight and the motion segment fulcrum moves dorsally.[32] Additionally, as the disk degenerates, it loses its biomechanical competence so that the facet joint becomes the primary restraint to translational and torsional moments across the involved motion segment.[33–35] This increased load concentration within the facet joints may accelerate facet degeneration and increase the likelihood of facet-mediated pain.[36,37]

Theoretically, an interspinous device should assist in the functioning of the diseased motion segment by providing stability and load-sharing the axial forces transmitted through the posterior elements. As such, if an elastic device is to be implanted to restore facet function its placement should be posterior.[16,17,32,38,39] The preloading of the implant should permit posterior tensioning restoring natural ligamentotaxis. An ideal shock absorber would be radiolucent and would display a nonlinear behavior in compression.[7,32,40]

◆ DIAM

Mechanism

The DIAM Spinal Stabilization System is a silicone "bumper" that is inserted between the spinous processes (**Fig. 35–1**). It acts as a shock absorber and displays nonlinear behavior.[17,40] The DIAM is designed to dynamically support the vertebrae while also maintaining distraction of the foramina. The DIAM will also restore posterior column height and share in load transmission, thereby theoretically relieving stresses on both the anterior and posterior elements of the spine. As a result of its interspinous position, the DIAM serves to realign the facet interface restoring its congruence (**Fig. 35–2A,B**). It is important to realize that the DIAM is designed to dampen the existing painful motion of the involved segment, whereas disk arthroplasty restores motion of a degenerated spinal segment.

The DIAM behaves as a pivot point for achieving spinal "balance."[7] With the DIAM implanted, resistance to flexion is controlled first by the stretching of the DIAM cable, followed by stretching of the posterior musculoligamentous structures. During extension, the DIAM continues to be loaded until reaching its limit of compressibility.[17,38,39] The deformability of the DIAM device allows for stress to be distributed evenly over the bony anatomy as opposed to a more rigid device. The deformability also serves to preserve motion in a passive capacity, reducing the potential for altered kinematics.

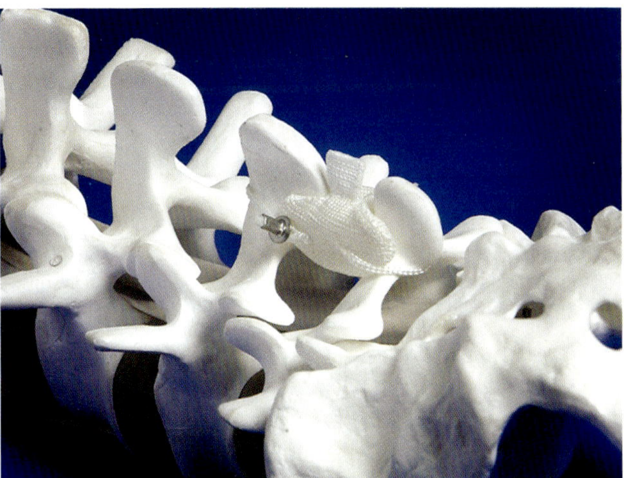

Figure 35–1   DIAM (Device for Intervertebral Assisted Motion) Spinal Stabilization System is a silicone "bumper" that is inserted between the spinous processes. (Image courtesy of Medtronic Sofamor Danek, Memphis, TN, 2004.)

Indications

Indications for the DIAM remain poorly defined and largely reflect individual surgeon biases. It would appear that the DIAM has been used in cases of disk herniation, spinal stenosis, and facet syndrome and disk dysfunction, and to dampen kinematic changes at levels adjacent to a fusion (known as topping off).

Disk Herniation

Hemilaminotomy and diskectomy are frequently used for the treatment of a symptomatic herniated disk. Although diskectomy is quite effective in relieving radicular symptoms, persistent mechanical low back pain is not uncommon.[33] Postdiskectomy back pain likely relates to underlying disk degeneration as well as the altered kinematics at the involved segment. Biomechanical studies have confirmed that a hemilaminotomy, partial diskectomy does indeed cause increased segmental angular motion over that seen in the intact state.[12,14] This nonphysiological motion may lead to altered stresses across the motion segment stabilizers, including the intervertebral disk, facet joints, and supporting musculoligamentous structures.[41] In a human cadaveric study, Phillips et al showed that the DIAM tends to normalize the altered motion segment kinematics seen after diskectomy.[14]

Spinal Stenosis

Acquired stenosis is the most frequent cause of neurogenic claudication. Retrolisthesis may worsen the stenosis. Implantation of the DIAM may effect indirect neural decompression by placing the motion segment in slight flexion, thereby increasing the spinal canal and neuroforaminal dimensions. In addition, the DIAM may mitigate dynamic stenosis by reducing motion of the involved segment. Although DIAM implantation may indirectly relieve foraminal stenosis or stenosis arising from soft tissue compression, it has been more typically combined with limited direct neural decompression.

Facet Syndrome and Disk Dysfunction

Dysfunction of the disk leads to posterior transfer of the loads to the facet joints.[19] The DIAM may play a role in preventing pain resulting from overloading of the facet joints by off-loading the facets and reducing motion.[15,16,38] Findings of facet dysfunction or overloading include the presence of hypertrophic facets, synovial cysts, and facet incongruity, which may also be inferred from laxity of the posterior interspinous ligaments with abnormal approximation of the spinous processes.[42,43] Taylor et al have described signs of posterior load transfer, including retrolisthesis and hyperlordosis, across the disk and have suggested these as possible indications for placement of DIAM at the time of diskectomy[14,32,40,44] (**Fig. 35–3A–C**).

Topping Off

Another potential application of the DIAM might be to dampen the changes in kinematics imposed at the levels

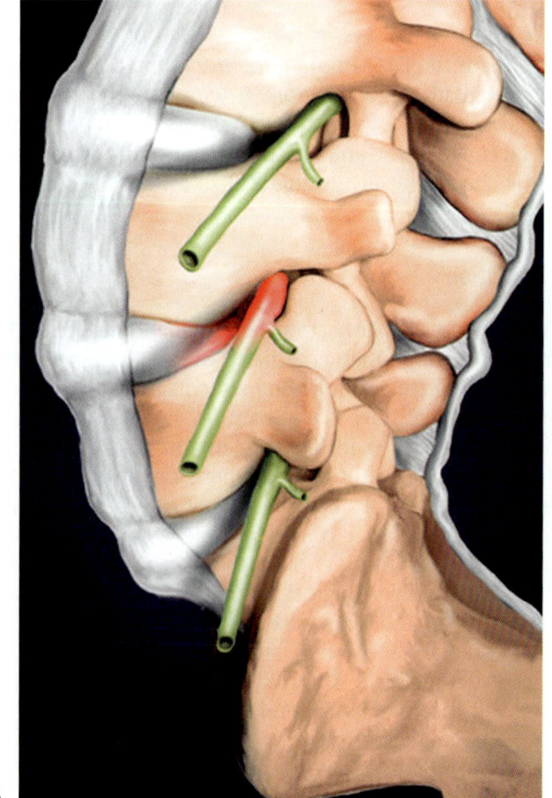

A

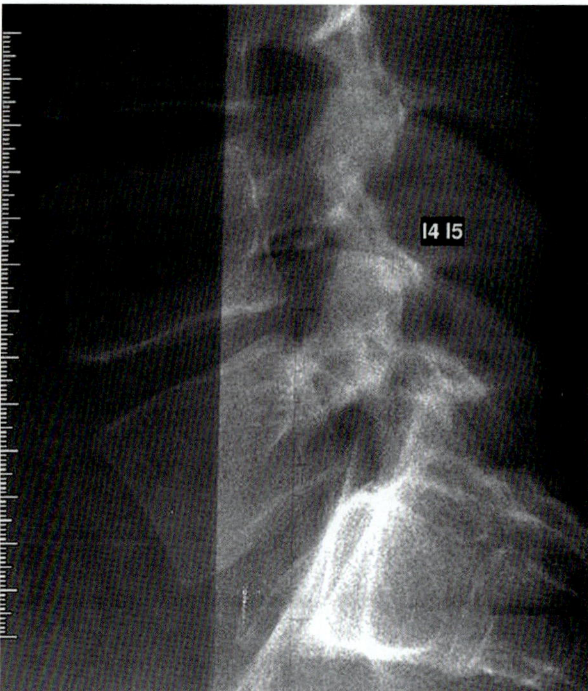

B

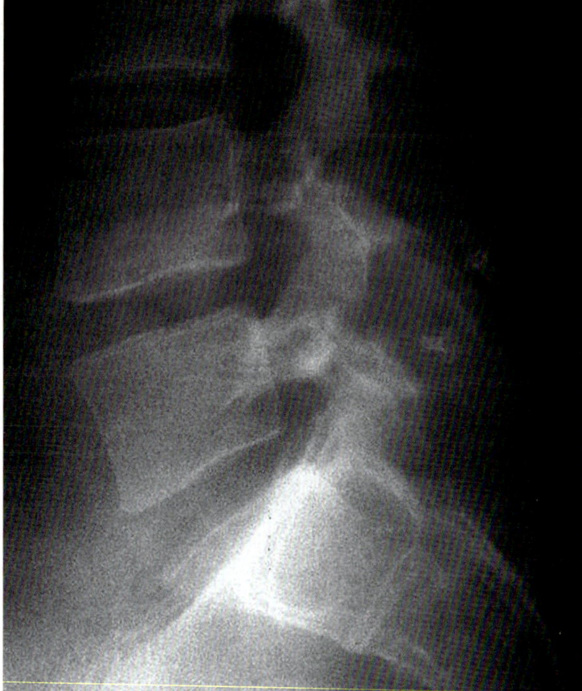

C

Figure 35–2   **(A)** A schematic of a patient with disk degeneration, loss of disk height and resultant facet subluxation causing foraminal stenosis. **(B)** A lateral radiograph demonstrating malalignment of the L4–L5 facets with **(C)** resultant correction and restoration of foraminal height after placement of the DIAM. (Image courtesy of Medtronic Sofamor Danek, Memphis, TN, 2004.)

adjacent to a fusion. Several authors have reported increased motion at the unfused segments above a fusion with the application of compressive and bending loads.[45] Similarly Shono et al reported significant increases in flexion-extension, axial rotation, and lateral bending at the segment adjacent to a single- or two-level pedicle screw construct.[46]

These studies along with clinical findings have contributed to the belief that the hypermobility and the altered kinematics at levels adjacent to a fusion predispose to accelerated degeneration of these levels that may become symptomatic. The ability of DIAM to stabilize the motion segment and at the same time not affect adjacent level kinematics may allow

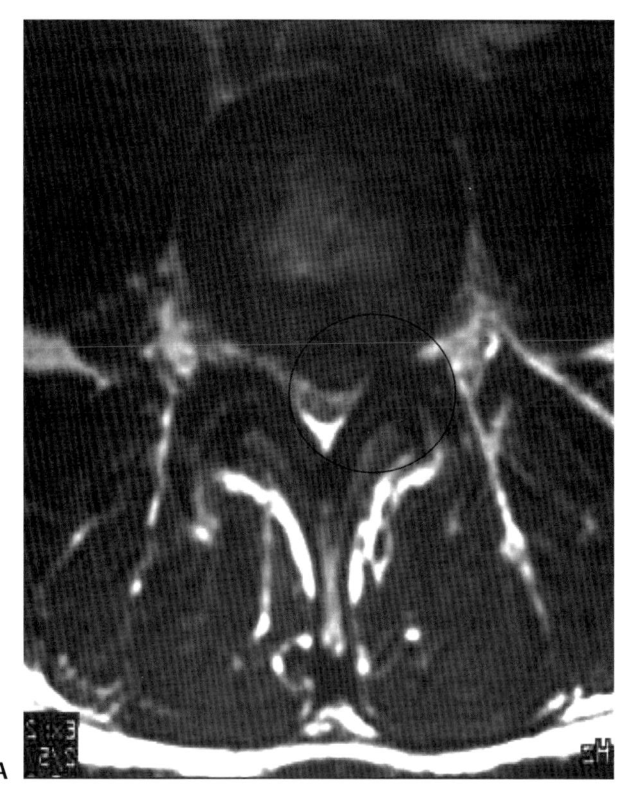

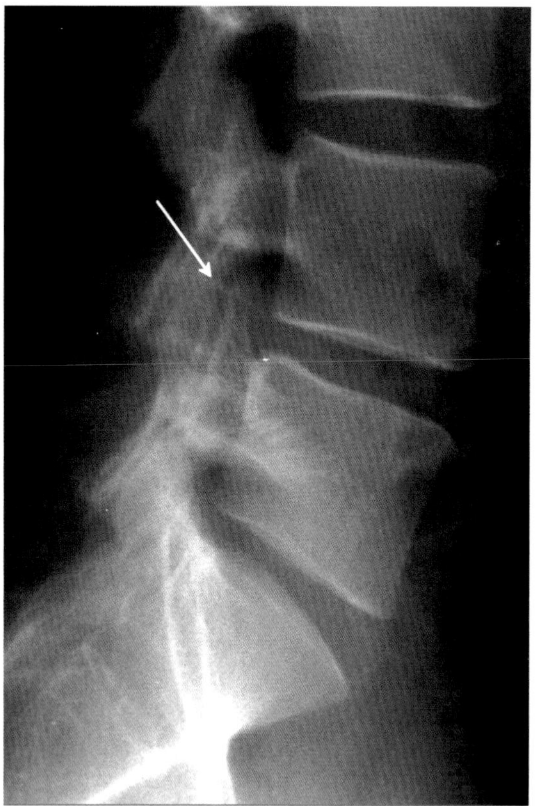

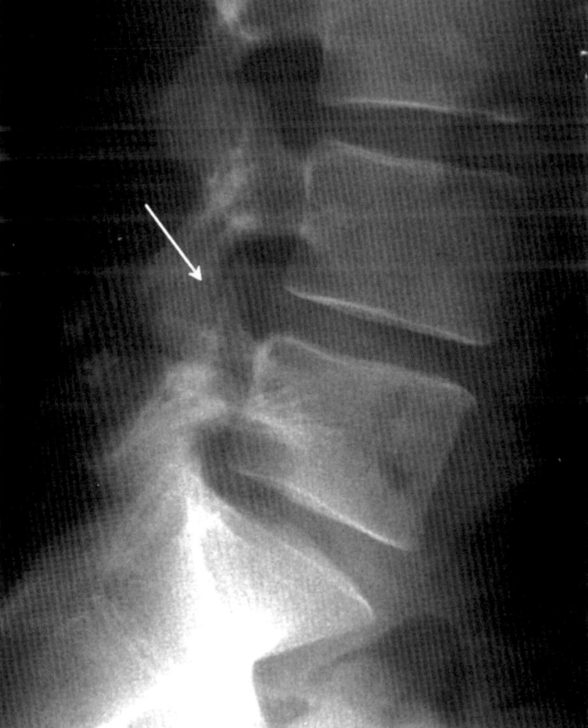

Figure 35–3 **(A)** Axial T2-weighted magnetic resonance imaging of the L4–L5 level demonstrating a left paracentral disk herniation. **(B)** A lateral radiograph of the same patient demonstrating subluxation of the superior facet. **(C)** A lateral radiograph of the patient after placement of the DIAM demonstrating reduction without kyphosis. (Image courtesy of Medtronic Sofamor Danek, Memphis, TN, 2004.)

for its use to gradually normalize load transfer across segments adjacent to a fusion and warrants further study.[14]

◆ Contraindications

Precautions

- ◆ Osteoporotic bone
- ◆ Stable degenerative spondylolisthesis (grade I)

Contraindications

- ◆ Isthmic spondylolysis
- ◆ Unstable spondylolisthesis ($>$ grade I)
- ◆ Neoplasia
- ◆ Fracture
- ◆ Significant scoliosis

◆ Surgical Considerations

Traditional fusion procedures disrupt the normal segmental paraspinal musculature, likely degrading the surgical outcome. As such, the DIAM conforms to the interspinous anatomy and allows placement with minimal disturbance of the paraspinal muscles through a simple midline approach with preservation of the segmental anatomy.

Surgical Technique

The most frequently involved anatomical level is L4–L5. The surgical approach is performed using a standard midline incision or a slightly lateral incision (10 mm lateral to the midline). First, anatomical lesions involving neurological compression are assessed. The use of a unilateral approach allows decompression of the nerve roots and spinal canal. A counterincision is necessary for insertion, preparation, and seating of the device.

Care must be taken to maintain continuity of the supraspinous ligament by preserving a band at least 10 mm wide and as thick as possible.[12] After identification of the interspinous space, resection of the interspinous ligament is carried down to the ligamentum flavum. A window is created in the interspinous space using a scalpel that is ideally curved upward; the window is then enlarged with a curved Kerrison taking care to preserve cortical spinous process bone (**Fig. 35–4**). This step is critical and requires caution. Using excessive force due to tissue entrapment may result in a fracture of the spinous process. In cases of overlapping and hypertrophic laminae (kissing laminae), trimming is recommended. Similarly, in cases of a kissing spine involving the spinous processes, trimming of the lateral hypertrophic aspects may be necessary. At this stage, the interlaminar distractor can be inserted as far anteriorly as possible at the junction between the base of the spinous process and the laminae (**Fig. 35–5**). It should be noted that during mechanical distraction, care should be taken to apply loads that do not exceed the bony stiffness. If resistance is felt, the

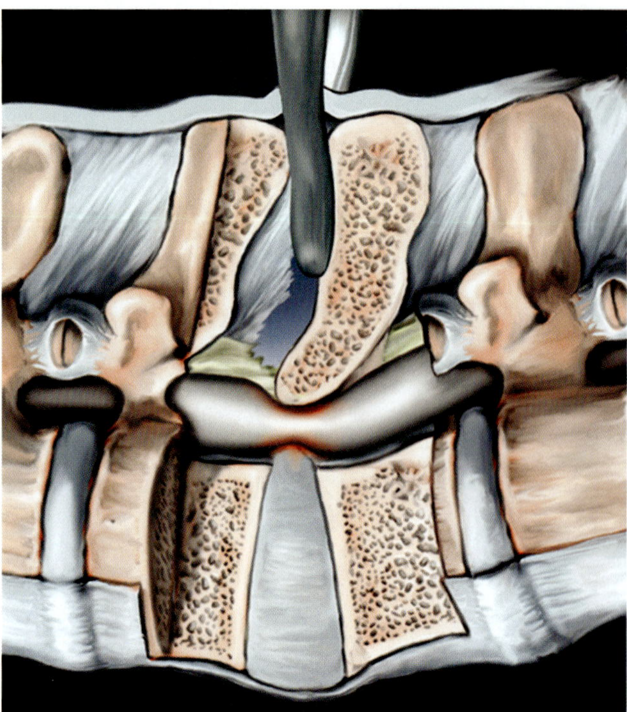

Figure 35–4 The interspinous space is prepared using a curved blade, curettes, and tissue resectors. (Image courtesy of Medtronic Sofamor Danek, Memphis, TN, 2004.)

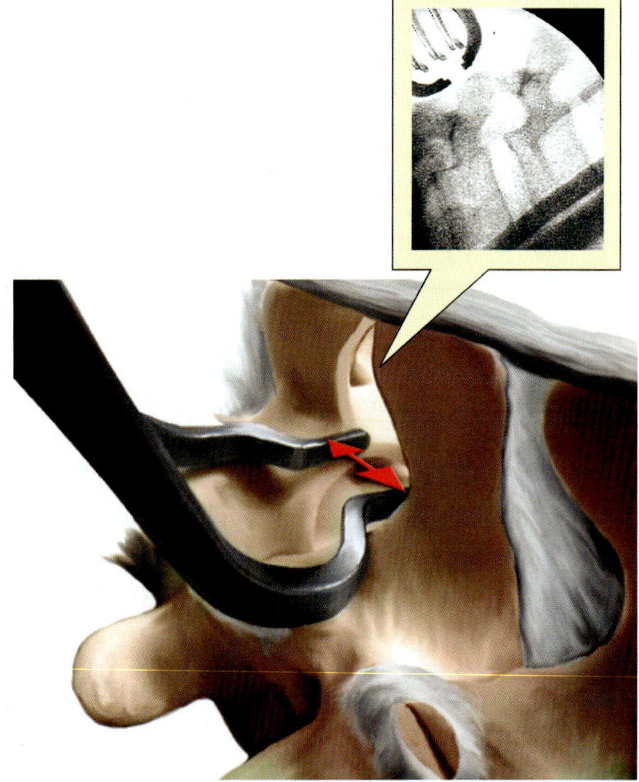

Figure 35–5 The distractor is positioned as far anteriorly as possible, ideally at the junction of the spinous process and lamina. The position of the end plates can be monitored by means of fluoroscopic imaging. The end plates should not go beyond parallel alignment. (Image courtesy of Medtronic Sofamor Danek, Memphis, TN, 2004.)

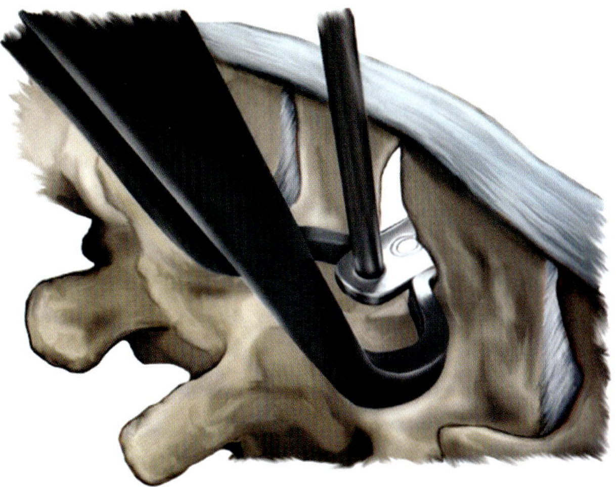

Figure 35–6   A series of templates is used to select the proper-size DIAM. The appropriate template should fit firmly within the interspinous process space. (Image courtesy of Medtronic Sofamor Danek, Memphis, TN, 2004.)

interlaminar bony bridges must be resected. Otherwise, fracture at the base of the spinous processes may occur, making implantation of the prosthesis impossible.

Implant Selection

The appropriate trial (sizes from 8 to 14 mm in 2 mm increments) is positioned between the grooves of the distractor to determine the implant size (**Fig. 35–6**). Proper fit of the DIAM should be based upon retensioning of the supraspinous ligament and realignment of the facets and articular capsule.[13] Excessive distraction might result in the creation of localized kyphosis and increased pressure on the disk. In situations where distraction cannot be accurately assessed visually, interlaminar distraction may be readjusted under fluoroscopic guidance. Parallel alignment of the end plates can be used as a reference for retensioning of the posterior longitudinal ligament.

Inserter

The implant is positioned into the claw of the inserter. Thus the implant can be easily inserted into the space previously created with the distractor. At this stage, the distractor may be used to temporarily overdistract the interlaminar space, facilitating insertion of the implant. While the implant is held firmly, the inserter is positioned in the interspinous space. Then the DIAM is passed beneath the supraspinous ligament. Next, the implant is inserted and driven to the opposite side with the claw. Pressing the trigger of the inserter both activates the claw and pulls back the arms of the inserter, allowing the wings to unfold and bringing them into contact with the spinous processes (**Fig. 35–7A–C**). The inserter can then be removed. In cases of spinal stenosis that have required a midline approach for decompression (partial laminectomy) with sacrifice of the supraspinous ligament, the implant is inserted from posterior to anterior without using the inserter.

Final Positioning

The impactor is placed on top of the implant and the DIAM is pushed down with gentle taps of the mallet. The distractor is then removed and the device is optimally seated as far anteriorly as possible close to the plane of the facets. Once the wings of the device are resting on the laminae, the tag is sutured to the supraspinous ligament.

Ligament Fixation

The posterior interspinous stabilizer is packaged with two independent ligaments that attach respectively to each adjacent spinous process. Each ligament is inserted into the adjacent overlying and underlying interspinous spaces and passed through the loop (**Fig. 35–8A,B**). The stiff portion of the ligament must be carefully sectioned obliquely with a scalpel to facilitate insertion of the titanium rivet. The rivet is brought down to the loop, tensioned, and secured with the crimper. The rest of the ligament is cut off and removed.

◆ Discussion

Although the DIAM has gained widespread popularity in Europe, the clinical indications for its use have been poorly defined. Few long-term studies and no prospective evaluations have been conducted thus far. Caserta et al evaluated its use in 61 patients with a mean follow-up of 20 months (minimum 12 months).[47] Preoperative diagnoses included degenerative disk disease, disk herniations, lumbar instability, spondylolisthesis, and spinal stenosis.[47] Because of the varied inclusion criteria, clinical conclusions are difficult to interpret. The authors reported that patients reported subjective pain relief that was noted postoperatively and continued to improve for a duration of 18 months.[47] No mention was given to the objective evaluation of pain.

Guizzardi et al implanted the DIAM in 50 young patients (< 40 years) who had undergone a simultaneous diskectomy for a herniated nucleus pulposus.[15] The authors noted that at 1-year follow-up, 45 patients (90%) demonstrated excellent results with no significant episodes of back pain and a return to work. Only five patients (10%) complained of back pain that caused them moderate discomfort. Retrospective studies were conducted by Schiavone and Pasquale and Barbagallo et al.[17,48] Barbagallo et al found a clinical improvement in 86% of patients (n = 26) at the 18-month final follow-up. Schiavone and Pasquale's findings were similar at 1-year follow-up, with patients reporting an 84% improvement in mechanical back pain without radicular findings.[17] It should be noted that all these studies were retrospective in nature with no clinical controls and no functional and pain outcomes assessments.

Taylor et al[44] recently presented a retrospective study of 104 patients who had the DIAM placed for mild, single-level stenosis. Patients were evaluated preoperatively and at 6 and 18 months postoperatively using the Dallas Self-Questionnaire. The authors noted a 6% (six patients) device-related failure rate, with five patients being revised with a new DIAM prosthesis, and one patient undergoing removal of the implant. Eighty-four percent of the patients had

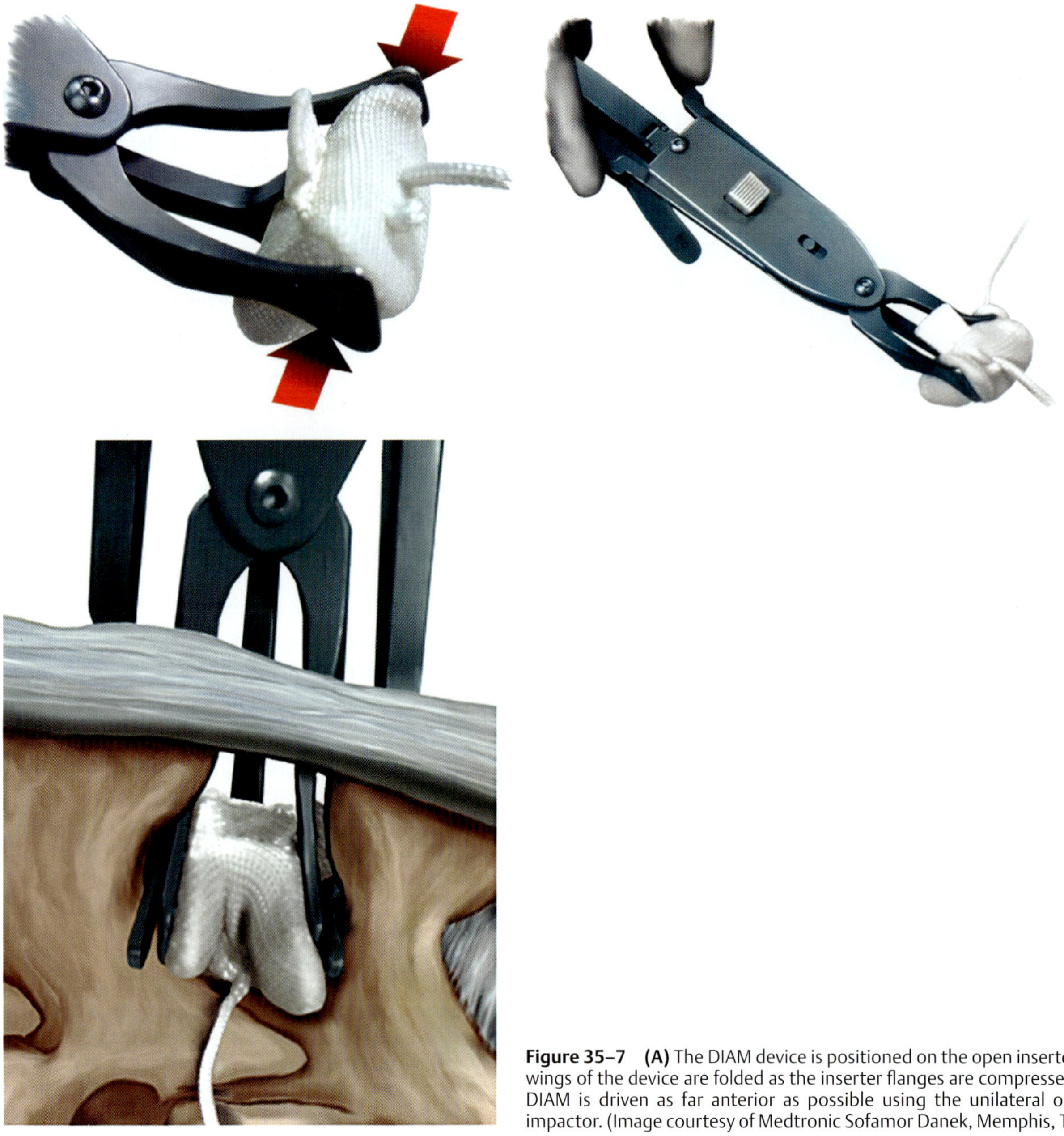

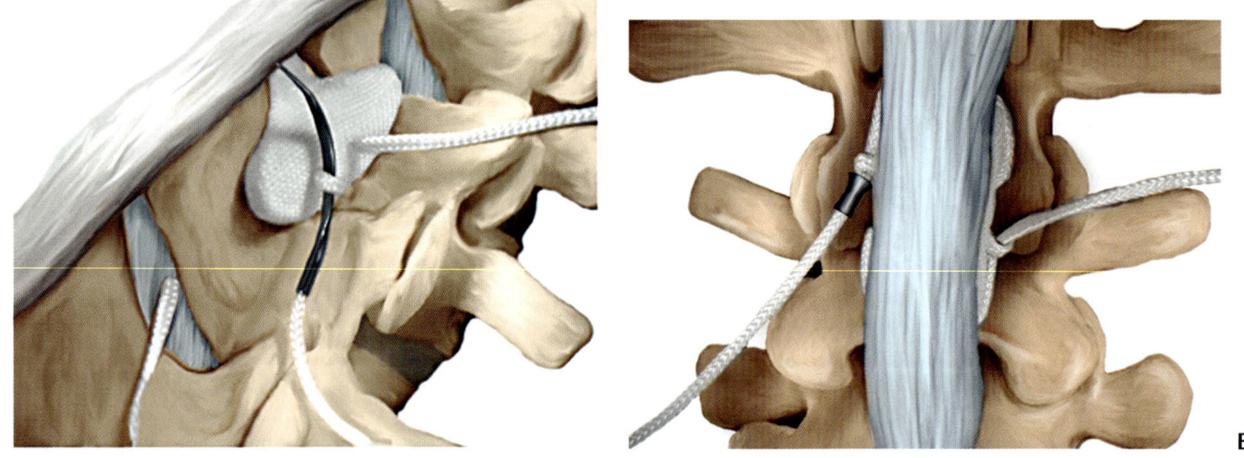

Figure 35–7 **(A)** The DIAM device is positioned on the open inserter. **(B)** The wings of the device are folded as the inserter flanges are compressed. **(C)** The DIAM is driven as far anterior as possible using the unilateral or bilateral impactor. (Image courtesy of Medtronic Sofamor Danek, Memphis, TN, 2004.)

Figure 35–8 **(A)** The DIAM is secured to the adjacent spinous processes by means of the tether. **(B)** Longitudinal tension is applied and a crimper is used to secure the rivets. The excess length is then cut. (Image courtesy of Medtronic Sofamor Danek, Memphis, TN, 2004.)

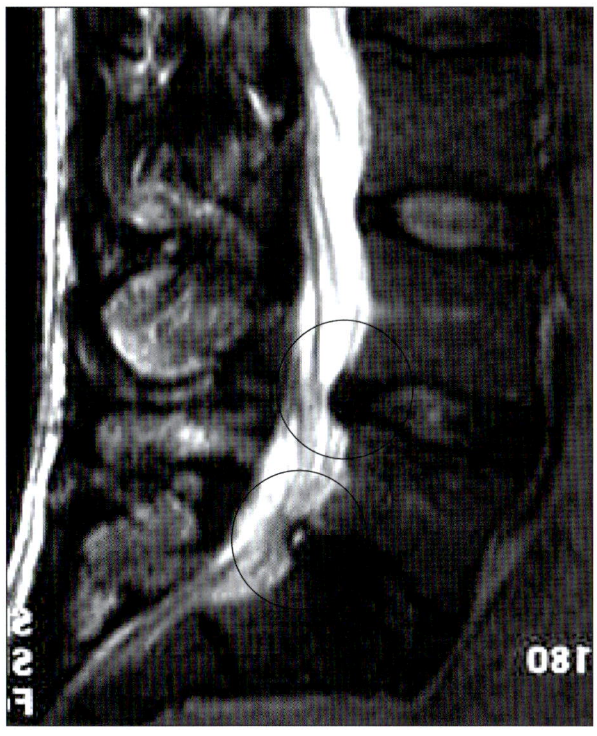

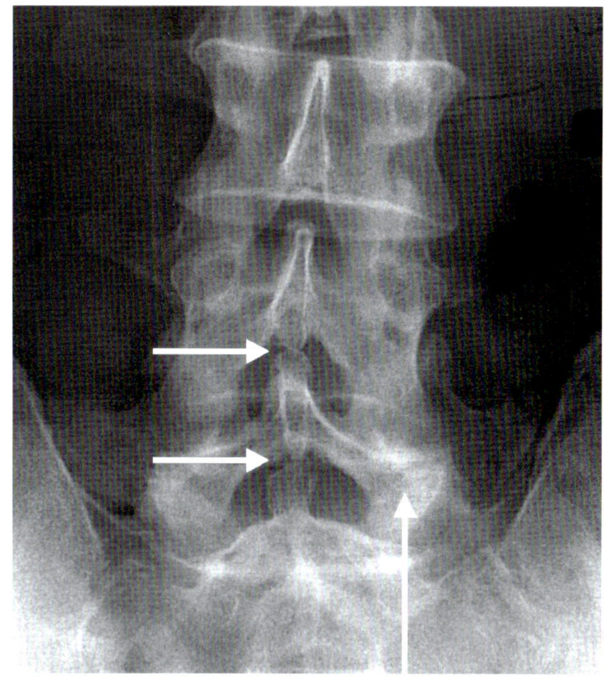

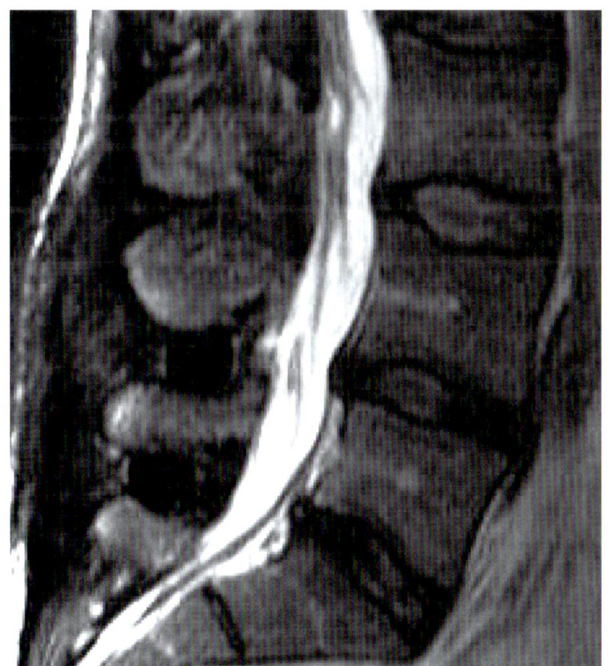

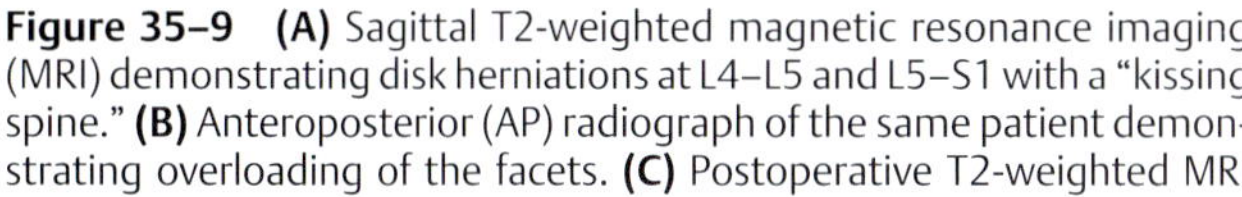

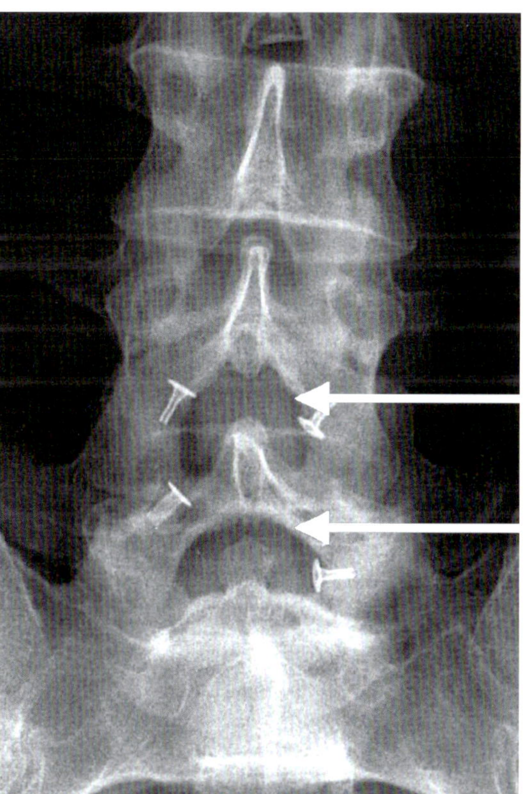

Figure 35–9 **(A)** Sagittal T2-weighted magnetic resonance imaging (MRI) demonstrating disk herniations at L4–L5 and L5–S1 with a "kissing spine." **(B)** Anteroposterior (AP) radiograph of the same patient demonstrating overloading of the facets. **(C)** Postoperative T2-weighted MRI demonstrating a two-level DIAM placement with off-loading of the facets. **(D)** AP radiograph demonstrating placement of the DIAM. (Image courtesy of Medtronic Sofamor Danek, Memphis, TN, 2004.)

Table 35–1   Total Flexion-Extension Range of Motion (deg) under 450 N Preload

	Intact	Facetectomy at L4–L5	Diskectomy at L4–L5	Diskectomy w/DIAM at L4–L5
L4–L5	8.8 (2.4)	9.1 (2.1)	9.7 (2.5)	3.9 (0.8)
P values (vs intact)[†]		*p* = .51	*p* = .12	*p* = .01
P values (vs diskectomy)				*p* = .01

The motion values are given as mean, with one standard deviation in parentheses, for flexion-extension moments of ± 6 Nm.

[†]Adjusted for four comparisons using Bonferroni correction.

Flexion-extension moments at L4–L5 were tested in the following sequence: (1) intact, (2) after unilateral hemifacetectomy, (3) after partial diskectomy, and (4) DIAM implanted.

improvement in pain relief as suggested by decreased medication usage and subjective self-evaluation. No implant migration and/or spinous fractures were noted at the final 18-month follow-up.

Phillips et al[14] tested the efficacy of the DIAM in stabilizing human cadaveric spines following unilateral hemifacetectomy and diskectomy using a follower-load construct. The results suggested that the DIAM stabilized the spines in both flexion and extension with behavior of the hemifacetectomy/diskectomy/DIAM group approaching motion of the intact spines (**Table 35–1**). Furthermore, the authors noted that in fatigue testing, the DIAM device survived at least 5 million cycles under physiological loads without generating harmful wear debris.

◆ Conclusion

Dynamic stabilization appears to be a useful technique in the management of degenerative conditions of the lumbar spine. Interspinous implants such as the DIAM may help reduce motion, widen intracanal dimensions, and off-load diseased painful facets. Clinical reports to date have been largely anecdotal but do suggest that the DIAM appears to provide symptomatic relief of degenerative back pain while also providing biomechanical stability (**Figs. 35–9A–D**). Interspinous implants will likely assume a specific role in a stepwise motion-sparing strategy in the management of the degenerating lumbar spine.

References

1. McLain RF. Instrumented fusion for degenerative spondylolisthesis: is it necessary? Spine 2004;29:170

2. Kuntz KM, Snider RK, Weinstein JN, Pope MH, Katz JN. Cost-effectiveness of fusion with and without instrumentation for patients with degenerative spondylolisthesis and spinal stenosis. Spine 2000;25:1132–1139

3. Hanley EN Jr. The indications for lumbar spinal fusion with and without instrumentation. Spine 1995;20(Suppl 24):143S–153S

4. Fischgrund JS, Mackay M, Herkowitz HN, Brower R, Montgomery DM, Kurz LT. 1997 Volvo Award winner in clinical studies: degenerative lumbar spondylolisthesis with spinal stenosis: a prospective, randomized study comparing decompressive laminectomy and arthrodesis with and without spinal instrumentation. Spine 1997;22:2807–2812

5. Fischgrund JS. The argument for instrumented decompressive posterolateral fusion for patients with degenerative spondylolisthesis and spinal stenosis. Spine 2004;29:173–174

6. Bridwell KH, Sedgewick TA, O'Brien MF, Lenke LG, Baldus C. The role of fusion and instrumentation in the treatment of degenerative spondylolisthesis with spinal stenosis. J Spinal Disord 1993;6:461–472

7. Taylor J. Nonfusion technologies of the posterior column: a new posterior shock absorber. Presented at: Spine Arthroplasty International Symposium. 2001, Munich, Germany

8. Tajima N, Chosa E, Watanabe S. Posterolateral lumbar fusion. J Orthop Sci 2004;9:327–333

9. Phillips FM. The argument for noninstrumented posterolateral fusion for patients with spinal stenosis and degenerative spondylolisthesis. Spine 2004;29:170–172

10. Bohnen IM, Schaafsma J, Tonino AJ. Results and complications after posterior lumbar spondylodesis with the "Variable Screw Placement Spinal Fixation System." Acta Orthop Belg 1997;63:67–73

11. Brinckmann P, Frobin W, Livbeth G, eds. Mechanical aspects of the lumbar spine. In: Musculoskeletal Biomechanics. 1st ed. New York: Thieme; 2002:105–206

12. Panjabi M, Goel V, Takata K. Physiologic strains in the lumbar spinal ligaments. An in vitro biomechanical study. Spine 1982;7:192–203

13. Ritland S, Petrini P., Phillips F. Rational and biomechanics of an interspinous shock-absorbing device in lumbar DDD. Presented at: The 11th International Meeting on Advanced Spine Techniques—Non-Fusion Techniques in Spinal Surgery. 2004, Milano, Italy

14. Phillips F, Voronov L, Gaitanis I. Biomechanics of posterior dynamic stabilizing device (DIAM) after facetectomy and discectomy. 2004 Conference on "Non-Fusion Technology." Chicago, IL

15. Guizzardi G, et al. The use of DIAM in the prevention of chronic low back pain in young patients operated on for large dimension lumbar disc herniation. Presented at: The 12th European Congress of Neurosurgery (EANS), 2003, Lisbon, Portugal

16. Iob I, et al. Axial-loaded CT scan and DIAM implants: an attempt to rationally approach instability in patients with failed back surgery syndrome. Presented at: The Congress of Neurological Surgeons—51st Annual Meeting. 2001, San Diego, CA

17. Schiavone AM, Pasquale. The use of disc assistance prosthesis (DIAM) in degenerative lumbar pathology: indications, techniques and results. Italian J Spinal Dis 2003;3:105–111

18. Sénégas J. Mechanical supplementation by non-rigid fixation in degenerative intervertebral lumbar segments: the Wallis system. Eur Spine J 2002;11(Suppl 2):S164–S169

19. Niosi CA, Oxland TR. Degenerative mechanics of the lumbar spine. Spine J 2004;4(Suppl 6):202S–208S

20. Oxland TR, Lin RM, Panjabi MM. Three-dimensional mechanical properties of the thoracolumbar junction. J Orthop Res 1992;10:573–580

21. Panjabi M, Abumi K, Duranceau J, Oxland T. Spinal stability and intersegmental muscle forces: a biomechanical model. Spine 1989;14:194–200

22. Panjabi M. Intrinsic disc pressure as a measure of integrity of the lumbar spine. Spine 1988;13:913–917

23. Panjabi MM, Krag MH, White AA III, Southwick WO. Effects of preload on load displacement curves of the lumbar spine. Orthop Clin North Am 1977;8:181–192

24. Panjabi MM, Oxland T, Takata K, Goel V, Duranceau J, Krag M. Articular facets of the human spine: quantitative three-dimensional anatomy. Spine 1993;18:1298–1310

25. Panjabi MM, Oxland TR, Yamamoto I, Crisco JJ. Mechanical behavior of the human lumbar and lumbosacral spine as shown by three-dimensional load-displacement curves. J Bone Joint Surg Am 1994; 76:413–424

26. Panjabi MM, Krag MH, Chung TQ. Effects of disc injury on mechanical behavior of the human spine. Spine 1984;9:707–713

27. Fujiwara A, Lim TH, An HS, et al. The effect of disc degeneration and facet joint osteoarthritis on the segmental flexibility of the lumbar spine. Spine 2000;25:3036–3044

28. Lorenz M, Patwardhan A, Vanderby R Jr. Load-bearing characteristics of lumbar facets in normal and surgically altered spinal segments. Spine 1983;8:122–130

29. Mimura M, Panjabi MM, Oxland TR, Crisco JJ, Yamamoto I, Vasavada A. Disc degeneration affects the multidirectional flexibility of the lumbar spine. Spine 1994;19:1371–1380

30. Yang KH, King AI. Mechanism of facet load transmission as a hypothesis for low-back pain. Spine 1984;9:557–565

31. Butler D, Trafimow JH, Andersson GB, McNeill TW, Huckman MS. Discs degenerate before facets. Spine 1990;15:111–113

32. Taylor J. Biomechanical requirements for the posterior control of the rotational centers (IAR). Presented at: The International Symposium Swiss Spine Institute, 2002, Berne, Switzerland

33. Dreyer SJ, Dreyfuss PH. Low back pain and the zygapophysial (facet) joints. Arch Phys Med Rehabil 1996;77:290–300

34. Fujiwara A, An HS, Lim TH, Haughton VM. Morphologic changes in the lumbar intervertebral foramen due to flexion-extension, lateral bending, and axial rotation: an in vitro anatomic and biomechanical study. Spine 2001;26:876–882

35. Fujiwara A, Tamai K, An HS, et al. The relationship between disc degeneration, facet joint osteoarthritis, and stability of the degenerative lumbar spine. J Spinal Disord 2000;13:444–450

36. Yamashita T, Cavanaugh JM, el-Bohy AA, Getchell TV, King AI. Mechanosensitive afferent units in the lumbar facet joint. J Bone Joint Surg Am 1990;72:865–870

37. Yamashita T, Minaki Y, Ozaktay AC, Cavanaugh JM, King AI. A morphological study of the fibrous capsule of the human lumbar facet joint. Spine 1996;21:538–543

38. Pupin P, Taylor J. Clinical experience with a posterior shock-absorbing implant in lumbar spine. Presented at: World Spine I, 2000, Berlin, Germany

39. Lindsey DP, Swanson KE, Fuchs P, Hsu KY, Zucherman JF, Yerby SA. The effects of an interspinous implant on the kinematics of the instrumented and adjacent levels in the lumbar spine. Spine 2003;28:2192–2197

40. Taylor J, Ritland S. Technical and anatomical considerations for the placement of a posterior interspinous stabilizer. In: Medtronic Sofamor Danek Technique Guide. Memphis: Medtronic Sofamor Danek; 2004;1–13

41. Kotilainen E, Alanen A, Erkintalo M, Valtonen S, Kormano M. Association between decreased disc signal intensity in preoperative T2-weighted MRI and a 5-year outcome after lumbar minimally invasive discectomy. Minim Invasive Neurosurg 2001;44:31–36

42. Iatridis JC, Setton LA, Foster RJ, Rawlins BA, Weidenbaum M, Mow VC. Degeneration affects the anisotropic and nonlinear behaviors of human anulus fibrosus in compression. J Biomech 1998;31:535–544

43. Ng HW, Teo EC. Nonlinear finite-element analysis of the lower cervical spine (C4–C6) under axial loading. J Spinal Disord 2001;14:201–210

44. Taylor J, Pupin P, Delajoux R. Retrospective study of the clinical results of implanting the DIAM spinal stabilization system. Presented at: Societe TEREO, 2004, Nice, France

45. Vuono-Hawkins M, Langrana NA, Parsons JR, Lee CK, Zimmerman MC. Materials and design concepts for an intervertebral disc spacer, I: Fiber-reinforced composite design. J Appl Biomater 1994;5:125–132

46. Shono Y, Kaneda K, Abumi K, McAfee PC, Cunningham BW. Stability of posterior spinal instrumentation and its effects on adjacent motion segments in the lumbosacral spine. Spine 1998;23:1550–1558

47. Caserta S, La Maida GA, Misaggi B, et al. Elastic stabilization alone or combined with rigid fusion in spinal surgery: a biomechanical study and clinical experience based on 82 cases. Eur Spine J 2002;11(Suppl 2):S192–S197

48. Barbagallo G, Alessandrella R, Barone F. DIAM: A new soft intervertebral implant for low-back pain treatment. Presented at: The 12th European Congress of Neurosurgery (EANS), 2003, Lisbon, Portugal

36

Tension Band System

Sang-Ho Lee, Ewy Ryong Chung, and Dong Yeob Lee

◆ **Components of Tension Band Systems**
   Artificial Ligament
   Artificial Ligament with Metal Interspinous Locker
   Biomechanics of the Tension Band System

◆ **Indications and Contraindications of the Tension Band System**
   Indications
   Contraindications

◆ **Surgical Techniques**
   Fixing the Artificial Ligament and Interspinous Locker
   Decompressive Laminotomy and Interspinous Locker
   Degenerative Spondylolisthesis and the Tension Band System
   Combination of Tension Band System and Other Soft Stabilization

◆ **Conclusion**

The spine can be considered a flexible, multicurved column. It has four major interrelated and somewhat disparate functions: to support, provide mobility, protect, and control. Mobility is required for the physical tasks of daily living, which affects the spine structures. The basic functional unit of the spine is termed the *motion segment*. The motions of the individual segments contribute to the total motion of the lumbar spine. A motion segment, also called a functional spinal unit, consists of two adjacent vertebrae with their shared intervertebral disk and facet joints.

The spine can be unstable. Instability may be a very specific diagnosis. Myriad biomechanical and clinical definitions have been developed to describe spinal instability.[1,2] At the most simplistic level, instability is a lack of stability, referring to decreased stiffness of the motion segment, excessive motion, abnormal motion, or, in some circumstances, simply painful motion. Instability of a motion segment is often called segmental instability. These descriptors are implicit in the definition given by the American Academy of Orthopaedic Surgeons, which states: Segmental instability is an abnormal response to applied loads, characterized by motion in motion segments beyond normal constraints.[3]

Segmental instability seems to be the cause of most of the problems that affect the vertebral column, whether they are fractures, fracture-dislocations, infections, tumors, spondylolisthesis, kyphoscoliosis, degenerative instability, or iatrogenic instability after decompressive surgery.[4] The goals of surgical management of segmental instability include stabilization of the spine, prevention of neurological injury, and relief of pain. Spinal fusion is the current gold standard in surgical management for lumbar spinal instability.[5–9] However, fusion with or without instrumentation has been shown to cause complications, such as damage to the spinal root caused by the pedicle screw, instrumentation failure, loss of lumbar curvature, new lesion development just above the area of fusion, and a higher incidence of wound infection.[10–14] In addition, the surgical procedure itself is complex and expensive. Motion preserving techniques will offer the opportunity to achieve intersegmental stabilization coupled with retained intersegmental mobility, a goal that is unattainable in fusion surgery. Dynamic posterior stabilization technologies have been reported in clinical studies since the 1980s.[15] Current dynamic posterior stabilization technologies fall into two main categories: interspinous process spacers and pedicle screw–based systems. The tension band system is an interspinous process spacer. There are two tension band systems: interspinous ligamentoplasty, originally documented by Senegas et al[16] and the artificial ligament with metal interspinous locker, developed by Lee et al.[19]

This chapter reviews the biomechanics of the tension band system, its indications, and surgical techniques used in tension band fixation.

◆ Components of Tension Band Systems

The tension band system is composed of an artificial ligament and interspinous spacer. Descriptions of the two tension band systems are described in the following sections.

Artificial Ligament

The artificial ligament (LIGANOVE Spine Ligament WSH Ba, Cousin Biotech, Wervicq-sud, France) is made of polyethylene terephthalate (polyester) and barium from polyethylene terephalate. It is 55 cm in length and 6.1 mm in diameter. Its

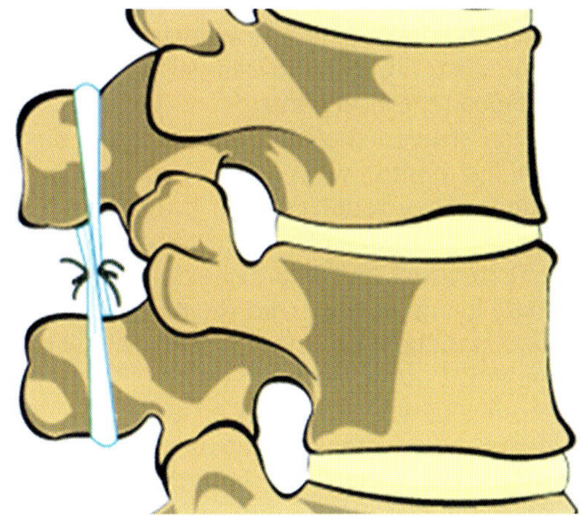

A

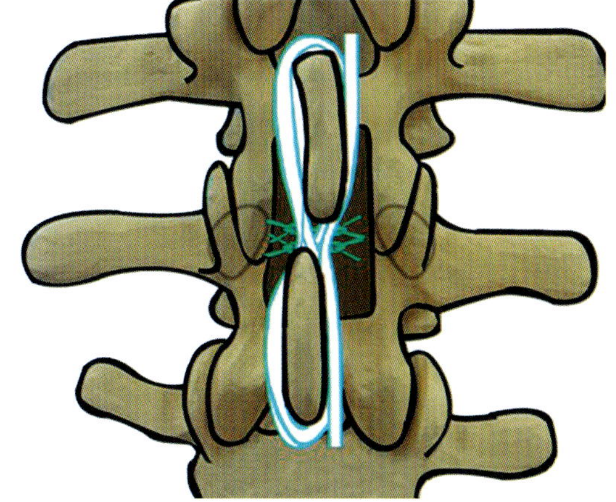

B

Figure 36–1 **(A)** Both upper and lower spinous processes are surrounded with an artificial ligament as a figure eight at the base of each spinous process. **(B)** After finishing bilateral partial micro-laminotomy and foraminal decompression, the waist of the figure eight is sutured several times just inferior to the upper spinous process and just superior to the lower spinous process with traction of the artificial ligament. This multiply sutured waist acts as an interspinous spacer.

extremities are prolonged with a traction thread and a needle. The artificial ligament is soaked in antibiotics mixed with saline before use. Both upper and lower spinous processes are surrounded with an artificial ligament as a figure eight at the base of each spinous process. The waist of the figure eight is sutured several times just inferior to the upper spinous process and just superior to the lower spinous process with traction of the artificial ligament. This multiply sutured waist acts as an interspinous spacer (**Fig. 36–1**).

Artificial Ligament with Ti-locker

This system combines artificial ligament with a Ti-locker. The interspinous locker is made of titanium. It is composed of four U-shaped flanges, a central hole, and a clip. The flanges enclose the spinous process, restricting the migration of the locker. The flanges also prevent the lateral translation of the locker. The artificial ligament passes through the central hole and surrounds both the upper and the lower spinous process as a figure eight. The clip tightens the artificial ligament to prevent loosening (**Fig. 36–2**).

Biomechanics of the Tension Band System

The spinal column complex consists of ventrally located vertebral bodies and intervening intervertebral disks that collectively assume most of the axial load–bearing responsibilities of the spine. The pedicle connects the ventral and dorsal components of each spinal segment. The laminae provide the roof for the spinal canal; the facet joints limit rotation, flexion, extension, lateral bending, and translation. The ligaments provide for and limit torso movement. The

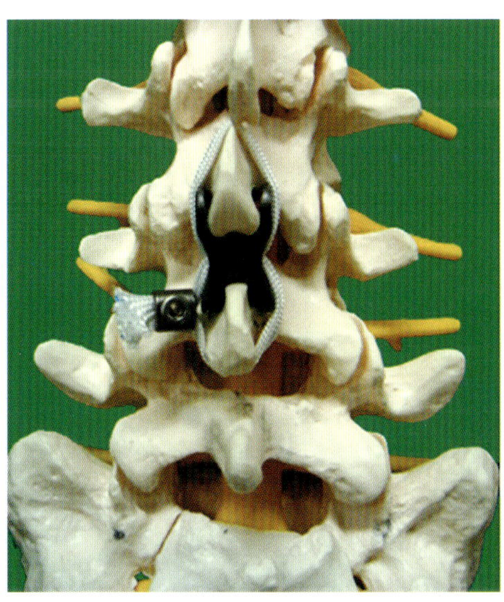

A

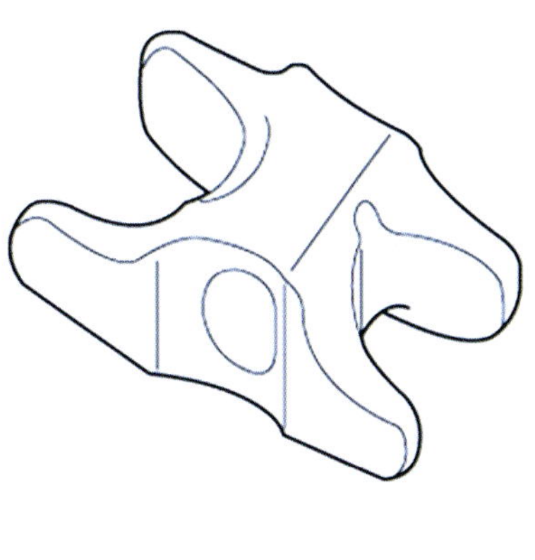

B

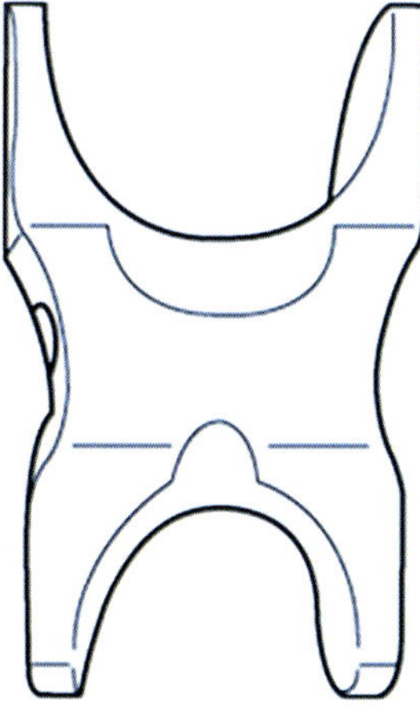

C

Figure 36–2 **(A)** Artificial ligament and titanium interspinous locker. **(B)** An oblique drawing showing a central hole and unique curve for creating lordosis. **(C)** An anteroposterior view presenting four U-shaped flanges.

ligaments also provide varying degrees of support for the spine.[20] The effectiveness of a ligament depends on the moment arm through which it acts.[21] Although the interspinous and supraspinatus ligament are not substantial, their attachment to a bone with a relatively long lever arm (spinous process) allows the applications of a significant flexion-resisting force to the spine by virtue of the significant distance between the instant axis of rotation and the point of the attachment of the ligament to the spinous process.

Many instability-definition schemes are based on a column concept to quantitate the extent of spinal integrity and to ultimately determine the presence or absence of spinal instability. The three columns of Denis[22] are conceptually useful. Denis's three-column theory, which adds the concept of a middle column to the anterior and posterior columns, allows specific assessment of that component of the spinal column in the region of the neutral axis. The neutral axis is the region of the spinal column about which spinal element distraction or compression does not occur with flexion or extension. Usually, the neutral axis is located in the region of the midposterior aspect of the vertebral body and the intervening disk; that is, the middle column.

The principle of the tension band system is borrowed from engineering (**Fig. 36–3**). If the spinal column is subjected to eccentric loading on the anterior column, we have not only the axial compressive stresses but also additional bending stresses that give rise to further compressive stresses on the anterior column and tensile stresses on the posterior column, which may contribute to the anterior sliding of vertebrae in degenerative conditions. These bending stresses can be neutralized by a chain (the posterior interspinous and supraspinatus ligaments) prestressed to exert a force equal and opposite to the weight. The tension band system can place an artificial ligament and its blocks in the posterior column, maintaining equilibrium when the anterior sliding is present. In some cases, degenerative changes of the intervertebral disk may result in the subsidence of the posterior part of the disk, which causes the posterior sliding of vertebra, referred to as retrolisthesis. In retrolisthesis, a repositioning

of facet joints has occurred and the facet joints bear abnormal loading. In the tension band system, an artificial ligament and its blocks in the posterior column can restore segmental alignment and unload the facet joints.

Voydeville et al studied the biomechanics of a similar type of artificial ligament in vitro on six functional human L4–L5 spinal units. They reported on a flexible, soft type of stabilization with artificial ligament–limited flexion-extension, axial rotation, and lateral flexion.[23,24] In addition, the artificial ligament corrected the narrowing of the spinal canal and stabilized the motion segment such that the canal remained at the appropriate width.[24,25] Papp et al studied the biomechanical effects of a flexible polyester artificial ligament.[22] Although their study used a hook system, the material used to construct the ligament is identical. Papp's study found that the ligament reinforced the posterior structure of the lumbar motion segment. Even though the material used to construct the ligament is soft and flexes with the patient's spine, it restricts 80% of the patient's motion and provides great stability through facet locking and through the retention of the body's own stabilization structures.

◆ Indications and Contraindications of the Tension Band System

The tension band system preserves the stabilization components[17]: the spinous process, the supraspinatus ligament, the posterior longitudinal ligaments, and the posterior annulus. The tension band system adds stability in these stabilizing components and restores the spinal alignment in the unstable spine, which can decompress the nerve roots by opening up the intervertebral foramen and spinal canal. The artificial ligament and Ti-locker in the posterior column can distract the affected spinal segment in lordotic posture, which allows unloading of the disk space and reduces the pressure on the facet joints,[26] resulting in the relief of back pain. However, the tension band system needs its bony anchor.

Indications

The tension band system can be applied in grade I degenerative spondylolisthesis without sagittal facet orientation, retrolisthesis, recurrent disk herniation, herniated disk with spinal stenosis, herniated disk with segmental instability, central canal stenosis, bilateral lateral recess stenosis, painful disk degeneration with segmental instability, adjacent lesion in instrumented fusion, and mild localized degenerative scoliosis or kyphosis.

Contraindications

The tension band system cannot work in postlaminectomy instability, degenerative spondylolisthesis with sagittal facet orientation, degenerative spondylolisthesis more than grade II, isthmic spondylolisthesis, retrolisthesis of more than 10 mm, severed disk collapse, spinal stenosis requiring total facetectomy, progressive or severe scoliosis or kyphosis, trauma, and tumors.

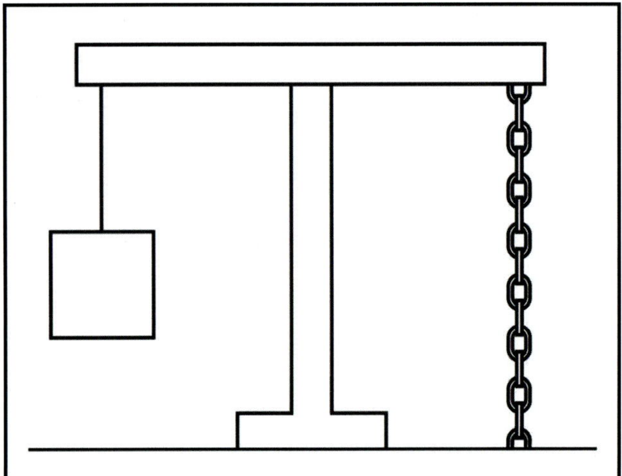

Figure 36–3   Tension band principle. The axial load, which gives rise to tensile stress on the opposite side, can be neutralized by a chain.

◆ Surgical Techniques

Fixing the Artificial Ligament and Interspinous Locker

Usually the tension band system can be applied from L1 down to L5. The L5–S1 stabilization requires the ligament fixing on the sacrum to be made with two intended staples because of the small or absent spinous process of S1.

The patient is initially placed in a prone position with flexion of the spinal column. Muscle stripping and retraction are limited from the lower half of the upper laminar to the upper half of the lower laminar and facet plane laterally. The interspinous ligaments are removed without violation of the two spinous processes. The supraspinatus ligament is detached from the tip of both spinous processes. An osteotomy of the spinous process tip can facilitate the detachment. Decompressive laminotomy can be done if needed. The interspinous locker is inserted between both spinous processes. After a soak in antibiotics mixed with saline, the artificial ligament is passed through the central hole, and both spinous processes are surrounded with an artificial ligament as a figure eight at the base of the spinous process. The interspinous locker and artificial ligament must be introduced as deep as possible, just level with the basis of the spine. After changing the position of the patient spine from flexion to extension, each traction thread is passed through the clip and pulled in opposite directions. The clip is locked, and both extremities of the ligament are additionally sutured, one next to the other, with nonabsorbable thread. The supraspinatus ligament is reattached onto both spinous processes with holding sutures (**Figs. 36–2** and **36–4**).

If the interspinous locker is not used, the posterior ligament complex should remain intact. The artificial ligament is introduced with a dissector under the interspinous ligament. Then both spinous processes are surrounded with an artificial ligament as a figure eight at the base of the spinous process. After changing the position of the patient spine from flexion to extension, each traction thread is pulled in opposite directions. The waist of the figure eight is sutured at least two times just inferior to the upper spinous process and just superior to the lower spinous process with traction of the artificial ligament. This multiply sutured waist acts as an interspinous spacer without bone erosion, which may be expected in a Ti-locker (**Figs. 36–1** and **36–5**).

Decompressive Laminotomy and Interspinous Locker

Lumbar stenosis is a common degenerative process among the elderly and can significantly limit their quality of life. Previously published data indicate that surgical decompression of stenosis can dramatically improve the patient's quality of life.[27] The traditional treatment of lumbar stenosis entails an extensive resection of posterior spinal elements such as the interspinous ligaments, spinous processes, bilateral lamina, portions of the facet joints and capsule, and the ligamentum flavum. However, such extensive open decompression is associated with significant pain, hospitalization, morbidity, a prolonged recovery period, and an increased incidence of medical complications in the elderly. Loss of the midline supraspinous/interspinous ligament complex can lead to a loss of flexion stability, thereby increasing the risk of delayed spinal instability.[28,29] Minimally invasive techniques may effectively reduce operative tissue damage and, therefore, prove to be an important tool in decreasing the risk of undesirable delayed spinal instability. Unilateral open laminotomy for bilateral decompression[30] can spare most of the lamina, spinous processes, and posterior ligament complex and help to preserve the biomechanical integrity of the spine while maintaining a good surgical outcome.[31]

The interspinous locker can facilitate this unilateral open laminotomy for bilateral decompression. After exposure, the interspinous ligament is removed and the supraspinous ligament is detached. The base of the spinous process is drilled out and extended laterally to unroof the lower laminar and

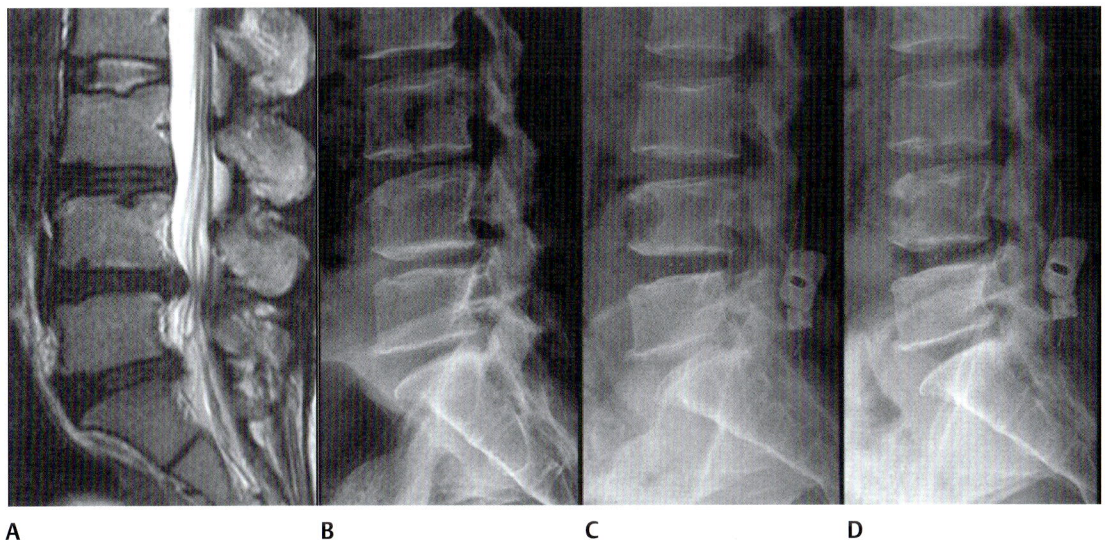

A   **B**   **C**   **D**

Figure 36–4   A 37-year-old female with intractable back pain for 8 years. She had disk degeneration with segmental instability. Combined surgery with a prosthetic disk nucleus to treat discogenic back pain and tension band fixation for instability was performed.   **(A)** Preoperative sagittal magnetic resonance imaging. **(B)** Preoperative lateral radiographs. **(C)** Postoperative flexion and **(D)** extension radiographs showing improovemnt of local kyphosis.

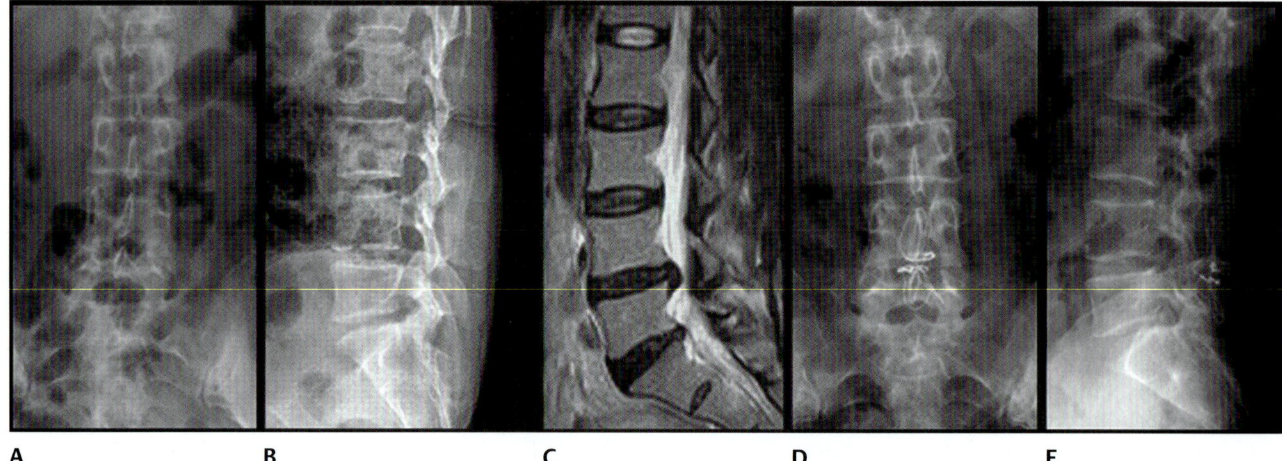

A   B   C   D   E

Figure 36–5 A 55-year-old female with a herniated disk and segmental instability at L4–L5. Microdiskectomy and the artificial ligament fixation were performed. **(A)** Preoperative anteroposterior and **(B)** lateral flexion radiographs. **(C)** Preoperative sagittal magnetic resonance imaging. **(D)** Postoperative anteroposterior and **(E)** lateral radiographs.

hypertrophied facets. A unilateral laminotomy, ipsilateral medial facetectomy, and foraminotomy are performed. Because the interspinous ligament is removed and the supraspinatus ligament is detached, complete ipsilateral foraminal decompression and ipsilateral decompression of an exiting nerve root as well as a traversing root can be obtained from the contralateral side without total facetectomy (**Figs. 36–6, 36–7, and 36–8**). The base of the spinous process is then undercut to permit progressive contralateral visualization. Once the contralateral pedicle is encountered, the bony decompression is deemed completed. The ligamentum flavum is resected, thereby exposing the neural elements. After decompressive laminotomy, the interspinous locker is inserted and fixed as described in the previous section.

Degenerative Spondylolisthesis and the Tension Band System

For several years, decompressive laminectomy has been performed either alone or with pedicle screw fixation to treat degenerative spondylolisthesis. Unfortunately, decompressive laminectomy alone for the treatment of degenerative spondylolisthesis with symptomatic spinal stenosis often leads to increased postoperative slip or segmental instability, which compromises the functional ability of the patient over time.[32-34] Consequently, fusion should be performed to improve the outcome for such patients.[35,36] As minimally invasive techniques are becoming increasingly important in the treatment of degenerative conditions and the applications of dynamic stabilization techniques are continually increasing, low-grade degenerative spondylolisthesis can be managed successfully without fusion (**Fig. 36–9**). Fassio et al encountered no complications in counteracting chronic instability due to degenerative disk disease.[37] Lee and Kim reported that the tension band system with an artificial ligament had a better clinical outcome in grade I degenerative spondylolisthesis compared with conventional rigid fixation such as posterior lumbar interbody fusion or posterolateral fusion with pedicle screw fixation. They concluded that soft stabilization with the tension band system

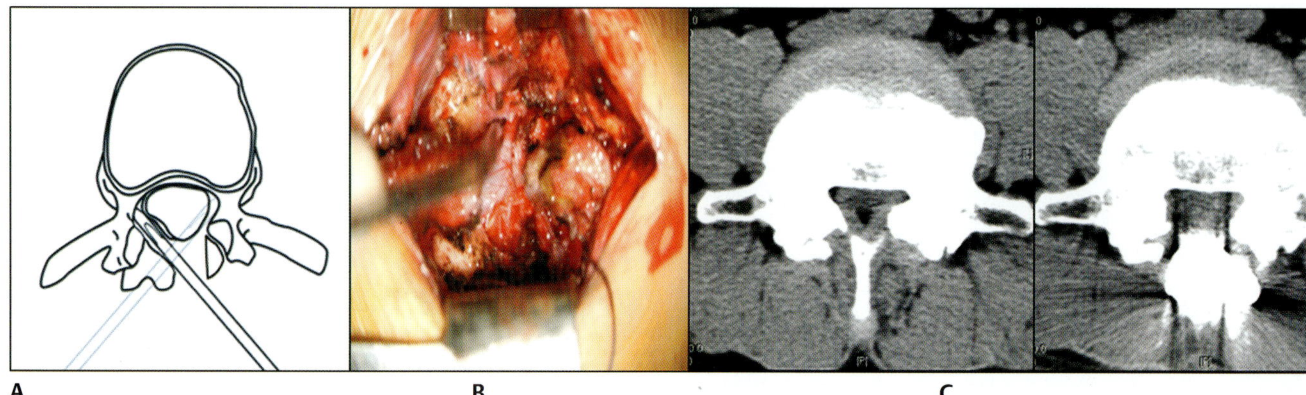

A   B   C

Figure 36–6 After the supraspinous ligament is detached and the interspinous ligament is removed, both ipsilateral and contralateral foraminotomy is performed, while preserving the contralateral facet joints. The removal of interspinous ligament can facilitate the unilateral open laminotomy for bilateral decompression through the existing physiological midline space. **(A)** Illustrative drawing. **(B)** Interoperative photograph. **(C)** Preoperative and **(D)** postoperative computed tomography scans.

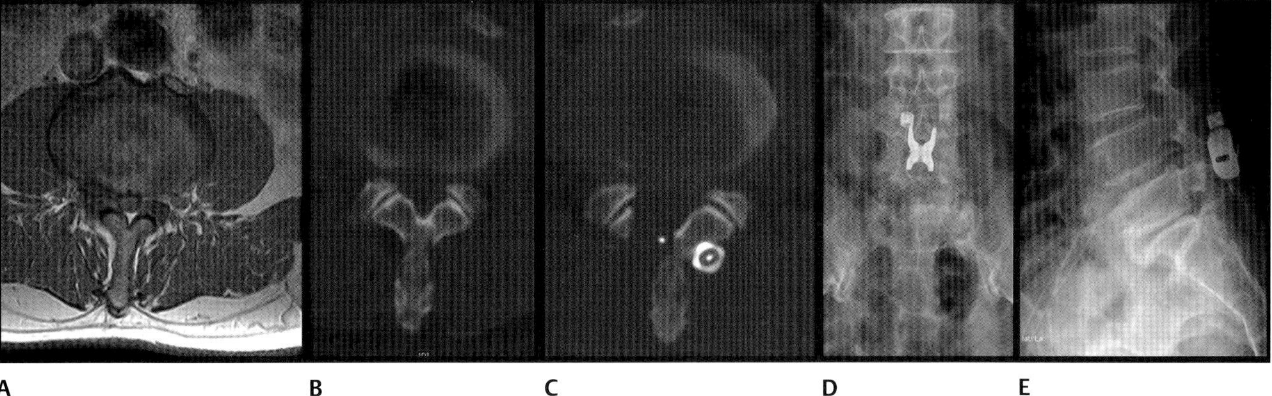

A B C D E

Figure 36–7 A 72-year-old male with central canal stenosis and foraminal disk herniation at L4–L5. Unilateral open laminotomy for bilateral decompression and foraminal diskectomy was done, and the tension band fixation was performed. **(A)** Preoperative axial magnetic resonance imaging showing the foraminal disk herniation. **(B)** Preoperative axial computed tomographic (CT) scan in a bone setting image. **(C)** Postoperative axial CT scan shows bilateral decompression. **(D)** Postoperative anteroposterior and **(E)** lateral radiographs.

A B C D

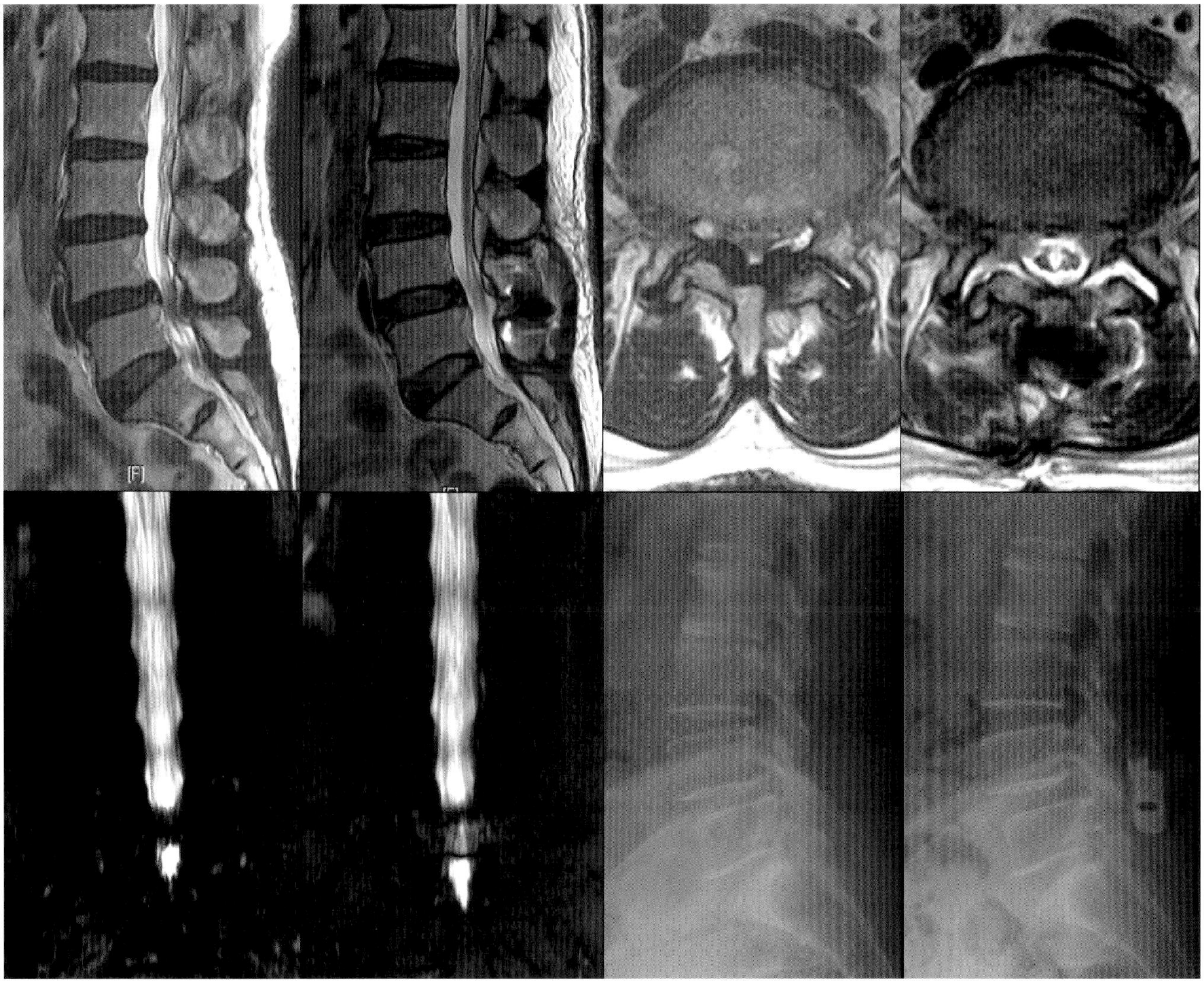

E F G H

Figure 36–8 A 67-year-old female with lumbar canal stenosis and degenerative spondylolisthesis at L4–L5. Unilateral micro-laminotomy for bilateral decompression by complete removal of interspinous ligament and ligamentum flavum without radical laminectomy and tension band fixation was performed. **(A)** Preoperative and **(B)** postoperative sagittal magnetic resonance (MR) imagings. **(C)** Preoperative and **(D)** postoperative axian MR imagings. **(E)** Preoperative and **(F)** postoperative MR myelograms showing recreating of normal spinal canal. **(G)** Preoperative and **(H)** postoperative lateral radiographs showing stabilization with interspinous locker fixation.

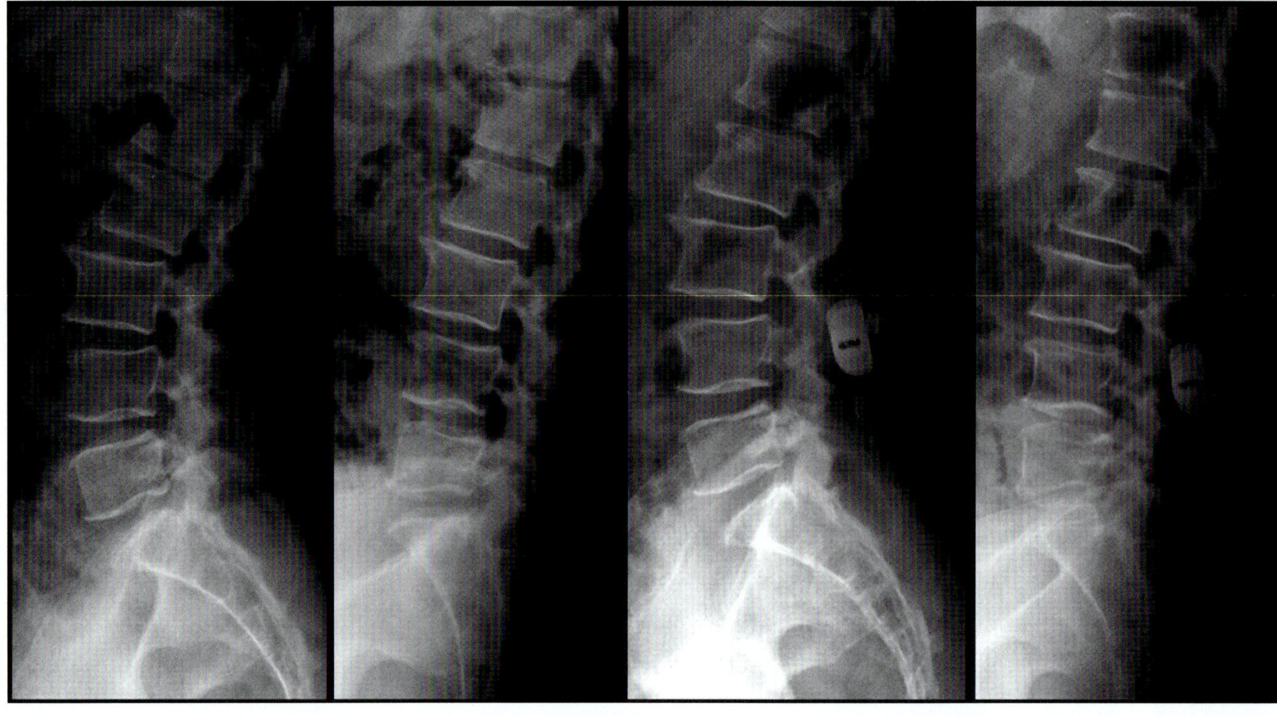

A   B   C   D

Figure 36–9 A 68-year-old female with degenerative spondylolisthesis with spinal stenosis. Unilateral open laminotomy for bilateral decompression and tension band fixation was performed. **(A)** Preoperative lateral radiographs in extension. **(B)** Preoperative lateral radiographs in flexion. **(C)** Postoperative lateral radiographs in extension. **(D)** Postoperative lateral radiographs in flexion.

would be more successful and easier for both the surgeon and the patient in mild degenerative spondylolisthesis and spinal stenosis.[38]

In degenerative spondylolisthesis and spinal stenosis, unilateral open laminotomy for bilateral decompression or bilateral partial laminectomy with foraminotomy should be performed to preserve the spinous processes, the supraspinatus ligament, and the facet joint. Because the procedure leaves so much of the surrounding area intact, only a small incision (~5 cm) is necessary. The interspinous locker can provide complete bilateral neural decompression even in this limited surgical exposure. For tension band fixation in degenerative spondylolisthesis, the interspinous ligament is removed and the supraspinous ligament is detached. As a result, complete ipsilateral foraminal decompression and ipsilateral decompression of the exiting nerve root as well as the traversing root can be obtained from the contralateral side without total facetectomy (**Fig. 36–6**).

There are various factors for and against tension band fixation in mild degenerative spondylolisthesis with spinal stenosis. Lee and Kim reported that when only an artificial ligament without interspinous locker was used and the disk height was less than 9 mm, the surgical outcome was very promising.[34] Facet morphology is another significant factor in the outcome of tension band fixation. Lee and Kim encountered successful outcomes in all patients suffering only from vacuum facet, without vacuum disk or facet destruction. If the patient had both a vacuum disk and a destroyed facet, half would have unsuccessful outcomes.[38] Clearly, this type of case merits the use of fusion with a pedicle screw.

The alignment of the facet joint also plays an important role in the outcome of tension band fixation. In Lee and Kim's report, if the joint has a more sagittal alignment ($>$ 52 degrees), the outcome tends to be unsatisfactory; if the alignment is coronal ($<$ 52 degrees) the outcome tends to be very good.[38] Grobler et al found that the reduced coronal dimension of the facet joint may be correlated to anterior slippage.[39] A more sagittal alignment of the facet joint means that the reduced coronal dimension of the facet joint could cause further postoperative anterior slippage.[40,41]

Combination of Tension Band System and Other Soft Stabilization

If the patient has painful degenerative disk with segmental instability, the tension band system might also be a useful augmentation method with a prosthetic disk nucleus or other disk replacement materials (**Fig. 36–4**). The tension band system is to other disk replacement materials for motion sparing what the pedicle screw fixation is to intervertebral cages.

◆ Conclusion

The management of degenerative spinal disorders has moved from its original focus, decompression, to the type of stabilization; soft versus rigid. With the development of minimally invasive techniques and the tension band fixation technique, soft stabilization with an artificial ligament and interspinous locker provides a highly successful surgical outcome.

Patients with degenerative spinal disorders are usually older, even medically compromised and osteoporotic. It is hazardous to do repeated surgeries like decompression alone followed by fusion, or to do fusion in an osteoporotic condition.

Given that the operative time is short, the procedure is less invasive, and fusion is not required, tension band fixation appears to be the best option to facilitate stabilization in treating degenerative diseases, especially in elderly patients.

References

1. Paris SV. Physical signs of instability. Spine 1985;10:277–279
2. Pope MH, Panjabi M. Biomechanical definitions of spinal instability. Spine 1985;10:255–256
3. American Academy of Orthopaedic Surgeons. A Glossary on Spinal Terminology. Chicago: American Academy of Orthopaedic Surgeons; 1981
4. Hazlett JW, Kinnard P. Lumbar apophyseal process excision and spinal instability. Spine 1982;7:171–176
5. West JL III, Bradford DS, Ogilvie JW. Results of spinal arthrodesis with pedicle screw-plate fixation. J Bone Joint Surg Am 1991;73:1179–1184
6. Zdeblick TA. A prospective, randomized study of lumbar fusion: preliminary results. Spine 1993;18:983–991
7. Bridwell KH, Sedgewick TA, O'Brien MF, Lenke LG, Baldus C. The role of fusion and instrumentation in the treatment of degenerative spondylolisthesis with spinal stenosis. J Spinal Disord 1993;6:461–472
8. Lorenz M, Zindrick M, Schwaegler P, et al. A comparison of single-level fusions with and without hardware. Spine 1991;16(Suppl 8):S455–S458
9. Vaccaro AR, Garfin SR. Internal fixation (pedicle screw fixation) for fusion of the lumbar spine. Spine 1995;20(Suppl 24):157S–165S
10. Davne SH, Myers DL. Complication of lumbar spinal fusion and transpedicular instrumentation. Spine 1992;16(Suppl 6):S184–S189
11. Deyo RA, Ciol MA, Cherkin DC, Loeser JD, Bigos SJ. Lumbar spinal fusion. Spine 1993;18:1463–1470
12. Fassio B, Cohen R, Beguin C, Jucopilla N. Treatment of degenerative lumbar spinal instability L4–L5 by interspinous ligamentoplasty. Rachis 1991;3:465–474
13. Steffee AD, Brantigan JW. The variable screw placement spinal fixation system: report of a prospective study of 250 patients enrolled in Food and Drug Administration clinical trials. Spine 1993;18:1160–1172
14. Yuan HA, Garfin SR, Dickman CA, Mardjetko SM. A historical cohort study of pedicle screw fixation in thoracic, lumbar, and sacral spinal fusions. Spine 1994;19(Suppl 20):2279S–2296S
15. Graf H. Lumbar instability: surgical treatment without fusion. Rachis 1992;412:123–137
16. Lee SH, Lee IM, Sung KH, Sung YS, Kim JS. Comparison of posterior interbody fusion, postorolateral fusion, and interspinous ligmertoplasty for degenerative lumbar instability. J Neurosurg. 1997;86:424A[abstr]
17. Lee HY, Chang SB, Lee SH. Interspinous ligamentoplasty. In: Soultz MH, Chiu JC, Rauschning W, et al (eds). The Practice of Minimally Invasive Spinal Technique 2005 Edition. New York: AAMISS Press; 2005: 551–554
18. Senegas J, Etchevers JP, Vital JM, Baulny D, Grenier F. Recalibration of the lumbar canal, an alternative to laminectomy in the treatment of lumbar canal stenosis [in French]. Rev Chir Orthop Reparatrice Appar Mot 1988;74:15–22
19. Lee HY, Chang SB, Lee SH, Shin SW. A modified technique of interspinous ligamentoplasty for lumbar stenosis or degenerative spondylolisthesis. Joint Diseases & Related Surgery 2005;16:146–152
20. Sharma M, Langrana NA, Rodriguez J. Role of ligaments and facets in lumbar spinal stability. Spine 1995;20:887–900
21. Panjabi MM, Greenstein G, Duranceau J, Nolte LP. Three-dimensional quantitative morphology of lumbar spinal ligaments. J Spinal Disord 1991;4:54–62
22. Denis F. The three-column spine and its significance in the classification of cute thoracolumbar spine injuries. Spine 1983;8:817–831
23. Voydeville G. Etude biomecanique d'une unite spinale L4/L5 saine, lesee puis stabilisee par une cale et un ligament. Presented at: the annual meeting of the Groupe International d'Etude des Approches du RACHIS, December 15, 1994, Paris, France
24. Voydeville G, Diop A, Lavsater F, Girard F, Hardy PH. Experimental lumbar instability and artificial ligament. Eur J Orthop Surg & Traumatol 2000;10:168–176
25. Papp T, Porter RW, Aspden RM, Shepperd JAN. An in vitro study of the biomechanical effects of flexible stabilization on the lumbar spine. Spine 1997;22:151–155
26. Swanson KE, Lindsey DP, Hsu KY, Zucherman JF, Yerby SA. The effects of an interspinous implant on intervertebral disc pressures. Spine. 2003;28:26–32
27. Atlas SJ, Keller RB, Robson D, Deyo RA, Singer DE. Surgical and nonsurgical management of lumbar spinal stenosis: four-year outcomes from the Maine Lumbar Spine Study. Spine 2000;25:556–562
28. Tsai RY, Yang RS, Bray RS Jr. Microscopic laminotomies for degenerative lumbar spinal stenosis. J Spinal Disord 1998;11:389–394
29. Tuite GF, Stern JD, Doran SE, et al. Outcome after laminectomy for lumbar spinal stenosis, I: Clinical correlations. J Neurosurg 1994;81: 699–706
30. Young S, Veerapen R, O'Laoire SA. Relief of lumbar canal stenosis using multilevel subarticular fenestrations as an alternative to wide laminectomy: preliminary report. Neurosurgery 1988;23:628–633
31. Aryanpur J, Ducker T. Multilevel lumbar laminotomies: an alternative to laminectomy in the treatment of lumbar stenosis. Neurosurgery 1990;26:429–432 discussion 433
32. Caputy AJ, Luessenhop AJ. Long-term evaluation of decompressive surgery for degenerative lumbar surgery. J Neurosurg 1992;77: 669–676
33. Feffer HL, Wiesel SW, Cucker JM, Rothman RH. Degenerative spondylolisthesis: to fuse or not to fuse. Spine 1985;10:287–289
34. Katz JN, Lipson SJ, Larson SG, McInnes JM, Fossel AH, Liang MH. Outcome of decompressive laminectomy of degenerative lumbar stenosis. J Bone Joint Surg Am 1991;73:809–816
35. Herkowitz HN, Kurz LT. Degenerative lumbar spondylolisthesis with spinal stenosis: a prospective study comparing decompression with decompression and intertransverse process arthrodesis. J Bone Joint Surg Am 1991;73:802–808
36. Rechtine GR, Sutterlin CE, Wood GW, Boyd RJ, Mansfield FL. The efficacy of pedicle screw/plate fixation on lumbar/lumbosacral autogenous bone graft fusion in adult patients with degenerative spondylolisthesis. J Spinal Disord 1996;9:382–391
37. Fassio B, Cohen R, Beguin C, Jucopilla N. Treatment of degenerative lumbar spinal instability L4–L5 by interspinous ligamentoplasty. Rachis 1991;3:465–474
38. Lee SH, Kim JS. Comparison of ligamentoplasty to rigid fixation for degenerative lumbar instability. J Minim Invasive Spinal Tech 2002;2:10–14
39. Grobler LJ, Robertson PA, Novotny JE, Pope MH. Etiology of spondylolisthesis: assessment of the role played by lumbar facet joint morphology. Spine 1993;18:80–91
40. Grobler LJ, Robertson PA, Novotny JE, Ahern JW. Decompression for degenerative spondylolisthesis and spinal stenosis at L4–L5: the effects on facet joint morphology. Spine 1993;18:1475–1482
41. Robertson PA, Grobler LJ, Novotny JE, Katz JN. Postoperative spondylolisthesis at L4–5: the role of facet joint morphology. Spine 1993;18: 1483–1490

37

Shape Memory Implant (KIMPF-DI Fixing) System

Young-Soo Kim and Ho-Yeol Zhang

◆ **Indications and Contraindications**

◆ **Description of System Components**

◆ **Operative Techniques for Loop Fixings (Type A)**
   Positioning
   Incision and Exposure
   Bony Preparation and Decision of Loop Size
   Deformation and Installation

◆ **Case Illustrations**
   Case 1
   Case 2
   Case 3

◆ **Conclusion**

Nitinol is an alloy of nickel and titanium that belongs to a class of materials called shaped memory alloys (SMAs). Nitinol was invented in 1962 by the U.S. Naval Ordnance Laboratory. The scientific team was seeking a nonmagnetic, high-hardness, noncorrosive material for hand weapons and tools. What they discovered was a relatively safer (nontoxic) SMA.[1]

The team named the new alloy nitinol. The name represents its elemental components and place of origin. *Ni* and *Ti* are the chemical symbols for nickel and titanium. The *nol* stands for the Naval Ordinance Laboratory where it was discovered.

SMAs have interesting mechanical properties. Nitinol for example contracts when heated, which is the opposite of what standard metals do when heated. Not only does the alloy contract but it also produces thermal movement (expansion, contraction) 100 times greater than standard metals.

Another interesting property of SMAs is their shaped memory effect (SME). The alloy can be heat treated to remember a particular shape. If the shape is later bent and distorted, the alloy may be heated to regain its original shape. These characteristics (**Table 37–1**) can be used for internal stabilization and prosthetics of bone and ligament–cartilage structures of the spine.

The KIMPF-DI Fixing (CJSC KIMPF Company, Moscow, Russia) shape memory implant system for spine surgery is both biologically and mechanically compatible.[2]

This system comprises five types: (**Fig. 37–1A–E**).

◆ Type A: Loop fixing type (Davydov shape memory loop)
◆ Type B: Vertebral fixing
◆ Type C: Intervertebral fixing
◆ Type D: Fixing without loop
◆ Type E: Endoprosthesis of intervertebral disks

Nitinol possesses a heterophase structure. This structure provides stable and appropriate characteristics and superelasticity, and it facilitates the shape memory effect.

Design of fixings ensures[2–4]:

1. Mechanical behavior that is similar to the behavior of ligament–cartilage structures replaced or reinforced by fixings. Fixings have the following characteristics: range of self-adjusting compression and stiffness of counteraction to the functional loads.

2. Rapid, low-traumatic installation and reliable functional stabilization of spine elements.

This system has unique temperature characteristics. Preliminary deformation is done at temperatures not exceeding +10°C. Deformed shape is kept unchanged up to +26°C. Shape recovery occurs under heating up to +35°C.

Table 37–1   Key Properties of Nitinol Alloys

Large forces that can be generated due to the shape memory effect
Excellent damping properties below the transition temperature
Excellent corrosion resistance
Nonmagnetic
High fatigue strength
Moderate impact resistance
Moderate heat resistance
Biocompatible

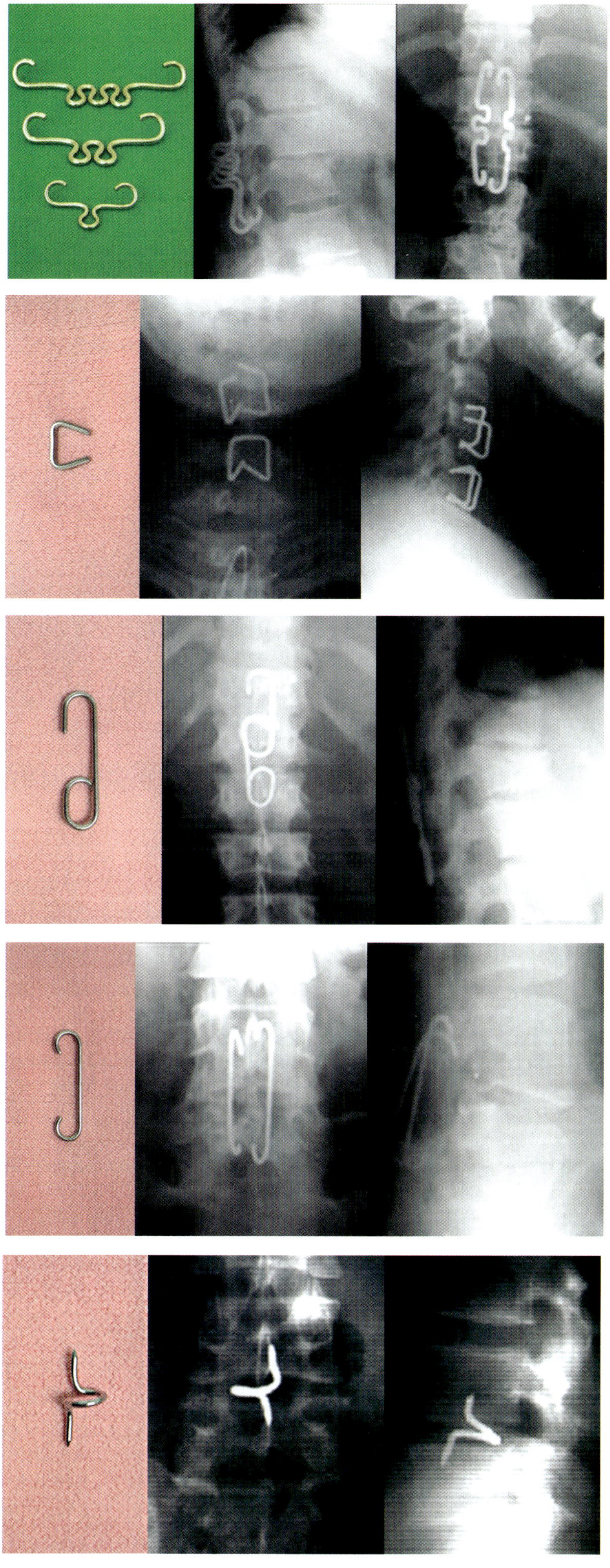

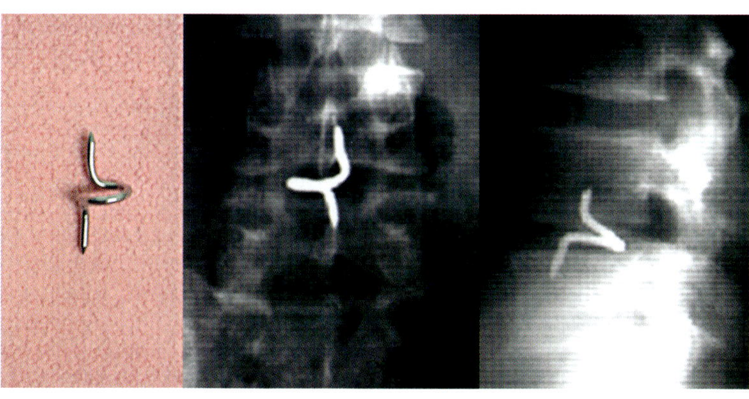

Figure 37–1 **(A)** Type A: loop fixing, intended for installation by vertebral arches of cervical, thoracic, and lumbar spine for the purposes of reinforcing posterior ligament–cartilage structures. These fixings are indicated for compression fractures of vertebral bodies, for degenerative-dystrophic affections, and after operations on spinal marrow related with resection of arches or spinous processes of vertebrae. **(B)** Type B: vertebral fixing, intended for osteosynthesis and fixation of bone implants. Characteristic features of the vertebral fixing are moderate compression and high stiffness compared with bone stiffness (1000 N/mm). **(C)** Type C: intervertebral fixing, intended for installation by spinous processes of the thoracic and lumbar spine to reinforce posterior ligament–cartilage structures in case of compression fractures of vertebral bodies and disruption of interspinous and supraspinous ligaments. **(D)** Type D: fixing without loop, intended for installation by the vertebral arches of the cervical, thoracic, and lumbar spine for reinforcing posterior ligament–cartilage structures. These fixings are indicated for compression fractures of vertebral bodies, for degenerative-dystrophic affections, and after spinal marrow operations for resection of arches or spinous processes of vertebrae. **(E)** Type E: endoprosthesis of intervertebral disks. The force of distraction is no less than 30 N at a temperature of 36.6°C. The stiffness of counteraction to axial and transverse displacement is no less than 15 N/mm. Spiral endoprosthesis of intervertebral cartilage is intended for the substitution of the cartilage or its parts. The fixing ensures stabilization of corresponding spinal-mobility segments in the horizontal plane and conservation of appropriate space between vertebrae. Meanwhile, the fixing does not interfere with vertebral inclinations in any direction and can easily be introduced between vertebral bodies after bringing together the stems of the fixing in the cooled state. The fixing recovers its spiral shape after heating.

◆ Indications and Contraindications

This shape memory loop system is extremely versatile and is indicated for a wide variety of posterior lumbar dynamic stabilization surgeries.

The indications include[2]:

◆ Type A: Installation by vertebral arches of the cervical, thoracic, and lumbar spine for the purpose of reinforcement of posterior ligament–cartilage structures. The use of fixing is indicated for compression fractures of vertebral bodies, degenerative-dystrophic affections, after operations on spinal marrow operations related with resection of arches or spinous processes of vertebrae (**Fig. 37–1A**) and for prevention of adjacent segment instability.

◆ Type B: The vertebral fixing is intended for osteosynthesis and fixation of bone implants (**Fig. 37–1B**).

◆ Type C: The fixing is intended for installation by spinous processes of thoracic and lumbar spine for reinforcement posterior ligament–cartilage structures in case of compression fractures of vertebral bodies and disruption of interspinous and supraspinous ligaments (**Fig. 37–1C**).

◆ Type D: The fixings are intended for installation by vertebral arches of the cervical, thoracic, and lumbar spine for the purpose of reinforcement of posterior ligament–cartilage structures. The use of fixings is indicated for compression fractures of vertebral bodies, for degenerative-dystrophic affections, and after spinal marrow operations related to the resection of arches or spinous processes of vertebrae (**Fig. 37–1D**).

◆ Type E: Spiral endoprosthesis of intervertebral cartilage is intended for substitution of the cartilage. The fixing ensures stabilization of the corresponding spinal-mobility segment in the horizontal plane and conservation of appropriate space between the vertebrae. Meanwhile, the fixing does not interfere with vertebral inclinations in any direction (**Fig. 37–1E**).

Relative contraindications for all types include:

◆ Profound osteoporosis
◆ Active infection

◆ Description of System Components

The key instruments featured in the KIMPF-DI System include:

◆ Containing box. All instruments and fixings are in the metal box for placement, transportation, storage, and sterilization (**Fig. 37–2**).

◆ Template retractor. Designed for deformation of fixings with loop (Type A) and fixings without loop (Type D) before installation (**Fig. 37–3A**).

◆ Intervertebral expander. Designed for increasing intervertebral space and conserving distraction under installation of the endoprosthesis of intervertebral cartilage (Type E) (**Fig. 37–3B**).

◆ Template conductor. Used for choosing the size and for puncturing holes (by straight awl) in the bodies of vertebrae under installation of fixings (Type B) (**Fig. 37–3C**).

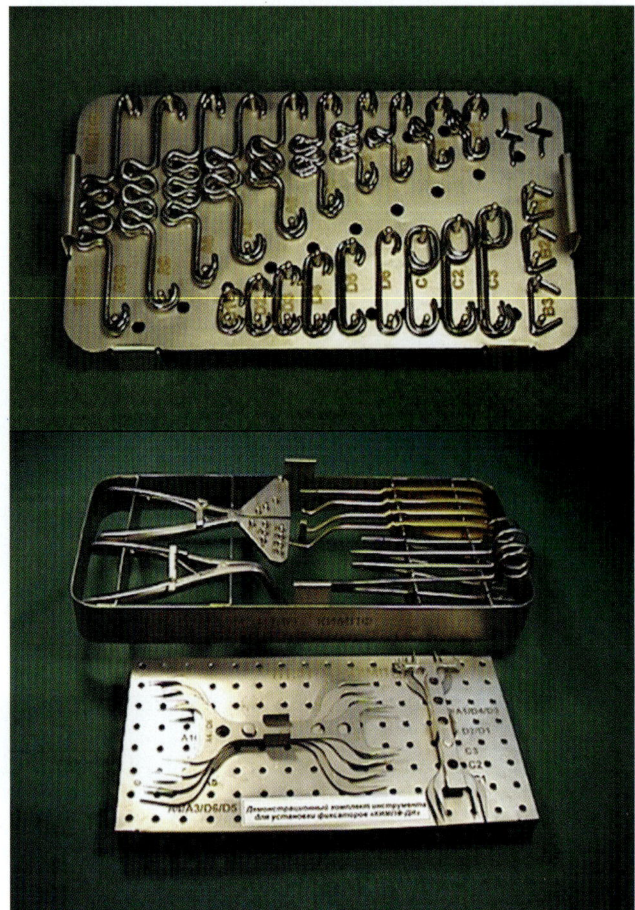

Figure 37–2   Container of instruments and fixings.

◆ Straight awl. Designed to puncture holes in the bodies of vertebrae under installation of fixing (Type B) (**Fig. 37–3D**).

◆ Curved awl. Designed to puncture holes in the bodies of vertebrae under installation of Type E (**Fig. 37–3E**).

◆ Template measures. One type is designed to measure the interval between the vertebral arches and choose the size of fixing with loops (Type A). Another type is designed to measure the interval between spinous processes and choose the size of intervertebral fixing (Type C) (**Figs. 37–3F,G**).

◆ Forceps. Designed to hold and install all fixing types (**Fig. 37–3H**).

◆ Deformator. Designed for the deformation of endoprosthesis of intervertebral cartilage (Type E) before installation (**Fig. 37–3I**).

◆ Guide raspatory. Designed for the skeletonization and cutting of vertebral arches and spinous processes before installation of Types A, C, and D fixings (**Fig. 37–3J**).

◆ Operative Techniques for Loop Fixings (Type A)

Appropriate preoperative evaluation and careful surgical planning are critical to a successful surgical outcome. This technique is used for the operation of L4–L5 stenosis and L3–L4 mild spondylosis[5] (**Fig. 37–4**).

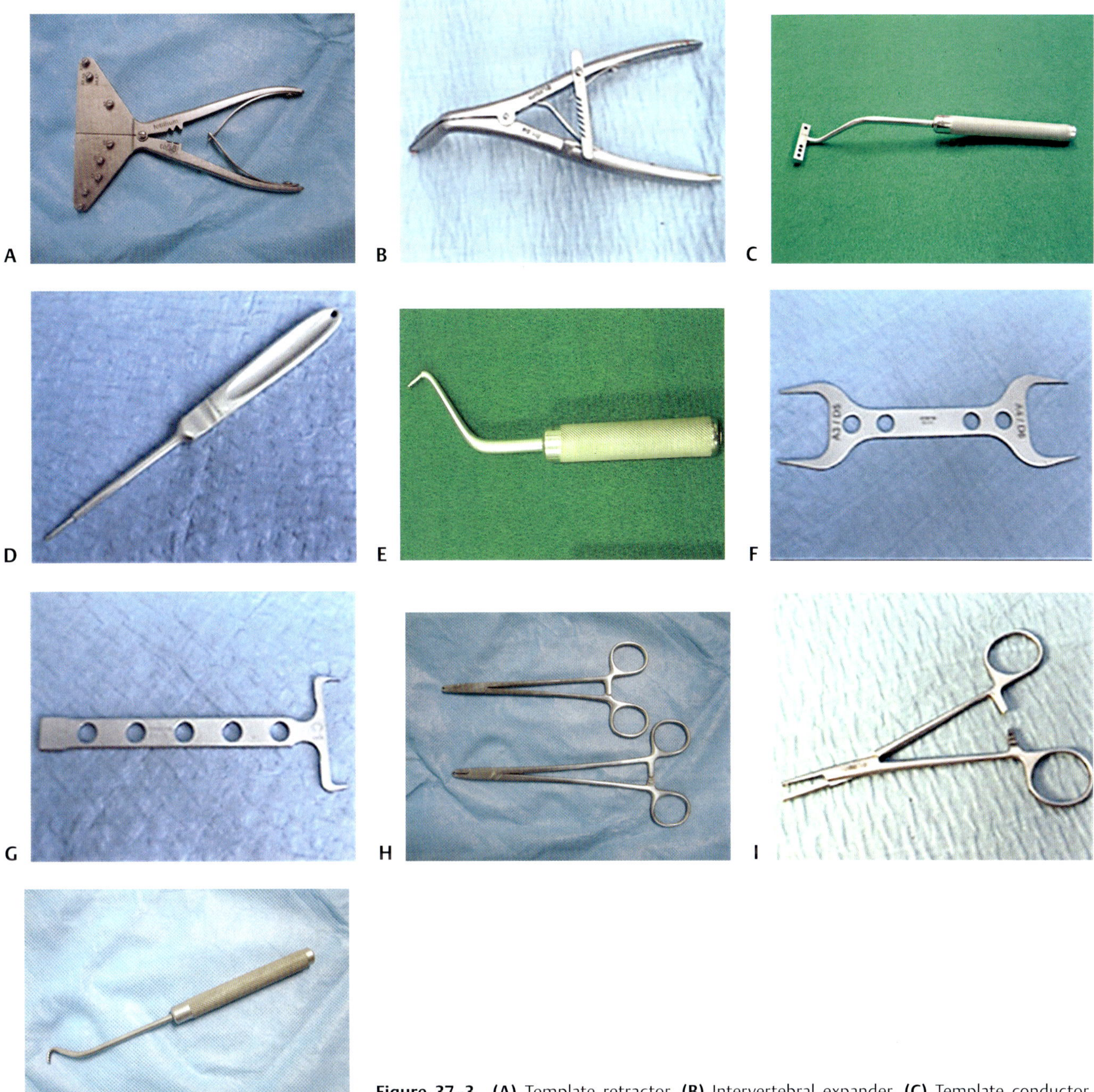

Figure 37–3 **(A)** Template retractor. **(B)** Intervertebral expander. **(C)** Template conductor. **(D)** Straight awl. **(E)** Curved awl. **(F)** Template measures for type A. **(G)** Template measures for type C. **(H)** Forceps. **(I)** Deformator. **(J)** Guide raspatory.

Positioning

Essentially, all cases requiring dorsal lumbar exposure can be managed adequately using a conventional operating table. After intubation and Foley catheter indwelling, the patient lies on gel rolls in the prone position. Care is taken to avoid undue pressure on bony prominences, genitalia, and neurovascular structures.

Incision and Exposure

A midline linear incision and exposure is made above L3 to L5 lamina. An L4 laminectomy is performed completely and the removal of ligamentum flavum of L3–L4 and L4–L5 is performed. The distance between the L3 upper lamina and L5 lower lamina will be shortened after loop application. If the ligamentum flavum remains during this shortening, it can bring about the dorsal compressed mass of the dural sac. Hence, complete removal of the ligamentum flavum is crucial. This is the first tip.[5] A diskectomy and posterior lumbar interbody fusion (PLIF) on L4–L5 is performed in the usual fashion.

Bony Preparation and Decision of Loop Size

The skeletonization of the lamina arches or spinous processes of the L3 upper end and L5 lower end provides the

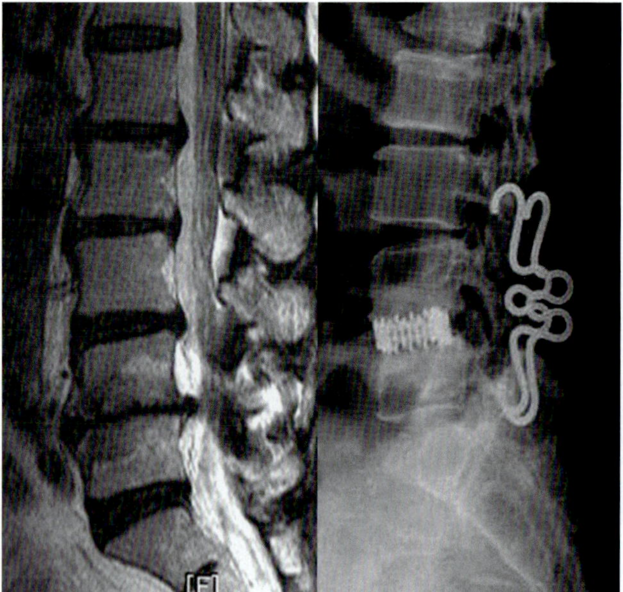

Figure 37–4 Case 1. L4–L5 stenosis +L3–L4 mild spondylosis. Preoperative magnetic resonance imaging and postoperative x-ray.

places to hook the fixing parts using the guide raspatory. Template measuring instruments are used to scale the exact size of the memory loop. When dynamic fixation for two motion segments is needed, we always use the loop 2 cm smaller than the distance between two laminae. The supine position during laminectomy can cause the disruption of lumbar lordosis and posterior ligamentous structures. This leads to pseudolengthening of the posterior column. If the size of the memory loop matches the distance between the two laminae, it can be loosened and dislodged. This is the second tip.[5]

Deformation and Installation

After selection of the proper fixing loop, the fixings are taken by forceps and cooled in sterilized physiological saline of 10–15°C for no less than 30 seconds (**Fig. 37–5**).

Each fixings has its own installation engineering features. The loopy fixings of Type A are deformed by the template-retractor. The deformed fixings are placed by one hook behind the lamina arch of the vertebra (or spinous process) so that the plane of its loops is parallel to the vertebral spinal alignments. The second hook of fixings is placed behind the lamina arch of another vertebra (or spinous process). Fixings for the lamina arches are bilateral to maintain uniformly distributed loading on vertebral segments.

After the fixing is installed, an irrigation of 45–50°C sterilized physiological saline is required. This enables the implant to accept the initial form, fixing the damaged segment of the spine. Hemostasis should be performed carefully and wound closure done layer by layer. Take note to leave a tubular drainage with an aspiration device.

◆ Case Illustrations

Case 1

Fig. 37–4 is of a patient with multiple lumbar stenoses. The main pathology is the L4–L5 stenosis, disk space narrowing, and asymptomatic L3–L4 mild spondylotic stenosis. Operations that were performed include L4 total laminectomy, diskectomy and PLIF at L4–L5, and shape memory loop application from L3 to L5. Rationales are as follows;

1. Enhancement of L4–L5 fusion rate due to compressive force of the shape memory loop

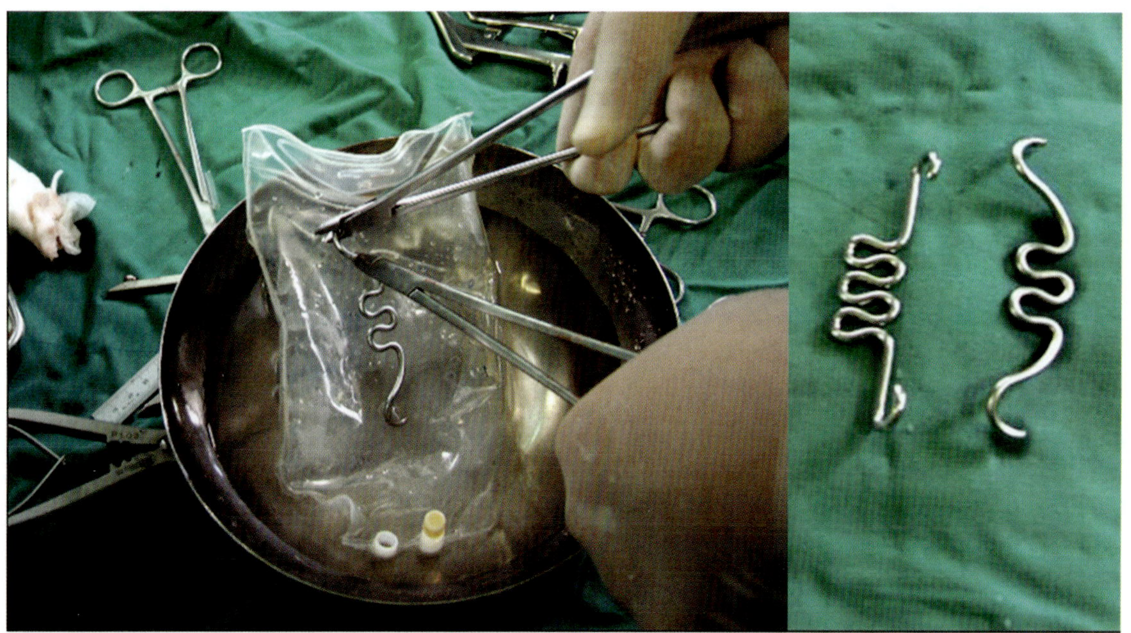

Figure 37–5 **(A)** Type A loop deformation after cooling. **(B)** Normal (left) and deformed (right) shape memory loop Type A.

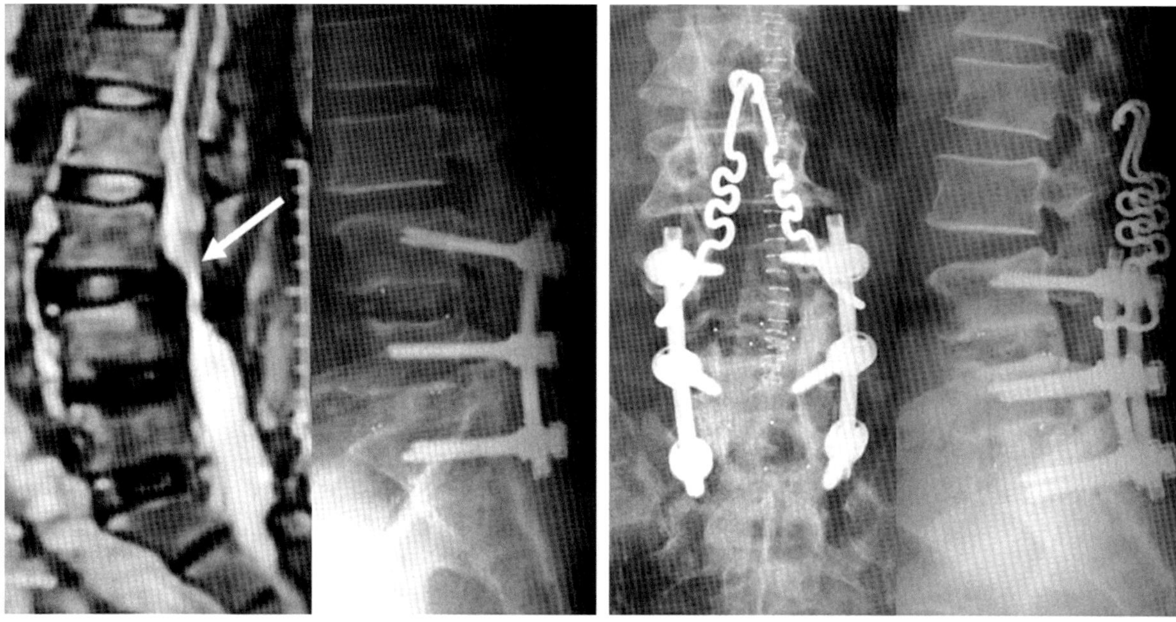

Figure 37–6   Case 2. L3–L4 topping-off stenosis after L4–L5–S1 360 degree fusion. **(A)** Preoperative and **(B)** postoperative radiological images.

2. Additional L4–L5 stability as the effect of a 360 degree fixation

3. Prevention of adjacent motion segment instability: L3–L4 has a more limited motion than its preoperative state due to the elasticity of the memory loop. This may prevent the degeneration of the L3–L4 motion segment. Also this motion can reduce the L2–L3 hypermotion when using the hard fixation at L3–L4–L5 and may reduce the adjacent segment (L2–L3) instability.[5]

Case 2

Fig. 37–6 is of a patient who underwent L3–L4 topping off stenosis after an L4–L5–S1 360 degree fusion. Operations that were done include L3 decompressive total laminectomy and the application of the shape memory loop between the L2 lamina and previously inserted L4 pedicle screw rod. The postoperative x-ray shows the reduction of the L3 spondylolisthesis and good alignment of the lumbar lordosis. This operation reduces L3 spondylolisthesis and prevents the expected upper segment (L2–L3 and L1–L2) from topping off.[5,6]

Case 3

Fig. 37–7 is of a patient with an L1 compression fracture with kyphosis. Preoperative (**Fig. 37–7A**) and postoperative (**Fig. 37–7B**) radiological images show the reduction of kyphosis. This idea initiated the development of the instrumentation system by Russian doctors.[3] The shape memory

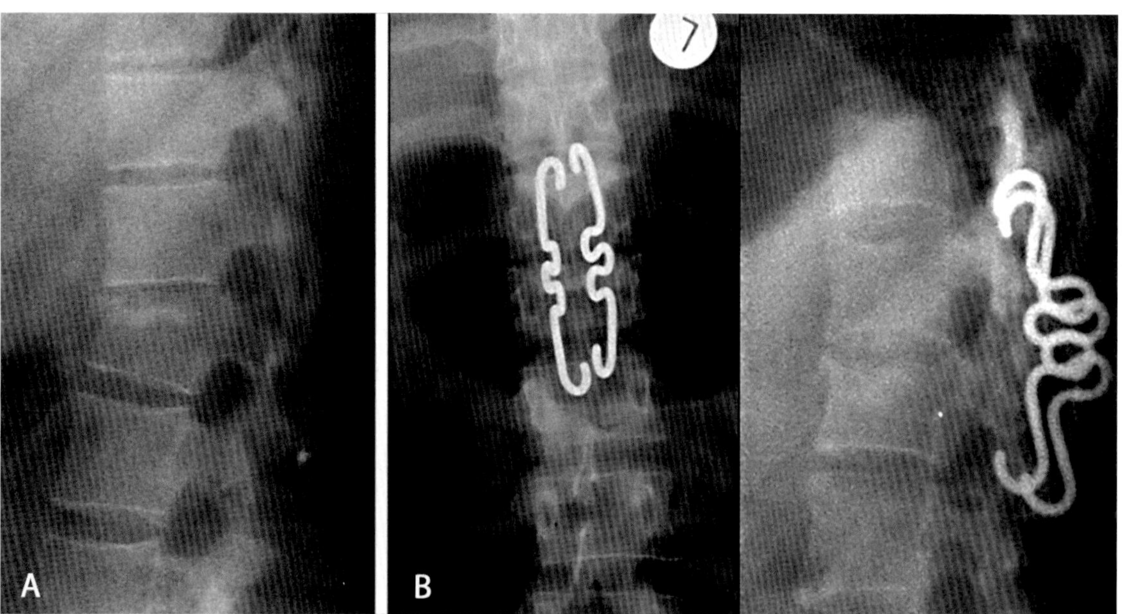

Figure 37–7   Case 3. Thoracolumbar kyphosis due to compression fracture of L1. **(A)** Preoperative and **(B)** postoperative radiological images.

Table 37–2   Patient Demographics

Operation periods: 8/30/2004–4/30/2005
·Patient: $N = 124$
M:F = 48:76
Mean age: 57.4 yrs
Mean follow-up: 4.6 months

Table 37–3   Operative Indications of Type A, C, D Loops

1. Posterior lumbar interbody fusion and posterior fixation
2. After decompressive laminectomy
3. Correction of degenerative kyphoscoliosis
4. Mild degenerative spondylolisthesis
5. Compression fracture with kyphosis
6. Prevention of adjacent segmental instability
7. Injury of ligamentous structure

Table 37–4   Operative Methods

Methods of Operations	No. of Patients
1. Decompression L3 and PLIF L4–L5 + loop (L3–L5)	38
2. PLIF L3–L4, L4–L5 + loop (L3–L5)	35
3. PLIF L4–L5 + loop (L4–L5)	27
4. Decompressive laminectomy + loop	12
5. Decompression of adjacent segment stenosis + loop	5
6. Correction to kyphosis	5
7. PLIF L1–L2 + loop	2
Total:	124

PLIF, posterior lumbar interbody fusion.

loop adds to the elasticity of the posterior ligamentous structures and returns the kyphotic angle to normal thoracolumbar alignment.[7,8]

◆ Conclusion

The shape memory implant (KIMPF-DI Fixing) system Type A, C, and D was employed to treat 124 patients from August 2004 to April 2005. The patients consisted of 48 males and 76 females with a mean age of 57.4 with 4.6 months follow-up[5] (**Table 37–2**).

Our operative indications were PLIF and posterior fixation, after decompressive laminectomy, correction of degenerative kyphoscoliosis, mild degenerative spondylolisthesis, compression fracture with kyphosis, prevention of adjacent segment problems (stenosis or instability), and injury of ligamentous structures (**Table 37–3**).

Operative methods were one-level PLIF + two-level loop, two-level PLIF + two-level loop, one-level PLIF + one-level loop, decompressive laminectomy + PLIF, loop to adjacent segment, and loop for kyphosis correction (**Table 37–4**). Postoperative results included a 93% satisfaction rate.

A Russian report of 32 patients' results is also satisfactory.[3] The patients were divided by categories according to fixings: Type A (19 patients), Type C (eight patients), and Type D (five patients). Fifteen patients (47%) experienced a satisfactory outcome. Seventeen patients (53%) experienced a good outcome. There were no further kyphotic deformations, or cracks and migrations of designs in any of the 32 patients.

Types B and E were used occasionally in the spine trauma cases. More case reports need to be presented to make a statistical analysis of the results.[9]

Despite the short-term results of these systems, we concluded as follows[5–8]: The nitinol-based SMA is flexible, which plays the role of a strong tension band to replace posterior ligaments. This semirigid fixation is more physiological and can reduce postoperative adjacent segment complications. Other advantages include ease of application, less tissue damage, and correction of kyphosis. If this system is combined with PLIF in selected cases, it can enhance the fusion rate and provide more stability, making it unnecessary to use pedicle screws.

References

1. http://mkalos.com/information.htm
2. http://www.implants.ru/ing-version/spinal/spinal-i.shtml
3. Il'in AA, Kollerov MJ, Sergeyv SV, et al. Biologically and mechanically compatible implants from titanium nickelide in the treatment of damaged chest and lumbar parts of the backbone. The Bulletin of Traumatology and Orthopedics (Moscow, Russia) 2002;2:19–26
4. Il'in AA, Kollerov MY, Khachin VI, Gusev DA. Medical Instruments and Implants of Titanium Nickelide: Physical Metallurgy, Technology, and Application. iAPC Nauku/Interperiodica 2002;3:296
5. Kim YS, Moon BJ, Park KW, Ryu KU, Lee WC. Posterior Interlaminar or Interspinous Processes Fixation Using Memory Loop Implant for Lumbar Disc Surgery. The 5th Biennial Japan–Korea Conference on Spinal Surgery, Sapporo, Japan, June 9–10, 2005
6. Kim YS. Dynamic Stabilization in Spine Surgery. The 5th Symposium of Yonsei University Spine Center, Seoul, Sep. 9, 2005
7. Kim YS, Moon BJ, Ryu KU, Lee WC. Experience of Thoracolumbar Posterior Fixation with Shape Memory Implant. The 2005 Annual Spring Meeting of Korean Neurosurgical Society, Jeju, Apr. 14–16, 2005
8. Kim YS, Moon BJ, Park KW, Ryu KU, Lee WC, Oh KS. Correction of Degenerative Thoracolumbar Kyphosis with Shape Memory Implant. 45th Annual Meeting of Korean Neurosurgical Society, Seoul, Oct. 12–15, 2005
9. Davydov EA, Il'in AA, Kollerov MY. Methods of Diskectomy with the Conservation of Biomechanics of the Vertebral Mobility Segment. The Third Scientific Practical Conference, Russian Spinal Cord Society, Saratov, Russia, Oct. 7–8, 2004

Treatment of Mobile Vertebral Instability with Dynesys

Gilles Dubois, O. Schwarzenbach, N. Specchia, and T. M. Stoll

- ◆ **Technical Aspects**
- ◆ **Indications**
- ◆ **Surgical Technique**
- ◆ **Performance**
- ◆ **Clinical Results**
- ◆ **Discussion**
- ◆ **Conclusion**

During the course of the natural evolution of vertebral disk degeneration starting from incipient diskopathy up to stenosis with fixed terminal deformation, the functional tripod (disk and facets) will experience a long period of destabilization with abnormal movements. Dynamic stabilization with the Dynesys Dynamic Stabilization System (Zimmer Spine, Inc., Warsaw, IN) provides distinct benefits (**Fig. 38–1**) in the phase of degeneration where symptoms are caused by diskovertebral dyskinesis; that is, between early stages of symptomatic degenerative changes of the spinal segment and structural deformities associated with spontaneous ossification.

The goal of dynamic stabilization with Dynesys is to realign and stabilize one or more intervertebral lumbar or lumbosacral segments in a position close to the normal anatomical position, with the intent of encouraging return to improved intervertebral physiology while enabling a certain degree of range of motion.

At the present time, more than 15,000 surgical procedures have been performed in over 15 different countries. The longest follow-up period is 10 years.

◆ Technical Aspects

To achieve this goal, Zimmer has developed a dynamic stabilization system called Dynesys (*D*ynamic *N*eutralization *Sys*tem for the Spine).

The Dynesys system consists of titanium alloy (Protasul 100) pedicle screws, polyester (Sulene-PET) cords and polycarbonate-urethane (Sulene-PCU) spacers. The cord and the spacer meet the International Standards Organization (ISO) 10993 international standards and the pedicle screws fulfill those of ISO 5822–11.

The cord controls the range of motion in flexion, whereas the spacer limits extension movements, enabling the posterior elements to be repositioned in accordance with a near normal anatomical situation.

All individual components and interconnections were tested for their static as well as for their dynamic behavior to assess the safety of the system. Fatigue testing of the complete assembly was performed to 10 million cycles, which is believed to represent a time in vivo of approximately 5 years. In an initial phase (1–2 million cycles), the system showed stress relaxation and remained stable at a substantial load level afterward.

Several biomechanical in vitro experiments were conducted to study the efficacy of the system. One recently published study tested six lumbar cadaver spines, loading them with pure moments in the three motion planes.[1] The spines were tested intact, with a defect of the middle segment, stabilized with Dynesys, and fixed with an internal fixator. For the

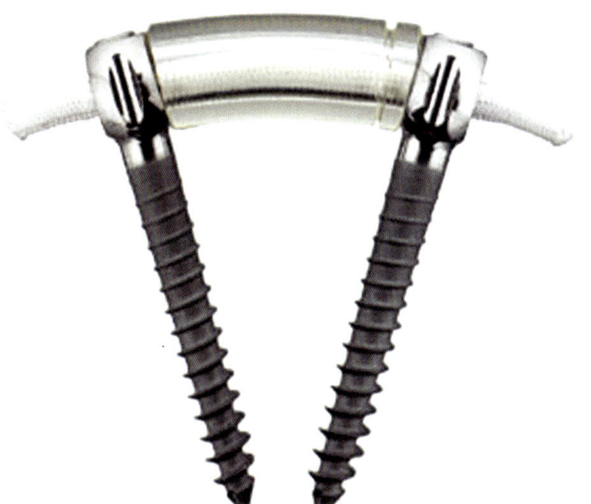

Figure 38–1 Functional model of Dynesys.

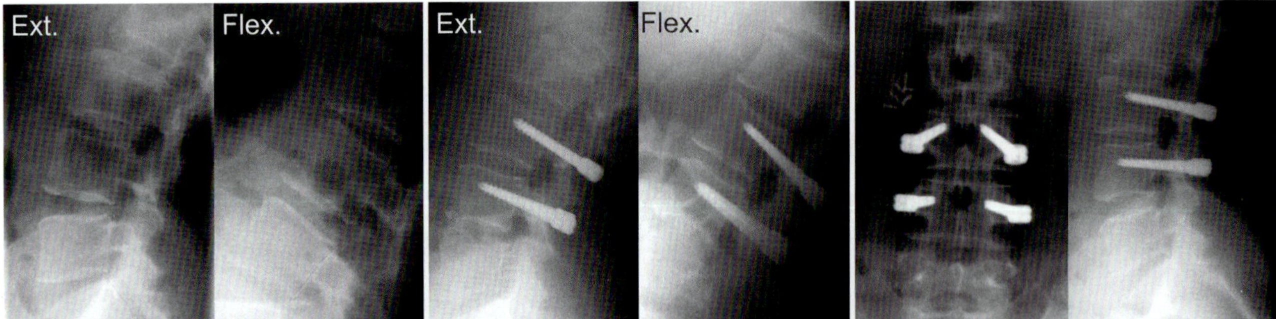

Figure 38–2   Female patient, 40 years old at time of surgery, presenting with degenerative disk disease in combination with spondylolisthesis. Dynesys was implanted without any additional surgical procedure. X-rays show preoperative and immediate postoperative functional x-rays and anteroposterior and lateral x-rays 9 years postoperatively.

instrumented segment, Dynesys stabilized the spine and was more flexible than the internal fixator, particularly in extension where Dynesys restored the range of motion to the intact condition. A second in vitro study found that increased spacer length increased the mobility in the segment.[2]

These biomechanical studies have confirmed that the stiffness of an instrumented segment was close to that of an intact spinal column. It therefore reinstates stiffness of the destabilized spinal segment on an experimental basis to a degree close to that of a normal and intact spine.

This internal bracing device enables the posterior elements, annulus, and posterior longitudinal ligament to be retensioned. It repositions the articulating surfaces to the areas in which they function normally, suppresses dyskinetic movements caused by loss of viscoelasticity of the disk, and restores the posterior pretensioning. It thus brings about anatomical conditions of the intervertebral joint that enable restoration of a better diskovertebral physiology, allowing a certain degree of freedom to be preserved due to the elasticity of the spacer. It limits the impact of the biomechanical stresses on the adjacent levels.

This device shows some potential for healing to take place in the disk space as well as in the end plates (see Performance).

◆ Indications

The indications for Dynesys are based upon their design and biomechanical effects. Dynesys addresses instabilities of all kinds: excessive or pathological motion and gradually developing deformity, including iatrogenic instability. This may involve low back pain as well as neurogenic pain.

The main goal of Dynesys is to address dynamic instability with autoreducible lesions in the early stages of degeneration as defined by Kirkaldy-Willis.[3] As a result of the instability, the patient may experience several types of clinical symptoms. These include dynamic stenosis or stenosis with degenerative olisthesis as evidenced by either or both neurogenic pain and low back pain (**Fig. 38–2**).Other indications for Dynesys are mono- or multisegmental degenerative disk disease (DDD) causing low back pain (**Fig. 38–3**) as well as iatrogenic instability following decompression.

In multilevel DDD, Dynesys may also be combined with a fusion procedure such as posterior lumbar interbody fusion (PLIF), depending on the severity of segmental disk disruption. Dynesys is not indicated as a primary stabilization method in lytic (isthmic) spondylolisthesis and severe degenerative scoliotic or kyphotic deformation.

◆ Surgical Technique

The surgical approach is along the median line, opening the lumbar aponeurosis, rasping the paravertebral muscles if the surgeon wishes to carry out intracanal activities aimed at associated decompression at the same time as the dynamic stabilization procedure. If no intracanal procedure is needed and if the lesion is of the dynamic stenosis type due to a soft lesion, then an intermuscular bilateral approach according to Wiltse or an intermuscular paraspinal approach can be

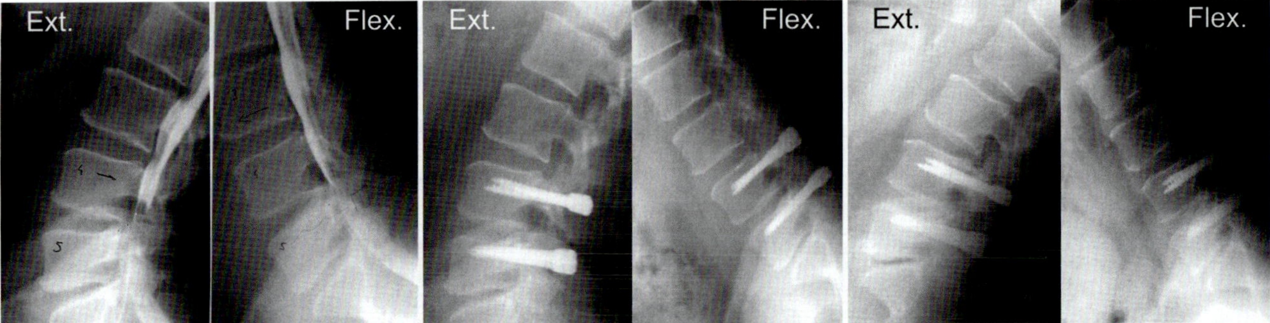

Figure 38–3   Male patient, 48 years old at time of surgery, presenting with permanent stenosis. Dynesys was implanted after recalibration of the affected level. Functional x-rays preoperatively, immediately postoperatively, and 6 years postoperatively.

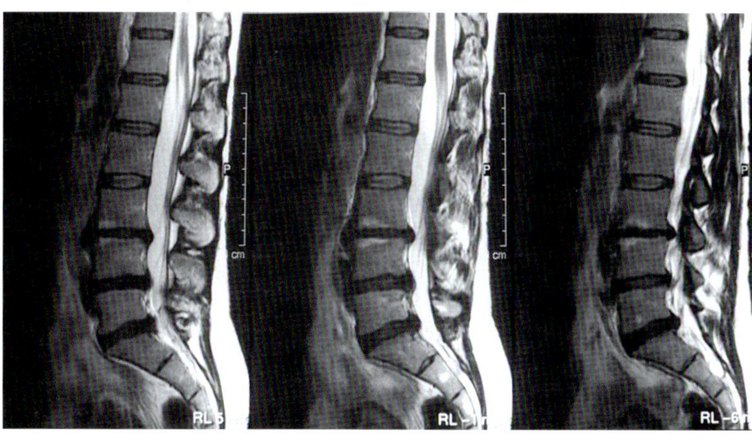

Figure 38–4 Female patient, 40 years old at time of surgery, presenting with Modic I signs at L3–L4, black disk on three levels, and positive diskogram at L3–L4 only. (Image provided by C. Crawshaw, Gloucester, U.K.)

performed. This approach does not interfere with the posterior muscles or the lumbar aponeurosis and provides direct access to the articular–transverse junction without interfering with the articulating surface and its capsule. It also enables the screw to be implanted at an angle that is almost always perfect.

Whatever approach is used, it is important not to interfere with the articular processes and their capsule. The point of intrapedicular penetration must be located at the external junction of the articular and transverse surfaces.

The steps for posterior compression or distraction of the heads of the screws enable determination of the exact length (6–45 mm) of the spacer that is required. This choice depends on the pathology being treated and on the degree of stabilization to be achieved.

With interpedicular distraction, the length of the spacer must ensure that the end plates of the level where Dynesys is implanted are perfectly parallel to avoid causing kyphosis of the segments. Restoration of lordosis of the segments may be left to the surgeon's discretion; however, hypercompression of the facet joints must be avoided under all circumstances because this may be detrimental to the appropriate functioning of the device as well as contrary to the underlying concept.

The assembly is completed with insertion of the cord and tensioning of the system.

◆ Performance

Treatment of unstable mobile diskopathies, in particular with restoration of stability, has previously consisted of medical and physical procedures. In cases of prolonged failure and as long as the displacements can be dynamically reduced, surgical stabilization, such as with the Dynesys, can be suggested.[4]

At best, the images accompanying clinical improvement clarify the contribution of dynamic stabilization toward restoring improved anatomy and physiology of the stabilized segment. The first effect is seen in postoperative myelograms, which show that the posterior annulus no longer bulges during flexion-extension movements. This is probably one of the reasons for the improvement of pain because the posterior longitudinal ligament is highly reflexogenic.[5]

In addition, various "regeneration" phenomena have been described anecdotally by Dynesys users. One prospective cohort study specifically addresses this.[6] In a consecutive series of 54 patients, Specchia found that after implantation of the Dynesys, Modic type I changes had disappeared at the time of follow-up. This has also been found in other hospitals (**Figs. 38–4 and 38–5**). Modic type I changes have been described as being a strong predictor of a painful disk[7] and also of having some correlation with pain and function in general.[8] Also, in 10% of the patients, a partial restoration of

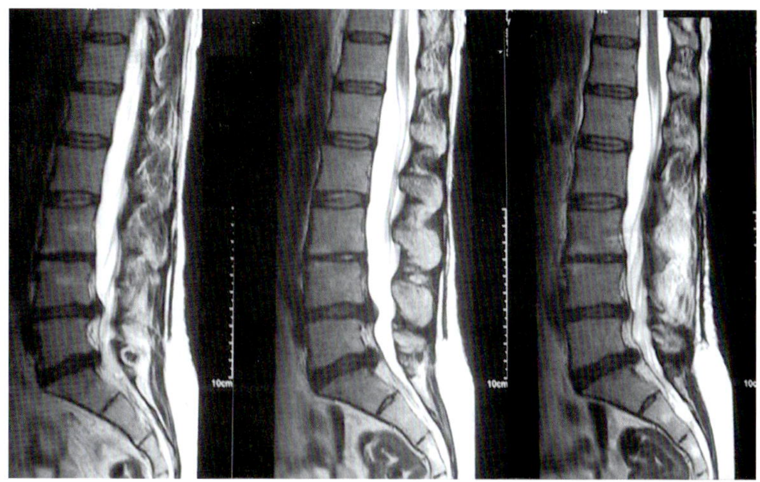

Figure 38–5 Dynesys implanted in L3–L4. Magnetic resonance imaging 11 months postoperatively shows recovery of Modic I signs at the Dynesys level. (Image provided by C. Crawshaw, Gloucester, U.K.)

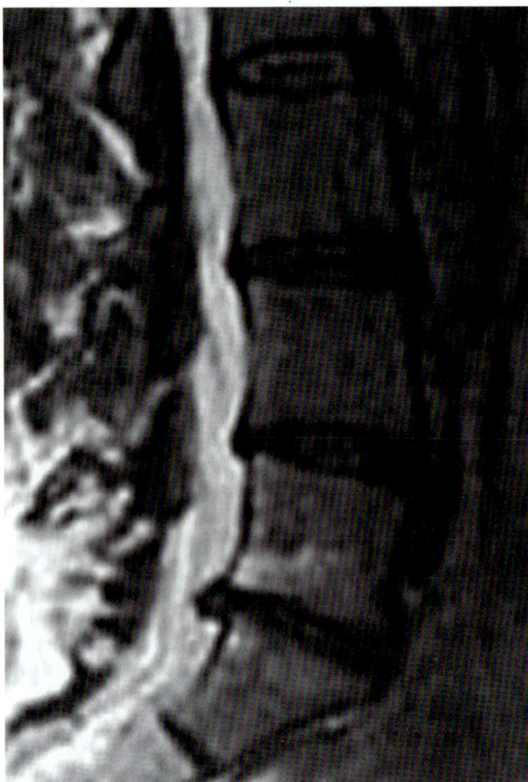

Figure 38–6   Female patient, 43 years old at time of surgery, with multilevel pathology necessitating diskectomy, foraminotomy, and posterolateral fusion in L5–S1 and Dynesys implantation in L3–L4.

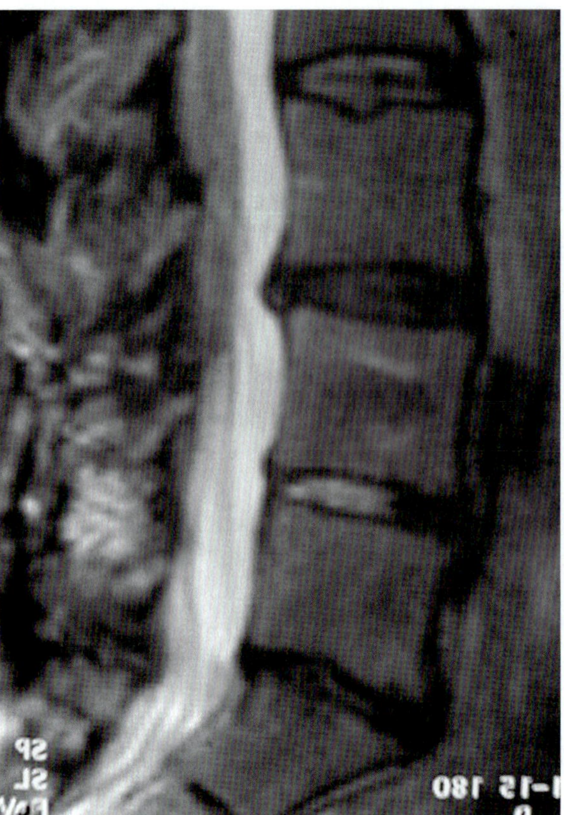

Figure 38–7   Magnetic resonance imaging 18 months postoperatively shows rehydration of the disk at the Dynesys level.

the T2-weighted magnetic resonance imaging (MRI) signal of the nucleus occurred (**Figs. 38–6 and 38–7**). The latter is a strong indicator for disk rehydration. This finding is in accordance with the results of an experimental study in New Zealand white rabbits[9] where it was found that degenerated dehydrated disks may regenerate after undergoing dynamic distraction.

As a whole, these observations suggest that the persistence of mechanical problems contributes to the biochemical phenomenon of degeneration. Due to the suppression of the intravertebral dyskinesis, an actual healing process of the annular and then of the intradiskal lesions may take place.

It is possible to imagine the following repair sequence:

◆ Suppression of the parasitic movements that cause the problems between the disk and the end plates (that may also interfere with nutrient exchange) to persist due to mechanical instability

◆ Mechanical neutralization which, due to suppression of the bulging, would enable healing with disappearance of the neovascularization at the level of the annular lesion

◆ Reestablishing new centers of rotation of the segment that suppresses segmental hyperpressure. This will foster the disappearance of neovascularization at the level of the end plates and will probably enable resumption of exchange between the subchondral bone and the intradiskal environment, which can enable rehydration in a later stage and, perhaps, reorganization of the nuclear structure.

Because the intradiskal liquid can be mobilized by the effect of pressure, and these pressures are redistributed and returned to a situation that resembles normality more closely, the alternating movements may be restored between the subchondral bone and the intradiskal environment. Given that this movement of liquid governs the balance between cell anabolism and catabolism, it will allow restoration of the fundamental substance, consisting of a highly hydrated proteoglycan gel inside the network of collagen (mainly type II). This interpretation was prompted by the clinical improvement of those patients who had benefited from dynamic stabilization and by the findings of the radiological follow-up. It currently remains, however, a purely intellectual construction to the extent that it is not supported by any histological or biochemical studies.

Research should be conducted in these areas.

◆ Clinical Results

Some high-quality studies are in progress, and several peer-reviewed journal publications on Dynesys are already available.

Stoll TM et al presented their first results with Dynesys[10] in 2002. Their prospective, multicenter study evaluated the outcome of a consecutive series of 83 patients treated with Dynesys for lumbar instability conditions, the pathology mainly involving lumbar stenosis (60% of patients) and degenerative diskopathy (24%). Thirty patients had had previous lumbar surgery. The mean age at operation was 58.2 (range, 26.8–85.3) years; the mean follow-up time was 38.1 months (range, 11.2–79.1). In 56 patients the Dynesys instrumentation was combined with a direct decompression procedure. Pain, function as measured by the Oswestry Disability Index (ODI), and radiological data were evaluated pre- and postoperatively and improved significantly from baseline to follow-up as follows: back pain scale from 7.4 to 3.1, leg pain scale 6.9 to 2.4, Oswestry Disability Index 55.4 to 22.9%. Most of the complications were unrelated to the implant. Additional lumbar surgery in the follow-up period included implant removal and conversion into spinal fusion with rigid instrumentation for persisting pain in three cases, laminectomy of an index segment in one case, and screw removal due to loosening in one case. In seven patients, adjacent segment degeneration necessitated further surgery.

The authors concluded that the study results compare favorably to those obtained by conventional procedures; however, mobile stabilization is less invasive than fusion. The natural course of polysegmental disease in some cases necessitates further surgery as the disease progresses. Dynamic stabilization with Dynesys proved to be a safe and effective alternative in the treatment of unstable lumbar conditions.

Cakir B et al published a retrospective comparative study in 2003[11] where they analyzed the functional outcome (ODI) and the quality of life [short form (SF)-36 Health Survey] of patients with degenerative lumbar instability with spinal stenosis who underwent decompression surgery with dorsoventral fusion or decompression surgery with posterior dynamic stabilization. In a small group of patients ($n = 20$), they showed a slightly better outcome for the Dynesys group. Furthermore, hospital stay and operation time were much shorter in the nonfusion group. They conclude that dynamic stabilization seems to be a promising alternative to fusion in patients with degenerative instability with spinal stenosis but point out the need for bigger studies.

Grob et al[12] published a retrospective study where 50 patients were implanted with the Dynesys and the results of 31 patients with a follow-up time of at least 2 years were presented. The pain and "patient-centered outcome" appears to be worse than in other publications. However, because no widely used standard outcome parameters enabling comparison with other studies are used, it is difficult to relate these findings to those in other publications.

Putzier et al compared the outcome after implantation of Dynesys in three different indication groups in 2004.[13] They compared patients with disk herniation ($N = 35$), spondylarthrosis/early osteochondrosis ($N = 22$), and severe degenerative changes (i.e., Modic II and III or spondylolisthesis up to grade II) ($N = 13$) using functional (ODI) and pain [visual analog scale (VAS)] outcome parameters. After a follow-up time of 33 months, they found that Dynesys yielded very good results in the first two groups but was not advisable for use in marked deformities.

The same group of researchers matched the subgroup of disk herniation patients of the previous study to a historical control group ($N = 49$) with the same pathology that had only received a nucleotomy.[14] In addition to the functional and pain outcome, they also analyzed the radiological outcome. At the time of follow-up (34 months), the patients who had received a Dynesys had a better functional (ODI) and pain (VAS) outcome than the other group. Besides this, progression of segmental degeneration was observed radiologically in 12% of the patients who had undergone sole nucleotomy and not in a single patient in the group where in addition Dynesys had been implanted. The authors conclude that Dynesys is useful to prevent progression of initial degenerative disease after nucleotomy.

Currently, our own series on patients with DDD and stenosis treated with Dynesys are being analyzed separately and will be published soon. Further publications on comparative studies are in preparation.

At present, 20 U.S. sites are participating in a Food and Drug Administration (FDA) Investigational Device Exemption (IDE) multicenter, prospective, randomized, clinical trial evaluating the safety and effectiveness of Dynesys. More than 400 Dynesys patients have been enrolled so far. The enrolment was completed at the end of 2004.

Moreover, several other randomized trials have been initiated to meet the demand for further high-quality research.

◆ Discussion

Dynamic stabilization with Dynesys is therefore indicated for mobile and self-reducible lesions when they occur during diskovertebral degeneration. The suppression of parasitic movements enables improvement of the pain symptoms and the appearance of healing at both the posterior and nuclear annular-ligamentary level and at the level of the end plates and articular processes. Due to the preservation of a certain degree of freedom in an area that functions normally from the anatomical point of view, this facilitates a return to local conditions that foster healing of the cartilaginous structures. Achieving this moderate postoperative intervertebral mobility is, moreover, the most important problem because it means that primary fixation of the pedicle implants must be absolutely perfect, with no technical error whatsoever and, in particular, no screw back-out during implantation.

The postoperative findings, based in particular on radiological examination of the patients, raised several questions and have encouraged us to envision other stages of research to achieve better histological understanding of the end plate lesions as described by Modic, and their possible reversibility. We should also consider studies on the disk, which appear to be even more complex, involving both histological and biochemical concepts.

In any case, healing phenomena do seem to exist, at least in the initial phase; that is, during the mobile phase of diskovertebral degeneration, and this should inspire great restraint in the future when faced with surgical choices. Irreversible procedures should probably be considered only when the lesions themselves are also irreversible.

◆ Conclusion

◆ At the present time, (2005) we believe it is possible to conclude that the concept of dynamic stabilization with Dynesys (**Fig. 38–8**) does have a place in the treatment of degenerative diskovertebral lesions. It deals in particular with the period of dynamic instability with mobile lesions that can still be self-reduced. The best example is probably dynamic stenosis and its clinical variants.

◆ The concept of dynamic stabilization is served well by the Dynesys system, which enables stabilization without fusion, preserves a controlled range of motion that facilitates local healing, and lowers the impact on the adjacent segments.

◆ It is advisable to analyze the true place of the Dynesys, in particular in the framework of subligament herniating diskopathy. This indicates local instability confirmed by abnormal intervertebral movements shown by dynamic imaging.

◆ Implanting pedicle screws constitutes the crucial point of the surgical procedure and requires technical perfection to optimize primary stability.

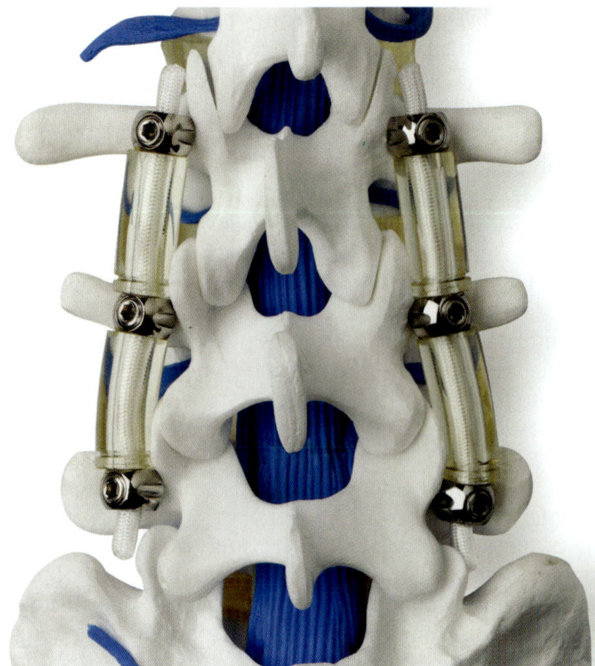

Figure 38–8   Dynesys mounted on a sawbone model.

References

1. Schmoelz W, Huber JF, Nydegger T, Claes L, Wilke HJ. Dynamic stabilization of the lumbar spine and its effects on adjacent segments: an in vitro experiment. J Spinal Disord Tech 2003;16:418–423

2. Niosi C, Zhu Q, Wilson D, et al. Does spacer length of dynamic posterior stabilization have an effect on kinematic behaviour? Paper presented at: SAS annual meeting, May 4–7 2005, Vienna, Austria

3. Kirkaldy-Willis SH. Managing Low Back Pain. 3rd ed. New York: Churchill Livingstone; 1992:49–74

4. Dubois G. Dynamic neutralization: a new concept for restabilization of the spine. Rivista di Neuroradiologia 1999;12(Suppl 1):175–176

5. Kuslich D, Ulstrom C, Michael C. The tissue origin of low back pain and sciatica: a report of pain response to tissue stimulation during operations on the lumbar spine using local anaesthesia. Orthop Clin North Am 1991;22:181–187

6. Specchia N. Disc regeneration after posterior lumbar dynamic stabilization. Paper presented at: Non Fusion Techniques in Spinal Surgery—international symposium, September 10, 2004, Milan, Italy

7. Braithwaite, White J, Saifuddin A, Renton P, Taylor BA. Vertebral endplate (Modic) changes on lumbar spine MRI: correlation with pain reproduction at lumbar discography. Eur Spine J 1998;7:363–368

8. Mitra D, Cassar-Pullicino VN, McCall IW. Longitudinal study of vertebral type-1 end-plate changes on MR of the lumbar spine. Eur Radiol 2004;14:1574–1581

9. Kroeber M, Unglaub F, Guegring T, et al. Effects of controlled dynamic disc distraction on degenerated intervertebral discs: an in vivo study on the rabbit lumbar spine model. Spine 2005;30:181–187

10. Stoll TM, Dubois G, Schwarzenbach O. The dynamic neutralization system for the spine: a multi-center study of a novel non-fusion system. Eur Spine J 2002;11(Suppl 2):S170–S178

11. Cakir B, Ulmar B, Koepp H, Huch K, Puhl W, Richter M. Posterior dynamic stabilization as an alternative in the treatment of degenerative lumbar instability with spinal stenosis. Z Orthop Ihre Grenzgeb 2003;141:418–424

12. Grob D, Benini A, Junge A, Mannion A. Clinical experience with the Dynesys semi-rigid fixation for the lumbar spine. Spine 2005;30: 324–331

13. Putzier M, Schneider SV, Funk J, Perka C. Application of a dynamic pedicle screw system (Dynesys) for lumbar segmental degenerations: comparison of clinical and radiological results for different indications. Z Orthop Ihre Grenzgeb 2004;142:166–173

14. Putzier M, Schneider SV, Funk JF, Tohtz SW, Perka C. The surgical treatment of the lumbar disc prolapse: nucleotomy with additional transpedicular dynamic stabilization versus nucleotomy alone [abstract]. Spine [journal online]. 2005;30:E109–114. Available at: http://www.spinejournal.com/pt/re/spine/abstract.00007632-200503010-00020.htm;jsessionid=CpkdD1RCCVsSQJLFHxYQYcxaZ-wOhcXOJzQJUmSoJUm41LJL4YAdw!-465889315!-949856031!9001!-1. Accessed July 29, 2005

39

Graf Soft Stabilization: Graf Ligamentoplasty

Young-Soo Kim and Dong-Kyu Chin

◆ **Concept and Rationale**

◆ **Indications and Contraindications**
   Indications for Graf Ligamentoplasty
   Contraindications for Graf Ligamentoplasty

◆ **Operative Techniques**
   Patient Operative Position
   Surgical Approach
   Implant Placement

   Band Placement
   Operative Precautions

◆ **Past, Present, and Future**
   Past: Graf Ligamentoplasty
   Present: Graf Ligamentoplasty with Anterior Column Support
   Future: Combination of Rigid and Soft Stabilization

Degenerative involution of the spine causes destruction of the spinal stabilizer, which consists of bone, ligament, joint capsule, and disk, which substantially leads to hypermobility and instability of the spine.[1,2] As the degenerative changes in the lumbar spine progress, the spinal canal is also compressed by a protruded disk, hypertrophied facet, and ligaments.[3,4] In the surgical treatment of such patients, decompression of the spinal canal is mandatory. But the structures, which are removed during decompressive laminectomy, are elements of a stable spine, and postlaminectomy iatrogenic spinal instability may become complicated.[5] In patients with preexisting instability or a high risk of postlaminectomy iatrogenic spinal instability, surgical insertion of an internal fixation device as well as spinal arthrodesis were the usual solutions.[6–9] The recent development of internal fixation devices such as the pedicle screw fixation system and interbody fusion cages has allowed rigid spinal stability and outstanding surgical outcomes.[6,9] However, acquiring stiffness and spinal stability has required the sacrifice of the unique physiological function (i.e., motion) of the spinal segment, which is, without doubt, a disadvantage.

Generally, the rigid fixation system has been used to treat lumbar instability. However, it can result in complications such as nonunion, screw loosening, screw fracture, and flat back syndrome.[10,11] Rigid fixation also increases the biomechanical stresses on the adjacent segments to the fusion level.[12,13] Clinically, the results of several long-term follow-up studies have suggested that spinal fusion might cause deterioration of the adjacent segment.[14–16]

The complications of rigid fixation have led to the invention of a nonfusion technology that is more physiological than any other fixation devices.[17–19] The concept of "dynamic stabilization" is to *restrict* the hypermobility of an unstable spinal segment rather than eliminating it. Among the types of soft stabilization systems, the Graf soft stabilization system (Sem Co., Montrouge France) was one of the first relatively widely practiced methods.[19]

◆ Concept and Rationale

The Graf soft stabilization system was invented by Henri Graf.[19] It consists of the surgical implantation of a titanium pedicle screw linked with polyester threaded bands as a ligament to connect the pedicle screws across the unstable

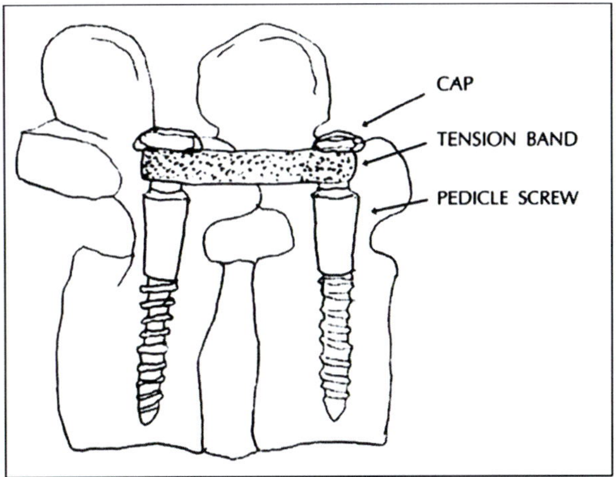

Figure 39–1 Graf pedicle screws and polyester bands. The Graf soft stabilization system consists of the surgical implantation of titanium pedicle screws linked with polyester threaded bands as a ligament to connect the pedicle screws across the unstable segment. (With permission from Sem Co., Montrouge, France.)

segment (**Fig. 39–1**). He believed that instability was related to the development of an abnormal rotatory movement. This abnormal rotatory movement and distraction at the facet joints might be a cause of low back pain. The basic concept is to dynamically stabilize abnormal rotatory movements in physiological lordosis using the Graf band, which results in the alteration of annular and end plate load bearing. This posterior immobilization in lordosis closes degenerative annular tears and degenerative gaps in the facet joint, allowing the healing of damaged tissues.[19,20]

Some biomechanical studies using cadavers show that Graf ligamentoplasty reduces the range of motion and provides flexibility under some loading conditions.[21–23] Strauss et al[21] found that Graf ligamentoplasty significantly reduced range of motion for flexion-extension but had little effect on the translation motion. This finding suggests that Graf ligamentoplasty had the potential to treat "flexion instability." The advantages of Graf ligamentoplasty are as follows: (1) less invasive, (2) more physiological, (3) reduced biomechanical stress on adjacent segments, (4) no risk of pseudarthrosis, and (5) no donor-site pain.[24]

The authors think the Graf soft stabilization system gave birth to the concept of dynamic stabilization, making surgeons realize the significance of the ideal stiffness. Undoubtedly, this progress is considered a big leap in the field of degenerative lumbar spine surgery.

◆ Indications and Contraindications

Our surgical indication for Graf ligamentoplasty is chronic degenerative lumbar disk disorders with or without segmental instability. Each patient has complained about chronic low back pain that has been resistant to conservative treatment over a 6-month or longer period. Initially, degenerative black disk and facet syndrome were included after a specific diagnostic protocol such as diskography and facetogram. However, the clinical outcomes in those entities were not as good. After gaining a certain amount of experience in Graf ligamentoplasty, degenerative black disk and facet syndrome, which Graf initially listed as indications, have been excluded from the indications.

In chronic degenerative disk disorder with canal stenosis, Graf ligamentoplasty can be used after decompressive laminectomy or diskectomy, which can prevent postoperative iatrogenic instability, and this turns out to be our major indication. Grade I spondylolisthesis and degenerative slipping (< 25%) of the vertebral body might be indications, too. However, we have to be aware that Graf ligamentoplasty is not a procedure that can completely replace spinal fusion and arthrodesis.

Indications for Graf Ligamentoplasty

1. Chronic degenerative disk disease with or without canal stenosis.

   ◆ When postoperative iatrogenic instability is anticipated, Graf ligamentoplasty may be indicated.

2. Multiple spondylotic lumbar spinal stenosis

   ◆ After wide decompressive laminectomy, Graf ligamentoplasty may prevent postoperative iatrogenic instability.

3. Lumbar instability syndrome

   ◆ Especially flexion instability is a good indication.

4. Stabilization of the adjacent segment above or below the main pathology.

   ◆ Graf ligamentoplasty may reduce the mechanical stress imposed on the adjacent segment.

5. Degenerative spondylolisthesis (< 25%) of the vertebral body.

6. Interbody fusion should be added in the following conditions:

   ◆ After diskectomy
   ◆ Modic degeneration
   ◆ Translational instability
   ◆ Narrowed disk height or neural foramen
   ◆ When anterior column support is indicated

Contraindications for Graf Ligamentoplasty

1. Isthmic spondylolisthesis
2. Retrolisthesis
3. Degenerative spondylolisthesis greater than grade I
4. Tumors, infection, or trauma
5. Scoliosis deformity
6. Rigid kyphotic deformity

◆ Operative Techniques

Patient Operative Position

The patient operative position is derived from one described by McNab. However, the trunk is placed in a horizontal position with pressure on the upper limbs to obtain an "on-all-fours" position. The cushion is mounted to the table to provide mild support of the rib cage so that it allows the abdomen to be dependent. In this position, the lumbar spine is left in a mean supple lordosis. Care is taken to avoid undue pressure on bony prominences, genitalia, and neurovascular structures. A radiological control allows detection of the involved vertebrae corresponding with the cutaneous guide.

Surgical Approach

A midline linear incision and exposure are made above the involved segments. The surgical approach is made in an assymetrical manner: fixed retractors are replaced by blunt retractors, held by an assistant. After having uncovered the articular area without opening the capsule, the transverse process is exposed. This allows the surgeon to identify the entry for implant insertion.

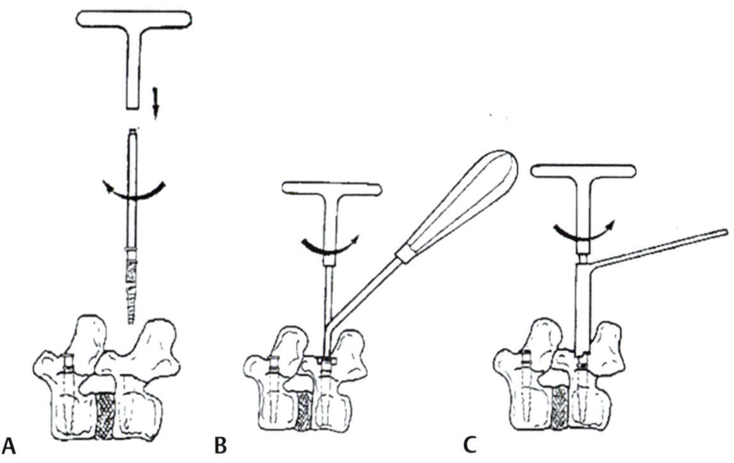

Figure 39–2   Implant placement. **(A)** Implant insertion is made with the male hexagonal screwdriver or the implant holder. **(B,C)** To unscrew the implant holder, one of the two implant holders is needed. (With permission from Sem Co., Montrouge, France.)

Implant Placement

The pedicular implant entry point is located approximately halfway between the superior and inferior edges of the transverse process at the junction of the articular processes. It is sometimes necessary to remove some of the external superior articular facet to free space between the implant and the vertebra. At the insertion point, the remaining bony crest should be removed using a gouge. The sacral implant entry point is located ~5 mm from the articular facet L5–S1 and halfway from the foramen S1. Great care should be exercised for sacral implant placement. It should follow a path parallel to the L5 implant in the direction of the sacral promontory. To reinforce insertion quality, it is recommended to secure the attachment by slightly perforating the anterior cortical promontory without penetrating the cortex wall completely.

The awl is used to perforate a 5 mm hole in the cortical bone. With gentle, twisting motions, the pedicular path is determined by using a graduated blunt curette. The appropriate screw length is determined by reading the graduation on the blunt curette. The implant placement follows the anatomical pedicular axis, which varies from one vertebra to another. Selection of screw size is based on the length measured in the preceding step and the diameter is determined on preoperative imaging studies. Implant insertion is made with the male hexagonal screwdriver or the implant holder. The length of these instruments allows the surgeon to insert screws through a skin counterincision. To unscrew the implant holder, one of the two implant holders is needed (**Fig. 39–2**).

Band Placement

Band size varies by 2.5 mm increments. The bands are measured with the band size measurer, which is used to grasp the head of the implanted pedicular screws. The measurer is used to calculate the desired tension and size of the band to be used. The tension chosen must be sufficient to eliminate local instability. For bands smaller than 25 mm, tension with graduation 5 is sufficient (read band size measurer). Over 25 mm, graduation 10 is suitable.

The band is placed on the implant head using the band tension forceps by making small rotational horizontal movements. Prior to band placement, the implants must be so that their upper collar is face to face. The band pusher may help to slip the band over the implant head and to control band tension. To secure band placement a one-half rotation is applied to position the screw top hemispherical flange in the opposite direction of the other screw. Such rotation retains the bands securely in position. For a two-level construction, a titanium screw cap is placed on the top of the middle implant to secure the band's positioning (**Fig. 39–3**).

Operative Precautions

It is important to protect the bands from abrasion by the facet joints. Therefore it is recommended:

◆ To check that sufficient space is left between the metallic implant and the external face of the articular facet

◆ To check that the band does not rub against the facet

◆ To prepare and correct the path of the band with a gouge forceps or a chisel

◆ Not to screw the metallic implant tight; this will cause band–bone contact

◆ Past, Present, and Future

Past: Graf Ligamentoplasty

Decompressive laminectomy is the most important part of the surgery for degenerative lumbar spine. The lamina, ligamentum flavum, medial facet and disk, all of which act as spinal stabilizers, may be removed during decompressive surgery. However, while performing multilevel laminectomy and foraminotomy, the facet joint may be damaged. In some cases, more than 50% of the facet is removed during the procedure, which results in postoperative iatrogenic instability. Controversies surround the concept of spinal fusion after decompressive laminectomy. On one hand, even after wide decompressive laminectomy, the possibility of spinal instability and slipping is low and therefore it is not necessary to perform the spinal fusion procedure.[25,26] On the other

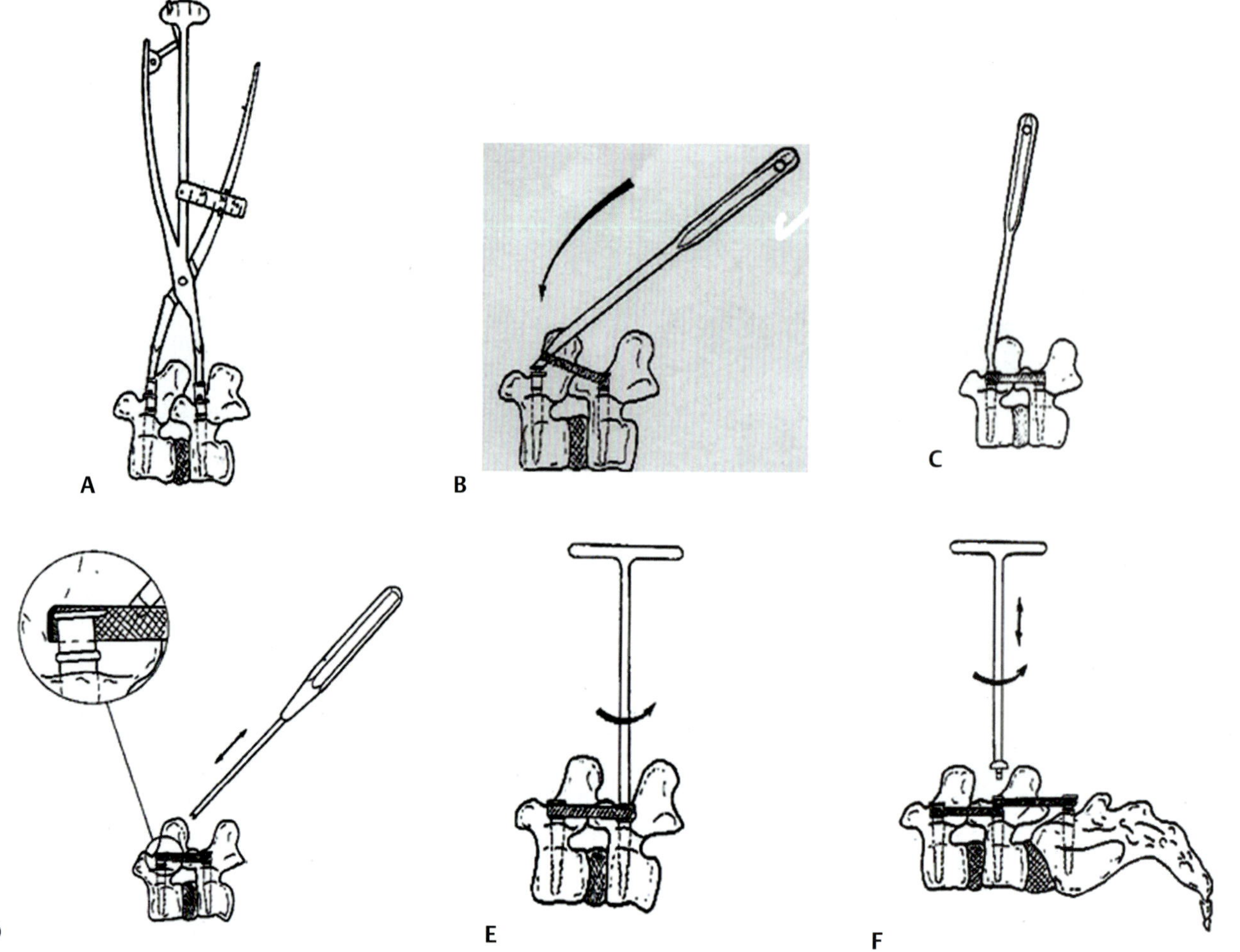

Figure 39–3   Band placement. **(A)** The band size measurer is used to grasp the head of the implanted pedicular screws. **(B,C)** The band is placed on the implant head using the band tension forceps by making small rotational horizontal movements. **(D)** The band pusher may help to slip the band over the implant head and to control band tension. **(E)** One-half rotation is applied to position the screw top hemispherical flange in the opposite direction of the other screw. **(F)** For a two-level construction, a titanium screw cap is placed on the top of the middle implant to secure bands positioning. (With permission from SEM Co., Montrouge, France.)

hand, there may be spinal instability up to 43% after decompressive laminectomy, and spinal fusion should be added after laminectomy.[27,28] Hanley and David suggest that spinal fusion should be done in the following conditions: facet injury more than 50%, total facetectomy on one side, multilevel laminectomy in young patients, and deformity cases.[29]

A total of 106 patients with lumbar spinal degenerative disk disease with canal stenosis were treated with the Graf soft stabilization system following decompressive laminectomies. Among them, 18 had degenerative spondylolisthesis, seven had recurrent disk protrusion, and 11 had failed back surgery syndrome (**Table 39–1**). Seventy-two patients showed segmental instability on preoperative dynamic radiograph: 60 angular instability and 21 translational instability (note that nine patients were redundant). Flexion instability changed from −6.9 degrees to 5.5 degrees on L3–L4, −7.45 degrees to 5.04 degrees on L4–L5, −2.09 degrees to 10.81 degrees on L5–S1; translation instability was corrected from 16.8 to 14.9% on L3–L4, 19.9 to 12.4% on L4–L5, 27.1 to 20.1% on L5–S1 after Graf ligamentoplasty.[30] Graf ligamentoplasty was particularly effective in patients with flexion instability due to degenerative facet loosening. These corrections of

instability were due to its role as an artificial ligament of the Graf soft stabilization system (**Fig. 39–4**).

However, Graf ligamentoplasty has not been used by the majority of spine surgeons because its long-term clinical outcomes are unsatisfactory. The main limitations of Graf ligamentoplasty are the lack of anterior column support and the production of joint overlocking. In our series of Graf

Table 39–1   Disease Classification

Disease	Graf Only	Graf with PLIF
Lumbar spinal stenosis	52	53
Chronic degenerative	33	48
Recurrent disk/FBSS	18	12
Spondylitic spondylolisthesis	0	7
Facet syndrome	3	0
Total	106	120

FBSS, failed back surgery syndrome; PLIF, posterior lumbar interbody fusion.

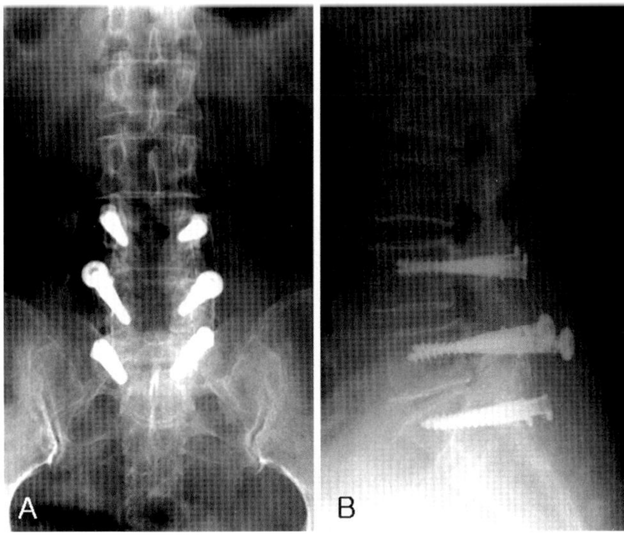

Figure 39–4 Radiographs showing Graf ligaments and pedicle screws. **(A)** Anteroposterior and **(B)** lateral radiographs were obtained after decompression at L4–L5 was performed and the Graf implant was inserted bilaterally.

ligamentoplasty, the radiological outcome was good but the clinical outcome was not satisfactory.

Present: Graf Ligamentoplasty with Anterior Column Support

The dynamic immobilization in physiological lordosis is the basic concept and the biggest advantage of the Graf soft stabilization system, but at the same time it can act as a disadvantage. The buckling of the ligamentum flavum and the joint capsule may compress the nerve root at the neural foramen. In cases with a narrowed disk height and foramen, immobilization in lordosis may be complicated in the foregoing radiculopathy. Graf ligamentoplasty after diskectomy may also result in nerve root compression at the neural foramen. The intervertebral disk is a key structure that supports the anterior column when applying compressive force to the pedicle screws, and the disk space should be preserved to avoid joint overlocking and iatrogenic neuroforaminal stenosis.

There may be an advanced loss of disk height and a loss of anterior column support with Graf ligamentoplasty in the following conditions: (1) after diskectomy, (2) Modic degeneration, (3) translational instability, and (4) narrowed disk height or neural foramen. So as already indicated, anterior column support with interbody fusion should be done in such conditions (**Fig. 39–5**).

Posterior lumbar interbody fusion (PLIF), which was established by Cloward,[31] has the best theoretical opportunity to achieve spinal fusion by way of the load-sharing effect of the anterior column, but it can also restore narrowed disk height and neural foramen. We modified the concept of Graf ligamentoplasty: the main pathological segment is stabilized with PLIF. The main pathological segment and the adjacent segment are stabilized with the Graf soft stabilization system to prevent adjacent segment degeneration. And also this posterior instrumentation with the Graf band can help the fusion process in PLIF (**Fig. 39–6**).

A total of 120 patients with lumbar spinal degenerative disk disease with canal stenosis were treated with PLIF and Graf ligamentoplasty (**Table 39–1**). Among them, there were 45 with degenerative spondylolisthesis and 79 with

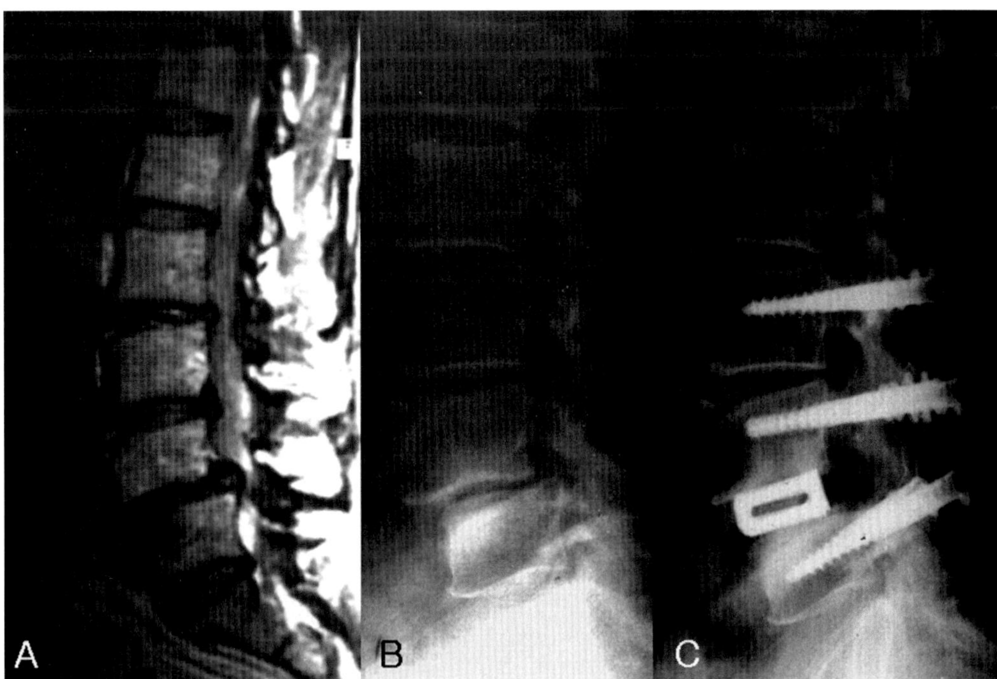

Figure 39–5 Radiographs showing Graf ligamentoplasty and anterior column support with interbody fusion. **(A)** Preoperative magnetic resonance imaging and **(B)** lateral radiograph showed degenerative slipping on L4–L5 level. There may be an advanced loss of disk height and a loss of anterior column support after decompressive laminectomy and Graf ligamentoplasty. **(C)** Postoperative lateral radiograph showed Graf ligamentoplasty and anterior column support with interbody fusion cages.

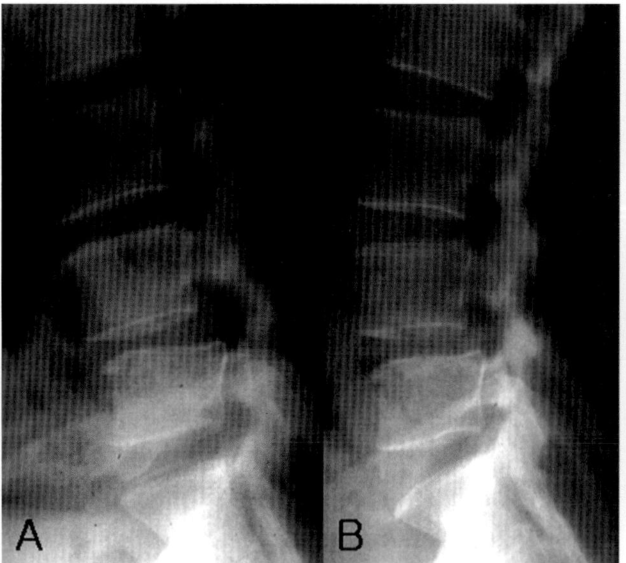

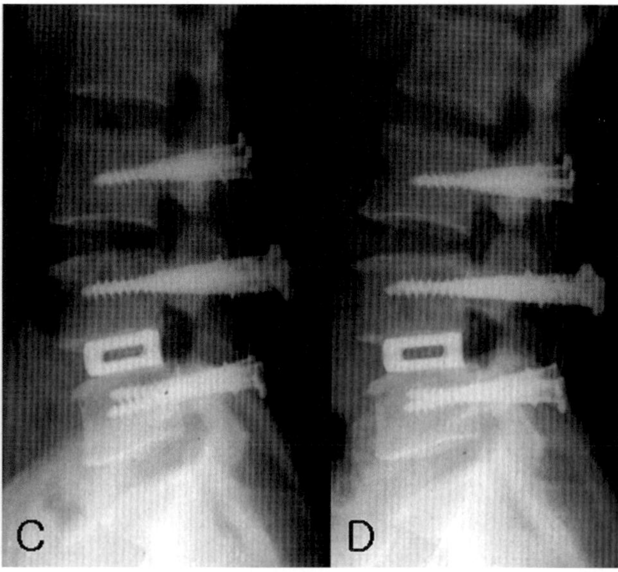

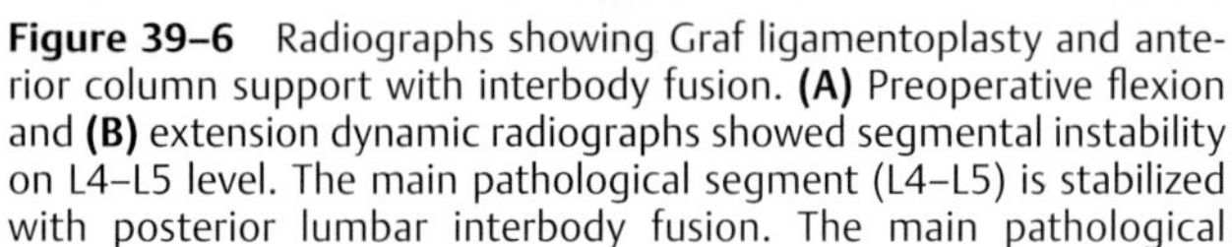

Figure 39–6   Radiographs showing Graf ligamentoplasty and anterior column support with interbody fusion. **(A)** Preoperative flexion and **(B)** extension dynamic radiographs showed segmental instability on L4–L5 level. The main pathological segment (L4–L5) is stabilized with posterior lumbar interbody fusion. The main pathological segment and the adjacent segment (L3–L4) are stabilized with the Graf soft stabilization system to prevent adjacent segment degeneration. **(C)** Postoperative flexion and **(D)** extension dynamic radiographs showed Graf ligamentoplasty and anterior column support with interbody fusion cages.

segmental instability on preoperative dynamic radiograph. The preoperative angular instability was 14.9 ± 6.4 degrees and it was significantly corrected to 3.4 ± 3.5 degrees after PLIF and Graf ligamentoplasty. The preoperative translational instability was 6.4 ± 1.9 mm and it was significantly corrected to 1.6 ± 1.1 mm after the operation. The disk height on the main pathological segment was also corrected from 9.8 ± 2.1 mm to 12.2 ± 2.4 mm. When compared with Graf ligamentoplasty without anterior column support, we had a satisfactory clinical outcome and 110 patients (88.7%) showed excellent or good outcome.[32]

Steffee reported on the ideal fusion rate and surgical outcome with PLIF and posterior pedicle screw fixation in a single incision.[9,33] Our modified concept of Graf ligamentoplasty is similar to Steffee's concept. One difference is that we used soft stabilization, whereas they used rigid stabilization. With this modified method of Graf ligamentoplasty, we can enable anterior column support and restore the narrowed disk height and neural foramen. We can also reduce the mechanical stress imposed on the adjacent segment, which can prevent transitional disease.

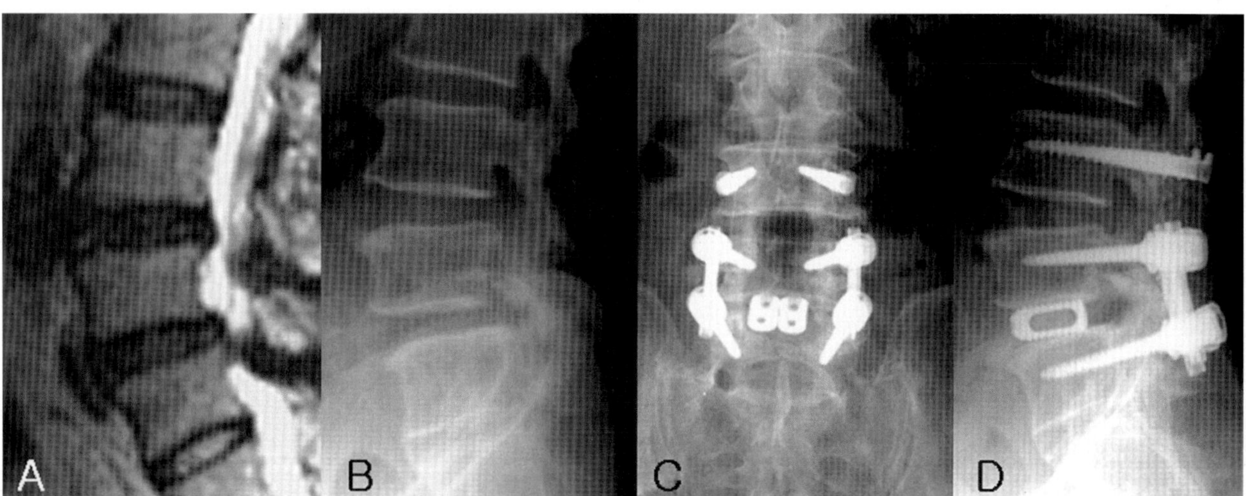

Figure 39–7   Radiographs showing hybrid stabilization, in which the main pathological segment is rigidly fused whereas the adjacent segment is softly stabilized with the Graf system. **(A)** Preoperative magnetic resonance imaging showed severe stenosis on L4–L5 and disk degeneration on L3–L4. **(B)** Lateral radiography showed degenerative slipping on L4–L5 and a traction spur on L3–L4. **(C)** Postoperative anteroposterior and **(D)** lateral radiographs showed hybrid stabilization.

Future: Combination of Rigid and Soft Stabilization

Traditionally, spinal fusion has been the mainstay of surgical procedures for the treatment of degenerative lumbar instability. However, rigid fixation increases the biomechanical stresses on the segments adjacent to the fusion level,[12,13] leading to transitional disease. This complication of rigid fixation has led to the invention of a more physiological fixation device with dynamic stabilization.

Even in dynamic stabilization, anterior column support is crucial. Because the intervertebral disk is a key structure to support the anterior column, dynamic stabilization without anterior column support is likely to fail. Although we can expect a better outcome with our modified Graf ligamentoplasty with anterior column support, this procedure cannot completely replace spinal arthrodesis.

We reported the new style Graf ligamentoplasty (which combined rigid and soft stabilization) at the 17th North American Spine Society meeting.[34] The main pathological segment was rigidly fused, whereas the adjacent segment was softly stabilized with the Graf system (**Fig. 39–7**). Gardner and Pande[35] referred to this combination of rigid and soft stabilization as *hybrid stabilization.*

We suggest that anterior column support is essential even in dynamic stabilization, and, furthermore, the combination of rigid and soft is a positive development for the future of dynamic stabilization.

References

1. Panjabi MM, White AA III. Basic biomechanics of the spine. Neurosurgery 1980;7:76–93
2. Schneck CD. The anatomy of lumbar spondylosis. Clin Orthop Relat Res 1985;193:20–37
3. Kirkaldy-Willis WH, Farfan HF. Instability of the lumbar spine. Clin Orthop Relat Res 1982;165:110–123
4. Kirkaldy-Willis WH, Wedge JH, Yong-Hing K, Reilly J. Pathology and pathogenesis of lumbar spondylosis and stenosis. Spine 1978;3:319–328
5. Posner L, White AA 3rd, Edward WT, Hayes WC. A biochemical analysis of the clinical stability of the lumbar and lumbosacral spine. Spine 1982;7:374–389
6. Roy-Camille R, Saillant G, Mazel C. Internal fixation of the lumbar spine with pedicle screw plating. Clin Orthop Relat Res 1986;203:7–17
7. Luque ER. The anatomic basis and development of segmental spinal instrumentation. Spine 1982 May–June;7(3):256–259
8. McGuire RA, Amundson GM. The use of primary internal fixation in spondylolisthesis. Spine 1993;18:1662–1672
9. Steffee AD, Biscup RS. Segmental spine plates with pedicle screw fixation. Clin Orthop Relat Res 1986;203:45–53
10. Deburge A. Modern trends in spinal surgery. J Bone Joint Surg Br 1992;74:6–8
11. Frymoyer JW, Hanley EN Jr, Howe J, Kuhlmann D, Matteri RE. A compression of radiographic findings in fusion and nonfusion patients ten or more years following lumbar disc surgery. Spine 1979;4:435–440
12. Schlegel JD, Smith JA, Schleusener RL. Lumbar motion segment pathology adjacent to thoracolumbar, lumbar and lumbosacral fusion. Spine 1996;21:970–981
13. Hilibrand AS, Robbins M. Post-arthrodesis adjacent segment degeneration. In: Vaccaro A, Anderson DG, Crawford A, et al, eds. Complications of Pediatric and Adult Spinal Surgery. New York: Marcel Dekker; 2003
14. Lee CK. Accelerated degeneration of the segment adjacent to a lumbar fusion. Spine 1988;13:375–377
15. Lehmann TR, Spratt KF, Tozzi JE, Fang D. Long-term follow-up of lower lumbar fusion patients. Spine 1987;12:97–104
16. Leong JC, Chun SY, Grange WJ, Fang D. Long-term results of lumbar intervertebral disc prolapse. Spine 1983;8:793–799
17. Ray CD. The PDN prosthetic disc-nucleus device. Eur Spine J 2002;11:(Suppl 2)S137–S142
18. Cinotti G, David T, Postacchini F. Results of disc prosthesis after a minimum follow-up period of 2 years. Spine 1996;21:995–1000
19. Graf H. Lumbar instability: surgical treatment without fusion. Rachis 1992;412:123–137
20. Kanayama M, Hashimoto T, Shigenobu K. Rationale, biomechanics, and surgical indications for Graf ligamentoplasty. Orthop Clin North Am 2005;36:373–377
21. Strauss PJ, Novotny JE, Wilder DG, Pope MH. Multidirectional stability of the Graf system. Spine 1994;19:965–972
22. Wild A, Jaeger M, Bushe C, Raab P, Krauspe R. Biomechanical analysis of Graf's dynamic spine stabilisation system ex vivo. Biomed Tech (Berl) 2001;46: 290–294
23. Hasegawa K, Takano K, Endo N, et al. A biomechanical study on the stabilizing effect of Graf ligamentoplasty in a graded destabilization model of porcine lumbar spine [in Japanese]. Rinsho Seikei Geka 2004;39:133–140
24. Gardner ADH. An alternative concept in the surgical management of lumbar degenerative disc disease flexible stabilization. In: Margulies JY, ed. Lumbosacral and Spinopelvic Fixation. Philadelphia: Lippincott-Raven; 1992:889–905
25. Shenkin HA, Hash CJ. Spondylolisthesis after multiple bilateral laminectomy and facetectomies for lumbar spondylosis: follow-up review. J Neurosurg 1979;50:45–47
26. Tsou PM, Hopp E. Postsurgical instability in spinal stenosis. In: Hopp E, ed. Spine: State of the Art Reviews. Philadelphia: Hanley and Belfus; 1987:533–550
27. Johnsson KE, Redlund-Johnell I, Uden A, Willner S. Preoperative and postoperative instability in lumbar sacral stenosis. Spine 1986;11:107–110
28. Nasca RJ. Rationale for spinal fusion in lumbar spinal stenosis. Spine 1989;14:451–454
29. Hanley EN, David SM. Who should be fused? Lumbar spine. In: Frymoyer JW, ed. The Adult Spine: Principle and Practice. Vol 2. 2nd ed. Philadelphia: Lippincott-Raven; 1997:2157–2174
30. Ha Y, Kim YS, Yoon DH, Jin DK, Park HW. Graf soft fixation for the treatment of degenerative lumbar disease. J Korean Neurosurg Soc 1998;27:1370–1378
31. Cloward RB. The treatment of ruptured lumbar intervertebral discs by vertebral body fusion, I: Indications, operative techniques after care. J Neurosurg 1953;10:154–163
32. Kim YS, Cho YE, Jin BH, Chin DK, Yoon DH. Soft graf fixation and posterior lumbar interbody fusion in multiple degenerative lumbar diseases. J Korean Neurosurg Soc 1998;27:229–236
33. Enker P, Steffee AD. Interbody fusion and instrumentation. Clin Orthop Relat Res 1994;300:90–101
34. Kim YS, Chin DK, Cho YE. An analysis of results of rigid and soft stabilization on degenerative lumbar instability. Presented at: the 17th Annual meeting of North American Spine Society, Montreal, Canada, October 29-November 2, 2002
35. Gardner A, Pande KC. Graf ligamentoplasty: a 7-year follow-up. Eur Spine J 2002;11(Suppl 2):S157–S163

40

Isobar TTL Dynamic Instrumentation

Antonio E. Castellvi, James J. Paraiso, and David Pienkowski

- ◆ **Dynamic Instrumentation and Adjacent Level Disk Degeneration**
- ◆ **Biomechanical Performance of the Isobar TTL System**
- ◆ **Finite Element Modeling and Analysis**
- ◆ **Indications**
- ◆ **Technical Notes for Placement of the Isobar TTL Dynamic Rods**
- ◆ **Summary**

It has been said that "necessity is the mother of invention" and in this new millennium of spine care, there is a need for finding a way to provide a better cure for back pain without predisposing patients to future spinal problems. Invariably, much of today's painful spinal conditions are centered on the functional spinal unit and the degenerative processes that occur to the intervertebral disk. Subsequently, before one could "invent" a theoretical instrumentation construct designed both to address spinal pain and to slow the process of disk degeneration, one must first understand the time-dependent cascade of events that leads to the physiological deterioration of the intervertebral disk.

There exists a certain group of people that will experience disk degeneration. As with any other degenerating joint, a specific subset of this group will become symptomatic from this degenerative process. Kirkaldy-Willis et al[1] was a pioneer in categorizing the three stages of this disk degeneration process. In stage one, there appears to be some unknown initiating event that causes end plate calcification of the vertebral body, limiting nutrient diffusion and subsequently causing adverse changes in the biochemistry and physiology of the nucleus pulposus (NP) within the intervertebral disk.[2] The nucleus is a thick and highly viscous gel-like substance consisting primarily of water-laden proteoglycans whose main function is to absorb shock and transmit loads. Age-related changes to the disk cause it to become a more fibrous material with abnormal viscoelastic properties. These property changes in turn lead to asymmetrical load distributions through the end plates and annulus, which in turn can cause pain as described by Henry Crock in 1970 as "internal disk disruption."[3] This may be the first source of pain experienced due to the abnormal loading pattern seen within the disk. It is theorized that as axial loads are applied, due to the altered material properties of the disk, asymmetrically distributed localized "high spot loading" occurs.[4,5] This "high spot loading" causes localized regions of excessive stress amplitudes and consequently excessive localized deformations, which in turn lead to pain. On a longer-term basis, load shifting (caused by the degenerated and abnormal NP)

asymmetrically shifts forces to both the vertebral end plates and the annulus fibrosus of the disk. This leads to end plate alterations and annular fissuring.[5] At this stage the radiographic appearance of the disk may essentially be normal, but magnetic resonance imaging (MRI) of the disk may show annular tears and be dark on T2 sequences, hence the name *dark disk disease.*

At this point the evolving failure of the disk transitions to the annulus fibrosus and its decreased ability to endure torsional, shear, and axial compressive loading. This subsequently heralds stage two of the degenerative cascade noted by Kirkaldy-Willis; namely, increasing instability of the functional spinal unit. Instability here means "a loss of spinal motion segment stiffness such that the application of force to a particular motion segment produces greater overall displacement(s) than would occur in a normal structure."[6] This forms the basis for another source of pain, as well as the potential for progressive deformity, and also puts selected neurological structures at risk. Furthermore, the inability of the nucleus to tolerate normal loads and subsequent abnormal motion leads to a compensatory response.

The previously described sequence of events (stages one and two) inevitably leads to Kirkaldy-Willis's third and final stage of the degenerative cascade. This stage begins with the musculoskeletal system's ultimate attempt at stabilization of the abnormally loaded, unstable, and nonprotective (of neural structures) functional spine unit. Evidence for this is clearly seen with ligamentum flavum hypertrophy, facet arthropathy, reduced disk height, and osteophyte formation. These biological responses collectively act to stabilize, or in some cases, pseudofuse the functional spine unit to limit motion and thereby reduce pain.

Recent literature[4] suggests that there may be a "safe window" in which a functional spine unit may be spared the degenerative cascade if the mechanical loads placed on it remain within a physiological range.[4] When load amplitude and motion are limited to an as yet incompletely understood physiologically benign "window" of load amplitudes, there is evidence that some regeneration of the disk may occur. Overloading may lead to additional tissue trauma or adaptive changes that initiate or exacerbate disk degeneration. Applied loads or motion outside this "window" may create damage exceeding the reparative abilities of the disk, and thus damage accumulation will occur faster than repair can occur. This rate of discrepancy (repair versus damage) will inevitably culminate in failure of the disk. This is the physiological basis of Stokes's working hypothesis describing the mechanobiological homeostasis of disk tissue.[4]

In addition to the various aspects of the degenerative cascade describing how the functional spine unit fails over time, the therapeutic options available to the spine surgeon to treat the aforementioned conditions also impose their own load and motion alterations on the functional spine environment. Thus, in a sense, surgical treatment can "add insult to injury," by destabilizing the functional spinal unit. It is particularly evident in the postlaminectomy patient who can experience as much as a 40% reduction in the stiffness of the functional spine unit and possibly back pain.[7]

Of more recent concern is the issue of postfusion adjacent level disk degeneration. Many articles have documented that the disk and end plate adjacent to a fusion, especially at the cephalad level, experience one or more of the following: increased stress, increased mobility or segmental displacement, and increased intradiskal pressure.[8–10] Because of the nonphysiological and apparently unfavorable environment induced at the cephalad level adjacent to a fusion, the literature reports increased rates of symptomatic degeneration that require surgery. As noted, there is good clinical evidence of disk degeneration in segments adjacent to the fusion. Complete removal of all stresses, loads, and motion at a disk segment suggests there are altered spinal column mechanics with increased stresses occurring at and concentrated in the adjacent levels. These increased loads, motion, and subsequent stresses and pressures in the adjacent disk are affected by the length, location, and stiffness of the fusion mass.[4] Gillet[11] reported that out of 37 subjects who had a one-level fusion, 32% experienced adjacent level degeneration and 11% needed a reoperation. In the same article, of the 26 subjects who had two-level fusions, 31% of them had degenerative changes and 27% required reoperation. Moreover, when they considered 27 subjects who had three- and four-segment fusions, 66% of them experienced adjacent-level degeneration and 33% required reoperation at the adjacent level. They concluded that we "need to find more reconstructive surgical procedures for the management of symptomatic degenerative spines that are resistant to conservative treatment." With regard to the transitional segment predisposed to degeneration, Gillet also stated that a possible solution to address that entity was to do some kind of "preventative reinforcement" of the adjacent level.

Fortunately, a paradigm shift in the approach to treating spinal problems is occurring that will help advance the technology of spinal treatments to become more on par with those used to treat other degenerated musculoskeletal joints. This paradigm shift is based upon the change in design philosophy from fusion and arresting spinal motion, toward instrumentation designs that decompress the stenotic motion segment and allow controlled movement of the functional spine unit while simultaneously unloading and protecting it from excessive forces or motion. The age of dynamic instrumentation of the spine has arrived.

◆ Dynamic Instrumentation and Adjacent Level Disk Degeneration

Dynamic instrumentation denotes the current physical embodiment of an implant designed with three contemporary realizations in mind. First, fusion changes the natural anatomy, eliminates motion, and may lead to adjacent-level degeneration. Second, due to these changes and the less than ideal successes that fusion confers, the spine community now recognizes that the methods of treating spinal degeneration and instability must change. Third, these changes are manifested in new methods of conceptualizing the surgical processes of stabilization, which in turn have inspired new instrumentation designs aimed at achieving enhanced clinical outcomes while simultaneously minimizing the drawbacks of current technologies.

The principal goal of dynamic instrumentation is to achieve stabilization while more closely replicating the natural function of the lumbar spine, as well as providing the patient with symptomatic relief. The instrumentation design allows a predetermined range of motion to achieve symptom relief yet preserve some of the anatomical load-bearing functions of a particular motion segment. Dynamic stabilization has been thought to be safe and effective in the treatment of lumbar degenerative disk disease through early clinical studies in Europe.[12] This instrumentation design is an effective means of decreasing the neohinge effect at the adjacent level by increasing the load and motion at the superior level of a fusion. This then led to the belief that dynamic stabilization may also be used to decrease the incidence or severity of adjacent level disk degeneration.

Dynamic instrumentation has two important design elements, one intended to change the loading, the other intended to change the motion. Both of these elements work hand in hand to achieve the intended effect. Practically, instability is defined as abnormal patterns of movement within the motion segment that cause altered loading to the spine unit such that pain, deformity, or neurocompromise occurs. It is the combination of both abnormal loading and abnormal motion that leads to a painful motion segment. Therefore, it is for this reason that the ideal design characteristics of dynamic instrumentation must address both abnormal loading and abnormal motion. Prior surgical treatment of lumbar degenerative disk diseases altered both load and motion in nonphysiologically relevant ways. Decompression procedures removed some of the anatomical motion constraints, whereas fusion eliminated all motion and shifted the loads to the adjacent level disk. This subsequently led to an increased likelihood for adjacent level disk degeneration because the stress amplitudes and distributions in the adjacent level disk were altered.

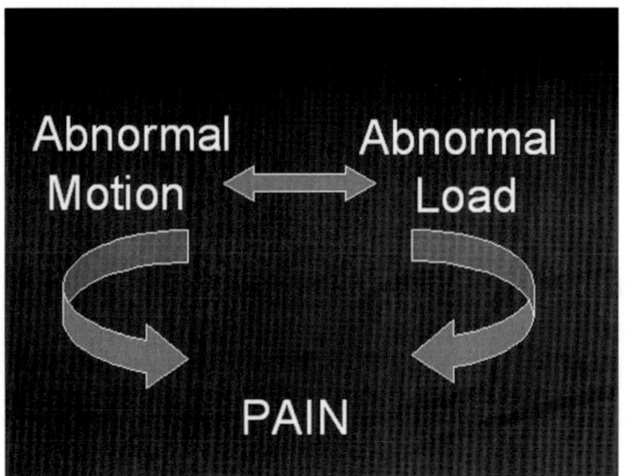

Figure 40–1   Pain generation in the lumbar spine.

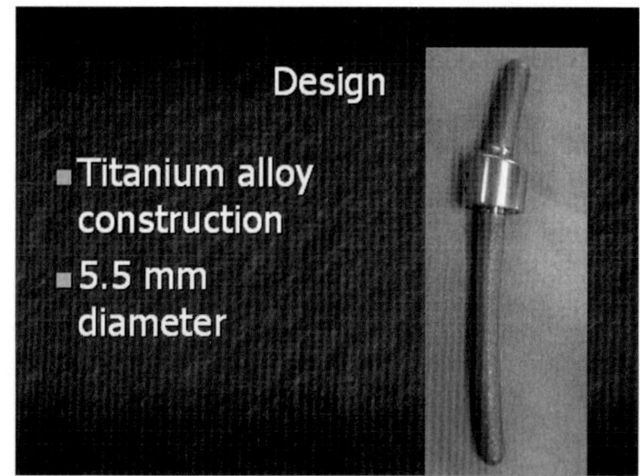

Figure 40–3   Isobar TTL design.

Furthermore, the loss of anatomical constraints of the motion segment allowed pathological displacement. The resulting altered loads and motions are the fundamental bases by which pain is generated in the lumbar spine (**Fig. 40–1**).

Thus the design goals of dynamic instrumentation are to: (1) provide adequate stability to provide symptomatic relief to a painful motion segment, (2) allow some controlled motion to the segment and thereby prevent substantial departure from the normal biomechanics of this segment, and (3) share the loads and stresses applied to that motion segment so that abnormally large loads are not created at the adjacent levels (**Fig. 40–2**).

The ideal dynamic system should unload the disk and provide adequate stability so that symptomatic relief is obtained, yet the system must also simultaneously distribute the load so that the adjacent-level disks are not excessively stressed and thus forced down the degenerative path, which culminates in their subsequent failure. As part of this designed stability with controlled range of motion feature, this ideal system would also preserve the natural anatomy by maintaining lordosis and would incorporate an instantaneous axis of rotation (IAR) that is more anatomically correct than rigid instrumentation techniques

provide. All of these features will act in concert to reduce significantly the morbidity and invasiveness of traditional fusion surgery. In addition, the design of the system should be such that the surgeon would find the approach familiar and easy to use. Finally, in the event of an undesirable outcome, the salvage surgery must be simple, with no "burning of bridges."

Today, the current embodiment of this system, developed as noted from the work of French engineer Albert Alby and subsequently refined in design and materials, is currently produced from titanium alloy (Ti6Al4Va) by Scient'x USA (Scient'x USA, Maitland, FL). This system, denoted Isobar TTL (**Fig. 40–3**), consists of a 5.5 mm diameter rod with an integral dampener element (**Fig. 40–4**). The dampener element contains stacked titanium alloy disk-shaped elements

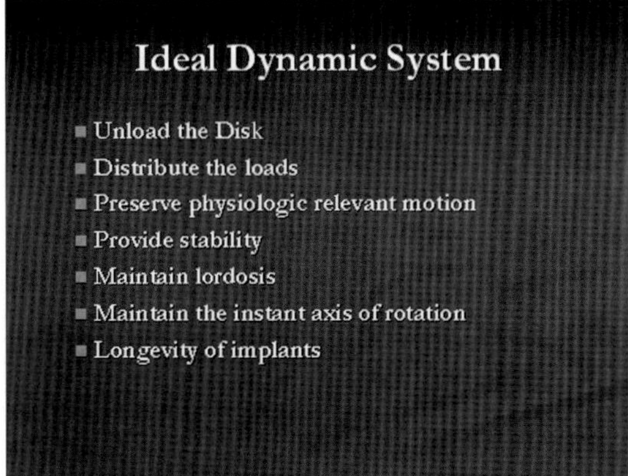

Figure 40–2   Ideal dynamic system.

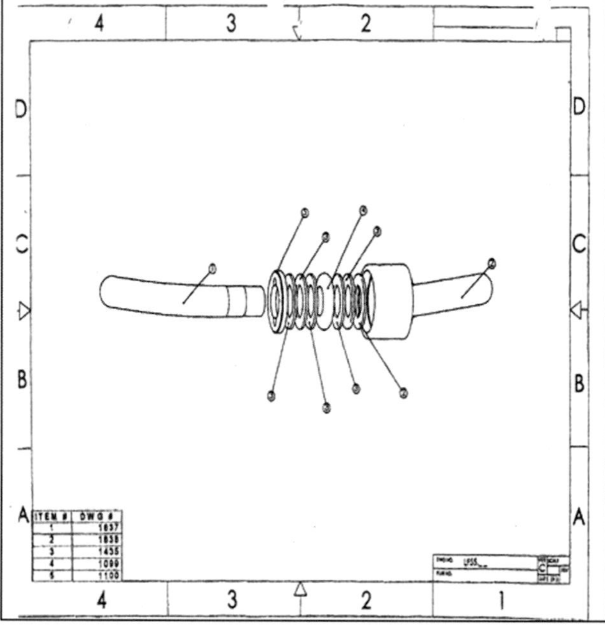

Figure 40–4   The dampener housing protects eight titanium O-rings treated with a nitrogen ion process to minimize wear. These provide the "shock absorber" dimension.

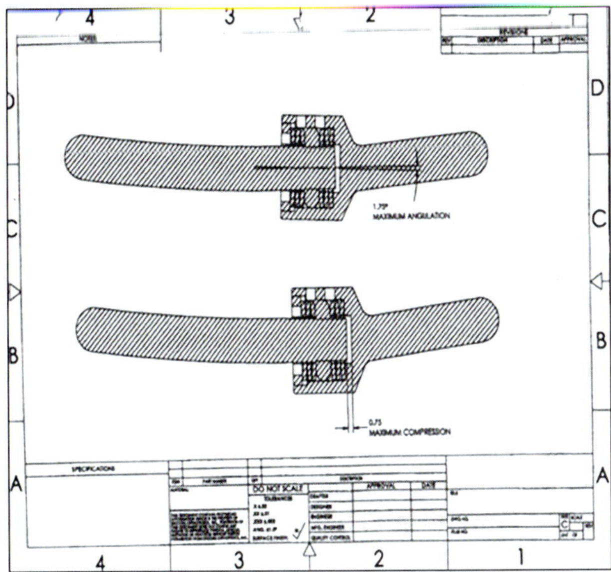

Figure 40–5   There are 0.75 mm of compression and 1.75 degrees of angulation built into the dampener mechanism.

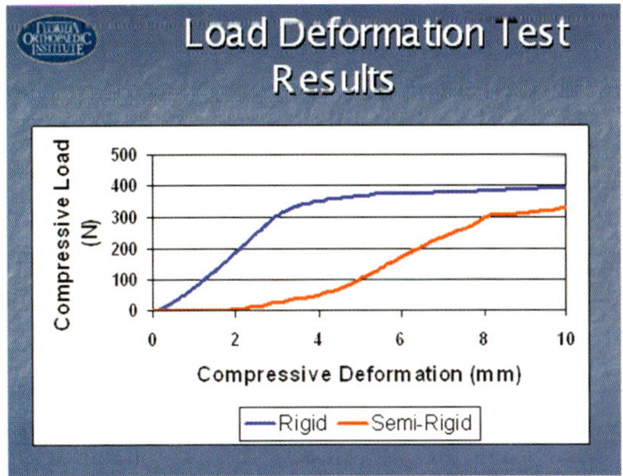

Figure 40–6   Load deformation test results.

that allow linearly elastic controlled axial and angular motions (**Fig. 40–5**). Each of these disks has a nitrogen ion surface treatment intended to substantially increase their wear resistance. This dampener feature of the rod results in a design-allowable 0.75 mm of maximum axial compression or distraction, as well as a maximal allowable 3 degrees of angular motion (in flexion-extension and lateral bending). Finally, the dampener feature also serves as a linearly elastic "shock absorber." In an assembled instrumentation system applied to a nonfused segment, only flexion-extension bending and axial motions are permitted (lateral bending is restricted due to the bilateral geometry of the device). This system also includes an approximate 15 degrees of lordosis built into the device.

◆ Biomechanical Performance of the Isobar TTL System

The technical design goals for the "ideal" system just described have been incorporated into this particular instrumentation system. Load bearing capabilities of this system were first studied by using standard production Isobar TTL posterior lumbar spinal fusion instrumentation as applied to a tried and tested, ultra high molecular weight polyethylene (UHMWPE) disk–based laboratory model of a lumbar spine functional unit. This model was originally developed by Cunningham et al[13] and was later formalized in an American Society for Testing and Materials protocol (F1717). Twelve such instrumented polyethylene lumbar spine functional unit models were tested; each of these had a fixed (fused) inferior level (L5–S1) but half of the L4–L5 levels were instrumented with rigid instrumentation and the other half of the L4–L5 levels were instrumented with Isobar TTL instrumentation. Thus there were six specimens in each of these two test groups. The instrumented lumbar spine models

were then axially compressed at a rate of 15 mm/minute (quasi-static rate of compression) in a servohydraulic materials testing system. The resulting load-deformation data were recorded and used to calculate the compressive "stiffness" of all constructs.

Mean elastic quasi-static compressive stiffness for the rigid constructs was 21,960 ± 8,034 Nm, whereas the corresponding mean elastic compressive stiffness for the dynamic construct was almost one fourth (specifically, $^1/_{3.6} \times$) this value (6169 ± 1298 Nm). These values were significantly ($p = .01$) different. The difference shows that the dynamic instrumentation segment (due to the dampener feature) at L4–L5 was 3.6 times less stiff than the rigid conventional instrumentation[14,15] (**Fig. 40–6**).

Single-load compressive stiffness testing was also performed. This was done at Ecole Nationale Supérieure d´Arts et Métiers (ENSAM) in Paris, France. This was a compressive bending test on 16 spinal rods. The test was performed on a Cunningham model made of UHMWPE vertebrae. Sinusoidal compressive loading was performed at a frequency of 5 Hz using an Instron 1331 (Instron Corporation, Norwood, MA) servohydraulic materials testing system. Over 5 million loading cycles without failure were completed.

◆ Finite Element Modeling and Analysis

Quantification of the quasi-static compressive stiffness testing of conventional and dynamic device designs was necessary to perform the next phase of instrumentation characterization. Because in vivo measurement of the stresses induced in the adjacent level disks is not a measurement option at this time, the best alternative is a mathematical—specifically, a finite element—model of these disks. For this purpose, a three-dimensional finite element model of the lumbar spine (L1–L5 including disks) was developed by obtaining a validated finite element mesh for the L4 vertebrae. The geometry of the vertebrae was developed based on a series of computed tomographic scans of L4 vertebrae of a 44-year-old male with no pathologies. The L4 mesh was then replicated to the model of the lumbar spine as well as the other (L1–L3 and L5)

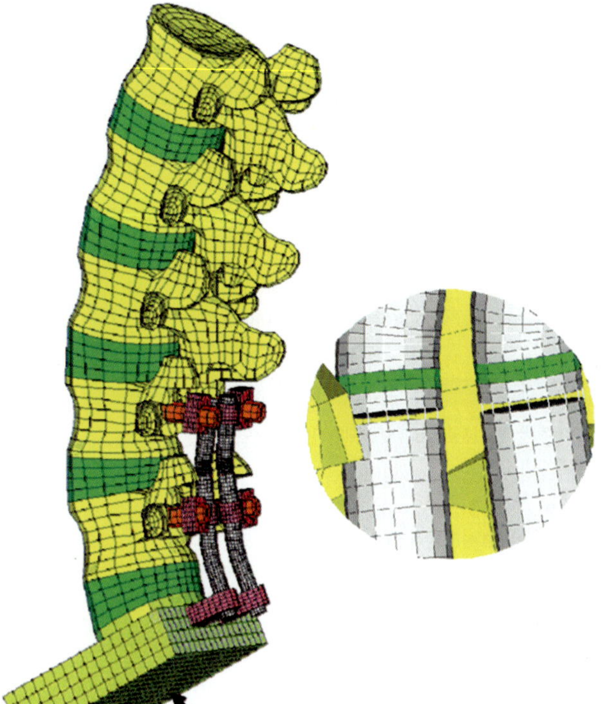

Figure 40–7   Isometric view of the finite element mesh of the lumbar spine and dynamic rods.

vertebrae. The resulting mesh of the L1–L5 vertebrae was positioned such that there was a 40 degree angle between the inferior surface of the L2 and the superior surface of the L5 vertebra (**Fig. 40–7**).

This finite element model consisted of a fused (totally rigid) L5–S1 segment, and an L4–L5 segment that was modeled to imitate rigid or dynamic fixation. The dimensions of the instrumentation used in the model were obtained from direct measurements of exemplar instrumentation of the Scient'x USA TTL rod. The fused segments between L5–S1 were modeled by setting the material properties of this disk so that they duplicated those of cortical bone. An adjacent pair of vertebrae was connected by a simulated intervertebral disk, which was modeled with a nucleus in the center and surrounded by three to four rings of annulus fibrosus. The entire finite element model contained 18,128 three-dimensional, eight-node linear brick elements. Loading of the model was accomplished by combining flexion (three discrete values) or extension (one value) plus axial loading. Specifically, the model simulated flexion at 15 degrees, 30 degrees, and 45 degrees, and extension at 15 degrees. The modeling process also incorporated the application of an axial compressive load of 400 N amplitude applied simultaneously with the applied flexions (noted previously). The dampener of the dynamic instrumentation permitted the upper segment of the rod to have a reduced ($^1/_{3.6}$ ×) stiffness in the model. This value was obtained from direct measurements obtained during the quasi-static biomechanical compressive testing stiffness. A limited and discretely variable (0, 0.2, 0.4, 0.6, and 0.8 mm) amount of axial

micromotion was also incorporated into the model. These two features of this dampener mechanism were modeled by employing a softer segment (with variable stiffness values, all of which were less than those of titanium alloy) placed in series with an axial motion connector.

The variable model parameters, R and G, were used to represent and quantify the reduced stiffness and axial micromotion, respectively, of the dampener element. The R parameter ($R = K_{rigid}/K_{dynamic}$) was calculated from the ratio of the stiffness obtained from the material properties of the rigid titanium alloy segment divided by the reduced stiffness of the constituent dynamic segment. The G parameter was defined as the maximum axial motion designed into the dampener mechanism. To study the effects of axial motion, five discrete maximum allowed axial displacements (0–0.8 mm in 0.2 mm increments) were studied.

Before reaching the maximum axial moment, the axial motion connector also functioned as an axial spring with a stiffness of 175 kN/m. This stiffness corresponds to 0.4 mm compression motion at an axial load of 70 N. The inferior portion of the sacrum was modeled as a block and the lower surface of the block was considered fixed. A static compressive load of 400 N was applied to the superior surface of L1. This level was maintained perpendicular to the superior surface of the L1 segment throughout the simulated axial load–induced deformation. All components were modeled by using linearly elastic materials. The material properties assigned to the components of this model are standard for Young's modulus and Poisson's ratio (**Table 40–1**).

Given the model built, the design features noted, and the material properties listed, the modeling and analysis were conducted to determine the:

◆ Kinematics

◆ Maximum stress amplitudes induced in the disks

◆ Distribution of stresses within the disks

◆ IAR

The resulting kinematic data showed that by allowing 2 degrees of rotation at the L4–L5 disk, less angular deformation will occur at the L3–L4 disk, and this will thereby

Table 40–1   Material Properties Used in the Lumbar Spine Finite Element Model

Material	Young's Modulus, GPa	Poisson's Ratio
Cortical bone	3	0.2
Cortex	12	0.3
Cancellous bone	0.5	0.2
Fibrous	0.03	0.45
Nucleus	0.001	0.49
Steel	190	0.3
Titanium	116	0.33

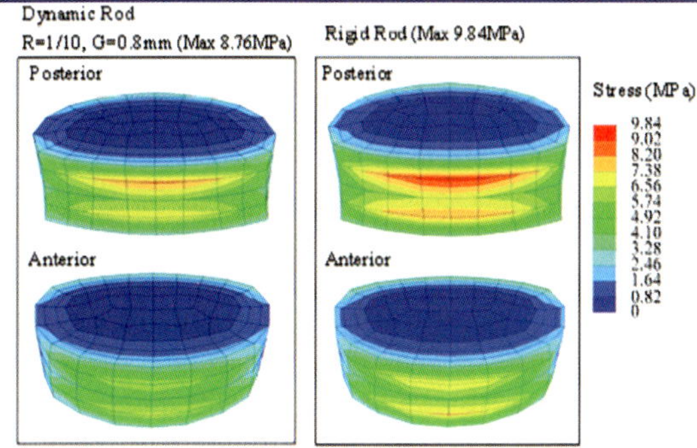

Figure 40–8 Finite element analysis (FEA) of stress distribution of L3–L4 demonstrating increased stress when using the rigid rod. Note the intensity of color.

generate less stress at this level (**Fig. 40–8**). There are two ways to generate 2 degrees of rotation: (1) create a posterior hinge effect, which would allow loading at the L4–L5 disk, or (2) move the IAR at the level of the disk to a more central and physiological position. For this to occur, we need to be able to allow axial extension and compression. This in turn allows a significantly smaller load that is needed to create the 2 degrees of rotation (**Fig. 40–9**).

Maximum stress values were calculated with a significant decrease in the Von Mises stress (i.e., the resultant stress obtained by combining the stresses induced in all three dimensions; finite element analysis stress results are typically presented as Von Mises stresses) at the L3–L4 disk of the spine having dynamic instrumentation at the L4–L5 disk. Also the volumetric distribution of maximum stresses experienced in the L3–L4 disk was decreased by 40% in the dynamic model.

A sensitivity analysis was performed with the dampener characteristics in an effort to determine the ideal biomechanical parameters of this device. Specifically, the model was analyzed for different values of axial displacement (G) and damper stiffness (R). The modeling demonstrated that decreased values of R made a slight reduction in the maximum stress induced in the L3–L4 (adjacent level) disk, but

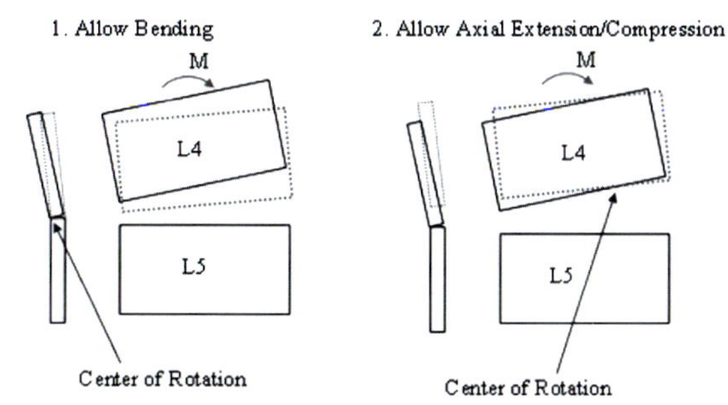

Figure 40–9 Centers of rotation.

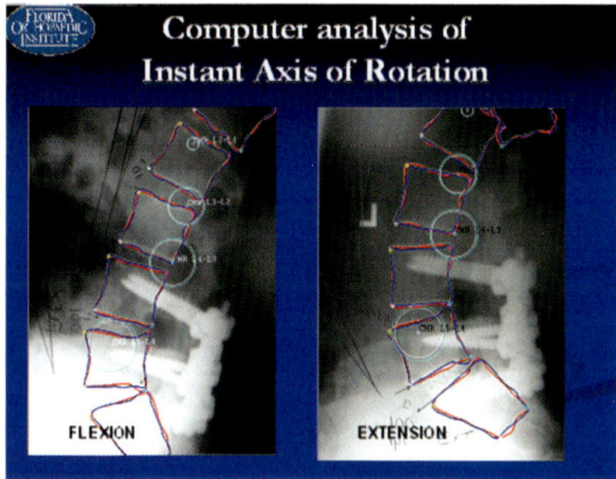

Figure 40–10 Computer-assisted analysis of the in vivo dynamic (flexion-extension) radiographs shows that motion is preserved at the dynamic level; there is no pathological motion at the adjacent level and the instantaneous angle of rotation (IAR) at the dynamic level is at a more physiological position. The IAR of the adjacent level is preserved in its physiological location. Early in vitro biomechanical analyses with cadaveric spines are in progress to confirm the biomechanical and finite element analysis (FEA) results.

increasing the value of G showed a larger reduction in this stress. Thus decreasing the rod stiffness and increasing the axial motion (especially) resulted in a decrease in the stress amplitude induced in the adjacent level disk, a decrease in the force necessary to create 2 degrees of rotation, and the preservation of the instantaneous axis of rotation into a more physiological position.

Biomechanical testing revealed that the mean elastic stiffness of the rigid instrumentation was 21,960 Nm and the mean elastic stiffness of the dynamic instrumentation was 6169 Nm. Using these data, the results of R and G values for the rigid rod were 1 and 0, respectively; whereas the R and G values for the dynamic rod were 3.6 and 0.4 mm, respectively (**Fig. 40–10**).

The stress reduction at the L3–L4 level caused by reduced stiffness of the dynamic rod and increased axial distraction associated with this particular type of instrumentation allowed the volume of disk tissue that is exposed to maximum stresses to be 47% less than the volume of disk tissue in the conventionally instrumented lumbar spine. The effects noted above were most prominent for the case of 45 degrees of forward flexion. Similar results were also observed at 15 degrees and 30 degrees of flexion and in 15 degree extension, but the magnitude of the disk loading was smaller in amplitude and smaller in relative difference between the rigid and dynamic instrumentation cases (**Figs. 40–8 and 40–11**).

◆ Indications

Disk decompression and fusion have constituted the historical surgical treatment for lumbar degenerative disk disease. All of these procedures create one type or another of abnormal loading or abnormal motion. The loss of anatomical constraints from decompression allows pathological displacement, creating further instability of the motion segment. Fusion causes

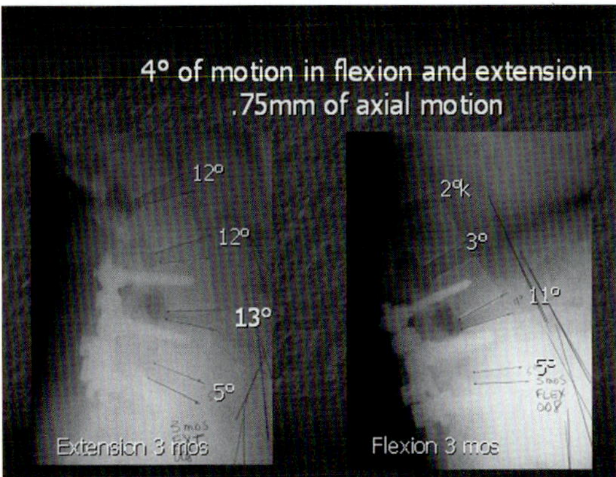

Figure 40–11 Four degrees of motion in flexion and extension and 0.75 mm of axial motion.

the stresses and angular motion to be transferred to the adjacent levels; the resulting abnormal loading refers not only to the maximum force amplitude but also to the force distribution in the disk.

These problems are addressed by the design of dynamic instrumentation (i.e., to provide stability of a painful motion segment and correctly distribute stress in the adjacent disk without overloading). In addition, a specific embodiment of this dynamic instrumentation, the Scient'x TTL system, is designed to maintain lordosis, stabilize the spine through its functional range of motion, and maintain the IAR while simultaneously guarding the disk from overloading. The built-in lordotic curve of the device is designed to preserve the natural anatomy of the lumbar spine, and this confers an additional important design feature of the TTL device. Unlike so many other orthopedic treatment options, use of the dynamic TTL system does not "burn the patients' bridge"—one can always return and perform a conventional fusion if by some chance the dynamic instrumentation is not satisfactory. Finally, the design of the TTL instrumentation offers a familiar surgical approach that requires only a brief learning curve and is mastered with relative ease.

Indications for use of dynamic instrumentation of the lumbar spine include:

1. Internal disk derangement
2. Grade I or II degenerative spondylolisthesis
3. Recurrent disk herniations
4. Massive diskectomies
5. Iatrogenic instability—unilateral facetectomy or decompressive laminectomy for spinal stenosis
6. Adjacent level degeneration prophylaxis

Contraindications for the use of dynamic instrumentation of the lumbar spine are:

1. Bilateral spondylolisis
2. Bilateral facetectomies
3. Grade III or IV spondylolisthesis
4. Greater than 50% disk space narrowing
5. Fractures
6. Scoliosis
7. Across thoracolumbar junction
8. Osteoporosis

(**Figs. 40–12, 40–13, and 40–14**)

◆ Technical Notes for Placement of the Isobar TTL Dynamic Rods

1. Use a lateral starting point for screw placement and do not violate facet joints (**Fig. 40–15**).
2. Utilizing the lumbar lordosis obtained by a Jackson frame, simply connect the rods to the screws in situ and be sure to have the writing on the dampener and the rod line up as well as facing dorsally (**Fig. 40–16A,B**).
3. Do not place rod connectors against the caudal aspect of the dynamic rod dampener because doing so will prohibit motion within the dampener (**Fig. 40–17A**). In the majority of cases, utilizing the off-set rod connectors can help

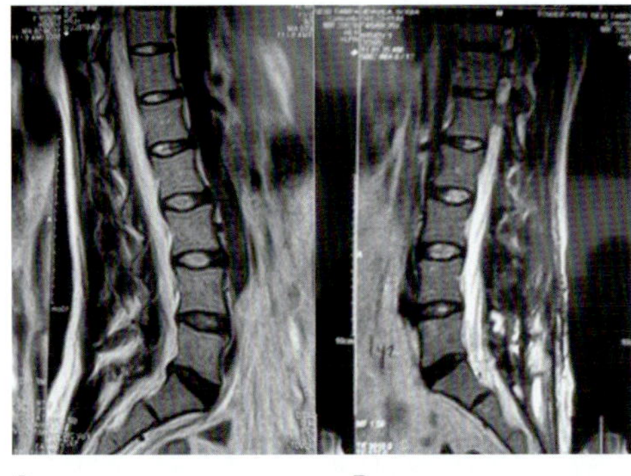
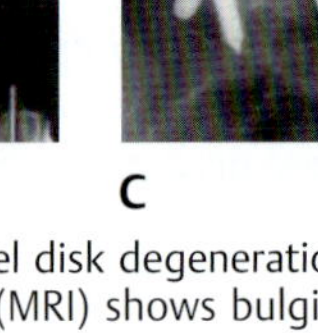
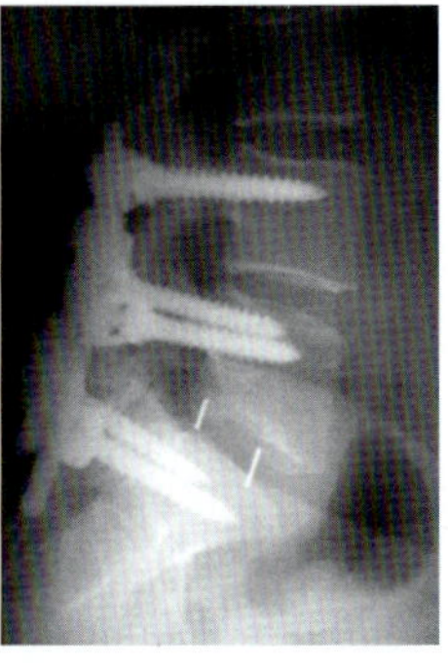

A   B   C   D

Figure 40–12 Case prevention of adjacent level disk degeneration. **(A)** Preoperative magnetic resonance imaging (MRI) shows bulging disks at L3–L4, L4–L5. A 35-year-old woman with low back pain and numbness and pain in left leg. **(B)** 1-year postop MRI shows no loss of disk height after fusion at L5–S1 and dynamic rod at L4–L5 with possible rehydration of that disk. **(C)** Postop anteroposterior and **(D)** lateral films demonstrate fusion with a poly-ether-ether-ketone (PEEK) cage at L5–S1 and dynamic rod at L4–L5 without fusion.

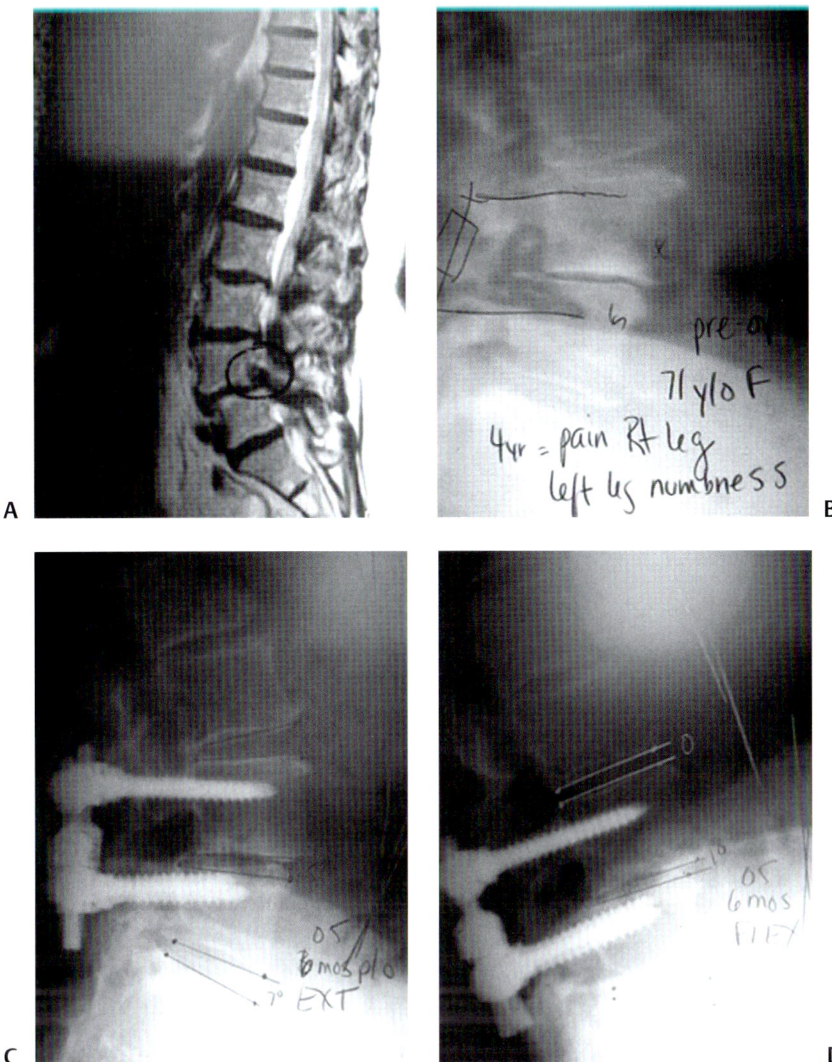

Figure 40–13 A 71-year-old woman with grade II spondylolisthesis with severe degenerative changes most prominent at L4–L5 with 8 mm anterolisthesis on L4–L5 and severe disk space narrowing. **(A)** Preoperative magnetic resonance imaging. **(B)** Preop lateral firm. **(C)** Postop extension and **(D)** flexion radiographs with dynamic rod at L4–L5 demonstrating 4 degrees of motion.

connect the dynamic rod to the closely placed screws and avoid dampener impingement (**Fig. 40–17B**).

4. Do not place a flexion moment or compress on the dynamic rod because in the motion segment at the level of the dynamic rod neuroforaminal narrowing will occur, asymmetric load will be placed onto the posterior aspect of the disk, and loss of flexion in the motion segment will result. Furthermore, do not place an extension moment or distract on the dynamic rod because doing so will place the motion segment into kyphosis, limit extension, and cause an increased load on the anterior portion of the disk.

◆ Summary

Reduced stiffness and increased axial motion of dynamic posterior lumbar spinal fixation instrumentation results in both lower maximum stresses and smaller volumes of tissue exposed to high amplitude stresses in simulated adjacent level disks. Although the stress reduction effect is considered by some to be small (~11% cumulatively for a single forward flexion), it is believed to be clinically important because this stress reduction benefit will be repeated over many loading and motion cycles. It is well known from conventional and biomechanical material and structural fatigue studies that when stress amplitudes are reduced by even a small amount, the increase in performance lifetime is usually substantial.

Although the reduced stiffness and increased axial motion conferred by dynamic instrumentation also increased the calculated maximum stress amplitude in the L4–L5 disk by up to 28%, this load increase needs to be considered in light of the overall maximum stress amplitude in the L4–L5 disks. There, the stress amplitude was only one half to one third the amplitude of the stresses that exist in the adjacent L3–L4 disks.

The reduced stiffness and increased axial motion of dynamic instrumentation designs also allow some rotation of the L4

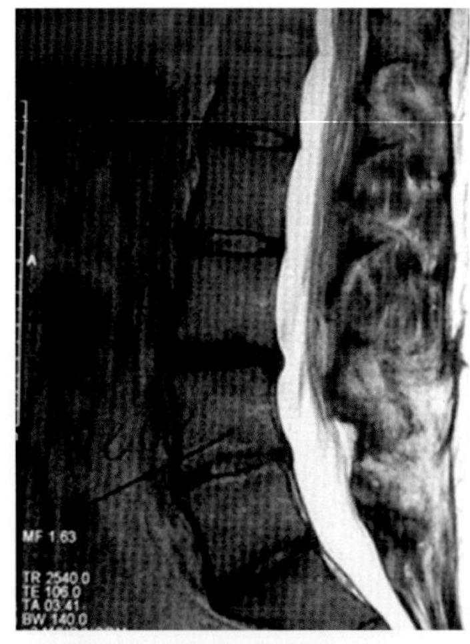
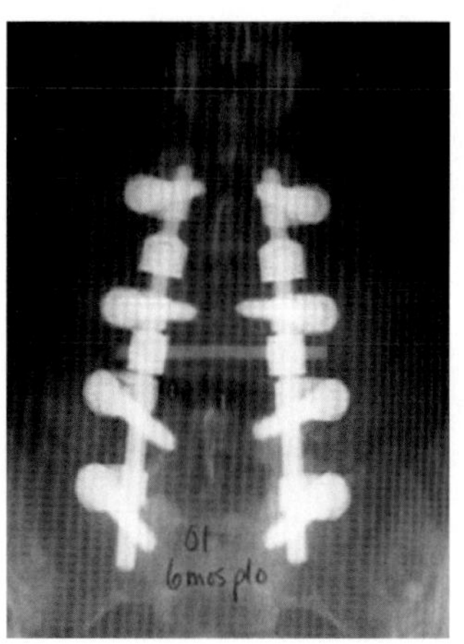
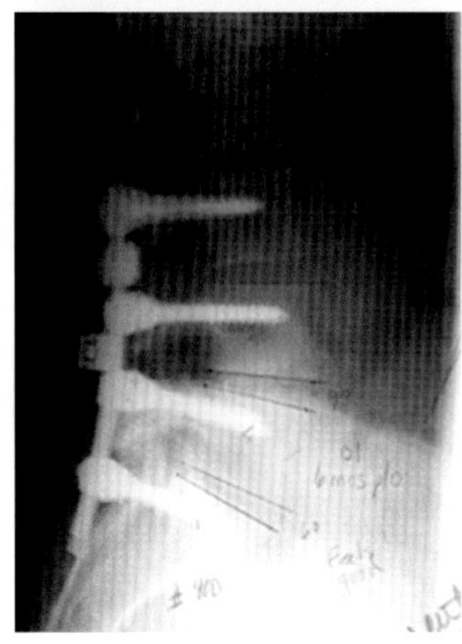

A

B

C

Figure 40–14   Postlaminectomy syndrome. **(A)** Preoperative magnetic resonance imaging demonstrates disk protrusion at L3–L4 with a prior laminectomy at L4–L5. A 30-year-old woman with low back pain and leg pain. **(B,C)** Postoperatively, fusion at L5–S1 and L4–L5 with transforaminal lumbar interbody fusion (TLIF), dynamic rod at L3–L4. Back to work at 3 months.

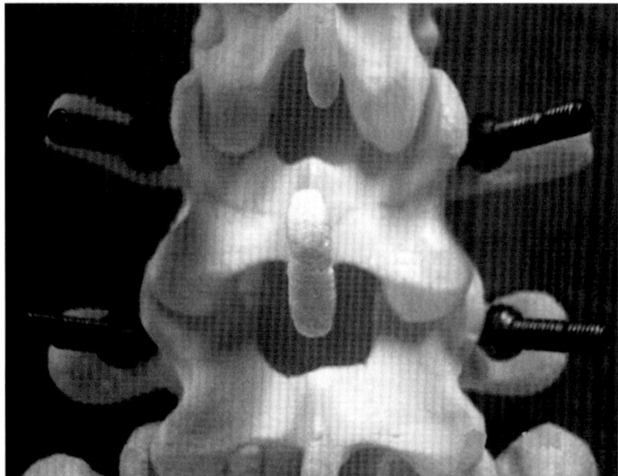

Figure 40–15   Surgical technique for placement of the Isobar TTL dynamic rods.

vertebra with respect to L5 (rotation that is not permitted by posterior hinge instrumentation designs). To achieve the same overall level of flexion when both types of devices are used, the L3–L4 disk enjoys smaller rotation demands when dynamic instrumentation is used. This reduced rotation is, of course, intimately coupled to the reduction in corresponding stress reduction in this disk.

Allowing axial motion confers an additional desirable benefit; that is, the location of the IAR is shifted anteriorly and thus is more physiological. Specifically, consider the two instrumented segments. If axial extension is permitted, then the center of rotation shifts and lies within the L4–L5 disk and not on the posterior side closer to the facets (**Fig. 40–9**). When no axial motion is allowed, the center of rotation lies at the junction of the two segments (**Fig. 40–9**). This shift in the center of rotation reduces the effective moment arm for L4 rotation, which in turn causes a reduced moment and hence lower stresses in the L3–L4 disk. The quantitative results obtained from the finite element analysis presented earlier in this chapter demonstrate that moving the center of rotation anteriorly (accomplished via allowed, but controlled, axial motion) is more effective in

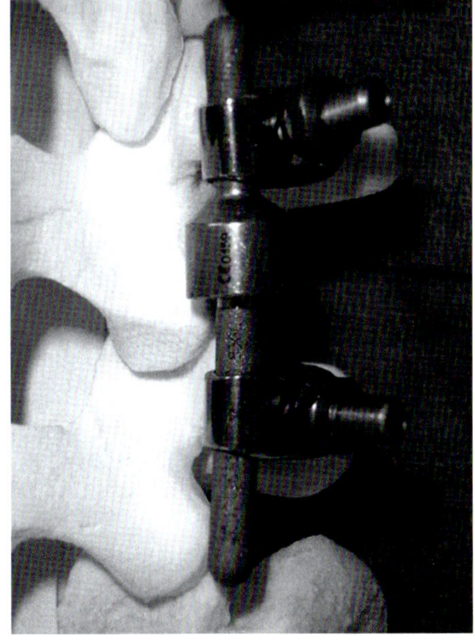
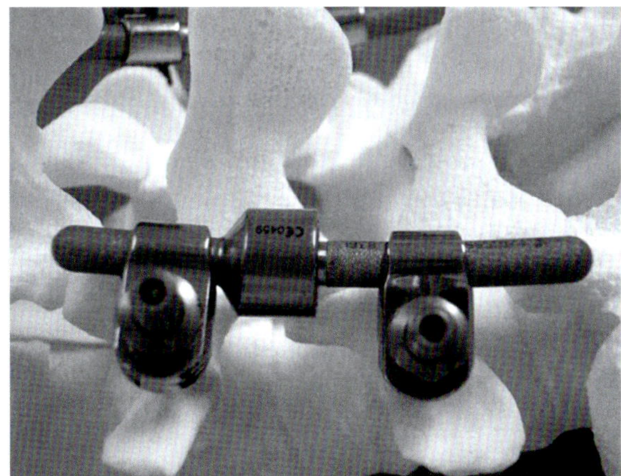

A   B

Figure 40–16   Surgical technique for placement of the Isobar TTL dynamic rods.

reducing the stress in the adjacent level disk than is reducing the elastic stiffness of the instrumentation.

Thus, by distributing loads and preserving motion, dynamic instrumentation is able to decrease pain, retain some motion in the pathological functional unit, and protect the adjacent level. By using dynamic instrumentation we are able to unload the disk and distribute the loads. We can preserve the sagittal alignment of the motion segment because the device has 15 degrees of lordosis. The device stabilizes the motion segment, preventing translation or abnormal motion, yet preserves a limited range of motion. By allowing axial distraction we maintain the IAR in a more physiological position. This should require less energy to move the motion segment and may be a valuable adjunct in total disk replacement.

The Scient'x TTL instrumentation meets the "ideals" noted earlier because it is:

- Easily implantable
- Burns no bridges
- Provides longevity
- Preserves motion
- Stabilizes the motion segment
- Shares the stresses or loads
- Preserves the IAR
- Maintains sagittal alignment–lordosis of the functional spinal unit

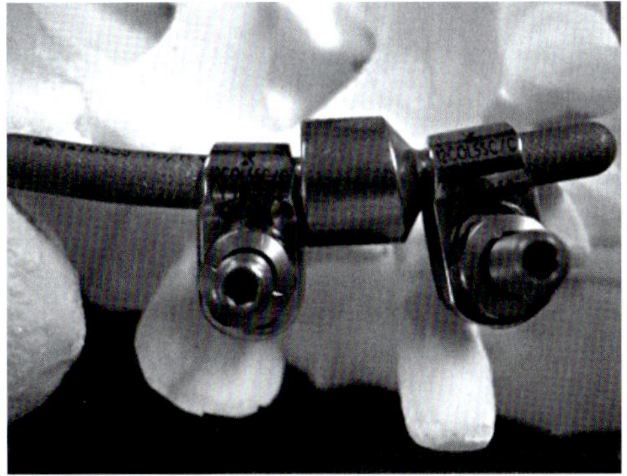
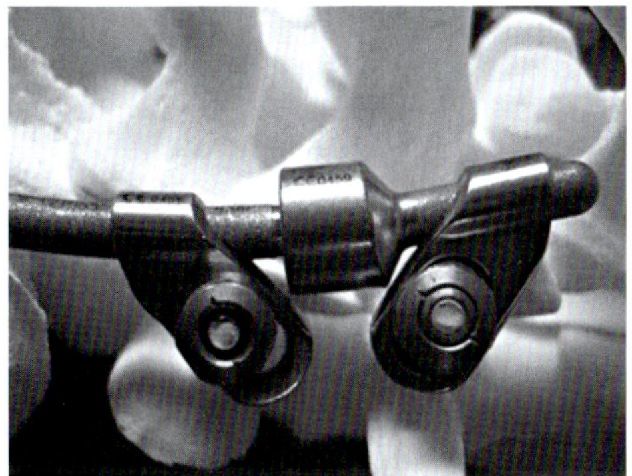

A   B

Figure 40–17   Surgical technique for placement of the Isobar TTL dynamic rods.

References

1. Kirkaldy-Willis WH, Farfan HH, Farfan HF. Instability of the lumbar spine. Clin Orthop Relat Res 1982;165:110–123

2. Benneker LM, Heini PF, Alini M, Anderson SE, Ito K. 2004 Young Investigator Award winner: vertebral endplate marrow contact channel occlusions and intervertebral disc degeneration. Spine 2005;30:167–173

3. Crock HV. Internal disc disruption: a challenge to disc prolapse fifty years on. Spine 1986;11:650–653

4. Stokes IA, Iatridis JC. Mechanical conditions that accelerate intervertebral disc degeneration: overload versus immobilization. Spine 2004;29:2724–2732

5. Mulholland RC, Sengupta DK. Rationale, principles and experimental evaluation of the concept of soft stabilization. Eur Spine J 2002;11(Suppl 2):S198–S205

6. Frymoyer. The Adult Spine: Principles and Practice. 2nd ed. Philadelphia: Lippincott-Raven; 1997

7. White AA, Panjabi M. Clinical Biomechanics of the Spine. 2nd ed. Philadelphia: Lippincott; 1990

8. Chen CS, Cheng CK, Liu CL, Lo WH. Stress analysis of the disc adjacent to interbody fusion in lumbar spine. Med Eng Physiol 2001;23:483–491

9. Eck JC, Humphreys SC, Hodges SD. Adjacent-segment degeneration after lumbar fusion: a review of clinical, biomechanical, and radiologic studies. Am J Orthop 1999;28:336–340

10. Weinhoffer SL, Guyer RD, Herbert M, Griffith SL. Intradiscal pressure measurements above an instrumented fusion: a cadaveric study. Spine 1995;20:526–531

11. Gillet P. The fate of the adjacent motion segments after lumbar fusion. J Spinal Disord Tech 2003;16:338–345

12. Perrin G. Prevention of adjacent level degeneration above a fused vertebral segment. Presented at: International Meeting for Advanced Spine Techniques, 2003, Rome, Italy

13. Cunningham BW, Sefter JC, Shono Y, McAfee PC. Static and cyclical biomechanical analysis of pedicle screw spinal constructs. Spine 1993;18:1677–1688

14. Huang H, Plenkowski D, Saigal S. Finite element analysis of dynamic instrumentation demonstrates stress reduction in adjacent level discs. Presented at: The 51st Annual Meeting of the Orthopaedic Research Society, 2005, Washington, DC

15. Castellvi AE, Huang H, Plenkowski D, et al. Finite element analysis of dynamic instrumentation demonstrates stress reduction in adjacent level discs. 2005; Journal of Spinal Disorders

41

Minimally Invasive Posterior Dynamic Stabilization System

Luiz Pimenta, Roberto C. Díaz, and Dilip K. Sengupta

◆ How Much Load Should be Shared and How Much Motion Restricted?

◆ How Will the Device Survive Fatigue Failure in the Presence of Continued Motion?

◆ The Design Rationale of the Dynamic Stabilization System

◆ Clinical Study with the Dynamic Stabilization System (DSS-II)

◆ Surgical Technique for Stabilization with the Minimally Invasive Dynamic Stabilization System

◆ Clinical Outcome

◆ Discussion

◆ Summary

The principles of dynamic stabilization in the treatment of activity-related chronic mechanical back pain has been described by one of the authors (DKS) in Chapter 31 of this book. An ideal dynamic stabilization system should prevent abnormal high-load transmission through the disk and the facet joints by sharing the load while permitting normal motion.[1,2] Load sharing is the principal mechanism of pain relief.[3,4] However, load sharing and motion preservation both need further clarification.[5,6]

◆ How Much Load Should be Shared and How Much Motion Restricted?

To maintain the nutrition and normal health of the disk and the articular cartilage of the facet joints, it is important that they bear a normal load and that motion is preserved. The device, therefore, should share only a partial load and allow a near normal load to be transmitted through the disk and the facet joints. Restriction of motion is neither the primary mechanism of pain relief nor is it desirable.[7] However, to achieve load sharing, the device almost invariably causes some restriction of motion. How much load should be shared and how much motion should be permitted for ideal pain relief have never been determined. Perhaps these two parameters vary among individuals and also among motion segments in the same individual. It may be hypothesized that around a 20 to 40% load may be shared by the device, permitting the rest of the load to be transmitted through the facet joints and the disk. Motion restriction should be minimal if at all. However, it is more important that the device prevent any abnormal, sharp load across the disk and

the facet joints throughout the range of motion (ROM), and that any abnormal quality of motion be prevented as well.[1,2]

◆ How Will the Device Survive Fatigue Failure in the Presence of Continued Motion?

Even a rigid fusion rod may fail if the segment does not fuse. How can the dynamic stabilization device survive fatigue failure in the presence of continued motion? The dynamic stabilization systems are inherently flexible and are designed to survive fatigue within a certain ROM and load. If at any stage during the ROM the device has to share a much higher load (say > 60% of the total load, when the device is meant to share only 30%) the device may undergo fatigue failure or loosening at the implant-bone junction. It is therefore important that load sharing be uniform throughout the ROM.[8,9]

The development of the Dynamic Stabilization System (DSS) (currently under development by the author (DKS), in collaboration with Abbott-Spine, Austin, TX) was based on these three principles: disk unloading by around 30%, minimal restriction of motion, and uniform load sharing throughout the ROM. The surgical principles dictating the design of the DSS were minimally invasive implantation and easy salvage in case of device failure.

◆ The Design Rationale of the Dynamic Stabilization System

The predecessor of the DSS design was the Fulcrum Assisted Soft Stabilization (FASS) (Neoligaments, Leeds, United

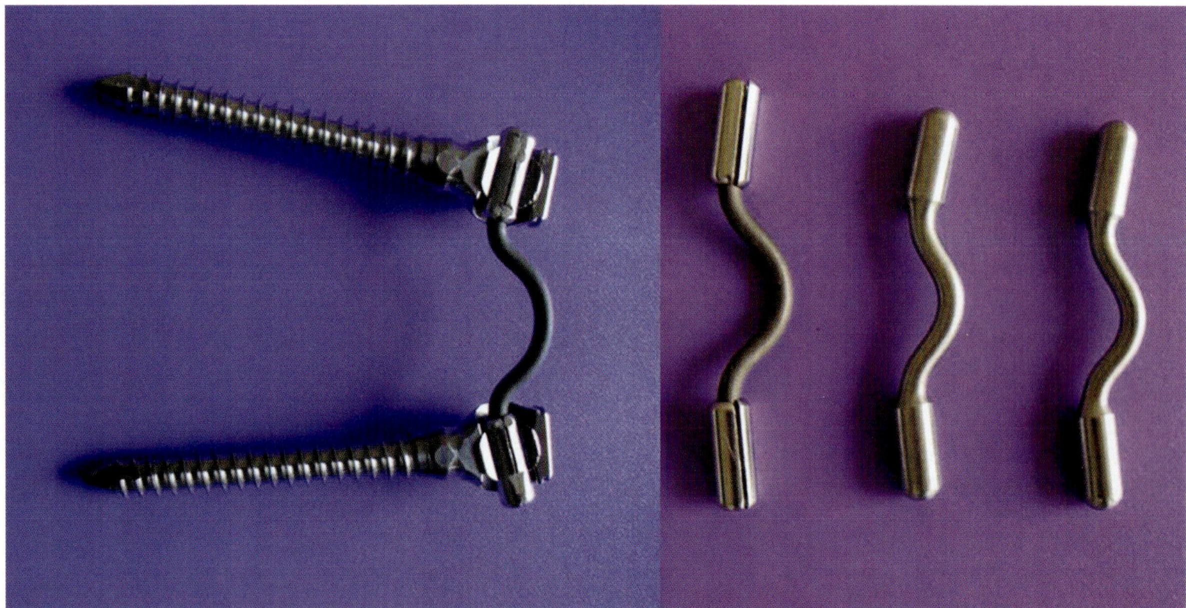

Figure 41–1   The first-generation Dynamic Stabilization System (DSS-I) was a C-shaped titanium spring, made of a 4 mm diameter spring-grade titanium. The ends were thickened to 6 mm or fitted with a 6 mm diameter bushing for easy fixation to the regular pedicle screws, which can take a 6 mm rod.

Kingdom) described by Sengupta and Mulholland.[10] The aim was to stabilize the spine and cause minimal restriction of motion, maintain a normal lordotic posture of the spine, and unload the disk. Biomechanical tests showed that, although the FASS system can unload the disk with minimal restriction of motion, the disk unloading and motion restriction were uneven. The FASS system produced restriction of flexion and too much unloading of the disk in flexion, whereas extension was unaffected. This predicted a possibility of excessive load being shared by the device in flexion, possibly resulting in early fatigue failure of the device or the implant-bone junction.[10]

The author (DKS) subsequently designed a C-shaped titanium spring device described as the Dynamic Stabilization System-I or DSS-I[11] (**Fig. 41–1**). Biomechanical tests with this device on cadaver spine showed a more favorable load-deformation curve and a uniform restriction of flexion and extension ROM by around 30% of normal range. This was important for fatigue resistance. An uneven restriction of motion in any particular direction would indicate excessive load sharing of the device in that direction of motion, which can lead to an early fatigue failure. However, when the effect of DSS-I was tested on cadaver spine, the disk pressure changes appeared to be unfavorable. The device unloaded the disk by ~30% in flexion, which was desirable, but a complete unloading of the disk in extension, creating a negative disk pressure at the maximum extension. Normally, the disk pressure rises in both flexion and extension and is lowest at the early phase of extension (**Fig. 41–2**). A progressively increasing negative disk pressure with DSS-I indicated that the device shares increasing load toward maximum sextension, which was not reflected in the load-deformation curve. Such excessive load sharing in extension would increase the possibility of an early device failure, and therefore this design was never implanted clinically (**Fig. 41–2**).

The DSS-II was designed (**Fig. 41–3**) to improve on the uniform load sharing during both flexion and extension motions. This consists of an a-shaped coil made of a 4 mm diameter spring grade titanium rod with an outer diameter of 25 mm. The coiled section is elliptical rather than circular, so that the instantaneous axis of rotation of the device simulates a normal motion segment to ensure more uniform load sharing as mentioned earlier.[8,9] The DSS-II device is attached to the pedicle screws, with a polyaxial screw head (Pathfinder system; Abbott Spine, Inc. Austin, TX) designed to accept 4 mm rod, as opposed to normal 6 mm rod used for fusion. The biomechanical tests on cadaver spine with the DSS-II system showed that the ROM was uniformly restricted by 30% in flexion-extension and lateral bending, and by 20% in rotation, compared with normal. A continuous pressure profile tracing from the center of the disk showed that the disk pressure was going up in both flexion and extension as in the intact spine, but the peak pressure at full flexion and extension was reduced by 25%. This indicates that the DSS-II system uniformly unloads the disk by sharing ~25% of the load off the disk at full flexion and extension. At the neutral position, the disk pressure remained unchanged, indicating that the DSS-II does not unload the disk at the neutral position (**Fig. 41–4**). Clinically, mechanical back pain due to degenerative instability is mostly experienced toward terminal ranges of flexion and extension. It is therefore expected that the DSS-II should be able to prevent such activity-related mechanical back pain. The disk pressure changes during lateral bending and rotation were minor even in the intact spine and therefore were not repeated with the DSS.

Fatigue testing in the laboratory showed that the DSS-II could survive 10 million cycles of motion with ±7.5 degrees of flexion and extension motion. It is expected that, because the DSS would produce 30% limitation of ROM, the expected ROM of the motion segment after stabilization with the DSS would not exceed this range. More importantly, the pressure

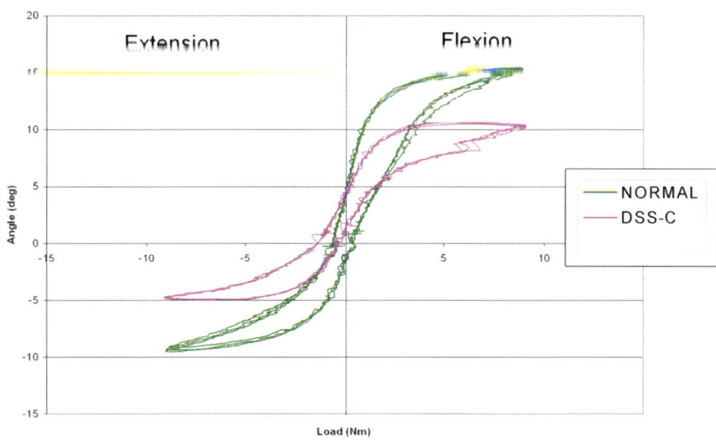

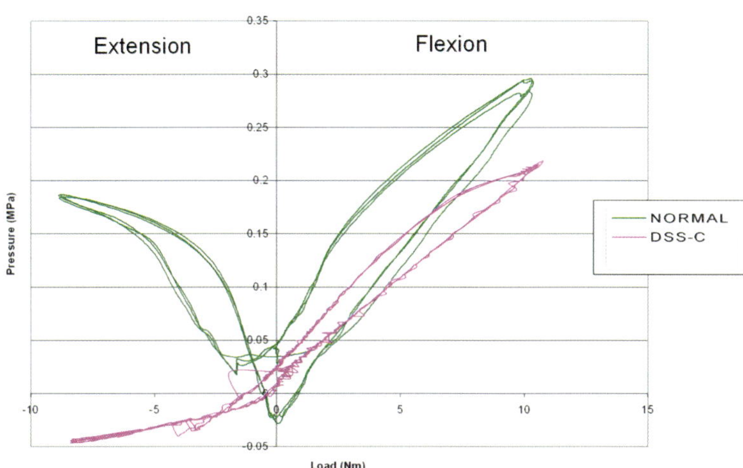

Figure 41–2 **(A)** The load–deformation curve in cadaver spine experiments with the first-generation Dynamic Stabilization System (DSS-I) shows around 30% of restriction of motion in both flexion and extension, compared with an uninstrumented segment. **(B)** A continuous tracing of the disk pressure at the center of the disk space shows that the pressure rises during both flexion and extension and is lowest at the early phase of extension. Following stabilization with the DSS-I, the final pressure at the end of flexion was reduced by around 30% but during extension the disk pressure was continuously decreasing and was the lowest at full extension. This indicates that the DSS-I was sharing 70% of the disk load in flexion but bearing nearly the full load during extension, leaving almost no load to be transmitted through the disk.

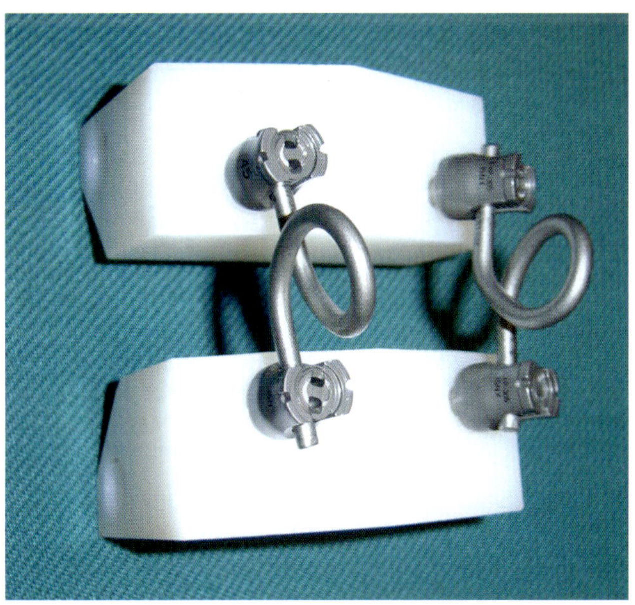

Figure 41–3 The second-generation Dynamic Stabilization System (DSS-II) was an α-shaped titanium coil made of a 4 mm diameter spring-grade titanium. This device can be attached to the pedicle screws (PathFinder system; Abbott Spine, Inc., Austin, TX), which can take 4 mm diameter rods.

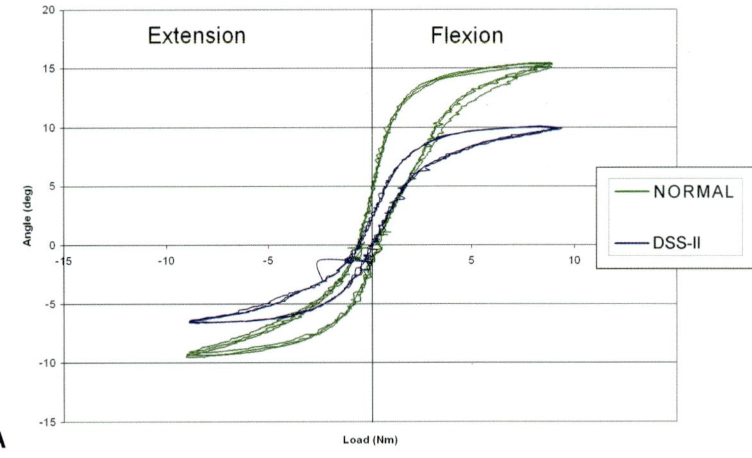

A

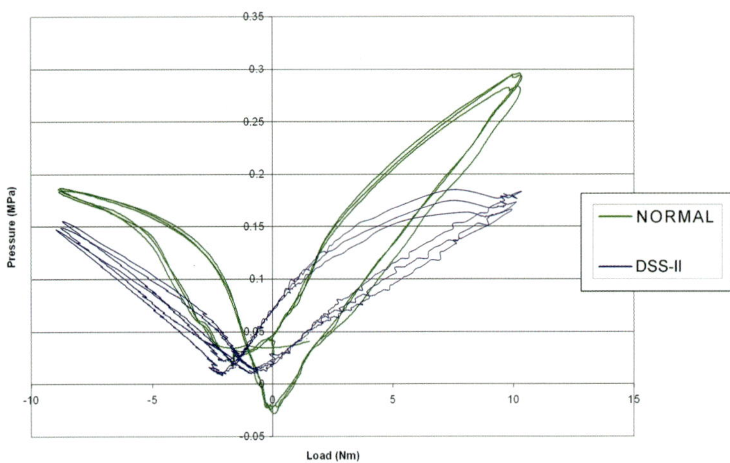

B

Figure 41–4 (A) The load–deformation curve in cadaver spine experiments with the second-generation Dynamic Stabilization System (DSS-II) shows around 30% of restriction of motion in both flexion and extension, compared with an uninstrumented segment. **(B)** A continuous tracing of the disk pressure at the center of the disk space shows that in an intact spine the pressure rises during both flexion and extension and is lowest at the early phase of extension. Following stabilization with the DSS-II, the final pressure at the end of both flexion and extension was reduced by around 25%, indicating a uniform unloading of the disk load at both of these two motions.

studies indicated that the DSS-II system was not expected to share more than 25% of the load off the disk during the entire range of flexion and extension. The bench tests therefore indicated a reasonable assurance that the DSS-II would survive a fatigue failure. It cannot be overemphasized that there is no ideal bench test available to simulate the complex motion of the device in vivo, which could predict a true fatigue life of the device after implantation.

◆ Clinical Study with the Dynamic Stabilization System (DSS-II)

Following the biomechanical studies, a pilot clinical study was undertaken to test the clinical efficacy and safety of the DSS device. The clinical study was performed in only one center (Santa Rita Hospital, São Paulo, Brazil) and all the cases were operated by one surgeon (Luiz Pimenta). The *inclusion criteria* were activity-related mechanical back pain for a duration of more than 6 months, associated with radiological evidence of a single level of disk degeneration [x-ray, magnetic resonance imaging (MRI), and positive diskography], and failure of conservative treatment. The cases with previous failed diskectomy and facet joint degeneration without causing significant stenosis were also included. *Exclusion criteria* included severe disk degeneration with disk collapse exceeding 50% of normal height, spondylolisthesis exceeding grade II, and significant osteoporosis. More importantly, patients requiring any other concomitant surgery like decompression or diskectomy at any level or fusion of an adjacent segment were excluded because these procedures may produce clinical improvement or deterioration, which may confound the outcome of dynamic stabilization. Patients with a body weight of more than 90 kg were excluded because only one size of the DSS-II system was used, which may not have been adequate for oversized patients. During 2002–2004, 19 cases were enrolled, of which 16 (7 M, 9 F) completed a minimum 1-year follow-up. Mean age was 52 years (range, 42–58). Primary diagnosis included disk degeneration (nine), disk degeneration with degenerative spondylolisthesis (four), failed nucleoplasty (two), and failed disk replacement (one). Operated segment included single level in 14 cases (L4–L5 in six, L5–S1 in eight) and two levels (L4–S1) in two cases. Preoperative diskogram was performed in all patients who did not have failed previous surgery.

◆ Surgical Technique for Stabilization with the Minimally Invasive Dynamic Stabilization System

The patients were positioned prone on rolls to create ideal lumbar lordosis, and this was checked by lateral fluoroscopy. The pedicle screws were inserted by percutaneous technique, using fluoroscopy, over guide pins and progressive dilators. Pedicle screws on the same side were inserted through the same longitudinal skin incision ~3 cm long. The track between the two pedicle screws was created by splitting the erector spinae muscles with a dissector. Each screw head was connected to a slotted extension tube projecting outside the skin. Once satisfactory screw positioning was confirmed, the DSS spring was slid down the slot in the extension tubes of the pedicle screws to sit into the screw heads. The coil of the DSS device was maintained in the sagittal plane and the locking nuts were tightened to the screw heads. No distraction or compression was applied. The procedure was repeated on the other side. The average operative time was 90 minutes and average blood loss was less than 50 mL. The patients were up and ambulatory within a couple of hours after surgery and usually discharged home the same day (**Fig. 41–5**).

◆ Clinical Outcome

The morbidity was very low and most cases could appreciate pain relief on the same day of surgery. At the 1-year follow-up, the mean visual analog scale (VAS) score was reduced from 7.3 to 3.5 and the mean Oswestry Disability Index (ODI) was reduced from 65 to 27. Fourteen of the 16 cases improved significantly from the preoperative pain and functional status. Twelve returned to their original job. Of the two cases who failed to experience significant improvement, one had a previous failed nuclear prosthesis (PDN, Raymedica, Inc., Minneapolis, MN), and two other cases had two previous diskectomies and a 50% collapse of disk height. In this small study group there was one case with persistent pain following disk replacement, and another case with failed PDN, and both these cases had significant pain relief following DSS stabilization. Postoperative standing lateral radiography showed well-maintained lumbar lordosis of the instrumented segment in all the cases. Flexion-extension radiographs showed mean 7.5 degrees of motion (68% of the motion observed in the proximal adjacent segment) at the operated segment. More importantly, the quality of flexion and extension was comparable to a normal motion segment (i.e., the anterior edges of the end plate opposing each other in flexion and posterior edges in extension) (**Fig. 41–6**). This indicated that the device was sharing the load in both flexion and extension,

allowing the remaining load to be transmitted through the disk. No radiographic loosening or implant breakage was seen. Postoperative MRI scan was obtained at 6 months in two cases, one of which showed increased signal intensity in the T2-weighted MRI scan in the operated level disk.[12]

◆ Discussion

The initial clinical results are encouraging. Most cases experienced significant pain relief, and there was no complication. The operative procedure is fairly simple and morbidity is low. The most important observation was that there was no implant failure. Considering these implants have to survive in the presence of continued motion, device failure in the form of breakage of the spring or screw loosening remains a matter of great concern. As mentioned earlier, the laboratory data regarding fatigue are inadequate because cyclical motion in the laboratory on a polyethylene American Society for Testing and Materials (ASTM) spine model does not replicate the complexity of the motion in vivo, and also the influence of the anatomical structures of the motion segment (i.e., the disk and the facet joints cannot be re-created in the laboratory). The uniform load sharing with the disk and the DSS device, as predicted by a normal quality of flexion and extension, endorses that the kinematics of the DSS is complementary to that of the intact motion segment. Therefore, the influence of the disk and the facet joints may not adversely influence the fatigue life of the DSS. Only long-term follow-up will deliver the true answer. Even if the DSS implant fails, it may be salvaged easily by revision or converting it into a fusion.

Although the present pilot clinical study did not enroll any patient who required concomitant surgery like decompression or fusion, it does not preclude the use of the DSS device as a concomitant procedure to supplement a diskectomy or decompression or fusion of an adjacent segment. The purpose of this clinical outcome study was to assess the efficacy of DSS without the confounding effect of other surgical procedures, particularly decompressive laminectomy, which has a high success rate in relieving leg pain secondary to spinal stenosis. In the previously reported clinical study with Dynesys,[13] 68% of cases had a concomitant decompression, making it difficult to assess whether the good result was due to decompression or to stabilization. Once the clinical efficacy of DSS is well established, the indications may be extended to include prophylactic stabilization of a segment adjacent to a fusion level, or to prevent instability following decompressive laminectomy.

The design of the DSS has been laboratory tested to match the kinematics of a normal lumbar motion segment. The kinematics may change after disk or nuclear replacement. As long as the kinematics remains reasonably close to that of a normal motion segment, the DSS may be a reasonable salvage operation for failed disk or nuclear replacement cases. Salvage of such cases with posterior fusion may not be easy in the presence of prosthesis in the disk space. However, ideally, the DSS should be tested together with such disk prostheses in the laboratory to observe whether they have complementary kinematics before the DSS may be recommended as a salvage procedure following disk replacement. Presence of a significant facet joint arthrosis remains a contraindication to disk replacement. If the kinematic property

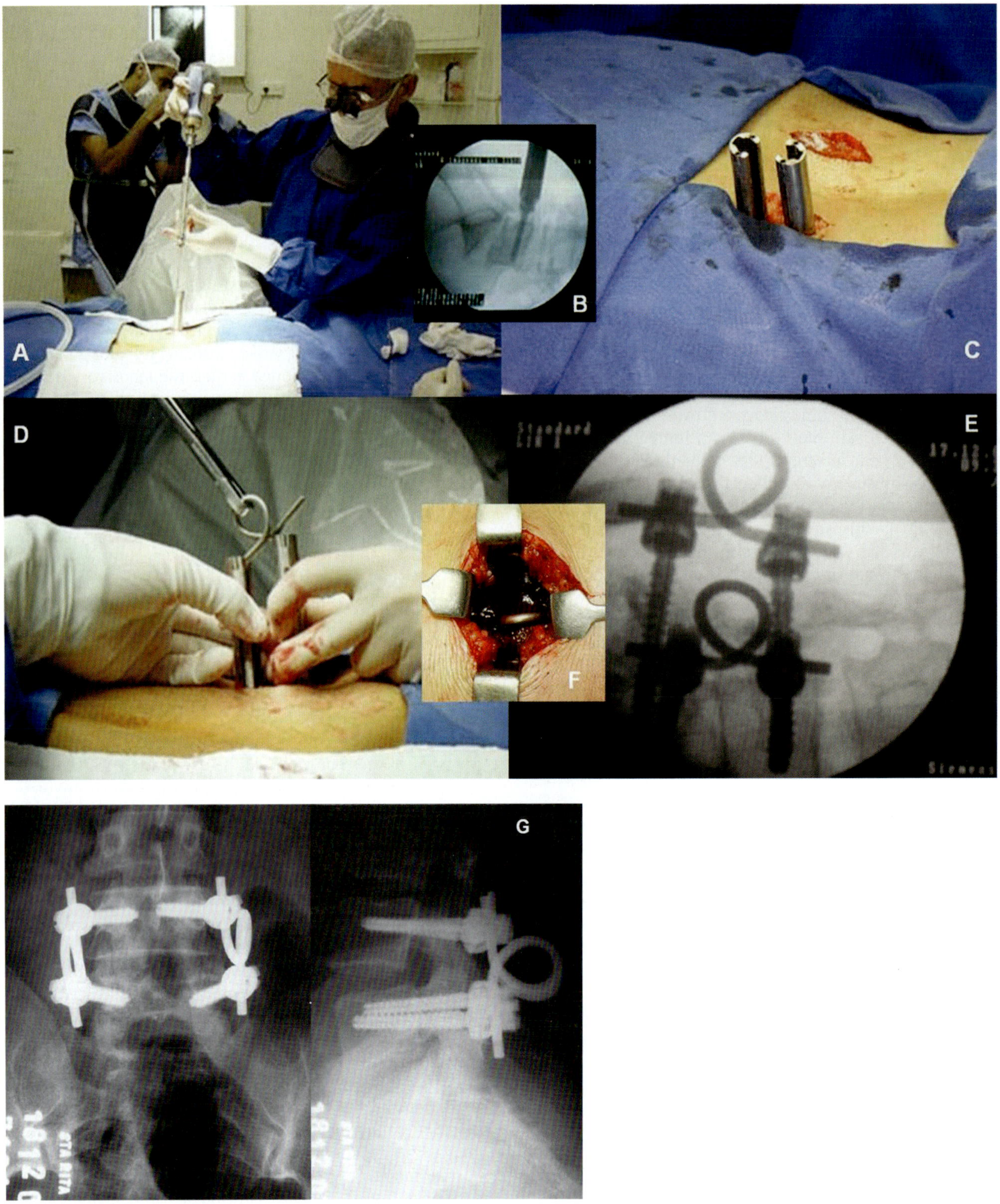

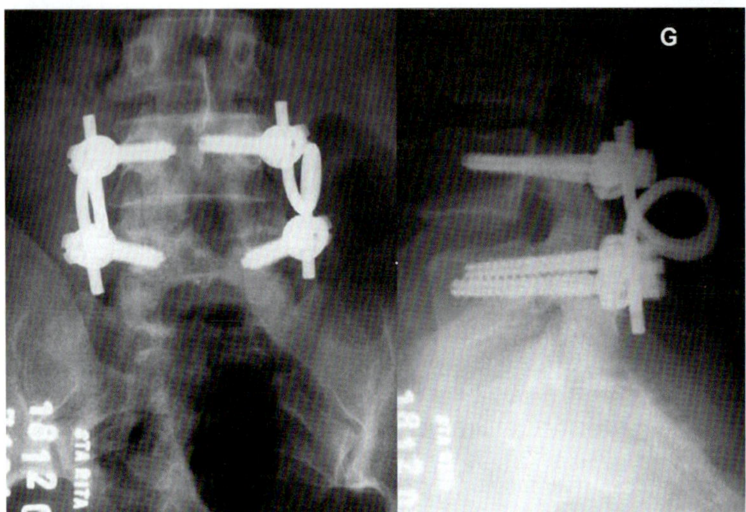

Figure 41–5 (A) The surgical technique for second-generation Dynamic Stabilization System (DSS-II) instrumentation. **(B)** The pedicle screws are inserted by a minimally invasive technique over guide pins, under x-ray control. **(C)** Two slotted outriggers, attached to the pedicle screw heads, project through the skin incision. **(D)** The DSS-II system is inserted along the slots of the outriggers into the pedicle screw heads. **(E)** Final x-ray after bilateral instrumentation. **(F)** The coil of the DSS-II system lies in the sagittal plane, well under the skin level, and does not stay prominent under the skin. **(G)** Postoperative anteroposterior and lateral radiographs after DSS-II instrumentation.

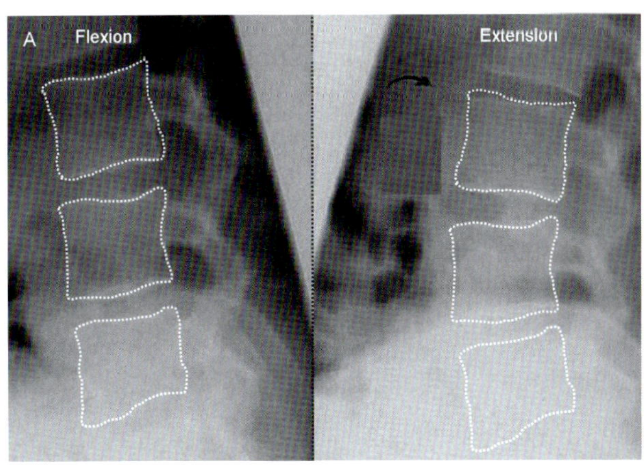

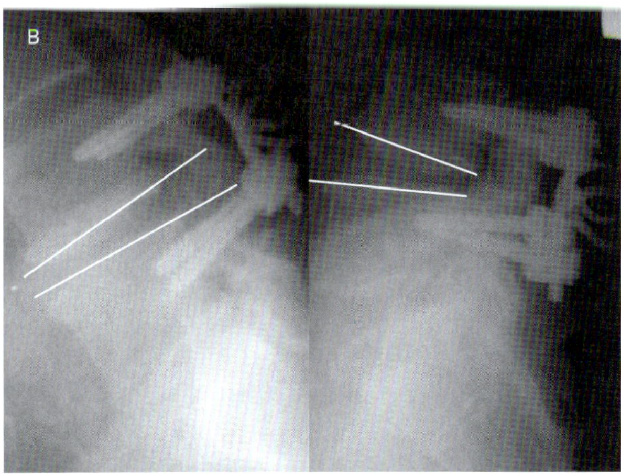

A   B

Figure 41–6 **(A)** Normally, the anterior edges of the vertebral bodies come closure to each other during flexion and the posterior edges come closure in extension, indicating that the center of rotation at these two stages of motion lies behind an anterior margin of the disk space in flexion and in front of the posterior margin of the disk space in extension. **(B)** This normal kinematic pattern of motion is also observed following second-generation Dynamic Stabilization System instrumentation.

of the DSS appears to be truly complementary to the disk prosthesis, the two procedures may be performed together as an elective procedure for degenerative disk as well as facet joint disease, making it a truly total joint replacement as opposed total disk replacement, which is equivalent to only a partial joint replacement.

◆ Summary

This pilot clinical study showed that the present design of the DSS appears to be safe and effective. The implantation is minimally invasive and postoperative morbidity is minimal.

From the results of the initial study it may be recommended that the DSS device can be used even in conjunction with decompressive laminectomy and to stabilize segments adjacent to fusion to prevent degeneration. However, several questions remain unanswered. Although the 4 mm device is appropriate in patients with average build, and at the L4–L5 or L5–S1 levels, what is the ideal size of the device for overweight or underweight patients? How many segments can be safely stabilized? Can it be used in conjunction with a disk or nuclear prosthesis in front? A long-term study will be required to answer the question of device failure with fatigue, and any effect on repair or regeneration of the degenerated disk following stabilization.

References

1. Sengupta DK. Dynamic stabilization devices in the treatment of low back pain. Orthop Clin North Am 2004;35:43–56
2. Sengupta DK. Dynamic stabilization in the treatment of low back pain due to degenerative disorders. In: Herkowitz HN, ed. The Lumbar Spine. Vol 1. 3rd ed. pp., 373–383. Philadelphia: LWW; 2004
3. McNally DS, Adams MA. Internal intervertebral disc mechanics as revealed by stress profilometry. Spine 1992;17:66–73
4. McNally DS, Shackleford IM, Goodship AE, Mulholland RC. In vivo stress measurement can predict pain on discography. Spine 1996;21:2580–2587
5. Panjabi MM. Clinical spinal instability and low back pain. J Electromyogr Kinesiol 2003;13:371–379
6. Panjabi MM. The stabilizing system of the spine, II: Neutral zone and instability hypothesis. J Spinal Disord 1992;5:390-396 discussion 397
7. Mulholland RC, Sengupta DK. Rationale, principles and experimental evaluation of the concept of soft stabilization. Eur Spine J 2002;11 (Suppl 2):S198–S205
8. Sengupta DK, Demetropoulos CK, Herkowitz HN. et al. Instantaneous axis of rotation and its clinical importance in a healthy lumbar functional spinal unit. Roundtables in Spinal Biomechanics 2004. St. Louis: Quality Medical Publishing, Inc. 1:2–12
9. Sengupta DK, Demetropoulos CK, Herkowitz HN, Mulholland RC. Instant centre of rotation and intradiscal pressure study to identify load-sharing property of dynamic stabilization devices in the lumbar spine without fusion: a biomechanical study in cadaver spine. Paper presented at: World Spine II, 2003, Chicago, IL
10. Sengupta DK, Mulholland RC. Fulcrum assisted soft stabilization system: a new concept in the surgical treatment of degenerative low back pain. Spine 2005;30:1019–1029 discussion 1030
11. Sengupta DK, Demetropoulos CK, Herkowitz HN, Hochschuler S, Mulholland RC. Loads sharing characteristics of two novel soft stabilization devices in the lumbar motion segments: a biomechanical study in cadaver spine. Paper presented at: Spine Arthroplasty Society Annual Conference, 2003, Scottsdale, AZ
12. Sengupta DK, Pimenta L, Mulholland RC. Prospective clinical trial of soft stabilization with Dynamic Stabilization System (DSS) in the treatment of chronic low back pain: results of minimum one-year follow-up. Paper presented at: Spine Arthroplasty Society Annual Meeting, 2005, New York, NY
13. Stoll TM, Dubois G, Schwarzenbach O. The dynamic neutralization system for the spine: a multi-center study of a novel non-fusion system. Eur Spine J 2002;11(Suppl 2):S170–S178

Nonfusion Stabilization of the Degenerated Lumbar Spine with Cosmic

Archibald von Strempel

◆ **Why Are Spondylodeses Performed in the Treatment of Degenerative Lumbar Vertebral Column Diseases?**

◆ **When Is a Correction Necessary?**

◆ **When Is a Fusion Necessary?**

◆ **When Will It Be Possible to Do without a Fusion?**

◆ **The Cosmic Implant System**

◆ **Indications for Dynamic Stabilization with Cosmic**

Symptomatic Lumbar Stenosis (Claudicatio Spinalis)

Chronically Recurring Lumbalgy in the Case of Diskogenic Pain and Facet Syndrome

Recurrent Disk Herniation

In Combination with a Spondylodesis

Extension of an Existing Spondylodesis in the Case of a Painful Adjacent Level Degeneration

◆ **Contraindications**

Stabilizations Extending beyond Three Segments

◆ **Surgical Technique**

◆ **Results**

◆ **Discussion**

The degeneration of the lumbar motion segment starts with a height loss of the disk caused by water loss of the nucleus pulposus. The facet joints lose their congruence, which may cause a consecutive spondylarthritis.[1] The fibers of the annulus fibrosus and the vertebral column ligaments lose tension so that a structural loosening occurs, complete with increased rotation instability.[2–4] To compensate for the instability, hypertrophy of the yellow ligament as well as the facet joints occurs very frequently, which may lead to a reduction of the cross-sectional surface of the central as well as the lateral spinal canal. At the same time, the motion segment may lose its original position, and scoliosis, flat back, rotation, and rotation sliding may develop. Further along the course of degeneration, lateral and frontal spondylophytes up to and including syndesmophytes may form, which in turn may lead to spontaneous stiffening of the segment.

The complaints depend on the stage of the vertebral column degeneration. In the first phase, with a reduction of the height of the vertebral disk and loss of the congruence of the facet joints, chronically recurrent lumbalgies may occur that increase under load stress. When the stenosis of the spinal channel increases, additional symptoms may occur in one or both legs, with the indications of a claudicatio spinalis. If spontaneous ankylosis of the segment occurs before a symptomatic spinal channel stenosis occurs, the frequency and intensity of lumbalgies decrease.

Leg symptoms can be caused by the compression of the neural structures, which results from a narrow spinal channel or recessus or neuroforamen. As a rule, adequate decompression of the neural structures leads to good clinical success. The etiology of the lumbalgy is less clear; also, clinical success does not occur in the same measure as the fusion rate of a spondylodesis. What is certain is that the instability in the motion segment caused by the vertebral disk shrinkage is a trigger for the frequency of lumbalgies. Nonphysiological movements that have become possible due to the vertebral disk shrinkage lead to shifting of the nucleus pulposus or nucleus pulposus fragments within the vertebral disk, with the vertebral disk itself experiencing increased ingrowth of pain-conducting nerve ends as a result of the degeneration.[5] This increased innervation of the degenerative vertebral disk is also responsible for the "memory pain" in the diskography.[6]

The term *instability* used in this context has been better defined by Panjabi as a "clinical instability" that leads to a pathological movement capability and to pain, deformities, and neurological failures.[7]

Operative treatment of the symptomatic lumbar vertebral column degeneration has thus far consisted of stabilizing, correcting, and adequately decompressing the diseased segment(s), always in connection with a spondylodesis. In recent years, the various forms of the spondylodesis [anterior and posterior lumbar interbody fusion (ALIF and PLIF), total lumbar interbody fusion (TLIF), posterior lumbar fusion (PLF)] were discussed intensively because 360 degree fusions were believed to provide the greatest clinical success rate.

This theory was disproved in a prospective, randomized, double-blind study. The clinical results were independent of the selected fusion form. Complications naturally increased with increased surgical effort (360 degree fusion). In this study, pseudarthroses did not have any influence on the clinical result.[8]

A possible disadvantage of spondylodesis in the treatment of degenerative lumbar vertebral column diseases is the increased risk of accelerating degenerative processes in the neighboring segment. Following a spondylodesis, 16.5% symptomatic vertebral disk degenerations after 5 years were expected in the neighboring segment, and 36.1% after 10 years.[9] Obviously there is a lower risk for spondylodeses without the use of pedicle screw systems.[10] It must be questioned whether the risk for the adjacent segment increases with the rigidity of the spondylodesis, which would above all concern the currently favored 360 degree fusions that use a cage in combination with a pedicle screw system.[11–13]

This does not appear to apply to spondylodeses that were performed for the correction of extended deformities. Thus, even after more than 20 years following a Harrington spondylodesis, low back pain was found in only 13% of cases.[14]

◆ Why Are Spondylodeses Performed in the Treatment of Degenerative Lumbar Vertebral Column Diseases?

Until recently, there were few alternatives to a standard spondylodesis. One important reason is that the surgery of the degenerative lumbar vertebral column is a relatively young chapter in spine surgery. The techniques of correction and fusion, so successful in scoliosis surgery, were transferred to this new area of spine surgery, increasing in usage since the early 1980s. An essential task of the spondylodesis consists of protecting the implants used against failure (dislocation, breakage).

◆ When Is a Correction Necessary?

In contrast to the treatment of adolescent scoliosis, where the correction of the deformity is also the objective of the treatment, there are not very many indications for correction of the degenerative lumbar vertebral column that actually serve the direct objective of the operation with pain release and restoration of neurological functions.

Positional deformities in the sagittal and frontal planes that in total do not lead to a loss of the body vertical plumb line need not be corrected. This concerns most lateral deviations. Therefore, the correction of a degenerative lumbar scoliosis is only necessary in exceptional cases.

The reduction of the vertebral disk always leads to flattening of the lumbar vertebral column, which also does not need to be corrected as long as the patient assumes an upright, well-balanced posture. True and degenerative olistheses at an adult age are not usually progressive. Stabilization and decompression without correction lead to the objective of the treatment. Therefore, it is not meaningful to transfer the principles of scoliosis surgery noncritically to the surgery of the degenerative lumbar vertebral column.

◆ When Is a Fusion Necessary?

A fusion is required when corrections (mostly in the sagittal plane) are necessary to treat pain.

◆ When Will It Be Possible to Do without a Fusion?

The precondition is a dynamic implant that does not require the protection of a spondylodesis. It must be possible to achieve the treatment objective (pain release, restoration of the neurological function) without correction. The stabilization does not need to include more than three segments.

◆ The Cosmic Implant System

A posterior nonfusion implant system, which can do without protection by a spondylodesis, should not have any rigid characteristics. However, to be able to control instabilities effectively, the system must also feature stable characteristics. The Cosmic Posterior Dynamic System (Ulrich GmbH & Co. KG, Ulm, Germany) is a stable, nonrigid implant. Stability is assured by the 6.25 mm rod, and nonrigidity is assured by the hinged screw head. The screw features a hinged joint between the head and threaded part, which causes the load to be shared between the implant system and the anterior vertebral column (**Fig. 42–1**). Laboratory tests show that

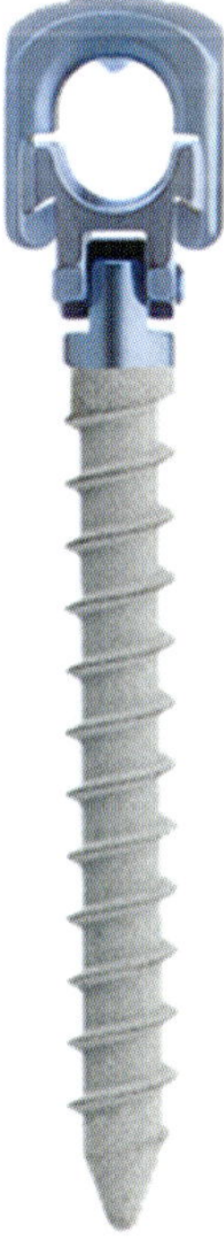

Figure 42–1   Cosmic screw.

Cosmic allows the same rotation stability as a healthy motion segment.[15] In a cyclic loading test with 0.3–3.0 kN/1Hz, we did not find an implant breakage or any debris after 10 million cycles.[16] Because Cosmic is used like a stability endoprosthesis, the bone healing of the pedicle screws is of major importance here. For this reason, the threaded part of the screw is coated with bonit. Bonit (Dot GmbH, Rostock, Germany) is the second generation of bioactive calcium phosphate coatings on implants. In 1995, it was originally used for the first time in oral surgery for dental implants.[17] In the area of vertebral column surgery, a study on the use of a first-generation bioactive calcium phosphate coating on Schanz screws found significantly improved fixation of the coated screws in comparison with uncoated screws.[18] Thus the screw is introduced transpedicularly into the vertebral body, similar to an orthopedic endoprosthesis. To achieve a sufficient press-fit, the pedicle is widened by drilling to 3.2 mm maximum; but only along ~50% of the screw. The screw has a self-tapping thread so that the tapping instrument is needed only in cases of extremely hard spongiosa. To prevent early loosening of the screw, the screw must not be manipulated in any major way. Before being implanted, the rods must be prebent such that they can be connected without any problems to the screw heads.

After the screw heads have been connected to the longitudinal rods, there remains only a micromobility in the hinges, which, without rod connections, are caudally and cranially mobile by ~20 degrees (**Fig. 42–2**).

Due to its good rotation stability, Cosmic is used not only for purely diskogenic pain conditions but is also combined with a conventional laminectomy or even a facetectomy. A transverse stabilizer is used for a monosegmental application in combination with a laminectomy. For two- or three-segmental applications, no transverse stabilizer is used.

The screws are implanted either by means of a conventional midline approach (point of entry lateral to the facet joint, angle ~15 degrees horizontal to the sagittal plane) or by means of the more laterally situated Wiltse access (a somewhat ventrally located point of entry close to the base of the transverse continuations, angle 20–25 degrees horizontal to the sagittal plane) (**Fig. 42–3**). A purely sagittal implantation direction is not recommended because this will lead to parallel positioning of the hinges and thus to increased mobility in the sagittal plane.

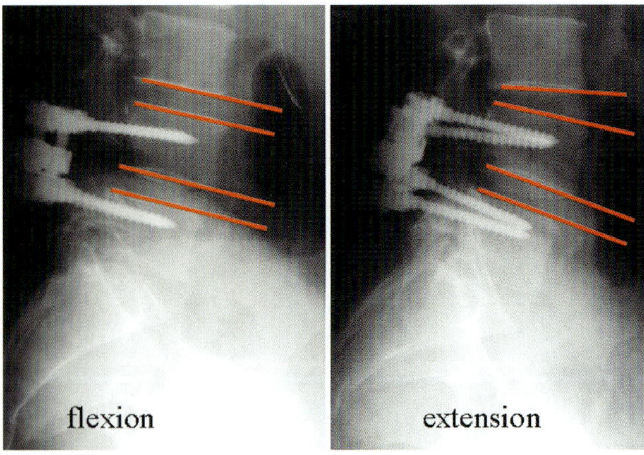

Figure 42–2   Flexion-extension view, 1 year postoperatively.

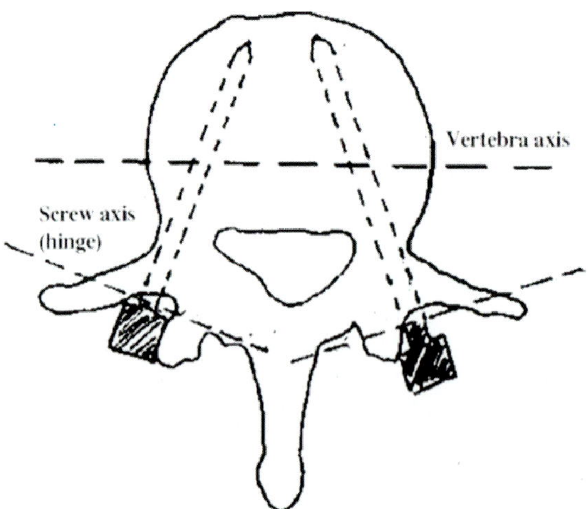

Figure 42–3   Angle of screw direction in the horizontal plan 15 to 25 degrees.

Before the rod is implanted, the correct positioning of the patient will be rechecked by means of lordosis that is as physiological as possible. To avoid any early loosening, correction forces must not be applied to the screw.

◆ Indications for Dynamic Stabilization with Cosmic

Symptomatic Lumbar Stenosis (Claudicatio Spinalis)

Stand-alone decompression of the spinal channel carries the risk of a recurrence of spinal narrowed because the instability that led to the hypertrophy of the yellow ligament and the facet joints is not taken into consideration. In addition, lumbalgies and deformities may increase as an expression of the increased clinical instability. For this reason, we always carry out an additional stabilization with Cosmic (**Fig. 42–4A–C**).

Chronically Recurring Lumbalgy in the Case of Diskogenic Pain and Facet Syndrome

Degenerated disk disease is present if, in the magnetic resource tomography (MRT), vertebral disk dehydration with height loss and positive Modic signs is detected. If there are further changed vertebral disks (black disk), we carry out an additional diskography. A positive memory pain confirms the suspicion of symptomatic vertebral disk degeneration.[19] In the case of a facet syndrome, we carry out a diagnostic local anesthesia under x-ray control, using 2 mL local anesthetic, respectively. If the pain subsides for some hours, the suspected diagnosis is confirmed. In such cases we carry out the Cosmic stabilization using a paraspinous transmuscular approach according to Wiltse[20] (**Fig. 42–5A–C**).

Recurrent Disk Herniation

In the case of a second recurrence of a disk herniation we carry out a stabilization with Cosmic in addition to the nerve root decompression.

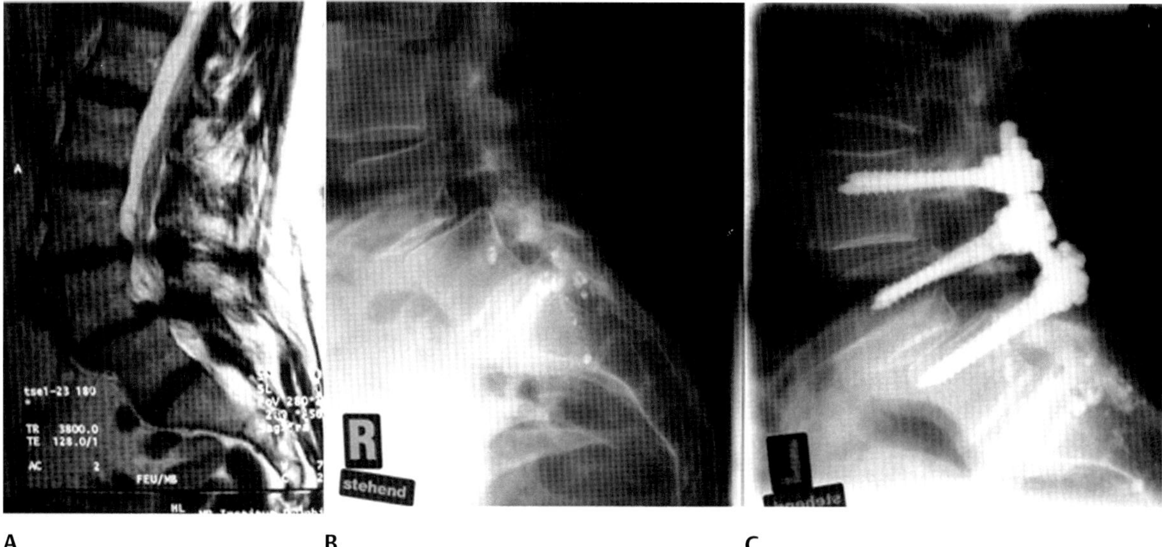

A   B   C

Figure 42–4   **(A)** Spinal stenosis, **(B)** pseudospondylolisthesis, **(C)** decompression and stabilization with Cosmic.

In Combination with a Spondylodesis

Cosmic can also be used if, in addition to the nonfusion stabilization, there is an indication of a spondylodesis in one or two segments. For example, if there is a spondylolisthesis with a clear shift in the function x-rays and, in addition, in a further segment a symptomatic vertebral disk degeneration. In addition to the Cosmic stabilization in situ, a posterolateral fusion is set up within the area of the spondylolisthesis. A laminectomy or facetectomy is performed if there is an indication for this purpose (**Fig. 42–6**).

Extension of an Existing Spondylodesis in the Case of a Painful Adjacent Level Degeneration

Typically, in the case of a rigid 360 degree spondylodesis with cage and pedicle screw rod or pedicle screw plate fixation, there is the risk of developing a painful connection instability. In these cases, we remove the pedicle screw rod or plate system and stabilize the adjacent segment with Cosmic together with a decompression, if indicated. We fill up the existing pedicle drilling holes with bone chips and use a 7 mm revision screw for this purpose (**Fig. 42–7**).

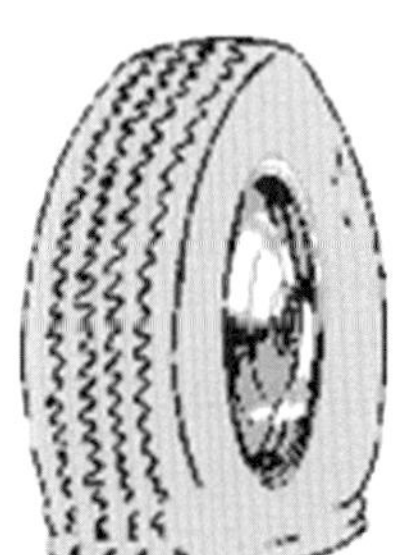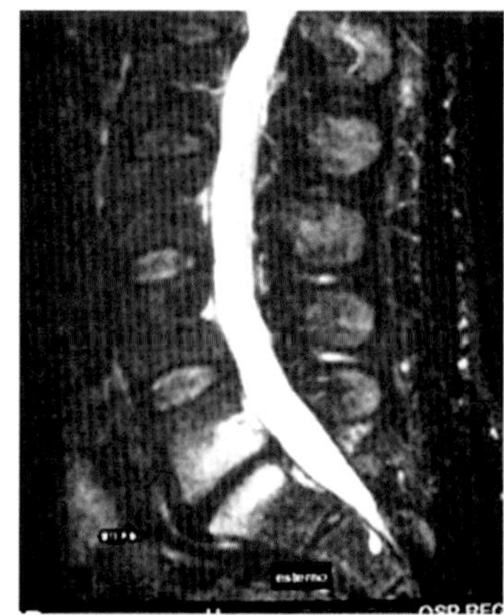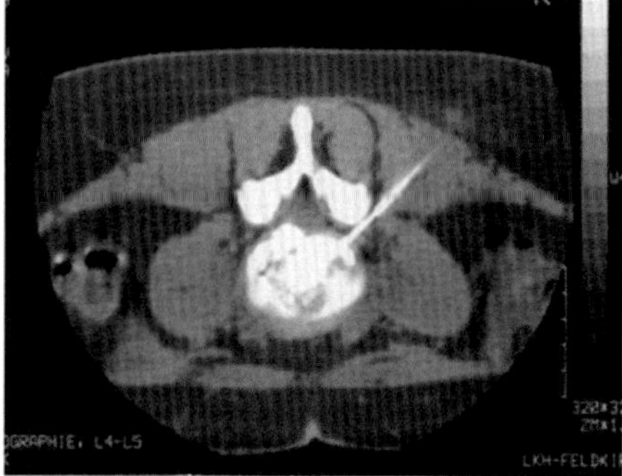

A   B   C

Figure 42–5   **(A)** Degenerated disk disease, (the "flat tire" disk) **(B)** positive Modic sign, **(C)** contrast computed tomography.

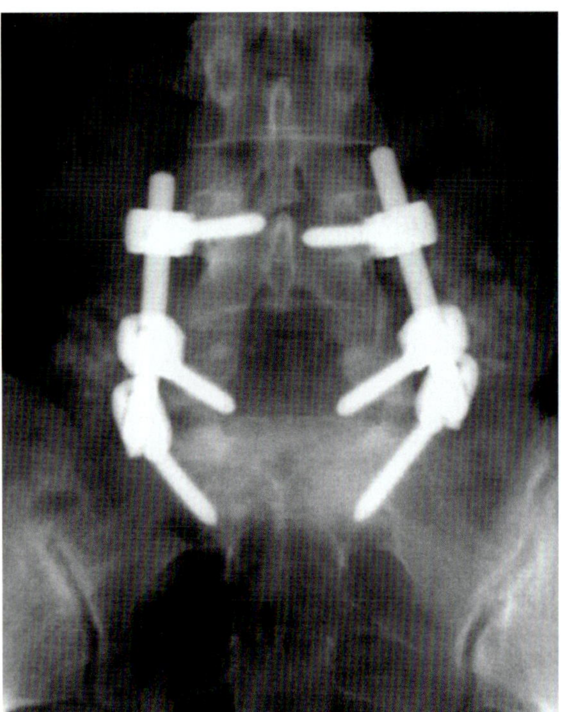

Figure 42–6   Unstable spondylolisthesis vera, stenosis L5–S1, degenerative disk disease L4–L5. Cosmic L4–S1, laminectomy L5, posterior fusion L5–S1.

◆ Contraindications

Cosmic should only be used for a maximum of three segments. If corrections are necessary, to influence the complaints of the patient (as already stated, in almost all cases of a degenerative deformity this is not indicated), a spondylodesis must be provided in addition to the Cosmic instrumentation. Such a case exists, for example, for a postfusion kyphosis where a correction such as a closing wedge–osteotomy is necessary to treat the pain. In adulthood, in the case of a spondylolisthesis vera, there is as a rule no significant shift in the lateral function x-rays. If this is the case, Cosmic is used in combination with a posterolateral fusion in situ. In cases of greater instability, as typically found in younger adults or youths, we carry out a posterior partial repositioning with Cosmic in combination with a posterolateral and interbody spondylodesis.

Stabilizations Extending beyond Three Segments

In the case of the degenerative lumbar vertebral column, extended instrumentations should in principle be avoided. If this is impossible, Cosmic may be used beyond three segments only in combination with a posterolateral spondylodesis. If, for example, there is a degenerative kyphoscoliosis with a loss of balance in the sagittal plane, where there is a necessity to correct the kyphotic part, longer extended instrumentations are required as a rule. Here, in the correction area, Cosmic can be used with a posterolateral spondylodesis, and in the further cranial segments in the nonfusion technology.

◆ Surgical Technique

Under general anesthesia, the patient is positioned in the knee-chest position with the hip joints flexed to 90 degrees to avoid any pressure on the abdomen. The lordosis is radiologically controlled and can be increased by lifting the leg section of the operating table. For pure stabilizations, two skin cuts are made paraspinally, each one in position located 4 cm laterally to the processus spinalis vertebrae. The fascia thoracolumbalis is split, and the finger is used to prepare the muscular system between the multifidus and longissimus, until the transverse processes can be felt. The screw implantation is effected under lateral imager control (C-arm). In the case of a monosegmental stabilization, only closed screws are used (**Fig. 42–8A–C**); two- or three-segmental stabilizations use closed screws at the caudal end of the instrumentation

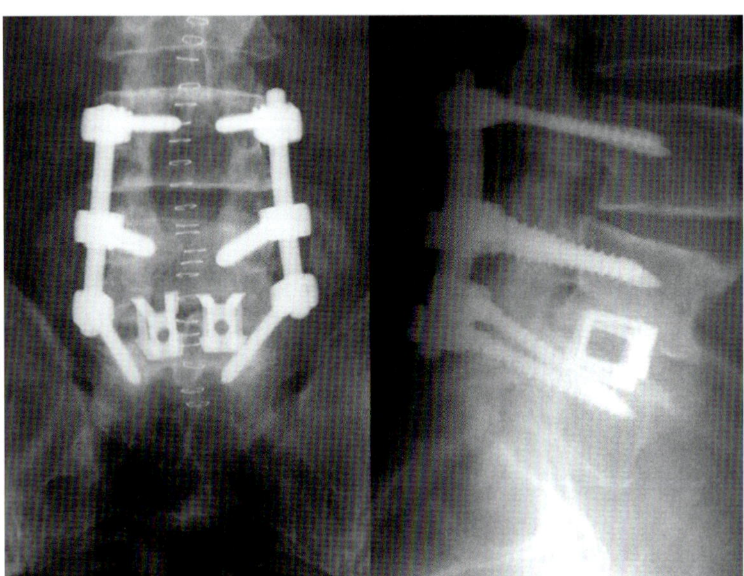

Figure 42–7   Cosmic L3–L5, laminectomy L3, preexisting fusion L4–L5.

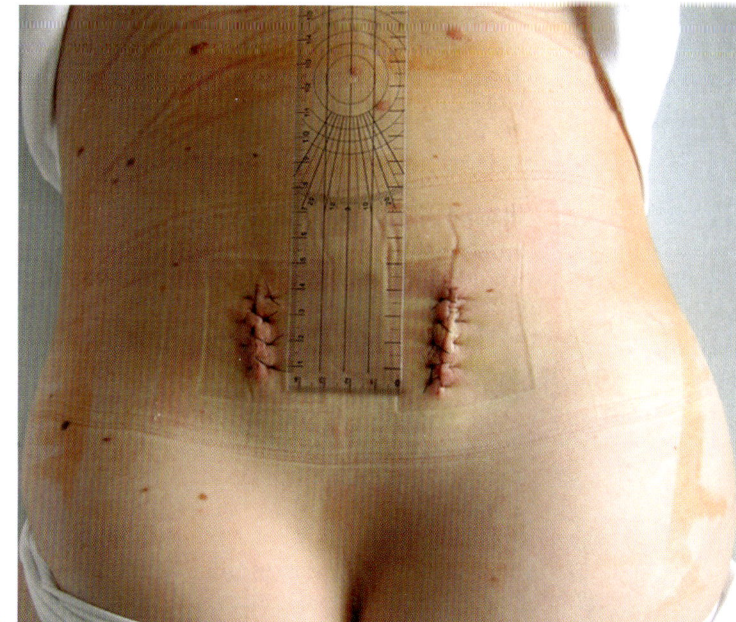

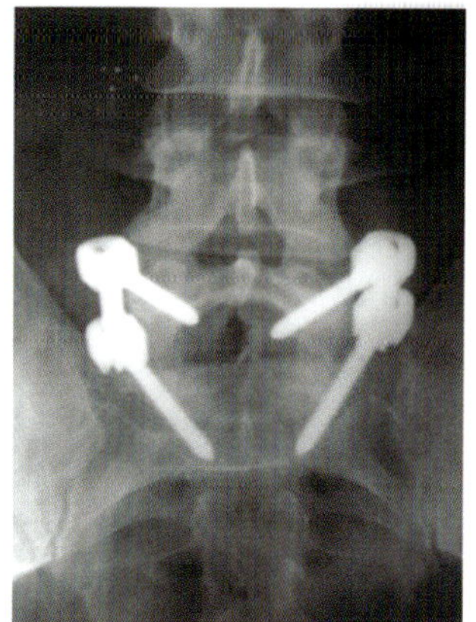

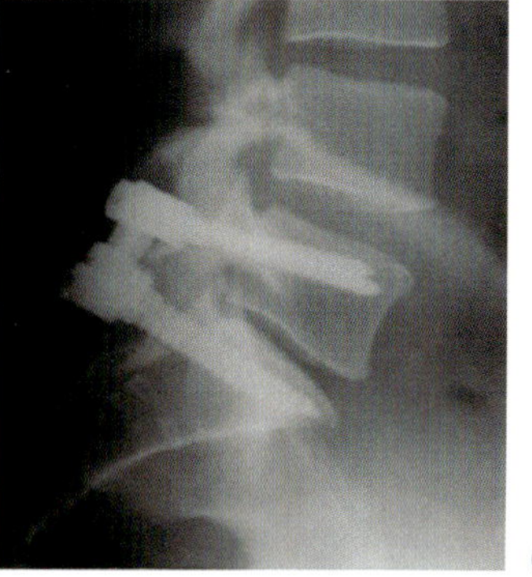

Figure 42–8   **(A)** Paraspinal approach L5–S1. **(B)** Single-level stabilization, anteroposterior and **(C)** lateral view at 2-year follow-up.

and, in all other respects, open screws (**Fig. 42–9**). In the sacrum we recommend a bicortical screw implantation if the screw length is 50 mm or shorter.

In the case of a monosegmental instrumentation, a straight rod is implanted, and in the case of two- and three-segmental instrumentations, the rod will first be bent in accordance with the profile. With open screws, the rod is fixed by a clamp to the screw base; the cap is then put on. The rod and screw base feature a thread for guaranteeing a high degree of rotation stability between the rod and screw (**Fig. 42–10**). Fixation is then effected by a small grub screw that is tightened by a force of 6 Nm. Lateral decompressions can also be performed from this access point. If a laminectomy is necessary, we carry out a midline incision from which either (1) the muscular system is then prepared beyond the joint continuations to carry out screw implantation and decompression from the same access point, or (2) the screws are first set, using the technique already described, followed by the economical preparation of the spinal muscular system from the processus spinalis vertebrae and the vertebral laminae to a medial position relative to the facet joints to make the decompression. The advantage of this latter procedure is that damage to the spinal muscles is reduced and there is less blood loss. In the case of pure stabilizations, the patient will be mobilized on the first postoperative day. In the case of a

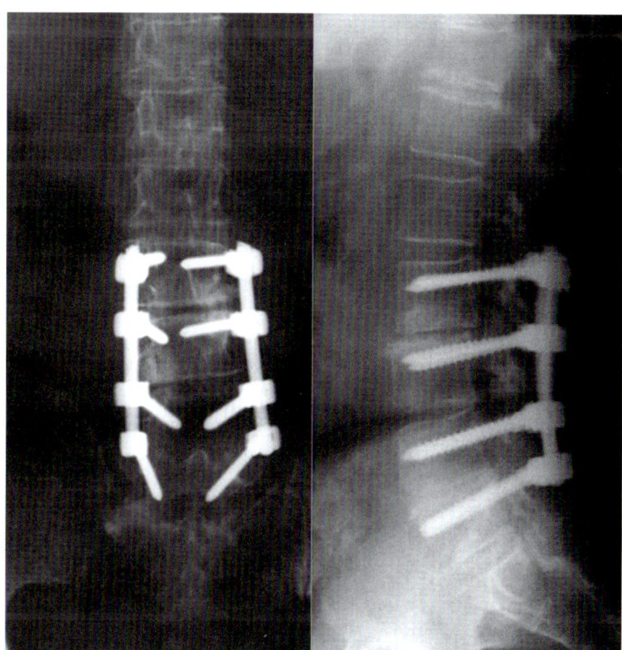

Figure 42–9   Three-level stabilization at 2-year follow-up.

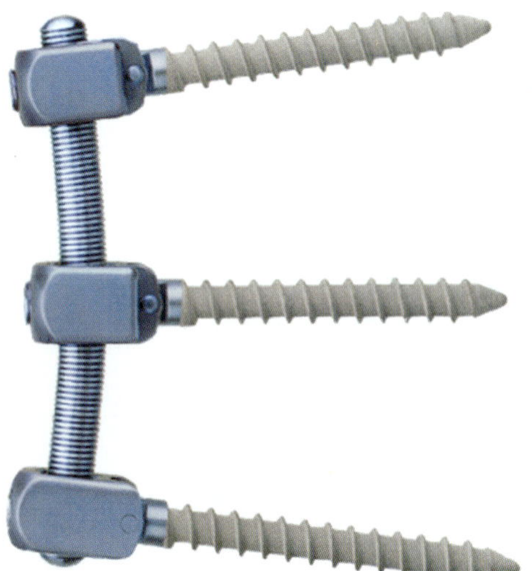

Figure 42–10   Cosmic screws and rod.

conventional midline approach with decompression, such mobilization will be effected on the second day. The redon drainage is removed on the first day. For infection prophylaxis, a dose of cephalosporin is given before the skin incision. The thrombosis prophylaxis is performed with a low molecular heparin for 2 weeks postoperatively. External support will not be used.

◆ Results

From January 2002 to June 2005, 203 patients were operated in Feldkirch (Austria). For 96 patients there is a 12-month follow-up course available, and for 38 patients of these 96 there is a 24-month follow-up course available. Preoperatively, there is conventional x-ray imaging for all patients, anteroposterior (AP) and lateral, in a standing position, and additionally, and where this was not possible (agoraphobia) a computed tomographic (CT) scan. The complaints are documented by a 10-part analog pain scale from 0 to 10 (0 = no pain, 10 = unbearable pain) and by the Oswestry Disability Index (ODI) score.

Three months, 12 months, and 24 months postoperatively conventional x-rays will be performed again, AP and lateral, in a standing position, and the clinical results documented by the pain scale and the Oswestry score. The x-ray images are studied for implant fractures, screw loosening, or screw dislocations. A screw loosening is defined as a loosening seam around the screw without any dislocation having occurred.

Of these 96 patients, 51 were female (53%) and 45 were male (47%). The age distribution was:

- ◆ 30–40 years 3 patients
- ◆ 41–50 years 8 patients
- ◆ 51–60 years 30 patients
- ◆ 61–70 years 19 patients
- ◆ 71–80 years 31 patients
- ◆ 81–90 years 5 patients

Four additional patients could not be examined for their 2-year check-up because they had died (three patients, the death having no connection to the operation) or had moved (one patient).

Fifty-one patients were stabilized in one segment, 35 patients in two segments, and 10 patients in three segments. In total, 494 screws, 192 longitudinal rods, and 23 transverse stabilizers were implanted.

The clinical results were compared with those from 75 patients with a follow-up of at least 24 months that, for the same indications, had been treated with the Segmental Spinal Correction System (SSCS; Ulrich GmbH & Co. KG, Ulm, Germany), which also contains a jointed head pedicle screw but without coating, and with a conventional posterolateral fusion. The SSCS has been used since 1989.

In both groups, the indications were comparable: symptomatic lumbar stenosis, painful olistheses, painful osteochondroses, painful spondylarthroses, recurring vertebral disk prolapses, and diskogenic pain.

The average age in the nonfusion group was 67.2 years, and in the fusion group 55.9 years. The reason for the increased age of the nonfusion group is that, during the first year, we predominantly used the nonfusion technique for the treatment of older patients to keep the surgery trauma as low as possible. With increasing experience we then used the nonfusion technique in the case of middle-aged adult patients.

In the nonfusion group, the visual analog scale (VAS) scores were 5.7 preoperatively and 2.9 postoperatively, and in the fusion group the pains were 5.8 preoperatively and 3.4.

The ODI in the nonfusion group was 25.4 points or 50.8% preoperatively and 17.0 points or 34% postoperatively. In the fusion group, the Oswestry activity score was 23.7 points or 47.4% preoperatively and 14.7 points or 29.4% postoperatively.

The hospital stay in the nonfusion group was 7.4 days (6–18 days), and in the fusion group 16.9 days (9-36 days).

The surgery time (skin to skin) in the nonfusion group was 118.8 minutes (62–200 minutes), and in the fusion group 172.4 minutes (120–215 minutes). Perioperatively, a total of 0.60 U of eryconcentrate were transfused (0–4 U), and, in the fusion group, 2.96 U of eryconcentrate (0–6 U) were transfused on average.

In the nonfusion group, revisions were performed in the case of four patients (4.2% of 96 patients) and, in the fusion group, revisions were performed in the case of six patients (8.0% of 75 patients). The revisions were caused by wound infections (one case in the nonfusion group as well as three cases in the fusion group), twice by symptomatic loosening of a screw in the nonfusion group, once by a screw break-off in the nonfusion group, and a total of three times due to a pseudarthrosis in connection with an implant fracture or implant loosening in the fusion group.

In the nonfusion group, a total of two broken screws were found in two patients, and in five patients a total of 10 screws with loosening edges (2.4% of 494 implanted screws) were found. In total, seven patients were affected; of these, three patients developed symptoms causing a revision to be performed.

In the case of the revision, the loosened or broken screws were removed, the pedicle bore holes were filled with bone chips (similar to matchsticks) from the spinous process, and 7 mm Cosmic revision screws were implanted. So far, there have been no new occurrences of renewed loosening or screw fractures in these patients. In one case, a rod fracture occurred without any symptoms. There was no record of any screw dislocations or the fracture of a transverse stabilizer. All implant failures observed so far occurred within the first year.

In June 2005 a multicenter study was started in cooperation with six international spine centers. So far, 215 patients have been documented; and for 100 of these 215, there is a 3-month follow-up available, and for 58 there is a 12-month follow-up. After 3 months no implant failures were found by this study, and after 12 months a screw fracture was found that led to a revision, as well as six loosening seams around the screws that, however, remained without symptoms and so far did not cause any revision. A screw dislocation was not observed.

◆ Discussion

Degenerative diseases of the lumbar vertebral column represent their own nosological entity. So far they have been treated primarily in accordance with the principles of deformities surgery and traumatology.

To achieve correction of existing deformities that is as complete as possible, rigid implants have been used that provide three-dimensional correction if at all possible. The experience that the fusion of individual segments of the degenerative lumbar vertebral column may cause painful connection instabilities—and this applies obviously in particular to the rigid 360 degree fusions—increasingly casts doubt over the use of such techniques for the treatment of degenerative diseases.[21-33] The postoperative sagittal profile of the lumbar spine did not have any influence on the development of adjacent instabilities.[34]

In addition, there is the problem that, in the case of older patients, the quality of the bone frequently does not allow any corrections, including secure fixation of rigid implants. Some patients at an advanced age also show additional secondary diseases that cause increased perioperative complications with more invasive operations on the vertebral column.

Fusion as the gold standard for the treatment of chronic pain within the area of the degenerative lumbar vertebral column must also be questioned because a 100% spondylodesis is not the equivalent of a 100% clinical success rate.[35,36]

The significance of patient selection is justifiably regarded as a decisive criterion for achieving a good clinical result.[37] For this reason it is not surprising that there is a search for different alternative operative techniques that prevent any fusion.[38] But what may be surprising is that it took so long to question fusion as the gold standard. However, for some time already, there have been individual efforts to develop alternative solutions in relation to the fusion concept. The Graf band is possibly the first pedicle screw–supported nonfusion system for the treatment of painful degenerative instabilities on the lumbar vertebral column. Biomechanically, it increases the use of dorsal tension chords and reduces painful movements in the facet joints and also in the disk. There are some reports of excellent clinical success.[39] [13]

What remains disadvantageous is surely the missing rotational stability and the risk of early failure of the cable. The Dynesys Dynamic Stabilization System (Zimmer Spine, Inc., Warsaw, IN) represents a further development of the Graf system. The band is provided with a plastic sleeve, and the band is tensioned against this sleeve. This causes increased stability but also an increased load on the interface between the vertebral bone and screw, which may cause loosening.[44] In relation to the rotational forces, the Dynesis system does not show any stability comparable to that of an intact vertebral column.[45]

The clinical reports that have been published on the Dynesys system are mostly positive.[46,47] In combination with decompressions, these two systems, Dynesys and the Graf, are used somewhat more rarely because even partial removal of the facet increases the rotational instability.[48]

Other nonfusion techniques not based on pedicle screws stabilize the motion segment by spreading the processus spinalis vertebrae, thereby expanding the spinal channel. The indications are limited to light spinal narrowing and facet syndrome. Interspinous spreaders can be implanted minimally invasively. At this time, major clinical studies are not yet available.

In contrast to the aforementioned posterior nonfusion systems, Cosmic is used for symptomatic spinal stenosis, in combination with decompressions, as well as in the case of purely diskogenic or facet joint–related pain.

The hinged screw provides a sufficient degree of dynamization and load sharing between the implant and the vertebral column and prevents any rotation and translation instability. The rotation stability corresponds to that shown by an intact lumbar vertebral column.[15]

Because nonfusion implants act like stability prostheses and must last permanently without the protection of a fusion, the Cosmic screw was additionally coated with Bonit to ensure better anchoring in the vertebral bone.[18] The clinical results found so far, when compared with conventional fusions, are equally good. The perioperative trauma was much lower. The careful transmuscular (between the musculus multifidus and musculus longissimus) access to the pedicles may further decrease the operative trauma.

Even when using Cosmic, careful selection of patients by the precondition for clinical success.

The radiological complex implant-related complications are in the lower range of those specified in the literature with regard to rigid implants in combination with a fusion. Here, between 2.5 and 15% screw fractures are specified.[49,50]

Radiological loosening seams, as documented in the present study, are not really considered in the literature, unless screw dislocations are noted. In fusion surgery as well as in nonfusion surgery, the meaning of implant-related complications cannot always be equated with a clinical failure. In those cases where a patient again develops pain after experiencing a temporary relief from complaints and where an implant-related complication can be radiologically detected, the revision is recommended in all cases. In principle, when using a nonfusion implant system, there is the option to carry out a conventional fusion in addition to the replacement of implants. The three patients revised in the present study due to symptomatic implant problems again received Cosmic revision screws without fusion.

So far, the results found with the Cosmic system are very encouraging. However, additional long-term observations are necessary. For this reason we started an international multicenter study in June 2004, which is Internet based.

◆ Conclusion

Posterior nonfusion stabilizations represent an alternative to spondylodesis in the treatment of painful degenerative diseases of the lumbar spine.

Cosmic is a dynamic nonfusion pedicle screw–rod system for the stabilization of the lumbar vertebral column. The hinged pedicle screw provides for the load being shared between the implant and the vertebral column and allows a high stability in relation to the rotational forces.

This report covers the clinical and radiological results of 96 patients with a follow-up of 12 to 24 months. The clinical results were compared with those from 75 patients who had been treated with hinged screws and a conventional posterolateral fusion. In both groups, the indications were comparable: symptomatic spinal stenosis, diskogenic pain, facet syndrome, and postdiskectomy syndrome. In both groups, the Oswestry score and the VAS showed a good improvement of the symptoms without any significant differences.

The perioperative morbidity in the nonfusion group was significantly lower. In the nonfusion group, with 494 screws implanted, two broken screws were found in two patients. In the case of five patients, 10 screws with radiological loosening were found. From these seven patients, three again developed symptoms that led to a revision. In the fusion group, three pseudarthroses with screw fracture were found that were also revised. All implant-related revisions occurred within the first year.

The early- and medium-term results found so far with the Cosmic system are very encouraging. Additional long-term observations are necessary.

References

1. Fujiwara A, Tamai K, Yamato M, et al. The relationship between facet joint osteoarthritis and disc degeneration of the lumbar spine: an MRI study. Eur Spine J 1999;8:396–401

2. Fujiwara A, Lim T-H, An HS, et al. The effect of disc degeneration and facet joint osteoarthritis on the segmental flexibility of the lumbar spine. Spine 2000;25:3036–3044

3. Krismer M, Haid C, Behensky H, Kapfinger P, Landauer F, Rachbauer F. Motion in lumbar functional spine units during side bending and axial rotation moments depending on the degree of degeneration. Spine 2000;25:2020–2027

4. Tanaka N, An HS, Lim TH, Fujiwara A, Jeon CH, Haughton VM. The relationship between disc degeneration and flexibility of the lumbar spine. Spine J 2001;1:47–56

5. Rauschning W. Pathoanatomy of lumbar disc degeneration and stenosis. Acta Orthop Scand Suppl 1993;251:3–12

6. Peng B, Wu W, Hou S, Li P, Zhang C, Yang Y. The pathogenesis of discogenic low back pain. J Bone Joint Surg Br 2005;87:62–67

7. Panjabi MM. Clinical spinal instability and low back pain. J Electromyogr Kinesiol 2003;13:371–379

8. Fritzell P, Hagg O, Nordwall A. Complications in lumbar fusion surgery for chronic low back pain: comparison of three surgical techniques used in a prospective randomized study: a report from the Swedish Lumbar Spine Study Group. Eur Spine J 2003;12:178–189

9. Ghiselli G, Wang JC, Bhatia NN, Hsu WK, Dawson EG. Adjacent segment degeneration in the lumbar spine. J Bone Joint Surg Am 2004;86–A:1497–1503

10. Park P, Garton HJ, Gala VC, Hoff JT, McGillicuddy JE. Adjacent segment disease after lumbar or lumbosacral fusion: review of the literature. Spine 2004;29:1938–1944

11. Chosa E, Goto K, Totoribe K, Tajima N. Analysis of the effect of lumbar spine fusion on the superior adjacent intervertebral disk in the presence of disk degeneration, using the three-dimensional finite element method. J Spinal Disord Tech 2004;17:134–139

12. Brantigan JW, Neidre A, Toohey JS. The Lumbar I/F Cage for posterior lumbar interbody fusion with the variable screw placement system: 10-year results of a Food and Drug Administration clinical trial. Spine J 2004;4:681–688

13. Rahm MD, Hall BB. Adjacent-segment degeneration after lumbar fusion with instrumentation: a retrospective study. J Spinal Disord 1996;9:392–400

14. Helenius I, Remes V, Yrjonen T, et al. Comparison of long-term functional and radiologic outcomes after Harrington instrumentation and spondylodesis in adolescent idiopathic scoliosis: a review of 78 patients. Spine 2002;27:176–180

15. Scifert JL, Sairyo K, Goel VK, et al. Stability analysis of an enhanced load sharing posterior fixation device and its equivalent conventional device in a calf spine model. Spine 1999;24:2206–2213

16. Ettinger C. Test report No. 27.011019.30.95. Rosenheim, Germany: Endolab Mechanical Engineering; 2002:1–7

17. Lacefield WR. Current status of ceramic coating for dental implants. Implant Dent 1998;7:315–318

18. Sanden B, Olerud C, Petren-Mallmin M, Larsson S. Hydroxyapatite coating improves fixation of pedicle screws: a clinical study. J Bone Joint Surg Br 2002;84:387–391

19. Guyer RD, Ohnmeiss DD. Lumbar discography: position statement from the North American Spine Society Diagnostic and Therapeutic Committee. Spine 1995;20:2048–2059

20. Wiltse LL, Bateman JG, Hutchinson RH, Nelson WE. The paraspinal sacrospinalis-splitting approach to the lumbar spine. J Bone Joint Surg Am 1968;50:919–926

21. Aota Y, Kumano K, Hirabayashi S. Postfusion instability at the adjacent segments after rigid pedicle screw fixation for degenerative lumbar spinal disorders. J Spinal Disord 1995;8:464–473

22. Esses SI, Doherty BJ, Crawford MJ, Dreyzin V. Kinematic evaluation of lumbar fusion techniques. Spine 1996;21:676–684

23. Kumar MN, Jacquot F, Hall H. Long-term follow-up of functional outcomes and radiographic changes at adjacent levels following lumbar spine fusion for degenerative disc disease. Eur Spine J 2001;10:309–313

24. Gillet P. The fate of the adjacent motion segments after lumbar fusion. J Spinal Disord Tech 2003;16:338–345

25. Etebar S, Cahill DW. Risk factors for adjacent-segment failure following lumbar fixation with rigid instrumentation for degenerative instability. J Neurosurg 1999;90:163–169

26. Eck JC, Humphreys SC, Hodges SD. Adjacent-segment degeneration after lumbar fusion: a review of clinical, biomechanical, and radiologic studies. Am J Orthop 1999;28:336–340

27. Chou WY, Hsu CJ, Chang WN, Wong CY. Adjacent segment degeneration after lumbar spinal posterolateral fusion with instrumentation in elderly patients. Arch Orthop Trauma Surg 2002;122:39–43

28. Booth KC, Bridwell KH, Eisenberg BA, Baldus CR, Lenke LG. Minimum 5-year results of degenerative spondylolisthesis treated with decompression and instrumented posterior fusion. Spine 1999;24:1721–1727

29. Axelsson P, Johnsson R, Stromqvist B. The spondylolytic vertebra and its adjacent segment: mobility measured before and after posterolateral fusion. Spine 1997;22:414–417

30. Sudo H, Oda I, Abumi K, et al. In vitro biomechanical effects of reconstruction on adjacent motion segment: comparison of aligned/kyphotic

posterolateral fusion with aligned posterior lumbar interbody fusion/posterolateral fusion. J Neurosurg 2003;99:221–228

31. Okuda S, Iwasaki M, Miyauchi A, Aono H, Morita M, Yamamoto T. Risk factors for adjacent segment degeneration after PLIF. Spine 2004;29: 1535–1540

32. Hilibrand AS, Robbins M. Adjacent segment degeneration and adjacent segment disease: the consequences of spinal fusion? Spine J 2004;4: 190S–194S

33. Wenger M, Sapio N, Markwalder TM. Long-term outcome in 132 consecutive patients after posterior internal fixation and fusion for grade I and II isthmic spondylolisthesis. J Neurosurg Spine 2005;2:289–297

34. Lai PL, Chen LH, Niu CC, Chen WJ. Effect of postoperative lumbar sagittal alignment on the development of adjacent instability. J Spinal Disord Tech 2004;17:353–357

35. Bohnen IM, Schaafsma J, Tonino AJ. Results and complications after posterior lumbar spondylodesis with the "Variable Screw Placement Spinal Fixation System." Acta Orthop Belg 1997;63:67–73

36. Tunturi T, Kataja M, Keski-Nisula L, et al. Posterior fusion of the lumbosacral spine: evaluation of the operative results and the factors influencing them. Acta Orthop Scand 1979;50:415–425

37. Fritzell P. Fusion as treatment for chronic low back pain: existing evidence, the scientific frontier and research strategies. Eur Spine J 2005;14:519–520

38. Huang RC, Wright TM, Panjabi MM, Lipman JD. Biomechanics of nonfusion implants. Orthop Clin North Am 2005;36:271–280

39. Sengupta DK, Mulholland RC. Fulcrum assisted soft stabilization system: a new concept in the surgical treatment of degenerative low back pain. Spine 2005;30:1019–1029

40. Kanayama M, Hashimoto T, Shigenobu K, et al. Adjacent-segment morbidity after Graf ligamentoplasty compared with posterolateral lumbar fusion. J Neurosurg 2001;95:5–10

41. Kanayama M, Hashimoto T, Shigenobu K. Rationale, biomechanics, and surgical indications for Graf ligamentoplasty. Orthop Clin North Am 2005;36:373–377

42. Kanayama M, Hashimoto T, Shigenobu K, Oha F, Ishida T, Yamane S. Non-fusion surgery for degenerative spondylolisthesis using artificial ligament stabilization: surgical indication and clinical results. Spine 2005;30:588–592

43. Brechbuhler D, Markwalder TM, Braun M. Surgical results after soft system stabilization of the lumbar spine in degenerative disc disease–long-term results. Acta Neurochir (Wien) 1998;140:521–525

44. Schwarzenbach O, Berlemann U, Stoll TM, Dubois G. Posterior Dynamic Stabilization Systems: Dynesys. Orthop Clin North Am 2005;36: 363–372

45. Schmoelz W, Huber JF, Nydegger T, Dipl I, Claes L, Wilke HJ. Dynamic stabilization of the lumbar spine and its effects on adjacent segments: an in vitro experiment. J Spinal Disord Tech 2003;16:418–423

46. Putzier M, Schneider SV, Funk J, Perka C. Application of a dynamic pedicle screw system (Dynesys) for lumbar segmental degenerations: comparison of clinical and radiological results for different indications. Z Orthop Ihre Grenzgeb 2004;142:166–173

47. Stoll TM, Dubois G, Schwarzenbach O. The dynamic neutralization system for the spine: a multi-center study of a novel non-fusion system. Eur Spine J 2002;11(Suppl 2):S170–S178

48. Zander T, Rohlmann A, Klockner C, Bergmann G. Influence of graded facetectomy and laminectomy on spinal biomechanics. Eur Spine J 2003;12:427–434

49. McAfee PC, Weiland DJ, Carlow JJ. Survivorship analysis of pedicle spinal instrumentation. Spine 1991;16:S422–S427

50. Marchesi DG, Thalgott JS, Aebi M. Application and results of the AO internal fixation system in nontraumatic indications. Spine 1991;16: S162–S169

43

BioFlex Spring Rod Pedicle Screw System

Young-Soo Kim and Byung-Jin Moon

◆ **Indications and Contraindications**

◆ **Advantage of System Components**

◆ **Description of System Component**
　BioFlex System Implants

◆ **Biomechanical Testing**
　Fatigue Strength Test
　Pullout Test
　Static Bending Compression Test

◆ **Operative Techniques**
　Patient Position
　Surgical Approach
　Screw Insertion
　Rod Insertion

◆ **Case Illustrations**
　Case 1
　Case 2

◆ **Discussion**

Rigid spinal fixation is the current gold standard in the surgical management of lumbar spinal instability. However, it can result in many complications such as nonunion, screw loosening, screw fracture, and flat back syndrome.[1,2] Rigid fixation also increases biomechanical stresses on segments adjacent to the fusion level.[3] Clinically, the results of several long-term follow-up studies have suggested that spinal fusion might cause deterioration of the adjacent segment.[4]

For 2 decades, the dominant surgical justification for fusing the painful motion segment has been the concept of instability. Spinal instrumentation has been continuously developing from a rigid system to the more physiological, flexible, and so-called dynamic stabilization.

Devices that have been developed for dynamic stabilization include artificial nucleus replacement, artificial disk replacement, and ligamentoplasty. Using ligaments across the pedicle screw system is thought to be the most effective method in dynamic stabilization because it allows for disk unloading and can correct sagittal plane imbalance of the spine.

The Graf ligamentoplasty system restricted flexion and was modestly successful, but it increased the load over the posterior annulus.[5,6] The Dynesys Dynamic Stabilization System (Zimmer Spine, Inc., Warsaw, IN) system reduced movement in both flexion and extension. However, the plastic cylinder of the Dynesys system is weak and it may prove difficult to unload the disk if the patient achieves a position of lordosis. This has resulted in a search for new material for flexible stabilization in spine surgery, or semirigid metallic dynamic stabilization.

Nitinol is an alloy of nickel and titanium that belongs to a class of materials called shape memory alloys. The properties of nitinol alloys are high elasticity and high tensile force, which means they can be used for tension bands posteriorly in the spine surgery.[7] Nitinol is biologically and mechanically compatible as an implant. The alloy has a particular propensity for temperature, being flexible at 10°C low and forms a shape at temperatures above body temperature.[8–10]

The BioFlex rod system has been developed by the author in our hospital. The system consists of a nitinol spring/straight rod and titanium screws. It is well suited for use in the posterior thoracolumbar spine. Currently, the BioFlex rod system is the only semirigid metallic device for dynamic stabilization with or without fusion available for clinical use in Korea.

◆ Indications and Contraindications

The BioFlex (Bio-Smart Ltd., Songnam-si, Korea) spring rod pedicle screw system is versatile and is indicated for a wide variety of posterior lumbar fusion and dynamic stabilization surgeries:

- Low back pain from symptomatic degenerative disk disease
- Spondylosis and spondylolisthesis in whole grade
- Segmental instability
- Following destabilizing decompression in a symptomatic canal or foraminal stenosis
- Pseudarthrosis
- Posterior lumbar interbody fusion and posterior fixation
- Correction of degenerative kyphoscoliosis
- Prevention of adjacent segment instability
- Injury of ligament structures

- Deformity correction, including postlaminectomy kyphosis and scoliosis
- Trauma
- Tumor

Relative contraindications for use include:

- Developmentally inadequate pedicles
- Active infection
- Profound osteopenia

◆ Advantages of System Components

Nitinol, the material of the rod in this system, behaves similarly to the ligament–cartilage structure of spinal elements. The nitinol rod is applied to the motion segment by pedicle screws. At rest, the system would share the loading and unloading of the disk. The flexible and high tensile characteristics of the rod restrict the flexion-extension of the motion segment like spinal ligaments. Therefore, this system is most suitable for dynamic stabilization biomechanically, to achieve the objectives of soft stabilization with optimum load sharing, disk unloading, and control of motion.

The BioFlex rod system achieves dynamic stabilization and at the same time functions as pedicle screw instrumentation. This semirigid segmental immobilization of the elements is necessary for spinal manipulation, reduction, and correction of spinal deformity. This system also enables compression and distraction of the disk space. It can increase the fusion rate if compression of the disk space with posterior or anterior interbody cage insertion is performed, and it can reduce the subsidence rate by posterior fixation.

The BioFlex rod system is built to suit attachment to each segment. If stabilization in the upper and lower segment is later compromised, an extension can be easily performed with a previous fixation segment. Rod insertion is easily achieved because the nitinol rod is flexible at low temperatures.

◆ Description of System Component

The key instruments featured in the BioFlex spring rod system include (**Figs. 43–1 and 43–2**):

- Modular awl and straight or curved pedicle probe
- Screwdriver with T-handle
- Rod holder
- Compressor and distractor pliers
- Countertorque wrench for maximal final nut tightening

BioFlex System Implants

BioFlex system implants (**Figs. 43–3 to 43–6**) include a straight and a spring rod (1, 2, and 3 coiling) with 3.5 to 4.3 mm diameter (in 3 mm increments) and 40 to 110 mm (in 5 mm increments) length made of Nitinol [American Society for Testing and Materials (ASTM F) 2063]. A fixed screw head (monoaxial) and a rotating screw head (multiaxial) provide two rod fixation holes: 4.0 to 8.5 mm diameter (in 5 mm

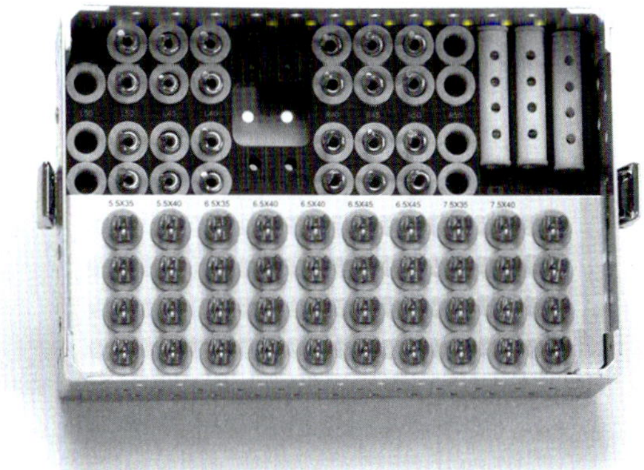

A

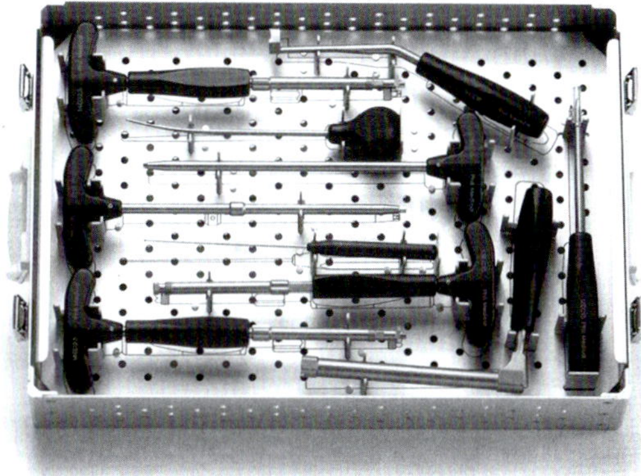

B

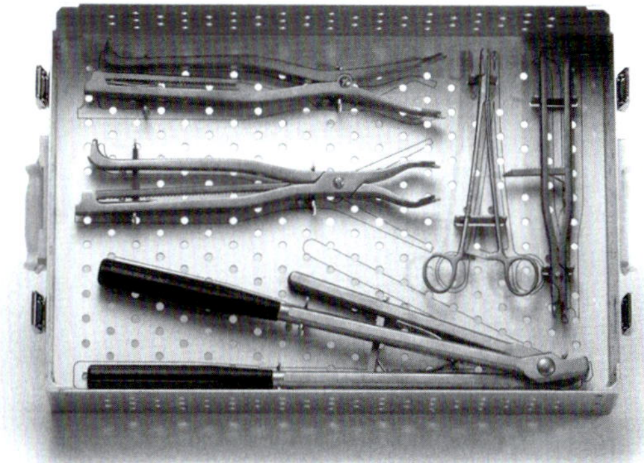

C

Figure 43–1 **(A–C)** Container of instruments.

increments) and 32 to 67 mm length (in 5 mm increments), and is made of Titanium (ASTM F-136).

◆ Biomechanical Testing

Fatigue Strength Test

The purpose of this testing was to determine the force required to fracture the BioFlex rod system flexible nitinol rods assembled in the titanium alloy pedicle screws. The test

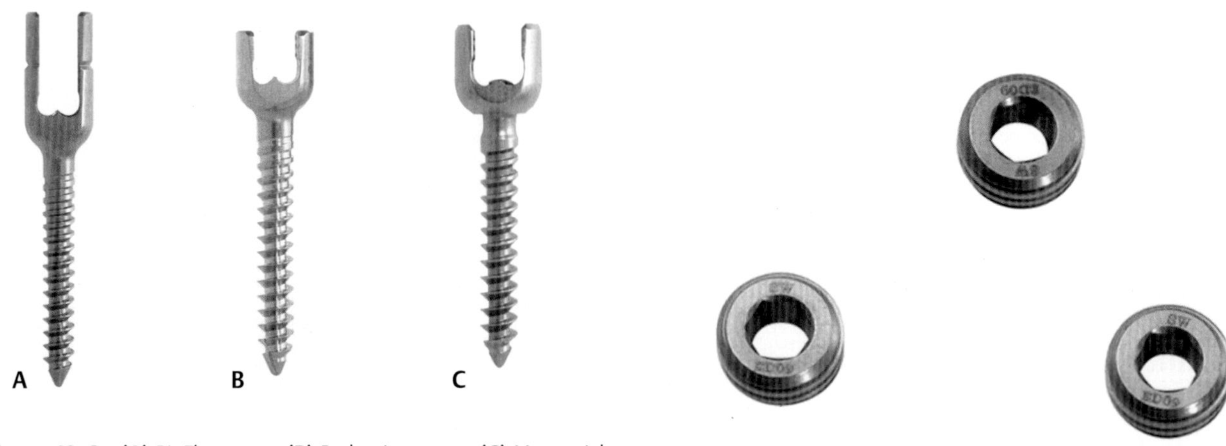

Figure 43–2 **(A)** BioFlex screw. **(B)** Reduction screw. **(C)** Monoaxial screw. Each screw head has two grooves.

Figure 43–4 Nut system.

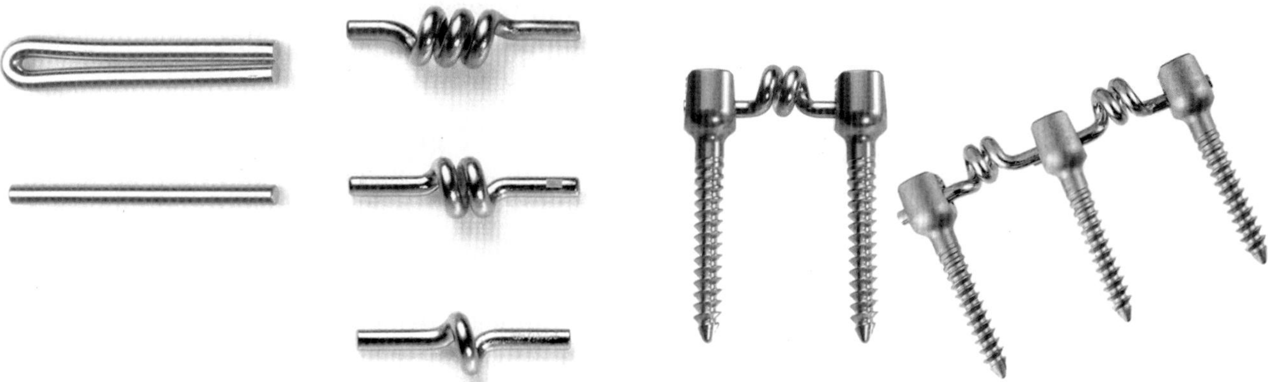

Figure 43–3 Nitinol rods, straight and coiled.

Figure 43–5 BioFlex rod pedicle screw systems.

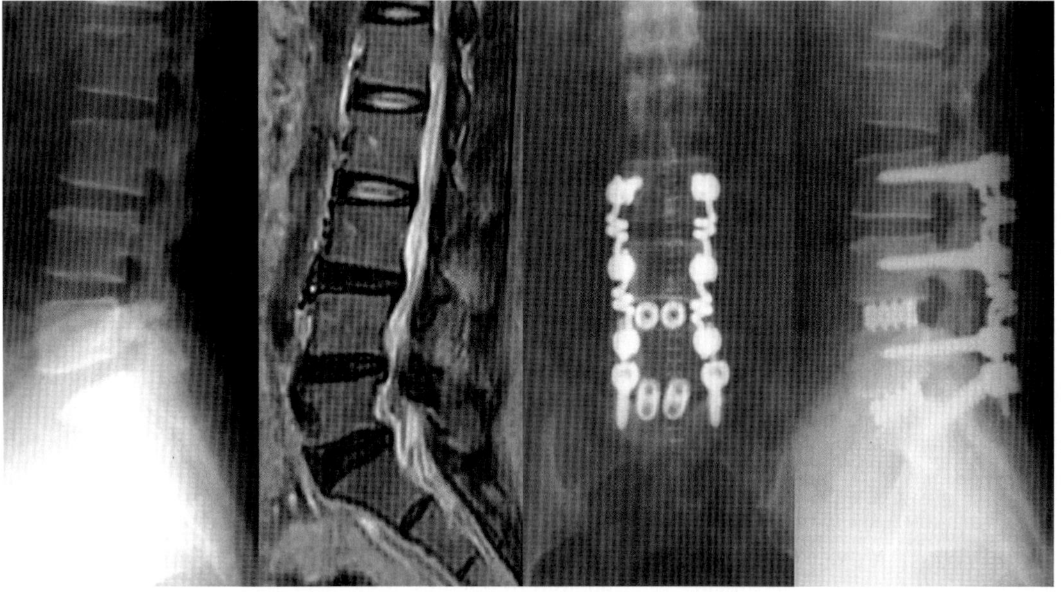

Figure 43–6 (Case 1) Spondylolitic spondylolisthesis L5–S1, L4–L5 instability and L3–L4 mild spondylolitic stenosis. Preoperative magnetic resonance imaging, x-ray, and postoperative x-ray.

conditions included displacement of 6 mm, velocity of 5 Hz, and 10,000,000 cycles. The result of the fatigue test was acceptable and without any failure or deformity.

Pullout Test

The purpose of this testing was to determine the force required to pull out the titanium alloy BioFlex pedicle screw. The result of the pullout test was more than 1000 N.

Static Bending Compression Test

The result of the static bending compression test was 130 N.

◆ Operative Techniques

Patient Position

Surgery is performed with the patient under general or epidural anesthesia and placed in the prone position. The hips are flexed, and the legs are adjusted to provide the desired sagittal and coronal alignment. The patient is placed so as to avoid abdominal compression, which eases the work of ventilation and reduced epidural venous plexus engorgement. Care should be taken to avoid pressure on the peripheral nerves. Sequential compressive stockings are also placed on the extremities for mechanical deep venous thrombosis prophylaxis.

Surgical Approach

A midline incision and approach are utilized in most dorsal exposures of the lumbar spine. The standard posterior midline incision and approach provide adequate exposure for virtually all posterior lumbar instrumentation systems.

After the skin incision and sharp dissection are carried to the lumbodorsal fascia, Bovie electrocautery is used for optimal hemostasis during subperiosteal dissection and paravertebral muscle elevation from the posterior elements. Working laterally in a subperiosteal fashion, exposure should include the pars interarticularis and facet joints. The facet branch of a segmental lumbar artery and corresponding vein is usually encountered. The facet joint complex should be preserved without disruption at the levels adjacent to the fusion site to minimize potential segmental instability. Exposure should be extended laterally to the tip of the transverse processes while avoiding the dissection anterior to the plane of the transverse process.

Screw Insertion

The pedicle entrance point is crossed by a vertical line that connects the lateral edge of the bony crest, which is the extension of the pars interarticularis, and the horizontal line that bisects the midline of the transverse process. This is at the junction point of the pars interarticularis, the lateral wall of the facet joint, and the transverse process.

Using a bone awl, the entrance of the pedicle is marked. The cancellous bone within the cortical tube of the pedicle is broached using a pedicle probe. The screws of the BioFlex system are self-tapping; however, tapping may be performed prior to screw insertion, based on the surgeon's preference and the bone quality.

At this point, the pedicle is prepared and ready to accept a screw. The screw diameter and length are appropriately selected and the screw is inserted into the pedicle. The medial border of the pedicle can be visually or tactically probed to make certain that the screws are well placed if a laminectomy has been performed at the same level.

Rod Insertion

Rods do not require cutting because they come in various sizes. Rods are inserted one by one into the segment. It is crucial to select the appropriate-sized BioFlex rod. Although left- and right-side rods are supplied, the direction is not important biomechanically. There are two grooves in each screw head. When the rod is inserted, each end of the rod should be situated along the same side of the groove. After the appropriate BioFlex rod is selected, lordosis may be obtained naturally without any rod bending because of the flexible coiled nature of the rod system. Carefully drive the chosen rod using the BioFlex rod holder and then insert the set screw into the screw housing. Tighten until it mechanically stops. After the rod and construct have been properly assembled, a final tightening should be administered until adequate torque is achieved. If rod insertion proves difficult, it can be made more manageable if the rod is soaked in cold water.

◆ Case Illustrations

Case 1

Fig. 43–6 is of a patient with multiple lumbar stenosis and spondylolitic spondylolisthesis of L5–S1. The main pathology is the instability of L5–S1 and L4–L5 and asymptomatic L3–L4 spondylotic stenosis. A total laminectomy of the L4 and L5 was done. Diskectomy and posterior lumbar interbody fusion (PLIF) L4–L5, L5–S1, and BioFlex spring rod pedicle screw insertion at L3–L4–L5–S1. The rationales are as follows: (1) 360 degree fusion of L5–S1 for spondylolitic spondylolisthesis. (2) Enhancement of L4–L5 fusion rate due to compressive force of the BioFlex screw system. (3) Prevention of adjacent motion segment instability: L3–L4 has a more limited motion than its preoperative state due to elasticity of the BioFlex rod system. This may prevent the degeneration of the L3–L4 motion segment. Also, this motion can reduce the L2–L3 hypermotion when using hard fixation at L3–L4 and may reduce the adjacent segment instability. (4) Maintain spinal sagittal balance.

Case 2

Fig. 43–7 is of a patient with an L2 compression fracture. Preoperative and postoperative radiological images show the reduction of kyphosis. The BioFlex rod system adds the elastic power of the posterior ligamentous structures and stabilizes the fractured vertebra, achieving normal alignment of the kyphotic angle.

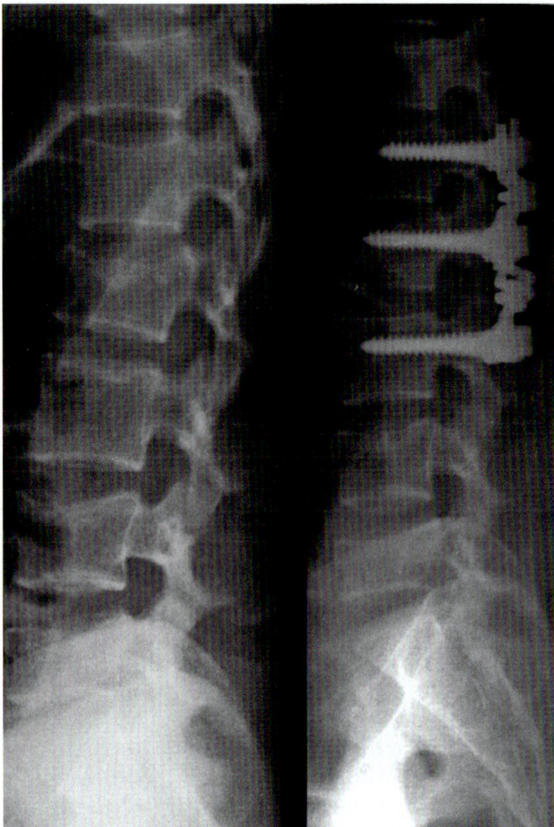

Figure 43–7   Compression fracture of L2 with kyphosis. Preoperative and postoperative x-ray.

◆ Discussion

Between January 2005 and August 2005, 75 patients underwent posterior spinal fusion using the BioFlex system. The average age of the 24 men and 51 women was 53.3 years (range, 18–72 years). Diagnosis included degenerative spondylolisthesis, degenerative stenosis, spondylolitic spondylolisthesis, spondylolitic spondylolisthesis and stenosis of adjacent level, pseudarthrosis, fracture, and adjacent segment stenosis. Thirty-two patients had single-level fixation, 37 patients had two-level fixation, and six patients had multilevel fixation.

The mean follow-up period was 3.5 months: short-term follow-up period. Visual analog scales (0–10) of low back pain and sciatic pain were 7.2 and 7.7 before surgery and 1.5 and 1.7 at the final follow-up, respectively. The BioFlex system as stabilization significantly improved symptoms of low back pain and sciatic pain. There was no instrumentation failure.

The BioFlex rod screw system refers to the semirigid metallic devices across the pedicle screw system. Nitinol flexible rods are applied to the motion segment by pedicle screws. Pretension of the rods during application ensures that the system will share the load and unload the disk at rest. The flexibility of the rods limits the flexibility of the motion segment, both flexion and extension, making this system physiologically sound.

References

1. Deburge A. Modern trends in spinal surgery. J Bone Joint Surg Br 1992;74:6–8

2. Frymoyer JW, Hanley EN, Howe J. A comparison of radiographic findings in fusion and non-fusion patients ten or more years following lumbar disc surgery. Spine 1979;4:435–440

3. Schlegel JD, Smith JA, Schleusener RL. Lumbar motion segment pathology adjacent to thoracolumbar, lumbar and lumbosacral fusion. Spine 1996;21:970–981

4. Lee CK. Accelerated degeneration of the segment adjacent to a lumbar fusion. Spine 1988;13:375–377

5. Ha Y, Kim YS, Yoon DH, Jin DK, Park HW. Graf soft fixation for the treatment of degenerative lumbar disease. J Korean Neurosurg Soc 1998;27:1370–1378

6. Kim YS, Cho YE, Jin BH, Chin DK, Yoon DH. Soft Graf fixation and posterior lumbar interbody fusion in multiple degenerative lumbar diseases. J Korean Neurosurg Soc 1998;27:229–236

7. Kim YS. Dynamic Stabilization in Spine Surgery. The 5th Symposium of Yonsei University Spine Center, Seoul, Sep. 9, 2005

8. Il'in AA, Kollerov MJ, Sergeyv SV, et al. Biologically and mechanically compatible implants from titanium nickelide in the treatment of damaged chest and lumbar parts of the backbone. The Bulletin of Traumatology and Orthopedics (Moscow, Russia) 2002;2:19–26

9. Il'in AA, Kollerov MY, Khachin VI, Gusev DA. Medical Instruments and Implants of Titanium Nickelide. Physical Metallurgy, Technology, and Application.

10. Davydov EA, Il'in AA, Kollerov MY. Methods of Diskectomy with the Conservation of Biomechanics of the Vertebral Mobility Segment. The Third Scientific Practical Conference. Russian Spinal Cord Society, Saratov, Russia, Oct. 7–8, 2004

Section III

**Restoration of Lumbar Motion Segment
D. Facet Replacement**

44

Facet Replacement Technologies

Moe R. Lim, Joon Y. Lee, and Todd James Albert

◆ Anatomy

◆ Facet Replacement as a Stand-Alone Device for Facet-Related Low Back Pain

◆ Facet Replacement as an Adjunct to Total Disk Replacement

◆ Facet Replacement for Posterior Dynamic Reconstruction after Wide Decompression

◆ Facet Replacements Currently in Development

◆ Conclusions

Motion-sparing or nonfusion technologies are becoming a part of the armamentarium of tools in the care of patients with degenerative disorders of the lumbar spine. Anterior nonfusion devices include total disk arthroplasty and nucleus pulposus replacements. Posterior nonfusion devices currently consist of three categories of devices: interspinous process spacers, pedicle screw–based soft stabilization systems, and facet replacements. This chapter focuses on facet replacements.

Devices intended to replace the function of the lumbar zygapophyseal or facet joints are still in the early stages of development. However, with the initial success of anterior total disk replacement devices, there has been much interest in the development of this technology. Potential indications for facet replacements include: (1) as a stand-alone device for treatment of facet-related low back pain (LBP); (2) as an adjunct to total disk replacement; and (3) as a posterior dynamic reconstruction device after wide decompression for lumbar spinal stenosis.

◆ Anatomy

The mobile spinal segment is composed of a three-"joint" complex, the intervertebral disk anteriorly and the paired zygapophyseal or facet joints posteriorly. The facet joints are true synovial joints with hyaline cartilage–bearing surfaces and synovial lining. The lumbar facet joints are oriented in an oblique plane with curved, saucer-shaped surfaces. On an axial view, the facet joints of the lower lumbar spine are medially angulated 30 to 40 degrees. On a sagittal view, the joints are angulated anteriorly 10 to 30 degrees (**Fig. 44–1**).[1–3]

The unique location and orientation of the facet joints contribute to segment stability in resisting rotation, extension, and anterior translation of the cephalad level.[4] Although the disk is the principal stabilizer of the motion segment, the facets are responsible for approximately half of the segmental torsional stability.[5] The two opposing articular surfaces serve a "blocking" function to limit the allowable extent of motion and serve a "guiding" function to control segmental kinematics.[6]

In a standing position, the lumbar facet joints accept ~15% of the compressive force of the body weight while the disk carries the remainder. The facets bear relatively less weight in flexed positions and relatively more weight in extended positions.[7] The relative load-bearing property of the facet joints increases with the progression of spinal segment degeneration.[8]

The facet joint capsule is capable of expressing high levels of inflammatory cytokines and pain-related neuropeptides.[9,10] The pain response is believed to be carried by nociceptive nerve fibers from the medial branch of the dorsal ramus. Each facet joint receives dual innervation from the dorsal rami of the level above the joint and the level of the joint. For example, the L4–L5 facet joint is innerved by the L3 medial branch (which courses over the L4 transverse process and downward to the joint) and the L4 medial branch (which courses between the superior articular process of L5 and the transverse process of L5, and curves upward to reach the L4–L5 joint) (**Fig. 44–2**). The medial branch also innervates the interspinous ligament and the multifidus and interspinal muscles. In contrast, the posterior margin of the intervertebral disk, the posterior longitudinal ligament, and the dura are innervated by the sinu-vertebral nerve off the ventral primary ramus.[11–16]

◆ Facet Replacement as a Stand-Alone Device for Facet-Related Low Back Pain

LBP is a ubiquitous condition with an annual incidence of 5% and a lifetime prevalence of 60 to 90%.[17] Despite the advances of modern medicine, the exact etiology of LBP is still poorly understood. The various anatomical candidates believed to contribute to LBP are the disk, annulus, facet joints, sacroiliac joints, ligaments, and muscles. Traditionally, the intervertebral disk had been considered the primary pathological structure. However, with advances in diagnostic

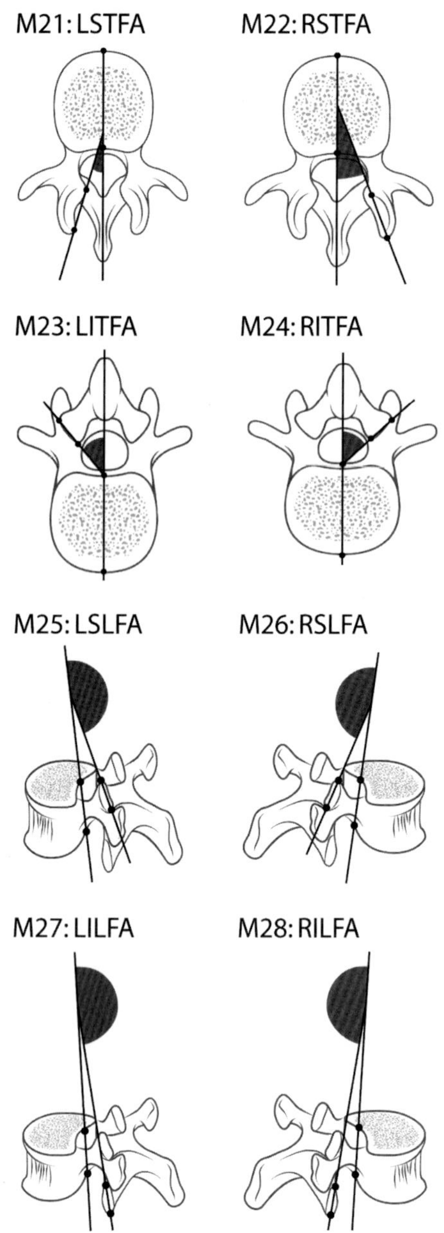

Figure 44–1 The facet joints are oriented obliquely in the sagittal and coronal planes. On an axial view, the facet joints of the lower lumbar spine are medially angulated 30 to 40 degrees. On a sagittal view, the joints are angulated anteriorly 10 to 30 degrees.

injection techniques, the facet joints have received recent attention as a pain generator.

Although few clinicians doubt the potential of the facet joints to cause pain, the relative contribution of facet-related (facetogenic) pain to chronic LBP is debated. Pathological facet joints are believed to contribute to pain in 8 to 70% of patients with chronic LBP.[18–22] This wide range results from the varied methods used to make the diagnosis of facetogenic pain. However, studies using more stringent diagnostic criteria have demonstrated that facet joints are the single or primary pain generator in < 10% of LBP patients.[19,23,24]

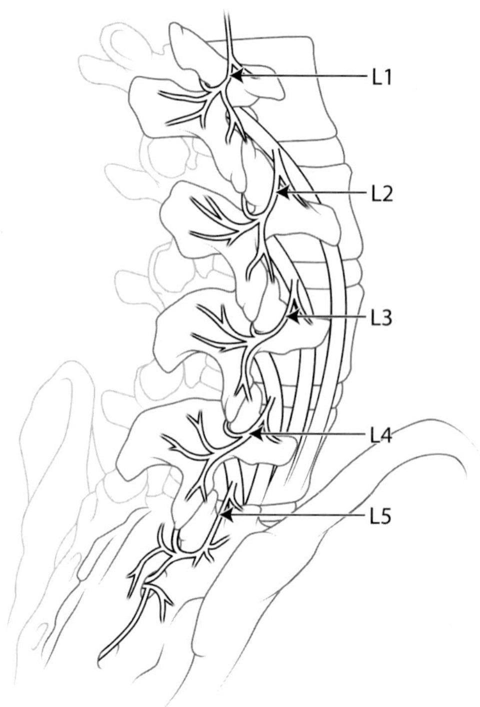

Figure 44–2 The anatomy of lumbar facet innervation. Each facet joint receives dual innervation from the dorsal rami of the level above the joint and the level of the joint. For example, the L4–L5 facet joint is innerved by the L3 medial branch (which courses over the L4 transverse process and downward to the joint) and the L4 medial branch (which courses between the superior articular process of L5 and the transverse process of L5, and curves upward to reach the L4–L5 joint).

A major difficulty in accurately diagnosing facetogenic pain stems from a lack of specific clinical features. Traditionally, facetogenic pain was felt to be elicited by lumbar extension and rotation, maneuvers that stress the facet joints.[23,24] However, studies using diagnostic injections as a gold standard have found that these maneuvers are nonspecific and refute the ability of any history or physical exam findings to identify primary facetogenic LBP.[25–27] Clinical findings are difficult to interpret because the facet joints do not function in isolation but act as part of the three-joint complex. Therefore, any movement that stresses the facet joints likely stresses multiple other structures, such as the disk and ligaments. Because patients with degenerated facet joints usually have degenerated disks as well, pain-eliciting maneuvers are entirely nonspecific.[28,29]

In addition to the nonspecific clinical findings, most studies also fail to find a correlation between any radiographic abnormalities and facetogenic pain. Imaging studies such as plain radiographs, computed tomography (CT), and magnetic resonance imaging (MRI) have very limited value in identifying the anatomical structure(s) responsible for LBP. This is due to the abundance of "abnormal" findings in asymptomatic patients.[30] Most persons over the age of 20 show radiographic evidence of age-related morphological changes of the spine, which are not necessarily pathological or causative of patient symptoms. Of the various modalities, CT is the best imaging test to visualize facet arthrosis.[29] However, CT evidence of facet degeneration is seen in more than half of asymptomatic patients over 40 years old.[31] In addition, there is no correlation between abnormal CT or MRI and relief of LBP by facet injection.[32,33] High-resolution single photon emission computed tomography (SPECT) shows promise in diagnosing facetogenic LBP. Focal facet uptake has been shown to correlate with pain relief from facet joint injections.[34,35]

Currently, the most effective means to identify patients with facetogenic LBP is via diagnostic facet injections. Significant relief of LBP with an intra-articular injection of a local anesthetic should indicate the facet as the source of pain. Most clinicians use fluoroscopic guidance to deliver a small volume (< 2 mL) of anesthetic into the joints after confirmation of the intra-articular location with radiopaque contrast. However, injection protocols vary considerably between published studies. Some authors consider a subjective 50% relief of pain as significant, whereas others use a subjective 80% relief as a cutoff. Protocols with a single anesthetic injection or a double anesthetic injection have also been used.[36,37] In a double injection technique, two separate injections using two different local anesthetics with different durations of effect are used. A positive only occurs when the duration of the patient's pain relief is concordant with the anesthetic used. Single-injection techniques have a false-negative rate of 38% when compared with double-injection techniques.[38] To improve specificity, other authors advocate even more stringent criteria such as: triple injections, identification of a negative control level, provocation of familiar symptoms with facet capsule distention,[39] and concordance of a facet joint injection with a medial ramus block.[40] Due to the lack of a true gold standard to diagnose facetogenic LBP, the sensitivities and specificities of these various diagnostic injection protocols remain unknown.

With such difficulty in diagnosing facetogenic LBP, treatment results are expectedly varied. In two randomized prospective trials, therapeutic intra-articular steroid injections failed to demonstrate any superiority in pain relief when compared with placebo.[36,41] Percutaneous radiofrequency ablation of the nerve supply to the facet joints was shown to be effective in many uncontrolled observational studies.[42–44] However, in a randomized, prospective trial, radiofrequency denervation failed to show any treatment effect when compared with sham therapy.[45] A similar randomized, prospective trial did show a therapeutic effect of radiofrequency ablation, but the patient numbers were small and the effect was modest and short-lasting.[37] Lumbar fusion has also been suggested to treat patients with presumed facetogenic LBP who respond favorably to facet injections.[46] However, a retrospective comparison demonstrated that the results of fusion in such patients were no better than nonoperative treatment.[47]

The ineffectiveness of currently available treatments for facetogenic LBP creates great potential for novel therapeutic approaches and technologies. Unlike the injection and neurotomy treatments, facet replacements can permanently remove the pain-generating articulation and capsule of the facet joints. Unlike fusion, motion and normal kinematics of the joint may be preserved. When used as a stand-alone device to treat facetogenic LBP, the prosthesis does not need to be anchored through the pedicles. Any design that removes the pain-generating portions of the facet joints and allows the remaining bone to anchor the prosthesis for bony ingrowth may be sufficient. Such a surface replacement design spares the pedicles to be used as spinal anchors in case a salvage revision procedure is necessary.

Facet replacement for isolated facetogenic LBP may have a relatively rare indication, however. In a series of 92 patients with chronic LBP who underwent diskograms and diagnostic double facet injections, only 5% of the patients were identified as having isolated facetogenic LBP (negative diskogram with positive facet injection).[19] There is ample clinical and basic science evidence to support the belief that the facet joints can be a source of LBP, either primarily or in conjunction with other anatomical structures. However, currently there is no single clinical feature, radiographic imaging modality, or diagnostic injection test that can discriminate facetogenic LBP over LBP originating from other structures. The biggest challenge to the use of facet replacements as a stand-alone device to treat facetogenic LBP will likely be in making an accurate diagnosis to correctly identify patients who may benefit from this technology.

◆ Facet Replacement as an Adjunct to Total Disk Replacement

The addition of facet replacements to total disk replacements (TDRs) for a 360 degree arthroplasty procedure could improve the outcome and expand the indications for TDRs. The facet joints are the most common source of theoretical contraindications to lumbar disk replacement.[48] Pathological facet joints have the potential to compromise the function of the TDR or lead to a failure to relieve symptoms after TDR. In a recent series of TDR complications, facet arthrosis was felt to contribute to TDR failure in over one third of the patients.[49] Facet replacement may serve as an adjunct to TDR in three clinical situations: (1) concomitant facetogenic and diskogenic LBP, (2) asymptomatic facet degeneration and diskogenic LBP, and (3) iatrogenic facetogenic pain secondary to TDR.

Concomitance of the facets and the disk as pain generators in chronic LBP is a relatively rare situation. In the aforementioned series of 92 chronic LBP patients who underwent diskograms and double facet blocks, only 3% of the patients had both positive diskograms and positive diagnostic facet injections. Patients with concomitant facetogenic and diskogenic pain thus likely represent a rare indication for a 360 degree arthroplasty procedure.

However, facet degeneration frequently accompanies disk degeneration, particularly in older patients with collapsed disks.[29,31,50] The availability of a facet replacement could widely expand the indications for TDR to include such patients with diskogenic LBP accompanied by asymptomatic facet degeneration. Degenerated facet joints are known to limit segmental mobility and have been considered a contraindication to TDR, partly due to the potential to inhibit TDR motion.[50] TDR motion is critical because long-term postoperative clinical outcome and incidence of adjacent level degeneration is likely related to the amount of segmental motion maintained.[51,52] Recently, in a cohort of patients implanted with the Maverick TDR (Medtronic Sofamor Danek, Memphis, TN), severe facet degeneration was shown to decrease TDR range of motion and adversely affect 2-year clinical outcome in a small subgroup of patients.[53] The addition of facet replacement in these patients with facet arthrosis may allow greater motion preservation and improve long-term clinical outcome after TDR.

Asymptomatic facet joints may also become symptomatic as a direct result of TDR implantation. TDR may cause iatrogenic facetogenic pain by two potential mechanisms. First, TDR implantation may cause lordotic disk space distraction with relatively greater anterior facet distraction than posterior distraction. This change in the relative positions of the facet joint surfaces may lead to point loading, and subsequent pain and accelerated degeneration. This altered facet loading may be more prominent if the postoperative position of the TDR is suboptimal. A finite element analysis demonstrated that anteriorly positioned ball and socket TDRs led to facet loads 2.5 times greater than normal.[54] Second, in patients with more severe facet arthrosis, the disk space is usually collapsed. The degenerated facets may have remained asymptomatic due to a lack of segmental motion. As a consequence of TDR implantation and the reintroduction of motion to that segment, the facet joints may experience motion and become a source of pain. Facet replacement technology has the potential to address these problems and provides a nonfusion salvage option for facet-related TDR failure.

The facet replacement designs intended to be used in conjunction with total disk replacements must incorporate design features to ensure biomechanical compatibility with the TDR. The two major TDR designs are the semiconstrained ball and socket of the ProDisc (Synthes, Inc.,West Chester, PA) and the nonconstrained sliding core of the Charité Artificial Disc (DePuy Spine, Raynham, MA). In the ball and socket design, flexion-extension of the TDR is obligatorily coupled to anteroposterior (AP) translation. As the TDR flexes, the cephalad end plate translates anteriorly on the caudal end plate. The amount of anterior translation relative to the degrees of flexion depends on the radius of curvature of the ball and socket.[55] The Maverick TDR has a smaller radius of curvature than the ProDisc and has less AP translation with flexion-extension. A facet replacement intended to be used in conjunction with a ball and socket TDR must also allow for AP translation with flexion-extension. In the absence of such a mechanism, the segmental range of motion will be severely limited, and attempted motion will lead to excessive stresses at the prosthesis–bone interface. In contrast, the sliding-core design of the Charité allows TDR flexion-extension to be independent of AP translation. As the TDR flexes, the sliding core translates posteriorly and the end plates remain stationary in the AP direction. A facet replacement intended to be used with a sliding core TDR needs only to allow cephalocaudal facet motion with TDR flexion-extension. Regardless of TDR designs, axial rotation in a 360 degree arthroplasty will be controlled exclusively by facet replacement because all current TDR designs allow unlimited axial rotation.

Although the idea of a 360 degree arthroplasty procedure is appealing, clinical application should be approached cautiously. Failure of implants or failure of the bone–implant interface in a 360 degree arthroplasty procedure has the potential to destabilize the entire segment with the possibility of disastrous neurological injury. The salvage options in the setting of implant failure or infection are also limited. Multilevel fusions with extension into the pelvis may be required to restore spinal stability.

◆ Facet Replacement for Posterior Dynamic Reconstruction after Wide Decompression

Facet replacement has the potential for its widest clinical application when used for dynamic posterior reconstruction in lumbar spinal stenosis. Hypertrophy of the degenerated facet joints plays a major role in the narrowing of the spinal canal and the subsequent symptoms of neural compression.[56] To achieve adequate decompression, partial or subtotal facet resection is necessary. Unfortunately, aggressive facet resection can induce segmental instability.[57] Thus surgical treatment of lumbar spinal stenosis requires balancing the opposing goals of achieving adequate decompression while preserving enough of the facets to maintain segmental stability. Patients who undergo an aggressive decompression or patients with degenerative spondylolisthesis[58] generally require a stabilization procedure in the form of instrumented fusion. Fusion, however, transfers stress to the adjacent segments and is associated with adjacent level degeneration.[59]

To avoid adjacent level degeneration and other morbidities related to fusion, the concept of pedicle screw–based dynamic soft stabilization was developed.[60] These soft stabilization systems use pedicle screws as spinal anchors that are attached to each other with elastic cords. The elastic cords are intended to re-create the posterior ligamentous tension band to eliminate pathological motion while preserving some physiological motion.

Facet replacements intended to be used for dynamic reconstruction in lumbar spinal stenosis would also need to be anchored in the pedicles because the facets will be resected. However, facet replacements may have several advantages. First, the complete removal of the facet joints provides a thorough decompression and eliminates a potential source of back pain. Second, facet replacements may better restore the normal kinematics of the spine. The elastic bands of the soft stabilization systems serve a "blocking" function to control the limits of motion, based on when the threshold tension on the elastic band is reached. However, the kinematics of the spinal segment within the allowed range of motion cannot be "guided" by the elastic bands. In contrast, the facet replacement can be designed with conforming articular surfaces to replicate the complex kinematics of the spinal motion segment throughout the entire range of allowed motion. This would replicate both the "blocking" and the "guiding" functions of the native facet joints.[6] Third, the elastic bands in soft stabilization cannot resist the anterior shear forces seen in degenerative spondylolisthesis. The facet replacement articular surfaces can be constructed to resist anterior shear forces. In the setting of degenerative spondylolisthesis, reduction of the slip can theoretically be achieved and maintained with a facet replacement.

These theoretical advantages of facet replacement over soft stabilization, however, require the addition of more intrinsic constraint to the prosthesis. Our experience with peripheral joint arthroplasty has taught us that greater inherent prosthesis constraint leads to increased stress at the prosthesis articulation and at the prosthesis–bone interface. Implant loosening has been the major clinical problem encountered with the use of the pedicle screw–based soft stabilization systems.[61] Facet replacement designs with greater inherent constraint may encounter even higher rates of implant failure or loosening at the prosthesis–bone interface.

◆ Facet Replacements Currently in Development

Four companies are currently known to be actively developing facet replacement devices: Facet Solutions (Logan, UT); Impliant (Netanya, Israel); Quantum Orthopedics (Carlsbad, CA); and Archus Orthopedics (Redmond, WA). The specifics of the Facet Solutions device are unknown. The Impliant device is composed of polyurethane bonded to two metal end plates anchored to the spine via four pedicle screws. The Zyre device from Quantum Orthopedics consists of a malleable spacer placed between the facet joints. The Zyre is a surface replacement intended to treat facetogenic LBP via a minimally invasive surgical approach.

The Total Facet Arthroplasty System (TFAS) of Archus Orthopedics represents the forefront in the field of facet replacement technology. The TFAS is intended to be used for posterior dynamic reconstruction after decompression for lumbar spinal stenosis, including grade I degenerative spondylolisthesis. This device is designed to serve as an alternative to instrumented fusion: to stabilize, to preserve motion, and to bear load. The system relies on a ball in trough, metal-on-metal articulation. Initial and long-term prosthesis–bone interface stability is achieved via polymethyl methacrylate cement fixation into the pedicles (**Fig. 44–3**).

The TFAS has undergone extensive development and pre-clinical testing. The fixation strength, biocompatibility, bearing surface durability, and kinematics of the TFAS have been tested successfully.[62] When compared with pedicle screw instrumentation, the TFAS experienced lower implant stresses and withstood greater ultimate fixation strength to bone. The interface strength between bone cement and TFAS was shown to withstand more than 2.5 times the projected maximum static in vivo loads. The TFAS construct and interconnection mechanisms withstood more than three times the projected maximum fatigue duty cycle loads for 10 million cycles in torsion, bending, and axial loading. The durability of the articulation and generated wear particle size/distribution were found to be comparable to those of metal-on-metal total hip arthroplasty. In a rabbit model, similar doses of wear particles did not cause neurotoxic effects and did not elicit a local or systemic histological response. In a cadaver injury model, the TFAS was shown to effectively restore the range and pattern of segmental motion in flexion, extension, axial rotation, and lateral bending.[6]

In March 2005, the TFAS received the CE marking to begin marketing in the European Union and received conditional Investigational Device Exemption approval by the U.S. Food and Drug Administration to initiate clinical trials. Archus Orthopedics plans to conduct a prospective, randomized trial comparing TFAS to instrumented fusion. In May 2005, the first TFAS was successfully implanted in Europe.

◆ Conclusions

Facet replacement technology represents an exciting new frontier in the treatment of the degenerated lumbar spine. For its use as a stand-alone device, it will be crucial to make an accurate diagnosis of primary facetogenic LBP. When used in conjunction with total disk replacement, facet replacements may eliminate facet pathology as a contraindication to disk replacement. Design feature modifications may be necessary to ensure biomechanical compatibility between the disk and facet replacements. When used as dynamic stabilization in lumbar spinal stenosis, the biggest clinical challenge of facet replacements will likely be related to implant loosening under repetitive loading conditions.

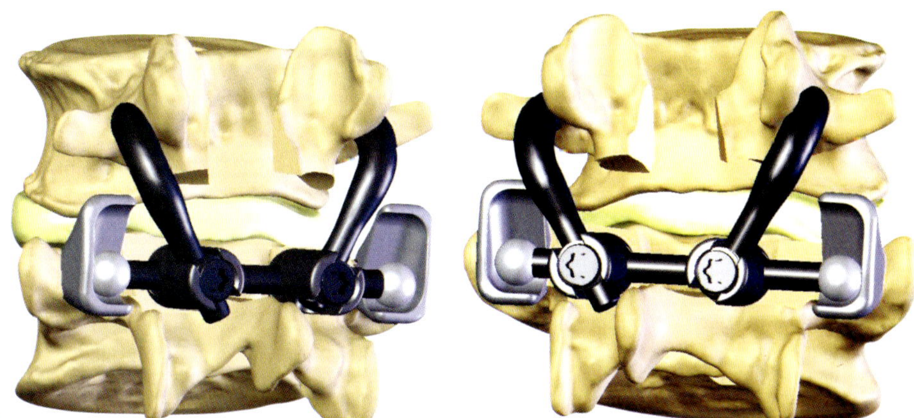

A   **B**

Figure 44–3 (A,B)   Two Perspectives of the Total Facet Arthroplasty System (TFAS) of Archus Orthopedics. The device has a ball in trough, metal-on-metal articulation. Initial and long-term prosthesis–bone interface stability is achieved via polymethyl methacrylate cement fixation into the pedicles.

References

1. Panjabi MM, Oxland T, Takata K, Goel V, Duranceau J, Krag M. Articular facets of the human spine: quantitative three-dimensional anatomy. Spine 1993;18:1298–1310

2. Masharawi Y, Rothschild B, Dar G, et al. Facet orientation in the thoracolumbar spine: three-dimensional anatomic and biomechanical analysis. Spine 2004;29:1755–1763

3. Tulsi RS, Hermanis GM. A study of the angle of inclination and facet curvature of superior lumbar zygapophyseal facets. Spine 1993;18:1311–1317

4. Twomey LT, Taylor JR. Sagittal movements of the human lumbar vertebral column: a quantitative study of the role of the posterior vertebral elements. Arch Phys Med Rehabil 1983;64:322–325

5. Farfan HF, Cossette JW, Robertson GH, Wells RV, Kraus H. The effects of torsion on the lumbar intervertebral joints: the role of torsion in the production of disc degeneration. J Bone Joint Surg Am 1970;52:468–497

6. Zhu QA, Larson CR, Sjovold SG, et al. Biomechanical Evaluation of the Total Facet Arthroplasty System (TFAS): An In Vitro Human Cadaveric Model. Presented at the Meeting of the Orthopaedic Research Society, Washington, DC, 2005

7. Adams MA, Hutton WC. The effect of posture on the role of the apophysial joints in resisting intervertebral compressive forces. J Bone Joint Surg Br 1980;62:358–362

8. Yang KH, King AI. Mechanism of facet load transmission as a hypothesis for low-back pain. Spine 1984;9:557–565

9. Kallakuri S, Singh A, Chen C, Cavanaugh JM. Demonstration of substance P, calcitonin gene-related peptide, and protein gene product 9.5 containing nerve fibers in human cervical facet joint capsules. Spine 2004;29:1182–1186

10. Igarashi A, Kikuchi S, Konno S, Olmarker K. Inflammatory cytokines released from the facet joint tissue in degenerative lumbar spinal disorders. Spine 2004;29:2091–2095

11. Sowa G. Facet-mediated pain. Dis Mon 2005;51:18–33

12. Kornick C, Kramarich SS, Lamer TJ, Todd Sitzman B. Complications of lumbar facet radiofrequency denervation. Spine 2004;29:1352–1354

13. Berven S, Tay BB, Colman W, Hu SS. The lumbar zygapophyseal (facet) joints: a role in the pathogenesis of spinal pain syndromes and degenerative spondylolisthesis. Semin Neurol 2002;22:187–196

14. Yamashita T, Cavanaugh JM, el-Bohy AA, Getchell TV, King AI. Mechanosensitive afferent units in the lumbar facet joint. J Bone Joint Surg Am 1990;72:865–870

15. Pickar JG, McLain RF. Responses of mechanosensitive afferents to manipulation of the lumbar facet in the cat. Spine 1995;20:2379–2385

16. Ashton IK, Ashton BA, Gibson SJ, Polak JM, Jaffray DC, Eisenstein SM. Morphological basis for back pain: the demonstration of nerve fibers and neuropeptides in the lumbar facet joint capsule but not in ligamentum flavum. J Orthop Res 1992;10:72–78

17. Frymoyer JW, Pope MH, Clements JH, Wilder DG, MacPherson B, Ashikaga T. Risk factors in low-back pain: an epidemiological survey. J Bone Joint Surg Am 1983;65:213–218

18. Moran R, O'Connell D, Walsh MG. The diagnostic value of facet joint injections. Spine 1988;13:1407–1410

19. Schwarzer AC, Aprill CN, Derby R, Fortin J, Kine G, Bogduk N. The relative contributions of the disc and zygapophyseal joint in chronic low back pain. Spine 1994;19:801–806

20. Schwarzer AC, Wang SC, Bogduk N, McNaught PJ, Laurent R. Prevalence and clinical features of lumbar zygapophysial joint pain: a study in an Australian population with chronic low back pain. Ann Rheum Dis 1995;54:100–106

21. Dreyer SJ, Dreyfuss PH. Low back pain and the zygapophysial (facet) joints. Arch Phys Med Rehabil 1996;77:290–300

22. Shih C, Lin GY, Yueh KC, Lin JJ. Lumbar zygapophyseal joint injections in patients with chronic lower back pain. J Chin Med Assoc 2005;68:59–64

23. Jackson RP, Jacobs RR, Montesano PX. 1988 Volvo award in clinical sciences. Facet joint injection in low-back pain: a prospective statistical study. Spine 1988;13:966–971

24. Helbig T, Lee CK. The lumbar facet syndrome. Spine 1988;13:61–64

25. Schwarzer AC, Aprill CN, Derby R, Fortin J, Kine G, Bogduk N. Clinical features of patients with pain stemming from the lumbar zygapophysial joints: is the lumbar facet syndrome a clinical entity? Spine 1994;19:1132–1137

26. Schwarzer AC, Derby R, Aprill CN, Fortin J, Kine G, Bogduk N. Pain from the lumbar zygapophysial joints: a test of two models. J Spinal Disord 1994;7:331–336

27. Jackson RP. The facet syndrome: myth or reality? Clin Orthop Relat Res 1992; 279:110–121

28. Butler D, Trafimow JH, Andersson GB, McNeill TW, Huckman MS. Discs degenerate before facets. Spine 1990;15:111–113

29. Fujiwara A, Tamai K, Yamato M, et al. The relationship between facet joint osteoarthritis and disc degeneration of the lumbar spine: an MRI study. Eur Spine J 1999;8:396–401

30. Boden SD, Davis DO, Dina TS, Patronas NJ, Wiesel SW. Abnormal magnetic-resonance scans of the lumbar spine in asymptomatic subjects: a prospective investigation. J Bone Joint Surg Am 1990;72:403–408

31. Wiesel SW, Tsourmas N, Feffer HL, Citrin CM, Patronas N. A study of computer-assisted tomography, I: The incidence of positive CAT scans in an asymptomatic group of patients. Spine 1984;9:549–551

32. Revel ME, Listrat VM, Chevalier XJ, et al. Facet joint block for low back pain: identifying predictors of a good response. Arch Phys Med Rehabil 1992;73:824–828

33. Schwarzer AC, Wang SC, O'Driscoll D, Harrington T, Bogduk N, Laurent R. The ability of computed tomography to identify a painful zygapophyseal joint in patients with chronic low back pain. Spine 1995;20:907–912

34. Dolan AL, Ryan PJ, Arden NK, et al. The value of SPECT scans in identifying back pain likely to benefit from facet joint injection. Br J Rheumatol 1996;35:1269–1273

35. Holder LE, Machin JL, Asdourian PL, Links JM, Sexton CC. Planar and high-resolution SPECT bone imaging in the diagnosis of facet syndrome. J Nucl Med 1995;36:37–44

36. Carette S, Marcoux S, Truchon R, et al. A controlled trial of corticosteroid injections into facet joints for chronic low back pain. N Engl J Med 1991;325:1002–1007

37. van Kleef M, Barendse GA, Kessels A, Voets HM, Weber WE, de Lange S. Randomized trial of radiofrequency lumbar facet denervation for chronic low back pain. Spine 1999;24:1937–1942

38. Schwarzer AC, Aprill CN, Derby R, Fortin J, Kine G, Bogduk N. The false-positive rate of uncontrolled diagnostic blocks of the lumbar zygapophysial joints. Pain 1994;58:195–200

39. Schwarzer AC, Derby R, Aprill CN, Fortin J, Kine G, Bogduk N. The value of the provocation response in lumbar zygapophyseal joint injections. Clin J Pain 1994;10:309–313

40. Manchikanti L, Pampati V, Fellows B, Bakhit CE. The diagnostic validity and therapeutic value of lumbar facet joint nerve blocks with or without adjuvant agents. Curr Rev Pain 2000;4:337–344

41. Lilius G, Laasonen EM, Myllynen P, Harilainen A, Gronlund G. Lumbar facet joint syndrome: a randomised clinical trial. J Bone Joint Surg Br 1989;71:681–684

42. Silvers HR. Lumbar percutaneous facet rhizotomy. Spine 1990;15:36–40

43. North RB, Han M, Zahurak M, Kidd DH. Radiofrequency lumbar facet denervation: analysis of prognostic factors. Pain 1994;57:77–83

44. Dreyfuss P, Halbrook B, Pauza K, Joshi A, McLarty J, Bogduk N. Efficacy and validity of radiofrequency neurotomy for chronic lumbar zygapophyseal joint pain. Spine 2000;25:1270–1277

45. Leclaire R, Fortin L, Lambert R, Bergeron YM, Rossignol M. Radiofrequency facet joint denervation in the treatment of low back pain: a placebo-controlled clinical trial to assess efficacy. Spine 2001;26:1411–1416 discussion 1417

46. Lovely TJ, Rastogi P. The value of provocative facet blocking as a predictor of success in lumbar spine fusion. J Spinal Disord 1997;10:512–517

47. Esses SI, Moro JK. The value of facet joint blocks in patient selection for lumbar fusion. Spine 1993;18:185–190

48. Huang RC, Lim MR, Girardi FP, Cammisa FP Jr. The prevalence of contraindications to total disc replacement in a cohort of lumbar surgical patients. Spine 2004;29:2538–2541

49. van Ooij A, Oner FC, Verbout AJ. Complications of artificial disc replacement: a report of 27 patients with the SB Charité disc. J Spinal Disord Tech 2003;16:369–383

50. Fujiwara A, Lim TH, An HS, et al. The effect of disc degeneration and facet joint osteoarthritis on the segmental flexibility of the lumbar spine. Spine 2000;25:3036–3044

51. Huang RC, Girardi FP, Cammisa FP Jr, Lim MR, Tropiano P, Marnay T. Correlation between range of motion and outcome after lumbar total disc replacement: 8.6-year follow-up. Spine 2005;30:1407–1411

52. Huang RC, Tropiano P, Marnay T, Girardi FP, Lim MR, Cammisa FP Jr. Range of motion and adjacent level degeneration after lumbar total disc replacement. Abstract from the SRS 2004 Annual Meeting, Sept. 6–9, 2004. Spine Journal 2005

53. Le Huec JC, Basso Y, Aunoble S, Friesem T, Bruno MB. Influence of facet and posterior muscle degeneration on clinical results of lumbar total disc replacement: two-year follow-up. J Spinal Disord Tech 2005;18:219–223

54. Dooris AP, Goel VK, Grosland NM, Gilbertson LG, Wilder DG. Load-sharing between anterior and posterior elements in a lumbar motion segment implanted with an artificial disc. Spine 2001;26:E122–E129

55. Huang RC, Girardi FP, Cammisa FP Jr, Wright TM. The implications of constraint in lumbar total disc replacement. J Spinal Disord Tech 2003;16:412–417

56. Hilibrand AS, Rand N. Degenerative lumbar stenosis: diagnosis and management. J Am Acad Orthop Surg 1999;7:239–249

57. Zander T, Rohlmann A, Klockner C, Bergmann G. Influence of graded facetectomy and laminectomy on spinal biomechanics. Eur Spine J 2003;12:427–434

58. Fischgrund JS. The argument for instrumented decompressive posterolateral fusion for patients with degenerative spondylolisthesis and spinal stenosis. Spine 2004;29:173–174

59. Kanayama M, Hashimoto T, Shigenobu K, et al. Adjacent-segment morbidity after Graf ligamentoplasty compared with posterolateral lumbar fusion. J Neurosurg 2001;95(1 Suppl):5–10

60. Hashimoto T, Oha F, Shigenobu K, et al. Mid-term clinical results of Graf stabilization for lumbar degenerative pathologies: a minimum 2-year follow-up. Spine J 2001;1:283–289

61. Stoll TM, Dubois G, Schwarzenbach O. The dynamic neutralization system for the spine: a multi-center study of a novel non-fusion system. Eur Spine J 2002;11(Suppl 2):S170–S178

45

TOPS—Total Posterior Facet Replacement and Dynamic Motion Segment Stabilization System

Larry T. Khoo, Luiz Pimenta, and Roberto C. Díaz

◆ **Rationale for Posterior Facet Replacement and Arthroplasty**

◆ **TOPS Implant Characteristics**
Design Parameters
Finite Element Analysis
Biomechanical In Vitro Motion Segment Analysis
Load on the Pedicle Screws

◆ **Surgical Technique for TOPS Posterior Facet Replacement System Implantation**

◆ **Clinical Data and Outcomes of TOPS Facet Replacement**

◆ **Conclusion**

The pathophysiological mechanisms of low back pain continue to be poorly elucidated and difficult to study effectively. Whereas pain resulting from neurological compression has been traditionally treated with great success via decompressive procedures, treatment of mechanical or diskogenic-type lumbar pain has proven far more problematic. For many patients who remain refractory to conservative or less aggressive modalities, spinal fusion continues to be the mainstay of surgical treatment for the relief of axial back pain.[1–7] Unfortunately, clinical outcomes have been variable and inconsistent with regard to the efficacy of spinal fusion in relieving lumbago as measured by standardized measures such as the Oswestry Disability Index, visual analog pain scale, and short form SF-36 Health Survey.[1] To compound the problem, accelerated degeneration of the adjacent segment has also been observed in biomechanical laboratory investigations, on long-term radiological studies, and in numerous retrospective clinical surgical series.[8–15] Although the exact incidence of this "adjacent segment disease" (ASD) remains poorly defined, it is clear that ASD is one of the most dreaded long-term clinical sequelae after successful fusion. From biomechanical investigations and clinical radiographic studies, it appears that there is an alteration of load sharing with an increase in mobility, shear, strain, and pressure at the intervertebral disk, uncovertebral joints, and facet joints of the adjacent segment(s) after rigid spinal fusion.[13,15] With this in mind, many postulate that preservation of either or both motion and load sharing at the index pathological level would help to mitigate or reduce the overall incidence of ASD.

◆ Rationale for Posterior Facet Replacement and Arthroplasty

In the hope of decreasing adjacent segment forces, total anterior disk replacement (TDR) devices such as the SB Charité III (DePuy Spine, Raynham, MA) and the ProDisc II (Synthes, West Chester) were developed in an attempt to preserve motion at the etiologic intervertebral disk. From the clinical Federal Food and Drug Administration (FDA) Investigational Device Exemption (IDE) study, the SB Charité III was able to provide equivalent relief of low back pain as compared with the randomized control arm of anterior fusion.[2,16] However, numerous authors have cited that severe facet arthropathy, spinal stenosis, neurogenic claudication, significant canal disease, spondylolisthesis, or translational instability are all relative or absolute contraindications to placement of an anterior TDR.[11,17] In a study by Huang examining the typical makeup of patients seen in a tertiary spinal clinic, there was a preponderance of such patients with dorsal disease, spinal stenosis, spondylolisthesis, and/or spinal instability. These patients were ideally suited for classical spinal decompression and, in many cases, posterior spinal fusion and were not candidates for TDR.[11] As such, it is clear that motion-preserving devices that can be used for patients requiring dorsal surgical treatment are needed.

When we examine the issue of posterior spinal disease and spinal stenosis, it is clear that we face not only the natural history of the disease process but also the iatrogenic instability that results from surgical decompression of these patients. Because a large majority of these patients are symptomatic from

"

radicular or central canal compression, they require decompression of the paramedian lamilna and at least the medial third or medial half of the facet complex. As a result, progressive resection for neural decompression can lead to progressive spinal instability in cases where the facet orientation is more sagittal than coronal.[1] In many patients with spinal stenosis who require aggressive decompression for extensive neural foraminal narrowing, spinal fusion is often necessitated after facet resection.[5,18] In Resnick et al. Fischgrund et al's analysis, patients with spondylolisthesis and stenosis overall did better with regard to their low back pain scores when they had a primary fusion in addition to decompression as opposed to those who had decompression alone.[6,7] However, it is also clear that many patients with either or both stenosis and stenosis with spondylolisthesis do well without fusion and do not go on to have gross or glacial spinal instability after decompressive surgery. As such, a motion-preserving technology that can be placed via a standard posterior approach can help to avoid fusion in the many stenotic patients who are either preoperatively only mildly unstable or made unstable after surgical decompressive destabilization of the facet complex.

With this in mind, the question remains as to the ideal nature of such a posterior motion-preserving stabilizer of the spine. Whereas numerous theories regarding the etiology of low back pain exist, perhaps the most developed of these is the concept of the biomechanical neutral zone as postulated by Panjabi.[19,20] In this useful heuristic system, a motion segment functions to share load and to move and impinge within a given set of mechanical parameters. During biomechanical testing, any given spinal motion segment will thus move a given amount per quantum of applied load as determined by the viscoelastic properties of the surrounding structures that bind the two vertebrae such as the intervertebral nucleus and annulus, facet joint and capsule, interspinous ligaments, spinal longitudinal ligaments, attached paraspinal muscles, and truncal musculature. Plotted in any of three dimensions, this leads to a classic load-displacement plot of the "neutral zone" (**Fig. 45–1**). Degeneration, acute injury, or other pathology thereby alters the biomechanical limiters of the system thereby leading to laxity, altered load sharing, and a widening of the load-displacement curves and altering of the neutral zone itself. As movement of the spinal segment begins to exceed its initial "setpoints," joint, nociceptive, and stretch receptors begin to activate and signal pain and injury in the area, which may lead to progressive pain and inflammation in that area. As such, induced injury of the ligaments or facets or disk complex will lead to a widened neutral zone as seen on load-displacement curves during biomechanical cadaveric testing (**Fig. 45–1B**). This model thus provides a useful point of reference as to the cause of mechanical back pain in patients.

Whereas decompression will help to relieve radicular pain, surgical restoration of proper load sharing and normalization of the neutral zone may help to decrease pain and inflammatory stimuli in the treated spinal segment(s). As such, the efficacy of rigid spinal fusion may ultimately result from its ability to radically correct the load-displacement characteristics of the motion segment to near-zero movement for any applied load after rigid fusion and instrumentation. With this in mind, a proper motion-preserving stabilizer device must also be able to correct the load-displacement curves back to an anatomically natural neutral zone while still preserving some degree of native spinal mobility above that of rigid fusion. Additionally, by preserving load sharing of the treated segment, it must also decrease the "stress-riser" effect on adjacent untreated levels to potentially minimize the incidence of ASD. Finally, the motion-preserving dorsal device must also be secured to the spine in such a way that the device–bone interface remains stable over several million cycles. For example, devices that are to be implanted through the vertebral pedicles must thereby minimize the stress at the screw–bone to prevent screw pullout. As such, the motion-preserving device must not only be able to provide motion but must also do so in a way that does not load the screws in any significant way.

◆ Total Posterior Facet Replacement System (TOPS) Implant Characteristics

Design Parameters

TOPS is a unitary device (**Fig. 45–2**) composed of a titanium "sandwich" with an interlocking polycarbonate urethane

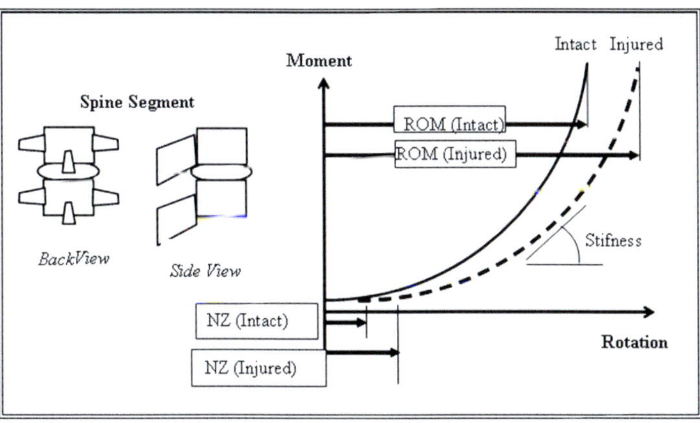

Figure 45–1   Mechanical properties of the intact and injured spine. ROM, range of motion.

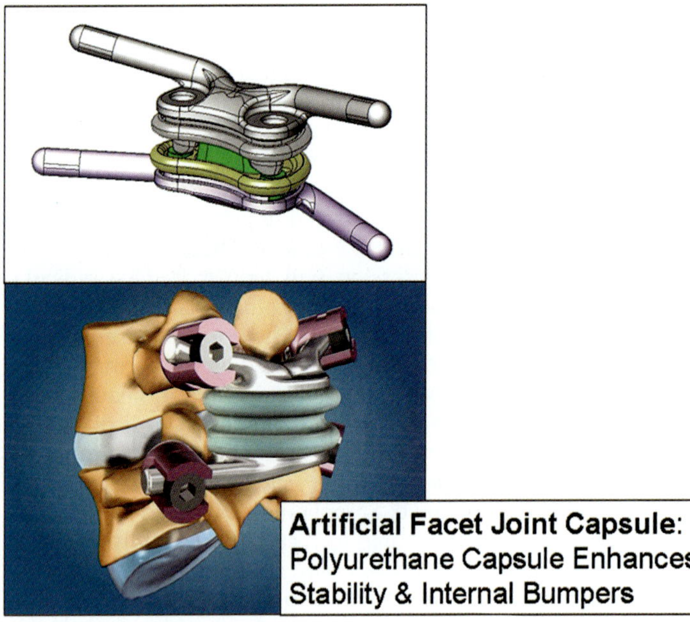

Figure 45–2   TOPS is a unitary device composed of a titanium "sandwich" with an interlocking polycarbonate urethane articulating construct.

(PcU) articulating construct. The flexible PcU elements within the construct allow relative movement between the titanium plates so as to create axial rotation, lateral bending, extension, and flexion. The internal construct mechanically restricts motion to ±1.5 degrees of axial rotation, ±5 degrees of lateral bending, 2 degrees of extension, and 8 degrees of flexion. The implant also blocks excessive posterior and anterior sagittal translation. The TOPS system uses four standard hydroxyapatite (HA)-coated polyaxial pedicle screws for fixation to the vertebrae (**Fig. 45–3**). Because the internal configuration of the PcU bumpers ultimately acts as the limiter of motion, the TOPS device has an inherent dampening property, which serves to dissipate energy that is passed through it during standard load sharing of the moving spinal motion segment. Furthermore, because the PcU elements also have some "shock-absorption" properties in the vertical axis, vertical load transmitted through the cross-bars through the centroid of the device is also somewhat dampened as well. These features not only serve to allow for near full spinal motion but also to decrease stresses at the adjacent levels and also at the screw–bone interface.

TOPS provides patients suffering from degeneration/hypertrophy of the facet joint, grade I degenerative spondylolisthesis, and spinal stenosis with three major advantages. The surgeon can perform a wide decompression to eliminate the pain generators. The procedure stabilizes the posterior spine. The procedure allows a controlled range of motion. The implanted device, made of flexible materials and titanium, allows for constrained bending, straightening, and twisting movements in the affected segment postsurgery. As such, the TOPS device serves to achieve the goals already detailed for restoring the physiological neutral zone, maintaining a degree of spinal motion over rigid fusion, decreasing abnormal load sharing at the adjacent levels, and minimizing screw–bone interface stresses through the dampeners of the PcU elements contained therein.

Finite Element Analysis

As part of the overall development program on early designs of the TOPS device, a finite element analysis (FEA) was performed on the implant using ANSYS computational software (Ansys, Inc., Canonsburg, PA). The original model developed

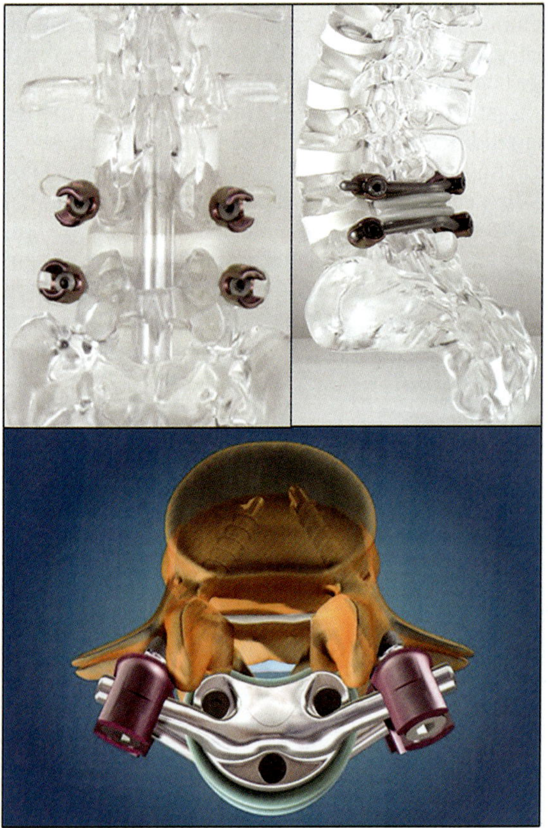

Figure 45–3   The TOPS system uses four standard hydroxyapatite-coated polyaxial pedicle screws for fixation to the vertebrae.

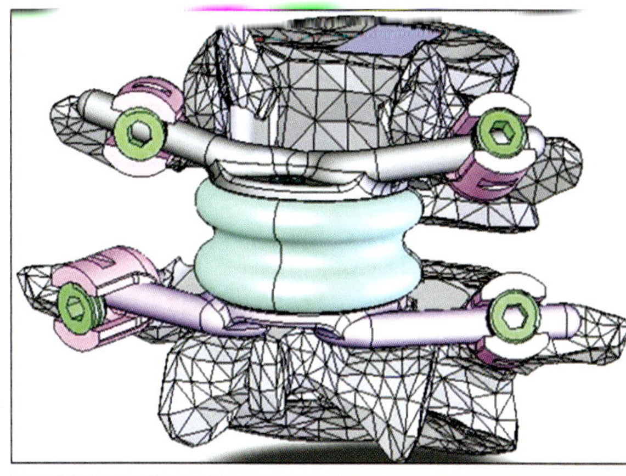

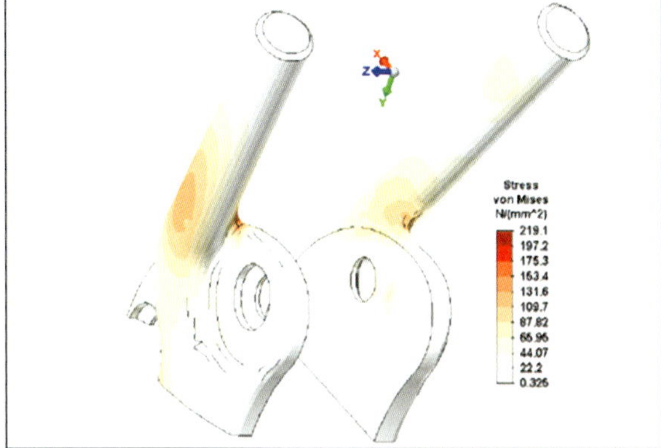

Figure 45–4 The principal stress generated in the device during maximum anticipated loading is well below the yield stress for the titanium alloy from which it is fabricated.

Dynesys Dynamic Stabilization System (Zimmer Spine, Inc., Warsaw, IN).[21] There was no effect shown on the adjacent segment. This, however, has to be interpreted carefully because this might be due to the loading condition with pure moments.

The intradiskal pressure data showed that the implant allows the disk to take part of the load, which is consistent with the natural biomechanics of the disk. However, the absolute values cannot be directly compared with the in vivo conditions because no preload could be simulated. Additionally, the hydrostatic pressure can only be determined accurately in a nondegenerated disk.

Load on the Pedicle Screws

To evaluate the efficacy of the polyaxial pedicle screws and the ability to fixate the TOPS device to the lumbar spinal vertebrae, a comparative test was performed. The examination was performed on cadaveric spine with the same polyaxial screws. Strain gauges were applied to the same four[4] screws so that the mechanical stress and resulting strains transferred to them from the leading competitor (Dynesys, Zimmer Spine, Warsaw, IN) and TOPS devices could be monitored while the spine simulator manipulated the spine segments (**Fig. 45–6**). Results of this study indicate that the load transmission to the pedicle screws is significantly less with the TOPS system than with the leading competitor.[21] As clinical results of the Dynesys have indicated a 6 to 8% screw loosening rate at 2- to 3-year clinical follow-up, it would be expected that the TOPS device will fare as well if not better after long-term clinical implantation.[8,22]

for this theoretical stress analysis was a half-section representation of the device. The model was chosen because the device itself and the loading conditions on it were found to be symmetric about the central plane. This hemimodel analysis allowed for faster computation without loss of precision. The results of this assessment show the principal stresses acting on the model as a result of the applied loading. The principal stress generated in the device during maximum anticipated loading is well below the yield stress for the titanium alloy from which it is fabricated[21] (**Fig. 45–4**).

Biomechanical In Vitro Motion Segment Analysis

The TOPS device was tested on six[6] frozen cadaver specimens to:

◆ Evaluate the capability of restoring motion to the intact spinal segment

◆ Evaluate the effects on motion to the adjacent spinal segment after stabilization

The test showed that the TOPS system almost ideally restores the motion behavior of a segment in left and right lateral bending (**Fig. 45–5A**) and left and right axial rotation (**Fig. 45–5B**) after facet removal compared with the intact segment. In flexion and extension (**Fig. 45–5C**), the range of motion was 55% of that of an intact segment. By way of comparison, these results are significantly better than the

◆ Surgical Technique for Total Posterior Facet Replacement System Implantation

The patient is positioned prone on the operative frame with either a four-poster or a double-roll configuration to simultaneously re-create the lumbar lordosis as well as to ensure that the abdomen is free and uncompressed. Preoperative biplanar fluoroscopic confirmation of the spinal alignment and the target level incision is obtained. Preinjection of the skin, fascia, and musculature with 0.25% lidocaine with 1:200,000 epinephrine is useful to decrease postoperative pain as well as to decrease intraoperative bleeding. The surgical field is then prepped and draped in the usual sterile fashion.

Using a no. 10 scalpel blade, a vertical incision is made down to the level of the lumbodorsal fascia. Subperiosteal dissection is then continued with the use of a Bovie cautery in combination with periosteal elevators to gradually tension and elevate the dorsal musculoligamentous complex off the spinous processes, lamina, and facets of the vertebrae above and below the target motion segment. As compared with classic spinal arthrodesis where exposure of the transverse processes is needed for future bone graft placement, exposure and retraction of the musculature for TOPS placement need to be carried only to the lateral aspect of the facet complex. Additionally, particular care should be paid to preserving the capsule and muscular attachments surrounding the superior facet complex above the target level.

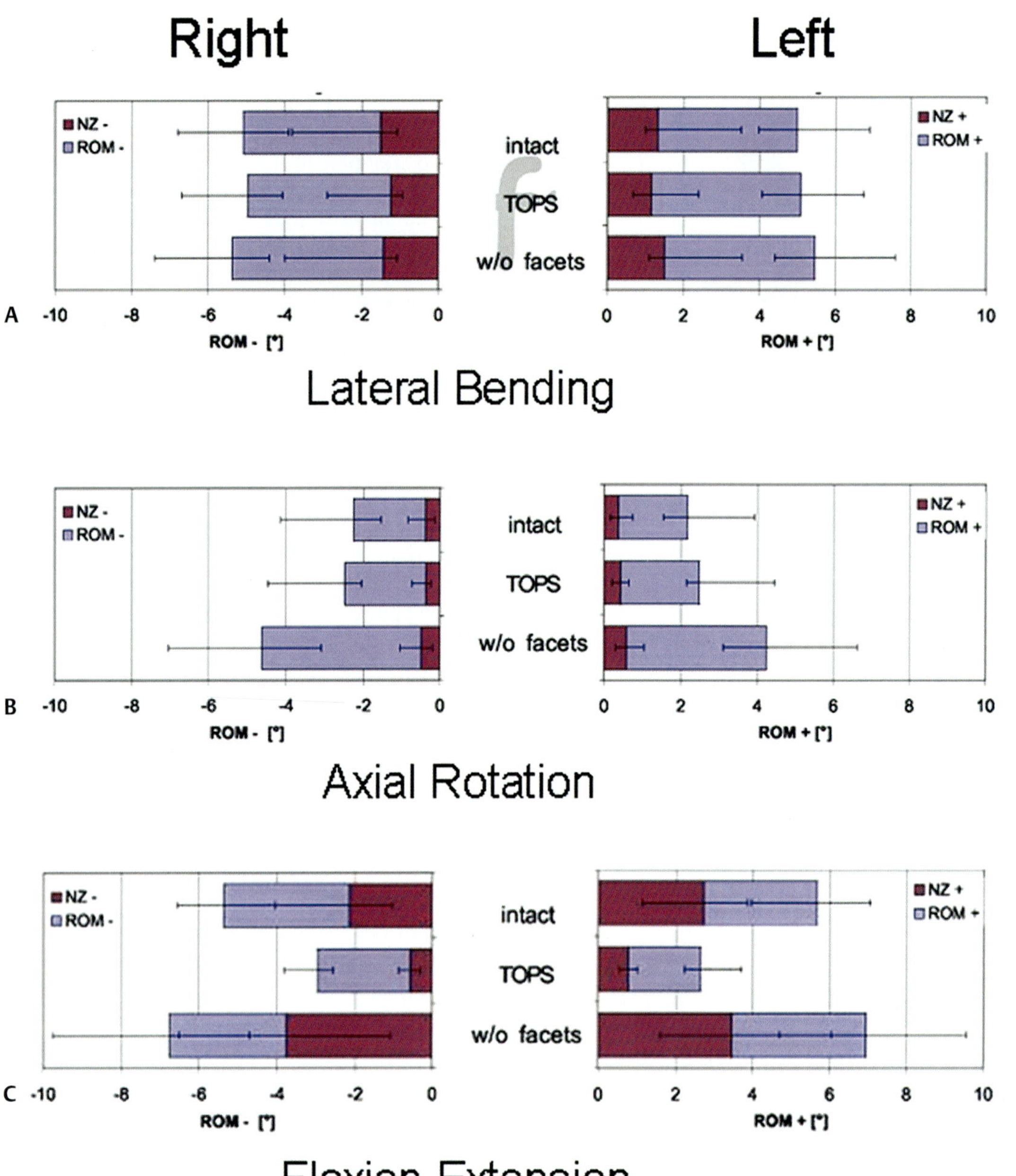

Figure 45–5   The test showed that the TOPS device almost ideally restores the motion behavior of a segment in **(A)** left and right lateral bending and **(B)** left and right axial rotation after facet removal compared with the intact segment. **(C)** In flexion and extension, the range of motion was 55% of that of an intact segment.

The surgical exposure is then secured using a self-retaining retractor system (**Fig. 45–7**).

Standard decompression of the index level is then completed via laminectomy and facetectomy techniques. Classically, spinal stenosis occurs at the central canal, lateral recess, and lateral neural foramen from a combination of disk herniation, dorsal uncovertebral joint spurring and lipping, facet osteophytes, and facet subluxation. Depending on the exact pathology of the individual case, the degree of bony, synovium, ligamentum flavum, and disk resection may thus vary accordingly. With specific regard to the TOPS implant, three unique points should be taken into account. First, it is recommended that aggressive resection of the intervertebral disk be avoided and that only herniated or bulging material be removed as needed to decompress the neural elements. Thermal annuloplasty with the bipolar forceps may be desired to stiffen and reinforce the annulus at the point of bulge or herniation.

Due to the specific design of the TOPS implant, total or near-total resection of the spinous process at the lower vertebrae of the index segment is needed to properly seat the four arms and centroid of the device. An implant trial is provided in the system and can be used to estimate the degree of laminar and spinous process removal that will be required (**Fig. 45–8**). Finally, because the TOPS implant serves to replace the motion restraint of the native facet complex, it is recommended that the facet joint be effectively decoupled. This can be achieved by aggressive resection through the

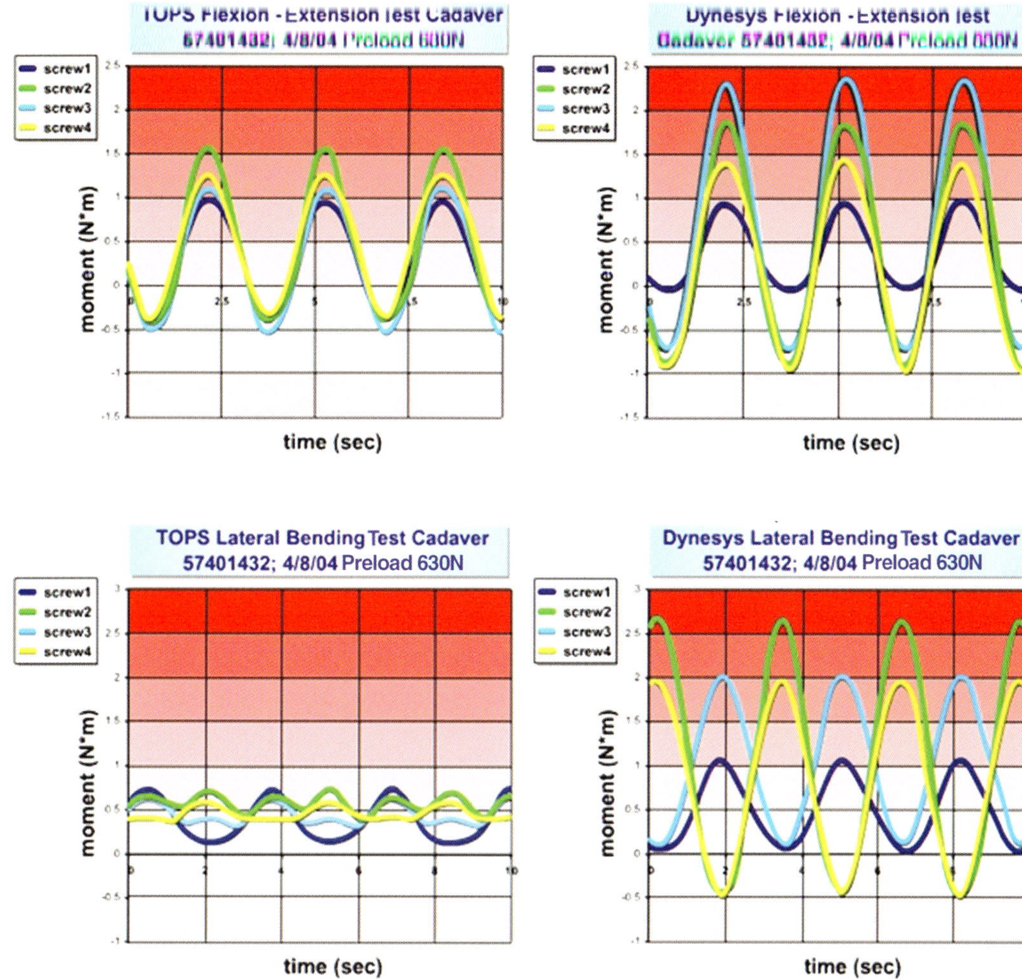

Figure 45–6 Strain gauges were applied to the same four[4] screws so that the mechanical stress and resulting strains transferred to them from the leading competitor (Dynesys, Zimmer Spine, Warsaw, IN) and TOPS devices could be monitored while the spine simulator manipulated the spine segments.

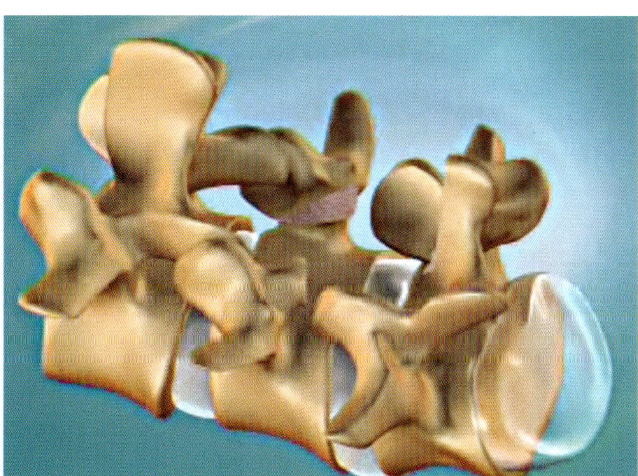

Figure 45–7 Particular care should be paid to preserving the capsule and muscular attachments surrounding the superior facet complex above the target level. The surgical exposure is then secured using a self-retaining retractor system.

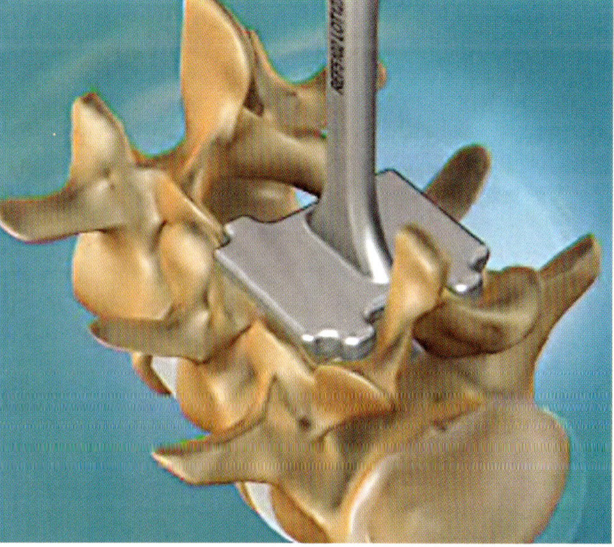

Figure 45–8 Due to the specific design of the TOPS implant, total or near-total resection of the spinous process at the lower vertebrae of the index segment is needed to properly seat the four arms and centroid of the device. An implant trial is provided in the system and can be used to estimate the degree of laminar and spinous process removal that will be required.

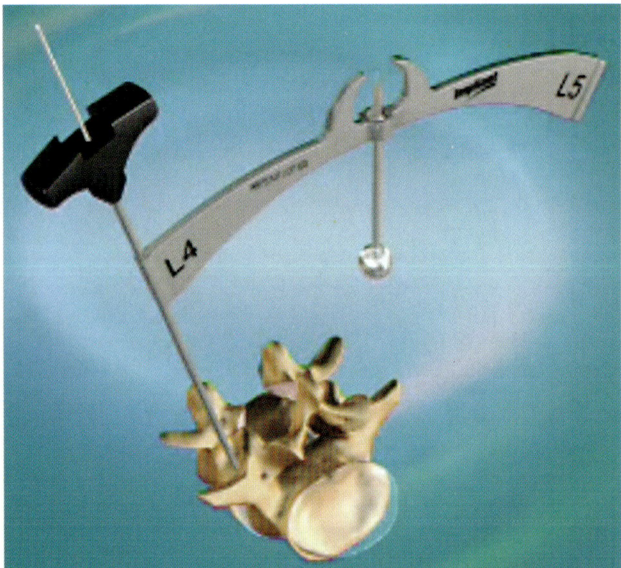

Figure 45–9 Because the TOPS implant serves to functionally replace the motion restraint of the native facet complex, it is recommended that the facet joint be effectively decoupled. This can be achieved by aggressive resection through the joint itself or by removing the superior articulating processes from the inferior vertebrae. This maneuver is often readily achieved by creating two surgical osteotomies at the level of the pars interarticularis with either an osteotome or a powered drill bit.

joint itself or by removing the superior articulating processes from the inferior vertebrae. This maneuver is often readily achieved by creating two surgical osteotomies at the level of the pars interarticularis with either an osteotome or a powered drill bit (**Fig. 45–9**). Once the necessary degree of bony resection has been achieved, adequate neural decompression is confirmed with a Woodson elevator bilaterally over the thecal sac, exiting and traversing nerve roots. Meticulous hemostasis should be obtained at this point with a combination of bipolar cautery, bone wax, Gelfoam with thrombin, and Surgicel as needed. Some of the authors also advocate placement of a collagen-barrier type material (e.g., DuraGen, Integra Neuro Sciences, Plainsboro, NJ) above the exposed neural elements to decrease the incidence of scarring and also to create a readily accessible surgical plane in case of revision or implant removal.

The pedicle screw entry points are then identified at the superior and inferior vertebral levels. Particular attention should be paid to obtain a more lateral to medial vector of pedicle cannulation such that more triangulation of the final screws can be achieved. Careful preservation of the superior facet complex is again desired. A cannulated system is provided with the TOPS implant for use via a semipercutaneous technique if desired. In this fashion, a Jamshidi needle can be used to cannulate the pedicles and then exchanged for a Kirschner wire once confirmation of the needle trajectory has been obtained on biplanar fluoroscopic guidance. A unique pendulum-type guide is provided in the TOPS system which will ensure that the angle of pedicle cannulation will remain within the acceptable range of angles which can be tolerated by the four-arm extensions of the implant. Then using the provided serial tissue dilator tubes, a working corridor is obtained through the lateral musculoligamentous

complex. In this fashion, excessive initial stripping and lateral exposure of the muscles can be minimized. A cannulated awl and tap can then be used to prepare the pedicle for instrumentation. It is recommended that a bicortical or near-bicortical triangulating passage be obtained to increase the pullout strength of the individual pedicle screw. Further, utilization of the largest diameter screw that can be accepted by the anatomy of the pedicle is recommended for similar reasons. Lastly, under-tapping by 0.5–1 mm will also serve to increase the ultimate strength of the screw threads purchase.

Once the desired length of screw has been determined, the pedicles are instrumented with the standard cannulated tulip-head polyaxial screws that are provided in the TOPS device. Snap-on slotted extension sleeves are available to facilitate final implantation of the TOPS device (**Fig. 45–10**). The pedicle screws can be placed with or without the sleeves attached according to the surgeon's preference. Whereas, the top two screws should be advanced to the end of their passage as low as desired, it is recommended that the bottom two screws be kept slightly more prominent initially. Using a separate four-armed targeting jig (**Fig. 45–11**), the cross-bars are first placed into the tulip heads of the superior screws. Using the adjustable sliding inferior arms of the targeting jig, the inferior screws can be advanced to the appropriate depth to ensure that it will readily accept the four-arm geometry of the TOPS implant. The authors recommend that the screws not be "backed up" if possible to again maximize their purchase and pullout strength.

At this point, the TOPS device is prepared for implantation. Earlier in the process, the exact profile (regular or low profile) has been determined using the sizing jigs already described. A small amount of sterile saline is injected through a small

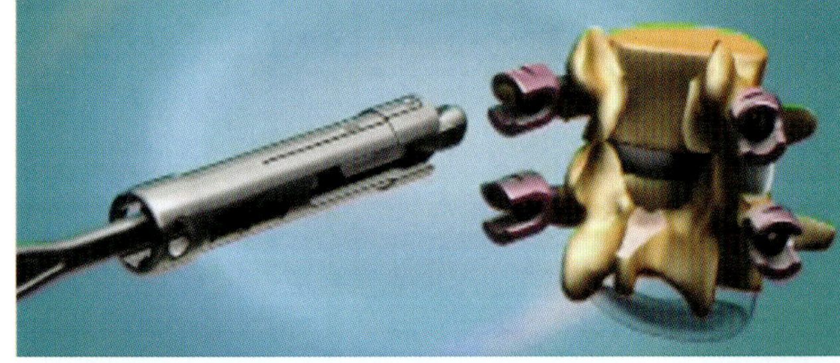

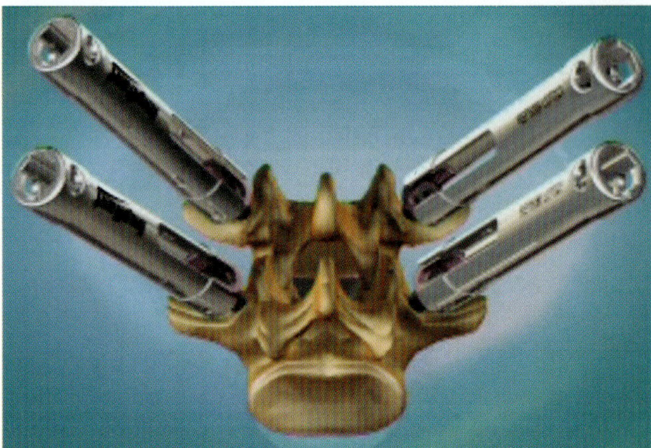

Figure 45–10 Snap-on slotted extension sleeves are available to facilitate final implantation of the TOPS device.

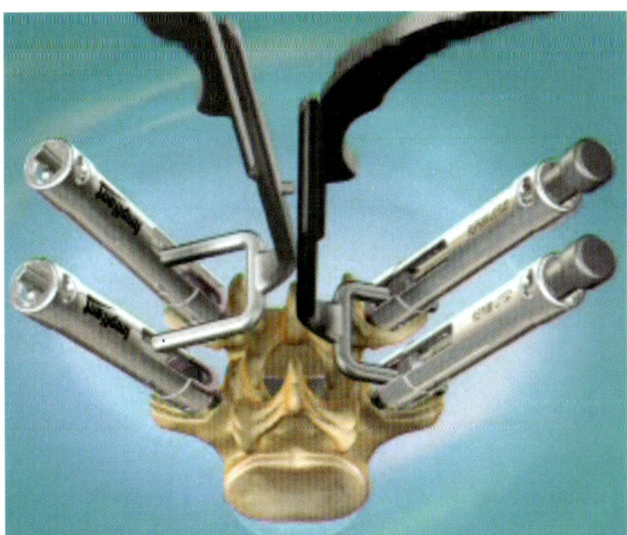

Figure 45–11 Using a separate, four-armed targeting jig, the cross-bars are first placed into the tulip heads of the superior screws. Using the adjustable sliding inferior arms of the targeting jig, the inferior screws can then be advanced to the appropriate depth to ensure that it will readily accept the four-arm geometry of the TOPS implant.

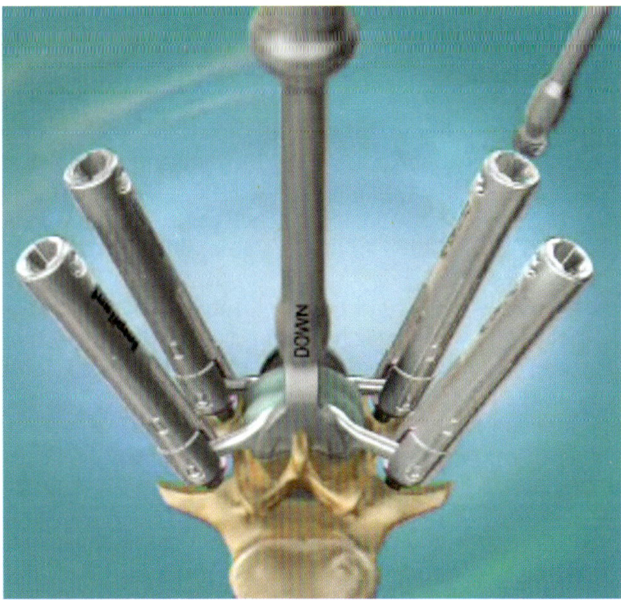

Figure 45–13 Once in place, each of the four crossbar arms is then secured using a standard locking nut and countertorqued to its final tightness.

port in the gasketed portion of the centroid of the implant to serve as a nonhydraulic lubricant. The device is then loaded on a specialized claw-armed holder (**Fig. 45–12**). The four arms of the TOPS implant are then passed into the tulip heads of the polyaxial screws. If the screw-extension sleeves were utilized, these can help to facilitate the passage of the arms at this point. Once in place, each of the four crossbar arms are then secured using a standard locking nut and countertorqued to their final tightness (**Fig. 45–13**). Careful inspection of the implant should confirm that all crossbars are well seated with no evidence of cross-threading or inadequate surface area of the bars within the tulip-head channels. If present, the extension sleeves are then unclipped from the tulip heads to complete the TOPS device implantation procedure. Biplanar fluoroscopic confirmation of the device and screw positions should be obtained prior to final closure to ensure good alignment and angle of the overall segment and construct (**Fig. 45–14**).

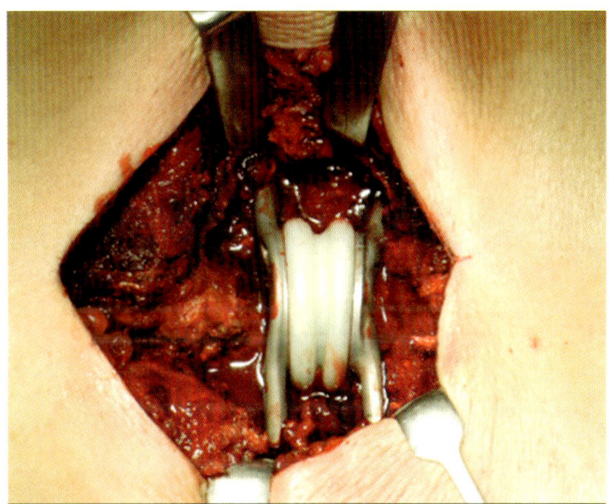

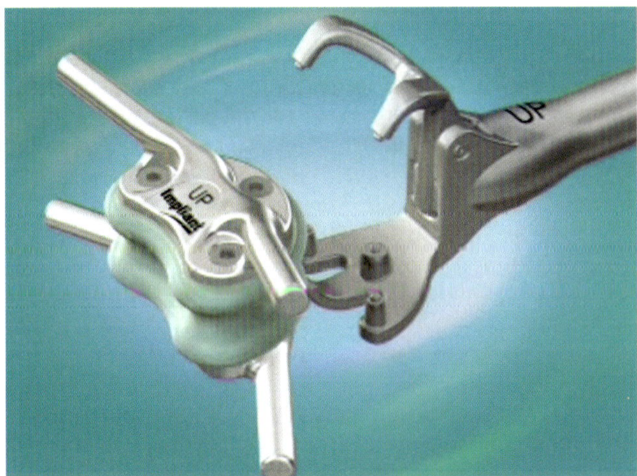

Figure 45–12 Claw-armed holder.

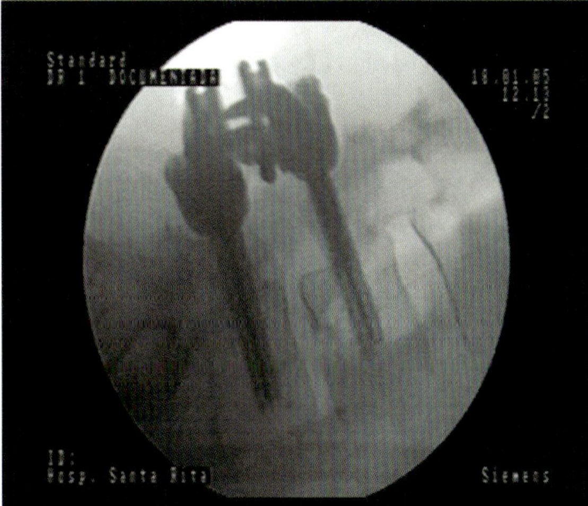

Figure 45–14 Biplanar fluoroscopic confirmation of the device and screw positions should be obtained prior to final closure to ensure good alignment and angle of the overall segment and construct.

Copious antibiotic-impregnated irrigation of the entire wound and implants is completed. A Davol or Jackson-Pratt wound drain should be placed at this time if there are concerns regarding hemostasis or seroma accumulation in the potential surgical dead space. Interrupted O Vicryl sutures are then used to appose and close the lumbodorsal fascia in a near-watertight fashion. Inverted 2–0 or 3–0 absorbable sutures are then used to appose the subcutaneous layer of the skin. Skin closure can proceed according to the preference of the surgeon.

Postoperatively, a rigid clamshell lumbar sacral orthosis (LSO) orthosis is generally not recommended due to the motion-preserving nature of the TOPS implant. However, a lumbar corset or semirigid brace is often useful in the early perioperative period for support and comfort of the patient. In comparison to spinal fusion patients, patients after TOPS implantation are encouraged to mobilize and ambulate early on in their recovery process.

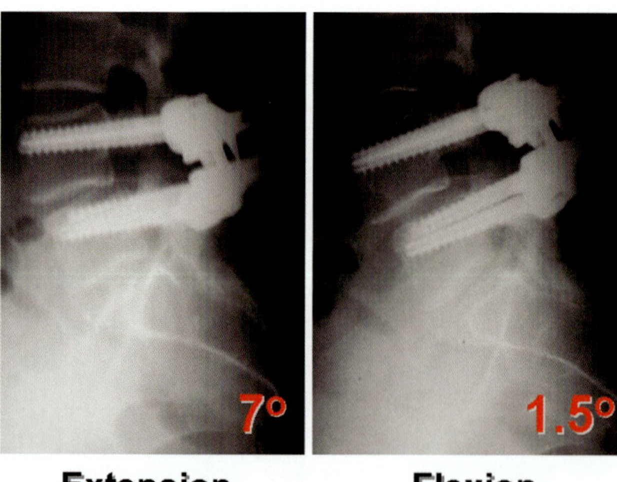

Figure 45–15   On flexion-extension, radiographs have demonstrated a preservation of 4 to 7 degrees of motion at the index level with no evidence of hypermobility at the adjacent levels to date.

◆ Clinical Data and Outcomes of TOPS Facet Replacement

Over a 1-year period, 10 patients with lumbar pain, radiculopathy, and/or neurogenic claudication were treated with decompressive surgery and TOPS placement at the L4–L5 level. This was due to the fact that the initial TOPS device crossbar geometries were designed primarily for single-level use at the L4–L5 level. Additional geometries and multilevel devices are now available as well. All 10 patients failed an extended period of conservative management including physical therapy, epidural injections, and other less invasive treatment modalities. On radiographic and magnetic resonance imaging evaluation, six patients had evidence of spondylolisthesis with superimposed spinal stenosis and radicular compression, whereas the remaining four patients had stenosis alone. In general, the primary indications for treatment of patients with the TOPS device have been: stenosis with evidence of instability of radiographic evaluation, stenosis with prior laminectomy induced instability, grade I to II spondylolisthesis with or without spinal stenosis, and severe mechanical diskogenic back pain with significant facet arthropathy or instability thereby excluding them from stand-alone TDR.

All patients underwent a surgical procedure at the L4–L5 level for their pathology that essentially involved a decompression and subsequent instrumentation as already described. The mean surgical time was 3.7 hours with an average blood loss of 200 mL. Early postoperative computed tomography and plain radiographs revealed excellent bony decompression of the central canal and lateral recess as well as the accuracy and triangulation of the screws. There were no intraoperative surgical or hardware-related complications. At the time of this chapter's submission, the follow-up has ranged from 5 to 12 months. Standardized flexion-extension radiographs as well as live-motion fluoroscopy has been obtained at 6 weeks, 3 months, 6 months, 9 months, and 12 months.

To date, there have been complications attributable to the primary index level operation or due to the TOPS implant itself. There has been one revision due to progressive disease and symptoms at the level L3–L4 above in one patient requiring additional fusion. In all 10 patients, there has been no evidence of device failure, radiographic lucency around the screws, screw migration, or implant device dehiscence. On flexion-extension, radiographs have demonstrated a preservation of 4 to 7 degrees of motion at the index level with no evidence of hypermobility at the adjacent levels to date (**Fig. 45–15**). On static neutral radiograph evaluation, an average of 30% reduction of spondylolisthesis cases was demonstrated.

Utilizing standardized outcomes measures, all patients have generally had good to excellent outcomes. The visual analog scale (VAS) pain scores were 82 mm on average initially with the following subsequent scores being 22.8 mm at 1 week, 23.3 mm at 6 weeks, 35.0 mm at 3 months, 26.5 mm at 6 months, and 22.5 mm at 9 months. The initial Oswestry Disability Index (ODI) scores averaged 72.4, indicating a significant degree of disability in the older stenotic study population. The subsequent scores were 57 at 6 weeks, 42 at 3 months, 39 at 6 months, and 31 at 9 months. Because clinical success for treatment in the ODI scale has been defined as more than a 15-point improvement, the TOPS device has clearly performed as a historical control for decompression and fusion for stenosis and spondylolisthesis.[5–7] With regard to the scores for the patient's neurogenic claudication, the Spinal Stenosis Scores (SSS) (modified Zurich stenosis scores) were 71.6 preop, 47.4 at 6 weeks, 41.2 at 3 months, and 38 at 6 months, thereby again indicating that there was good relief with regard to the patient's neurological compressive symptoms.

◆ Conclusion

The total facet replacement system (TOPS) is a novel posterior stabilizing device that is able to preserve motion, restore the biomechanical neutral zone, and prevent abnormal load sharing at the treated and adjacent spinal motion segments. Within the limited clinical study, it appears that decompression combined with implantation of the TOPS device is able to achieve functional outcomes as favorable as historical control arms for fusion for stenosis and spondylolisthesis. ODI, VAS, and SSS results indicate that the device is effective in treating the back pain component of these patients as well as rigid spinal fusion in prior studies. Whereas the device itself has been tested for over 10 million cycles with no functional failures and a minimum of wear debris, questions concerning screw purchase and pullout will require far more extensive follow-up and study. Because the device appears to have less screw–bone interface stresses than other predicate devices, it would be reasonable to expect a failure rate less than or equivalent to previously published predicate screw pullout rates of 6 to 8%.[8,22] Additional long-term studies will also be required to examine the effect this device has on the incidence of ASD as well. Overall, the TOPS device represents a novel means of treating back pain while still preserving the native motion of the pathological spinal segment.

References

1. Abumi K, Panjabi MM, Kramer KM, Duranceau J, Oxland T, Crisco JJ. Biomechanical evaluation of lumbar spinal stability after graded facetectomies. Spine 1990;15:1142–1147

2. Blumenthal S, McAfee PC, Guyer RD, et al. A prospective, randomized, multicenter Food and Drug Administration investigational device exemptions study of lumbar total disc replacement with the CHARITE artificial disc versus lumbar fusion, I: Evaluation of clinical outcomes. Spine 2005;30:1565–1575 discussion E387–391

3. Resnick DK, Choudhri TF, Dailey AT, et al. Guidelines for the performance of fusion procedures for degenerative disease of the lumbar spine, V: Correlation between radiographic and functional outcome. J Neurosurg Spine 2005;2:658–661

4. Resnick DK, Choudhri TF, Dailey AT, et al. Guidelines for the performance of fusion procedures for degenerative disease of the lumbar spine, VII: Intractable low-back pain without stenosis or spondylolisthesis. J Neurosurg Spine 2005;2:670–672

5. Resnick DK, Choudhri TF, Dailey AT, et al. Guidelines for the performance of fusion procedures for degenerative disease of the lumbar spine, IX: Fusion in patients with stenosis and associated spondylolisthesis. J Neurosurg Spine 2005;2:679–685

6. Resnick DK, Choudhri TF, Dailey AT, et al. Guidelines for the performance of fusion procedures for degenerative disease of the lumbar spine, X: Fusion following decompression in patients with stenosis without spondylolisthesis. J Neurosurg Spine 2005;2:686–691

7. Fischgrund JS, Mackay M, Herkowitz HN, et al. 1997 Volvo Award winner in clinical studies: degenerative lumbar spondylolisthesis with spinal stenosis: a prospective, randomized study comparing decompressive laminectomy and arthrodesis with and without spinal instrumentation. Spine 1997;22:2807–2812

8. Gamradt SC, Wang JC. Lumbar disc arthroplasty. Spine J 2005;5:95–103

9. Geisler FH. Surgical technique of lumbar artificial disc replacement with the Charité Artificial Disc. Neurosurgery 2005;56(Suppl 1):46–57 discussion 46–57

10. Grob D, Benini A, Junge A, Mannion AF. Clinical experience with the Dynesys Semirigid Fixation System for the Lumbar Spine: surgical outcome and patient oriented outcome in 50 cases after an average of two years. Spine 2005;30:324–331

11. Huang RC, Lim MR, Girardi FP, Cammisa FP Jr. The prevalence of contraindications to total disc replacement in a cohort of lumbar surgical patients. Spine 2004;29:2538–2541

12. Hunter LY, Braunstein EM, Bailey RW. Radiographic changes following anterior cervical spine fusions. Spine 1980;5:399–401

13. Kostuik JP. Complications and surgical revision for failed disc arthroplasty. Spine J 2004;4(Suppl 6):289S–291S

14. Lee CK. Accelerated degeneration of the segment adjacent to a lumbar fusion. Spine 1988;13:375–377

15. Lee CK, Langrana NA. Lumbosacral spinal fusion: a biomechanical study. Spine 1984;9:574–581

16. Lu WW, Luk KD, Holmes A. Pure shear properties of lumbar spinal joints and the effect of tissue sectioning on load-sharing. Spine 2005;30:E204–E209

17. Olsewski JM, Garvey TA, Schendel MJ. Biomechanical analysis of facet and graft loading in a Smith-Robinson type cervical spine model. Spine 1994;19:2540–2544

18. McAfee P. Biomechanics and results of implant testing of the TOPS Facet Replacement Device. Luncheon symposium presentation-TOPS Device. Presented at: the 5th Annual Spine Arthroplasty Society Meeting, New York, New York, May 9, 2005

19. Panjabi MM. Clinical spinal instability and low back pain. J Electromyogr Kinesiol 2003;13:371–379

20. Panjabi MM. The stabilizing system of the spine, II: Neutral zone and instability hypothesis. J Spinal Disord 1992;5:390–396 discussion 397

21. Stoll TM, Dubois G, Schwarzenbach O. The dynamic neutralization system for the spine: a multi-center study of a novel non-fusion system. Eur Spine J 2002;11(Suppl 2):S170–S178

22. Yone K, Sakou T, Kawauchi Y, et al. Indication of fusion for lumbar spinal stenosis in elderly patients and its significance. Spine 1996;21:242–248

46

Total Facet Arthroplasty System (TFAS)

Scott Webb

◆ **The Role of Total Facet Arthroplasty in Restoration of Spinal Biomechanics**

◆ **Facet Biomechanics**

◆ **Design Rationale**

◆ **Product Performance**

◆ **Surgical Technique**

◆ **Total Facet Arthroplasty System Investigational Device Exemption Clinical Study Inclusion Criteria**

◆ **Facet Arthroplasty versus Dynamic Stabilization**

◆ **Conclusion**

The Total Facet Arthroplasty System (TFAS) (Archus Orthopedics, Inc., Redmond, WA) is designed as a total joint replacement of the facets, employing proven technologies and approaches used successfully in total hip and total knee arthroplasty. It is a pedicle-based system that replaces the articulating zygapophyseal joint. The TFAS (**Fig. 46–1**) was invented by Mark Reiley, M.D., and designed in conjunction with Archus Orthopedics, Inc., as a patented, articulating joint prosthesis intended to provide stabilization of spinal segments in skeletally mature patients as an adjunct to laminectomy, laminotomy, neural decompression, and facetectomy in the treatment of several acute or chronic instabilities or deformities of the lumbar spine, including degenerative disease of the facets, degenerative disease of the facets with instability, grade I degenerative spondylolisthesis with objective evidence of neurological impairment, or central or lateral spinal stenosis. Although stability in all of these cases can be restored surgically with a properly designed implant, as in the case of pedicle rod fusion technologies, to provide a better outcome to the patient in terms of functionality and reduced incidence of complications, a "motion restoring" device that dynamically stabilizes and restores normal motions to the spine (TFAS) has been designed.

With the advent of motion-preserving technology in the treatment of spinal disorders, many new products are positioning themselves as treatment alternatives to instrumented fusion. Many of these concepts are incremental line extensions of current fusion applications, as compared with TFAS, which represents a significant advancement in the treatment of posterior lumbar pathologies. Today, these pathologies are most frequently addressed via wide decompression procedures, which often lead to instability at the affected levels. Currently, instrumented fusion hardware is most commonly applied to address these iatrogenic instabilities. Adjacent level disease will be impacted at some level by motion-preserving technologies such as TFAS. The goal of these motion-preservation devices should be to re-create segmental function while attempting to restore stability and physiological motion to improve the biomechanics of the patient's spine over the short and long term.

◆ The Role of Total Facet Arthroplasty in Restoration of Spinal Biomechanics

With the advent of motion preservation devices for spine arthroplasty such as total disk and nucleus prosthetic replacements, the role of the facet joints in the etiology of spinal pathology, as well as the effect of surgical intervention on its temporal changes in physiology, contribution to biomechanics, and effect on the natural trajectory of spine disease, has been newly scrutinized.[1–3] In the context of the functional spinal unit (FSU) segment biomechanics, the intervertebral disk, facets, and ligaments all play a key role. In general these structures have three main roles: to stabilize the vertebrae relative to each other and protect the nerves through a range of motion and loads; to provide proper motion for each FSU and the spine as a whole; and to transfer and share loads in the spinal column.

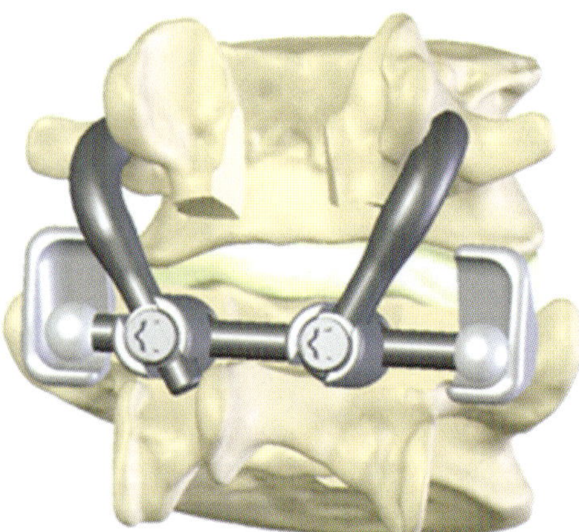

Figure 46–1 Schematic of the Total Facet Arthroplasty System (TFAS).

The balance of these three biomechanical imperatives is disrupted by surgical procedures such as decompression for stenosis in the lumbar spine, which is often accompanied by adjuvant stabilization through rigid fixation with metallic hardware or fusion or both. This surgery removes all or part of the posterior spine elements, including the lamina, ligaments, and facets, to enlarge the neural foramina to free either or both the spinal cord and the offended nerve root. This concurrent fusion is solely intended to stabilize the spine and prevent motion until fusion is complete. Although stability is obtained, the two other elements—motion and load sharing—generally are not met.

◆ Facet Biomechanics

The FSU motion segment consists of two vertebral bodies and the intervening facet joints, intervertebral disk, posterior elements, and spinal ligaments. Each vertebral body interacts with its adjacent vertebrae by means of three articulating joints (**Fig. 46–2**). The major joint, in terms of load transmission and kinematic guidance, is the intervertebral disk joint. The disk and its components (annulus fibrosus, nucleus pulposus, and vertebral end plates) maintain the stiffness of the disk against compressive loading and allow for some degree of movement between vertebral bodies. Besides enabling bending movements between vertebral bodies, the intervertebral disk allows for twisting and small sliding movements. The posterior elements (pedicles, facets, transverse processes, superior articular processes, laminae, and spinous process) control the position of the vertebral bodies. These several processes serve as sites of attachment for muscles and ligaments that stabilize the lumbar vertebral column. The fine balance of all of these elements is usually disrupted by surgical procedures, such as decompression of stenosis in the lumbar spine, and is many times accompanied by adjuvant stabilization through rigid fixation with either or both metallic hardware and fusion. While stability is obtained, the additional elements: motion and load sharing, generally are not met. Lastly, damage to and pain from the diarthrodial facet joints and their corresponding capsular ligaments independent of surgical intervention for other causes can precede or coexist with spinal stenosis and deformities such as spondylolisthesis.

The ability of spinal segments, from individual FSUs to multivertebral segments, to bear and transmit load while allowing for motion has been measured in the laboratory, characterized through mathematical modeling, and predicted through physiological loading regimes and ranges of motion. Unfortunately, up to this point, the study of the mechanics of the intervertebral joints has been reserved almost exclusively for the intervertebral disk joint, especially in the shadow of the design and development of artificial disk replacement hardware.

Historically the facet joints have been attributed the role of motion limiters, which complement by their shape, size, location, and orientation the individual contributions of each anatomical spinal segment to the total role of the spine. The location of the facet joint along the spine determines its function (**Fig. 46–3**). In the cervical spine the loads transmitted across the facet joints are the lowest. However, the cervical spine exhibits the most freedom in lateral bending, extension, and axial torsion. The facet joints are located laterally almost in the coronal plane and are tilted in abduction to allow these motions. The cervical area is the region of lowest effective transmitted loads in the spine, but the region with most freedom in lateral

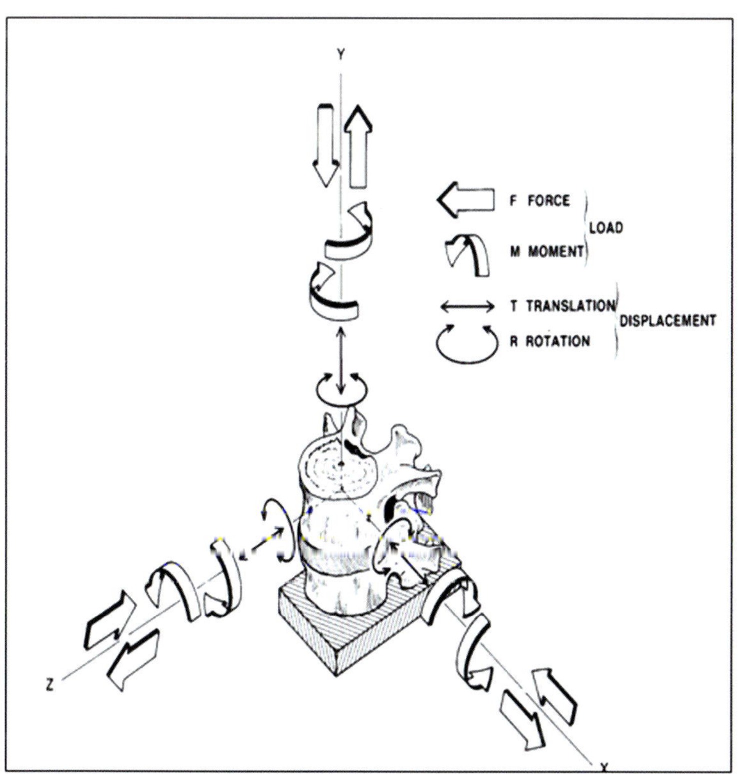

Figure 46–2   Degrees of freedom and motions of a functional spinal unit. (With permission from White and Panjabi, Clinical Biomechanics of the Spine, 2nd ed. Lippincott, Williams, and Wilkins, Philadelphia, PA).

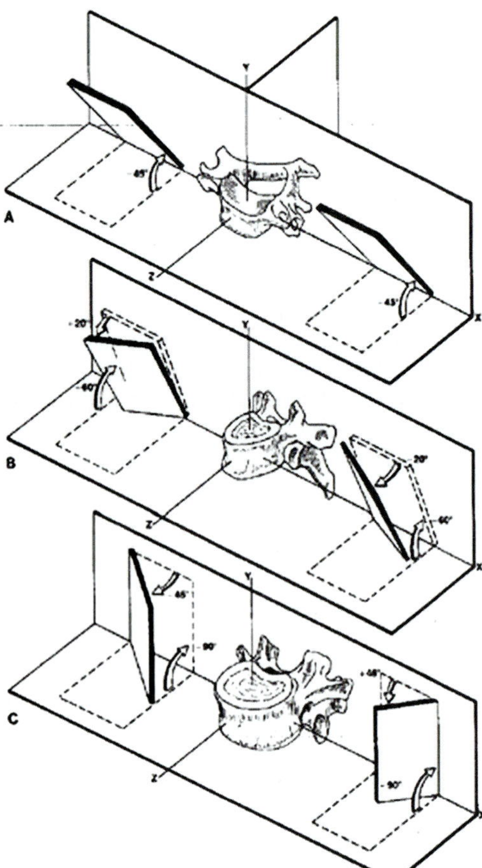

Figure 46–3 Variation in facet orientation and location within vertebral regions. (With permission from White and Panjabi, Clinical Biomechanics of the Spine, 2nd ed.)

bending, extension, and axial torsion, the facets, are located laterally, almost in the coronal plane, and are "tilted" in abduction to allow for these motions. In the lumbar spine, where axial rotation and lateral flexion are limited, the facets act like kinematic stops in these motions because most of the lumbar spine's role is that of allowing flexion-extension in the sagittal plane, and the facets are subjected to the highest load magnitudes. As such, the facets are large, more centrally located, and oriented in a more sagittal (adducted) manner. In fact, they are almost parallel along that sagittal plane, allowing maximum flexion-extension while acting as "cam-like" stops for hyperextension and axial torsion. We know that the FSU has a documented "neutral zone" where the axial force transmitted by the spine is such that it is stiffer at the extreme ranges of motion and less so near the neutral position. A study of instrumented facet joints indicates that the facet joints have a similar dwell point or neutral zone (**Fig. 46–4**). Although its biomechanical activity and pathology can be as important and painful as those of the intervertebral disk, the zygapophyseal joint has been the subject of marginal attention.

Furthermore, because facets are synovial joints, damage to and pain from these diarthrodial joints and their corresponding capsular ligaments can present themselves independently of

surgical intervention, such as from degenerative causes like arthritis. The ability to remove and replace the diseased joint and associated pain generators in the cartilaginous surfaces and synovial capsules and ligaments is analogous to the current treatment for major joints in the appendicular skeleton. Finally, because arthropathy and even trauma can also precede or coexist with spinal stenosis and deformities such as spondylolisthesis, the ability of the implant to remove and replace the zygapophyseal joints must be able to, at least in less severe cases, account for slipping and relative motion of the vertebral bodies. Therefore, the TFAS was designed to provide a better outcome to the patient in terms of functionality and reduced incidence of complications—a device that dynamically stabilizes and restores normal motions to the spine.

◆ Design Rationale

The potential clinical benefits of TFAS are particularly evident. With respect to symptom relief, complete versus partial removal of facets and even a wide decompressive laminectomy allows for safer, more comprehensive decompression, eliminates the possibility of further degeneration and recurrence, and removes a potential source of low back pain. When considering that motion is restored to normal levels because no fusion is effected, the patient gets full range of back motion and normal spinal biomechanics are restored, preventing future adjacent segment issues (by minimizing stress on adjacent levels), and, because there is no bone graft harvest procedure, the associated pain is eliminated from the procedure. Therefore, all three kinematic imperatives of stabilizing the vertebrae relative to each other and the nerves through a range of motion and loads, providing proper motion for each FSU and the spine as a whole, and transferring and sharing loads in the spinal column can be achieved while eliminating pain and other neurological symptoms. Finally, with the high incidence rate of contraindications (89% of candidates for nonfusion surgery) in total disk replacement,[1,2] where the most common are related to stenosis and facet arthropathy, a viable option to restore posterior column biomechanics, especially after surgical decompression, can be a prime enabler for the use of anterior column arthroplasty devices, such as total disk and nucleus replacements.

Although anterior (total disk and nucleus) and posterior (dynamic stabilizers) nonfusion devices have been clinically used, in general they do not address all three key functional elements of restoring proper stability, motion, and load sharing. These implants "preserve" motion in whatever limited form it exists postsurgery (decompression) or as allowed by a disease state (arthritis, stenosis, spondylolisthesis) and focus mostly on achieving stability. For the posterior elements of the spine, only one approach, TFAS, has been able to incorporate and validate that all three functional biomechanical elements are restored.

The advent of nonfusion spinal implants has necessitated the accurate characterization of the biomechanics of the anterior (disks) and posterior elements of the spine (facets). This has been methodically undertaken in recent years, with the development of techniques to assess their contributions to the stability, load transfer/sharing, and overall kinematics of the spine. The ability to characterize

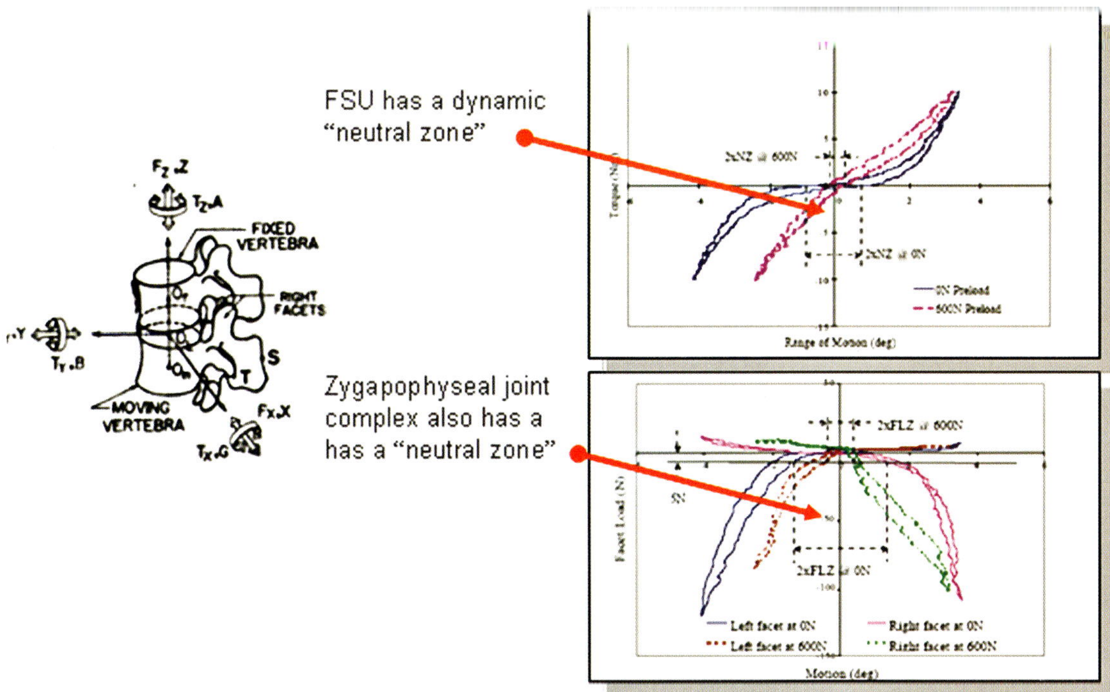

Figure 46–4   Facets exhibit a neutral zone similar to that of the disk within a functional spinal unit. (With permission from Zhu QA, et al. 50th ORS, March 2004:1125.)

these functions completely is important because their understanding becomes the foundation for the design inputs for nonfusion orthopedic implants that can account for and ultimately reestablish stability, motion, and load sharing in a surgically altered, diseased spine. The same techniques can then be utilized to validate the design performance of motion-preserving implants.[4–6] Furthermore, as artificial disk, nucleus, and facet replacements make their way to the market, their biomechanics must be better understood and characterized, with a special focus on the effect of such implants on the biomechanics of adjacent segments as well

their individual interaction. This should be done in an effort to ensure that postoperatively, their function will be clinically successful, and that additional potential failure modes have not been created at the complementary joints.[7–9]

The TFAS implant has been designed to accommodate a high degree of anatomical variability. It has also been designed to allow surgeons to continue using their normal technique for decompression and implantation of pedicle instrumentation. The system does not require surgeons to change surgical approach to accommodate the implant due to its unique design and high degree of modularity (**Fig. 46–5**).

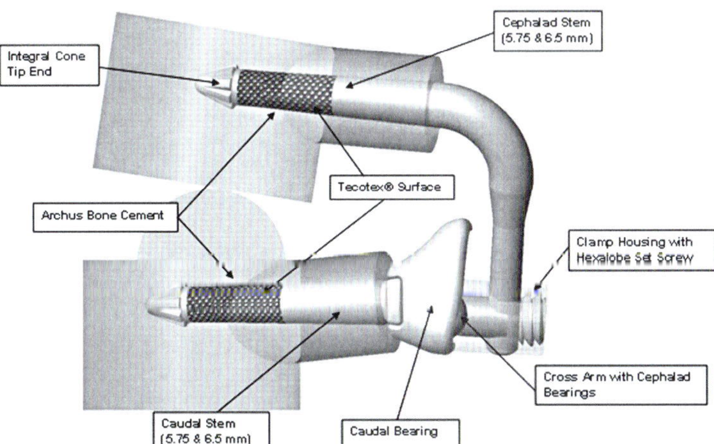

Figure 46–5   Schematic of the modular options available in the Total Facet Arthroplasty (TFAS) implant system.

Range of Motion	Natural[*]	TFAS™
Flexion/Extension	L3-L4 $\approx 11.2° \leq \theta \leq 15.3°$ L4-L5 $\approx 14.5° \leq \theta \leq 18.2°$	15° (+13°/-2°)
Lateral Bending	L3-L4 $\approx \pm 5.7° \leq \theta \leq \pm 12.4°$ L4-L5 $\approx \pm 5.7° \leq \theta \leq \pm 12.4°$	±7.5°
Axial Rotation	L3-L4 $\approx \pm 1.5° \leq \theta \leq \pm 2.6°$ L4-L5 $\approx \pm 1.5° \leq \theta \leq \pm 2.2°$	±2°

[*]White and Panjabi <u>Clinical Biomechanics of the Spine</u>, 2nd Ed., 1990, J.B. Lippincot Philadelphia

Figure 46–6 Motion design specifications for the Total Facet Arthroplasty (TFAS) implant system compared with natural intervertebral motions of the lumbar spine.

TFAS allows flexion of 13 degrees and extension of 2 degrees. Lateral bending is allowed up to 7.5 degrees and axial rotation up to 2 degrees. The instant axis of rotation is in the posterior third of the vertebral body (**Fig. 46–6**).

◆ Product Performance

Exhaustive testing of the intact as well as surgically destabilized posterior elements has resulted in a set of performance criteria that have been incorporated into a pedicle-based total joint replacement for the facets and posterior elements that extrinsically restores stability, kinematics, and load sharing through a patented, metal-on-metal articulation.[10,11] The TFAS components have been shown to effectively stabilize motion in flexion and lateral bending, restore the motion in extension, and appropriately limit the motion in axial rotation. In summary, TFAS restores the motion of an unstable FSU to that of an intact FSU, restoring a natural range of motion in all directions when compared with the intact condition[11] (**Fig. 46–7**). Additionally, it has been shown that a TFAS-treated FSU shares load with the intervertebral disk in a manner similar to that of an intact FSU.

The intrinsic elements of performance of TFAS—fixation, biocompatibility, and bearing couple durability—have been tested and their safety verified. When compared with a commercially available pedicle-based fusion system, under identical applied moments, the structural loads on the TFAS components experienced significantly lower implant stresses than the fusion system and withstood more than two times the ultimate fixation strength of pedicle screw-based fusion systems in vertebral bone. Because TFAS is fixed in the body with polymethyl methacrylate (PMMA) bone cement, the interface strength with the PMMA was tested and shown to withstand more than 2.5 times the maximum static in vivo loads with no dissociation or failure between the PMMA and anchor under maximum static loading; TFAS withstood more than three times the maximum fatigue duty cycle [activities of daily living (ADL)] loads for 10 million cycles of load application in torsion, bending, and axial loading.

When tested under a facet replacement-specific, modified American Society for Testing and Materials (ASTM) F-1717 test regime, the construct was able to support load levels of two to three times the maximum projected static in vivo loads with no dislocation, dissociation, or failure under static loading, while the integrity of the construct and interconnection mechanisms was shown to support more than two times the maximum projected fatigue in vivo ADL loads to 10 million cycles.

The durability of the articulation was validated through multiple tests in a custom-designed and fabricated wear simulator (**Fig. 46–8**). The tests were run in isolated chambers lubricated in bovine serum, the wear debris was

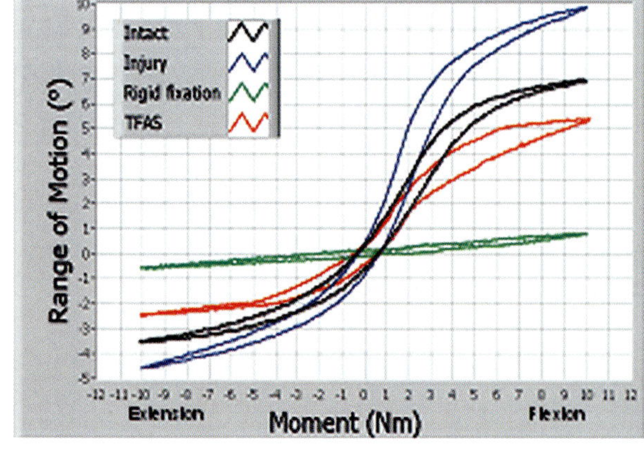

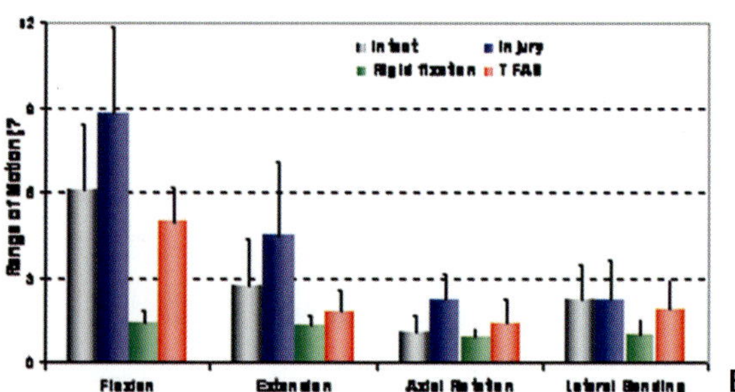

Figure 46–7 **(A)** Flexion-extension range of motion (ROM) for intact, decompressed, and Total Facet Arthroplasty (TFAS) treated and fused cadaveric spines. **(B)** ROM in flexion, extension, axial rotation, and lateral bending for TFAS ROMs in axial rotation and lateral bending are average of left and right directions. (With permission from Moumene M. Roundtables Spine Surg 2005;1:38–4.)

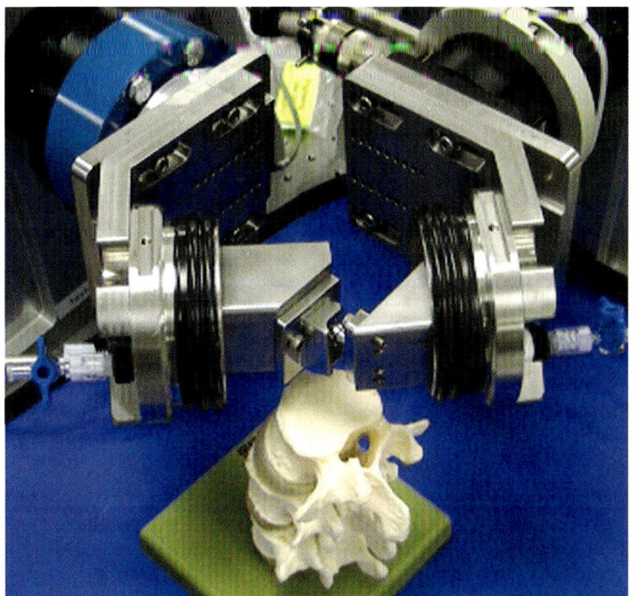

Figure 46–8 The Archus Wear Tester System.

collected and analyzed, and bearing surfaces were characterized. The wear surfaces and volume of cobalt-chromium (CoCr) debris was comparable to that reported in literature for the low end of metal-on-metal total hip arthroplasty (THA) at 10 million cycles. The wear particle size and distribution were also comparable to state of the art metal-on-metal hips, and therefore these findings were unremarkable. In addition, doses of CoCr particulate of the same size and distribution to those produced during wear testing were applied to the dura at L2–L3 of New Zealand white rabbits and the toxic reaction to wear debris was compared between the termination intervals in subjects sacrificed at 48 hours and 2, 4, 12, 24, and 32 weeks. No neurotoxic effect was observed in the test subjects and gross necropsy and histological evaluation demonstrated no cellular or tissue response in comparison to the control group locally or systemically in this model.

Biocompatibility in this first embodiment was achieved by selection of materials with a long history of use in implantable medical applications: CP titanium per American Society for Testing and Materials International (ASTM) F-67; Ti-6Al-4V per ASTM F-136; CoCr per ASTM F-75, F-799, and F-1537; and PMMA per ASTM F-451.

◆ Surgical Technique

Positioning is important and the Jackson table is preferred so that physiological lordosis can be obtained during surgery. The decompression is performed in the usual fashion. At the level to be instrumented (L3–L4 or L4–L5) the inferior articulating facet is removed, assisted in decompression of the neuroforamen, at the cephalad pedicle. The pedicles are entered according to the surgeons' preference. The pedicles are reamed to 4 mm and the templating trial is placed into the caudal pedicle, one on each side. They are labeled left and right. Once placed anteroposterior (AP) and lateral fluoroscopy images are obtained to determine the caudal implant to be used. Sagittal and coronal angles are noted under fluoroscopy by placing the transparent templates over the fluoroscopic image (**Fig. 46–9**). After the caudal implant is chosen the trial is assembled and inserted into the pedicles. A spring-loaded gauge is used to determine the angle and length of the cephalad implants as well as the angle of the housing connectors. Once the implant dimensions are determined the final implant is assembled. The pedicles are then reamed to their final diameter allowing for insertion of the final implant into the pedicle while providing a known cement mantle. The cement is injected first into the caudal pedicles and the caudal implants are inserted. When the cement has hardened a crossarm measurement is taken, the construct is assembled, and the final crossbar is inserted with the tulip heads in place to receive the cephalad arms. Cement is injected into the cephalad pedicles and the implants are placed into the pedicle such that the arms from the cephalad implants drop into the tulip heads on the crossbar, and the final assembly is locked into place with the torque wrench while the articulating

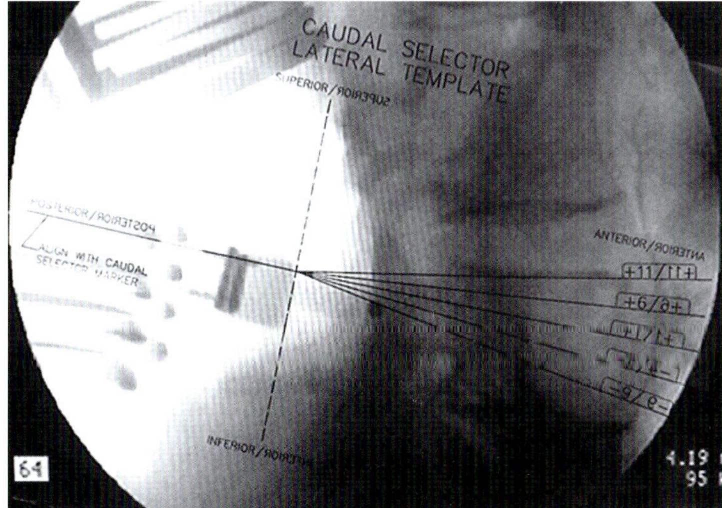

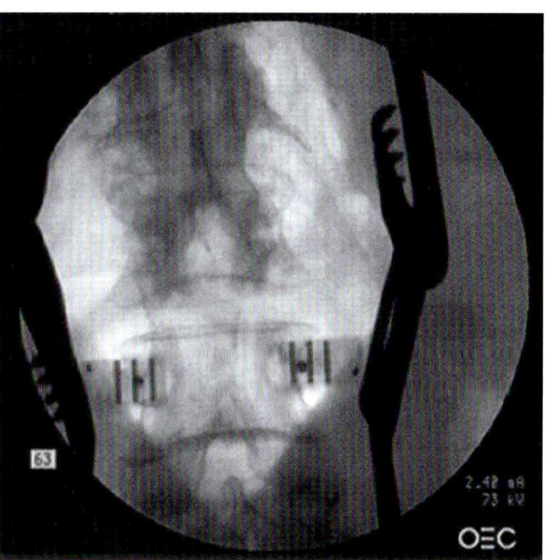

A **B**

Figure 46–9 **(A,B)** Anteroposterior and lateral fluoroscopic images of instrumentation used to size the Total Facet Arthroplasty (TFAS) caudal implants.

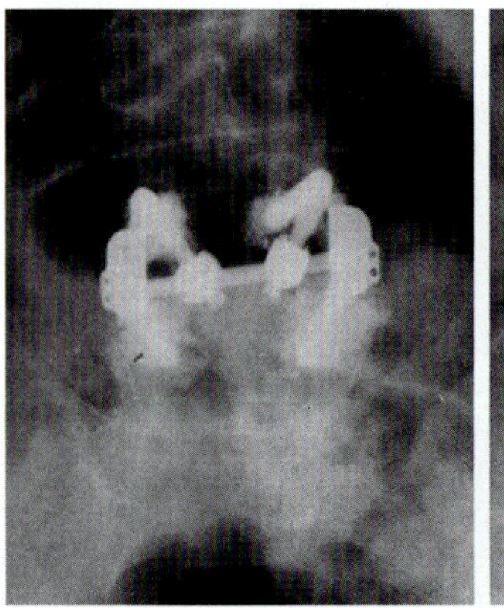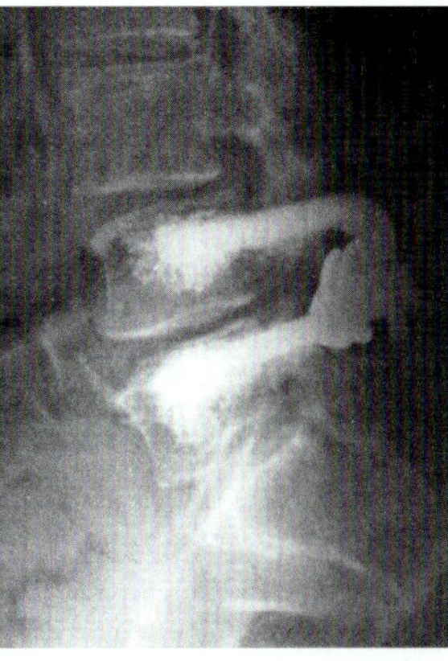

Figure 46–10 Postoperative radiographs of the Total Facet Arthroplasty (TFAS) implant in situ.

balls are held in the neutral position in the caudal cups. Final x-rays are then obtained (**Fig. 46–10**). Closure is performed in the usual fashion.

The patient begins rehab the following day.

◆ Total Facet Arthroplasty System Investigational Device Exemption Clinical Study Inclusion Criteria

◆ Degenerative spinal stenosis, central or lateral, at spinal levels L3–L4 or L4–L5, with radiographic confirmation of any one of the following by computed tomography (CT), magnetic resonance imaging (MRI), plain film, or myelography:

  ◆ Evidence of thecal sac and/or cauda equina compression

  ◆ Evidence of nerve root impingement by either osseous or nonosseous elements

  ◆ Evidence of hypertrophic facets with encroachment into the central canal or lateral recess

◆ No greater than grade I degenerative spondylolisthesis at the stenotic level

◆ Neurogenic claudication, indicated by the presence of persistent leg symptoms, marked by posterior or anterior thigh or calf discomfort, pain, numbness, paresthesia, weakness, tiredness or heaviness, buttock or lower back symptoms including pain, numbness, burning or tingling, that is aggravated by walking or standing and is relieved only after resting in a flexed lumbar spine position

◆ Skeletally mature male or female between the ages of 50 and 80 years of age inclusive

◆ Operative candidates with no more than three levels of degenerative lumbar spinal stenosis requiring decompression (up to three contiguous levels of decompression is allowed; however, only one level is eligible for instrumentation with the TFAS system or control)

◆ Willing and able to sign the informed consent document

◆ Experienced symptoms of neurogenic claudication or functional deficit or both for a minimum duration of 6 months

◆ Failed to respond to nonoperative treatment modalities for a minimum duration of 6 months

◆ Facet Arthroplasty versus Dynamic Stabilization

Currently other technologies being considered for indications similar to those of TFAS can be classified into three categories: interspinous spacers, pedicle-based stabilizers, and facet arthroplasty. Interspinous spacers, although easy to implant and potentially providing the most tissue-sparing "burns-no-bridges" approach, can at most provide some foramen widening and relative positioning of the vertebral bodies but have little to no effect on stenosis caused by encroachment of the foramina due to facet hypertrophy or herniated disks. They can act as an extension stop but are not operational through the whole range of motion, and most importantly they, in general, do not address the disease pathology, are not appropriate for severe stenosis or instability, and provide minimum benefit in lateral bending, axial rotation, or translation due to spondylitic slip, all the while creating potential segmental kyphosis.

Pedicle-based stabilizers are composed of elastomeric cushions and bands, polymeric tethers and pseudoligaments, and metallic constructs that are fixed with the familiar pedicle screw technique. Although they can offload the disk and restore disk height, somewhat limit motion in the case of instability, and can be easily converted to fusion, they don't fully restore natural kinematics. They require a long learning curve and patient-specific surgical techniques to obtain proper stability or dynamization. In addition they are a fairly stiff construct, do not address spondylolisthesis, and are at risk of loss of fixation through screw loosening. In summary, current dynamic stabilizing nonfusion device alternatives do not address all three key functional elements of restoring proper stability, motion, and load sharing. They only preserve whatever motion and stability is available due to the pathology or that is present postsurgery.

Facet replacement devices that are more akin to surface replacements that have small footprints may be useful when replacing an arthritic facet and ligaments specifically for pain, but because of their inherent size and location they offer limited options for fixation. If using currently available biomaterials, due to scale effects brought on by the size of such devices, unacceptably high contact stresses and wear debris would be generated and are a major consideration in the design and performance of such devices. There are also limited means through which to stabilize, transfer loads, and affect the kinematics of the FSU through a full range of motion. Therefore, long-term fixation, restoration of natural motion, and physiological load sharing are a much higher bar to meet for such devices.[12]

◆ Conclusion

Dynamic stabilization makes conceptual sense but the associated biomechanical science is sparse except in the case of TFAS. Clinical experience is the key to determining and expanding proper indications for facet arthroplasty devices, and although the proper kinematic imperative for "posterior stabilization" (i.e., stabilize the structure, preserve existing motion, or restore natural kinematics and load sharing) can be debated, for the posterior elements only the Total Facet Arthroplasty System incorporates all three functional biomechanical elements. Because TFAS is a first-generation device, development efforts are under way to incorporate alternative fixation modes, multiple level applications, as well as conservative and minimally invasive product line extensions. Regardless, one must stay vigilant to determine how these implants may affect the natural trajectory of spinal disease, and what, if any, are the unintended consequences of dynamic stabilization—in an effort to ensure that postoperatively, their function will be clinically successful, and that an additional potential failure mode has not been created at the other locations along the spine.

References

1. Schellinger D, Wener L, Ragsdale BD, Patronas NJ. Facet joint disorders and their role in the production of back pain and sciatica. Radiographics 1987;7:923–944
2. Fujiwara A, Tamai K, Yamato M, et al. The relationship between facet joint osteoarthritis and disc degeneration of the lumbar spine: an MRI study. Eur Spine J 1999;8:396–401
3. Grobler LJ, Robertson PA, Novotny JE, Pope MH. Etiology of spondylolisthesis: assessment of the role played by lumbar facet joint morphology. Spine 1993;18:80–91
4. Huang RC, Lim MR, Girardi FP, Cammisa FP Jr. The prevalence of contraindications to total disc replacement in a cohort of lumbar surgical patients. Spine 2004;29:2538–2541
5. Zhu, et al. Trans. 50th Annual ORS, San Francisco, CA, 2004:1125
6. Zhu, et al. Trans. 51st Annual ORS, Washington, DC, 2005:1125
7. Cripton, et al. Trans. 5th Combined ORS, Banff, Canada, 2004:320
8. Cripton, et al. Roundtables Spine Surg 2005;1:22–29
9. Panjabi. Goel Roundtables Spine Surg 2005;1:45–55
10. Little JS, Ianuzzi A, Chiu JB, Baitner A, Khalsa PS. Human lumbar facet joint capsule strains II: Alteration of strains subsequent to anterior interbody fixation. Spine J 2004;4:153–162
11. Moumene M. The effect of artificial disc placement on facet loading: mobile core us fixed core In Goel VK, Panjab MM, eds. Roundtables on Spine Surgery, Spine Biomechanics: Evaluation of motion preservation devices and relevant terminology. 2005, vol 1, No. 1:38–4
12. Shaw, et al. Trans. 51st Annual ORS, Washington, DC, 2005:1263

Section III

Restoration of Lumbar Motion Segment
E. Annular Repair

47

Indications and Techniques in Annuloplasty

Michael Y. Wang

◆ **Treatment Indications and Strategy**

◆ **Annular Anatomy and Function**

◆ **Treatment following Microdiskectomy**
  The Rationale for Preventing Reherniations
  Surgical Strategies

◆ **Treatment of Symptomatic Annular Tears**
  The Argument for Treating Annular Pathology
  Interventional Strategies

◆ **Treatment after Placement of Intervertebral Prostheses**

◆ **Conclusion**

◆ Treatment Indications and Strategy

Although annular repair techniques are in their infancy, this area has been the subject of intense recent investigation. Reconstruction or restoration of this component of the lumbar spine is appealing for several reasons. The annulus fibrosus gives the intervertebral disk its mechanical integrity. As such, disruption of its architecture, whether through degenerative processes or surgical intervention, has significant implications for the mechanical function of the lumbar spinal column. Currently, there are three major areas where annular repair may find clinical utility:

1. Prophylactic treatment following microdiskectomy to prevent subsequent degeneration or reherniations

2. Treatment of fissures and tears believed to be causing axial back pain symptoms

3. Replication of connective tissue barriers and mechanical structures following insertion of intervertebral prostheses

◆ Annular Anatomy and Function

The annulus fibrosus is a fibrous ring composed primarily of type I collagen and elastin. Its fibers are oriented in a lamellar pattern around the circumference of this ring in roughly a dozen distinct layers. The fibers within each layer are organized in a parallel fashion oriented at 70 degree angles to the adjacent layers. These fibers have a high tensile strength and serve to contain the nucleus pulposus. The nucleus is composed primarily of type II collagen and proteoglycans, which retain a high water content to give it a deformable jellylike consistency. The annulus and nucleus thus work in concert like an inflated radial tire.

In the healthy intervertebral disk axial, compressive forces transmit pressure to the nucleus, resulting in annular tension. The two structures are thus well designed to handle these physical forces. However, progressive disk degeneration leads to mechanical incompetency of the disk. Early degeneration involves loss of nuclear water content. The decreased turgor within the disk causes slackening of the annulus. Axial compressive forces then result in compression and deformation of the annular tissue instead of tension, forces that the annulus withstands poorly. A cascade of pathology can then result, including fissuring of the annulus, nonuniform loading of the vertebral end plates, irritation of local nerve fibers, herniations of disk materials outside the annulus, abnormal facet joint loading, and loss of spinal alignment.

In addition, the annulus is intricately associated with the anterior longitudinal ligament (ALL) and posterior longitudinal ligament (PLL) to constrain motion in multiple planes. Both degenerative and iatrogenic events will frequently involve these ligamentous structures as well.

Attempts at annular repair thus focus on restoring one or more of the functional roles of the annulus. Specifically, annuloplasty can be directed at (1) repairing defects to appropriately retain nuclear material; (2) treating symptomatic, painful disruptions in the connective tissues; and (3) restoring the biomechanical functions of the annulus.

◆ Treatment following Microdiskectomy

The Rationale for Preventing Reherniations

Approximately 500,000 lumbar diskectomies are performed each year in the United States. Although some of these procedures involve an intervertebral fusion or total disk replacement, most are for the removal of frank herniations causing nerve root compression.[1] In this setting the herniations can be either contained within the annulus and result in a large, broad-based mass impinging on the nerve root, or the herniations may have ruptured through the annular ring and lie in proximity to the thecal sac and nerve root. One of the concerns regarding surgery for symptomatic disk herniations

"

is the recurrence of symptoms from reherniation. This can result from defects in the annular wall from rupture and extrusion of free fragments or may be due to an annulotomy created at the time of surgery to remove a contained herniation. Several strategies have thus been developed to minimize the risk of reherniations. One approach is to reduce trauma to the annulus by limiting the surgical dissection to removal of only the free fragment, leaving the remainder of the disk undisturbed. This conservative approach, the Williams' sequestrectomy, theoretically causes less annular disruption at the time of surgery, reducing reherniations.[2] An alternative approach is to clean the disk space thoroughly at the time of surgery to ensure that there are no loose fragments that are prone to later herniation.

Despite these efforts, symptomatic disk reherniations are not infrequent, occurring in 5 to 15% of patients. In one study by Carragee et al, lumbar disk herniations were classified into four categories based on intraoperative findings: fragment-fissure herniations, fragment-defect herniations, fragment-contained herniations, and no fragment–contained herniations. As expected, annular competence was found to be associated with the rate of reherniation. Patients in the fragment-fissure group with small annular defects had the lowest rates of reherniation (1%), and patients in the fragment-defect group, with extruded fragments and large posterior annular defects, had a 27% rate of reherniation.[3] These findings suggest that repair of the annulus may serve functionally to contain any reherniations.

Surgical Strategies

Annular repair strategies to combat this phenomenon have taken two pathways. The first involves the instillation of a replacement nuclear material that binds to the native disk. This theoretically fills the diskectomy void to maintain nuclear bulk and mechanically adhere any and connective tissue fragments. In addition, the annular defect is sealed to prevent reherniations. The NuCore Injectable Nucleus (SpineWave, Inc., Shelton, CT), consisting of injectable nuclear protein, was primarily developed as a nucleus replacement but also seals the annulus. In the clinical setting, the gel is utilized after completion of the microdiskectomy. The proprietary injectate is then instilled into the center of the disk space through a double-barrel syringe catheter. The two injectates mix in situ to form a semisolid adhesive gel. Although not yet available in North America, clinical experience is being developed in Europe, and NuCore is due to begin investigational trials in the United States in 2006. Another polymeric injectable that has the potential to repair annular defects is the BioDisc (Cryolife, Kennesaw, GA). This device is currently starting to be used in the United Kingdom, but no trials in the United States have been scheduled.

The second strategy for annular reconstruction involves placement of a suturable or anchored patch to repair the defect in the annulus. One device consists of a flexible polymeric sheet that is secured in place over the annular defect using sutures, which are anchored to the vertebral end plates (Annulex Technologies, Inc., Maple Grove, MN) (**Fig. 47–1**).[4] In this fashion, any reherniated tissue will be retained within the disk space. Although not yet commercially available, these devices will likely be available for use in the United States in 2006.

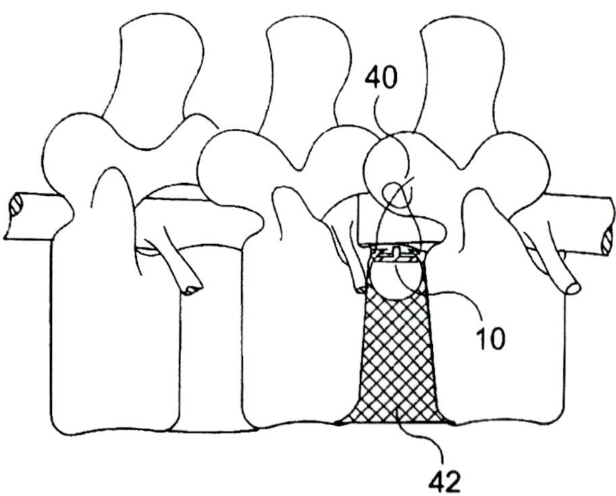

Figure 47–1   Anchored annular repair patch device (U.S. Patent no. 6,592,625 B2).

◆ Treatment of Symptomatic Annular Tears

The Argument for Treating Annular Pathology

The diagnosis and treatment of diskogenic back pain has advanced greatly over the past decade, but substantial controversy still surrounds this area. The notion that damage to the intervertebral disk can result in axial back pain, independent of spinal nerve root compression, is intuitive. The lumbar disks are subject to substantial cyclic mechanical loading with resultant degeneration consisting of dehydration of the central nucleus pulposus and reduced elasticity of the annular fibers. The abnormal degenerated disk is then prone to trauma-induced disruption of the annulus. Pain can then result from several mechanisms. Nociceptive nerve endings in the disk or vertebral end plate can be mechanically irritated, chemical irritants from within the nucleus can be released, and abnormal spinal biomechanics may trigger remote pain generators.

Early stages of disk degeneration can be appreciated radiographically. Reductions in nuclear water content cause a loss in intervertebral height and changes in the signal characteristics on magnetic resonance imaging (MRI). This is most commonly appreciated as a "black disk" on T2-weighted MRI reflecting the loss of the normal nuclear signal characteristics (**Fig. 47–2**). Abnormalities in the annulus can also be appreciated as "high intensity zones," believed to represent disruptions in its highly organized architecture.[5,6] First described by Aprill and Bogduk in 1992, this appears as a high signal intensity (white) area within the posterior disk space.[7] However, the significance of these MR findings is still a topic of debate.

Diskography, which involves the direct injection of radiocontrast dye into the nucleus pulposus, provides direct visualization of disruptions in the annular architecture. Fissurelike cracks in the posterior annulus result in mechanical incompetence and dye leakage through the outer ring and even into the spinal canal (**Fig. 47–3**).

Interventional Strategies

Even surgeons who believe in the concept of diskogenic pain from annular injury will frequently disagree over the proper

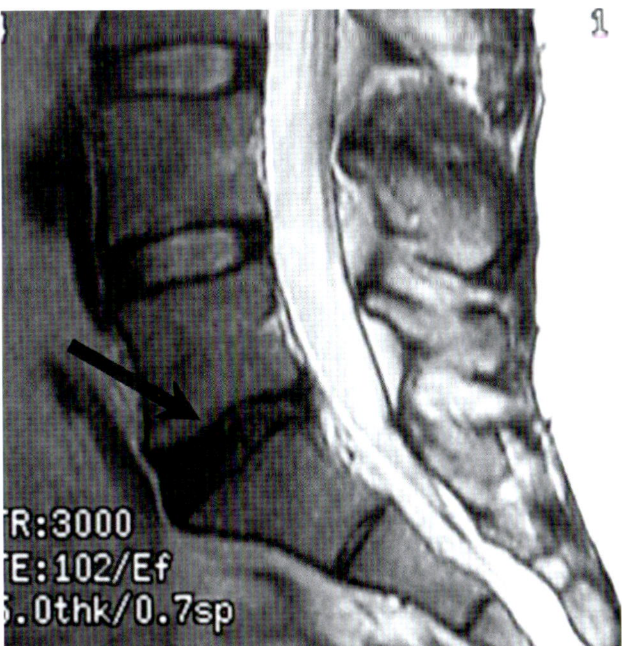

Figure 47–2 Isolated "black disk" at the L5–S1 level on T2-weighted sagittal magnetic resonance imaging (arrow).

diagnostic criteria and treatment measures. Surgical correction of the pathology is performed with a lumbar interbody fusion or total disk replacement. However, the morbidity of these surgical procedures for the treatment of relatively early degenerative changes can be prohibitive, particularly for young adult patients. For these reasons, less destructive and minimally invasive procedures have been developed to target the pathology directly.

Intradiskal electrothermy (IDET) (Smith & Nephew, Memphis, TN) was innovated in the late 1990s to treat this population of patients. The procedure involves percutaneous parapedicular insertion of a radiofrequency catheter into the intervertebral disk space. The lead is then coiled under fluoroscopic guidance through the disk and into the posterior annulus. The tip of the probe is then activated, heating the surrounding disk tissues (**Fig. 47–4**). The mechanism of action by which IDET exerts its clinical effect is poorly understood. Proposed mechanisms include the contraction of collagen with "tightening of the annulus" to improve the biomechanics of the disk, the coagulation and denervation of annular nociceptors, and the reduction in size of disk herniations impinging upon the nerve roots.

Heating of the annulus fibrosus to treat annular degeneration has been studied by Freeman et al in an ovine model. The study involved creating surgical incisions in the lumbar disks of sheep to mimic the annular tears seen in humans. Radiofrequency electrothermy was then performed 12 weeks later in an attempt to denervate and repair the annular lesion. During the procedure the mean maximum temperature in the posterior annulus was 64°C, and the mean maximum temperature in the nucleus was 67°C. Histological analysis demonstrated thermal necrosis of the inner annulus and nearby nucleus, sparing the peripheral disk, but there was no change in the number of nerve fibers in the posterior annulus.[8] Shah et al's cadaveric study showed that IDET effected increased temperatures in the outer annulus, gross macroscopic changes, and circumferential tissue alterations localized to the posterior annulus but not extending to the end plates. Histological changes included posterior lumbar disk denaturation, shrinkage, and coalescence of annular collagen. Electron microscopy showed collagen disorganization, decreased collagen quantity and fibril shrinkage, and chondrocyte damage.[9] Pollintine et al's cadaveric study

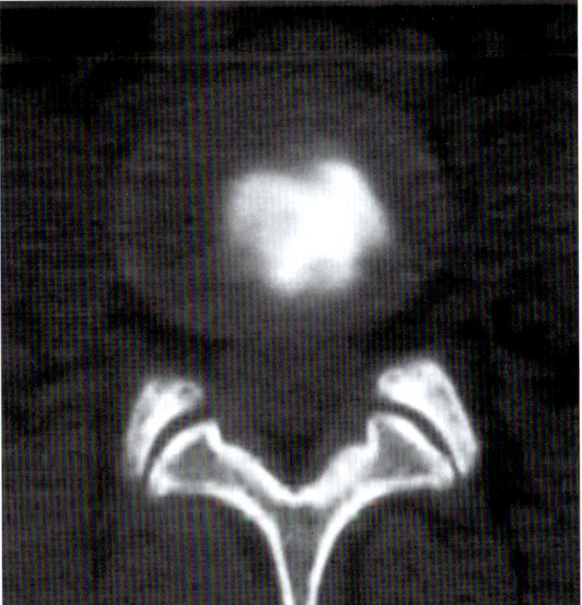

A

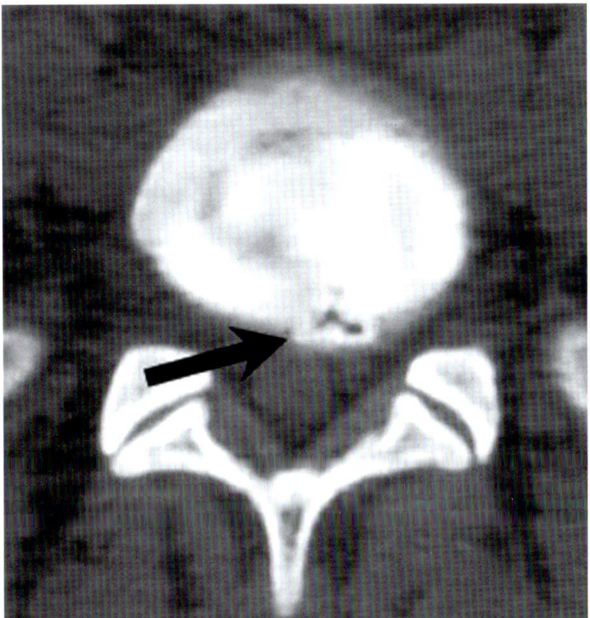

B

Figure 47–3 Same patient as in **Fig. 47–2** with a postdiskogram computed tomographic (CT) scan. **(A)** L4–L5 showing contrast distribution in a healthy disk postinjection. **(B)** Axial CT image of L5–S1 showing contrast leakage through annular fissures to the spinal canal (arrow).

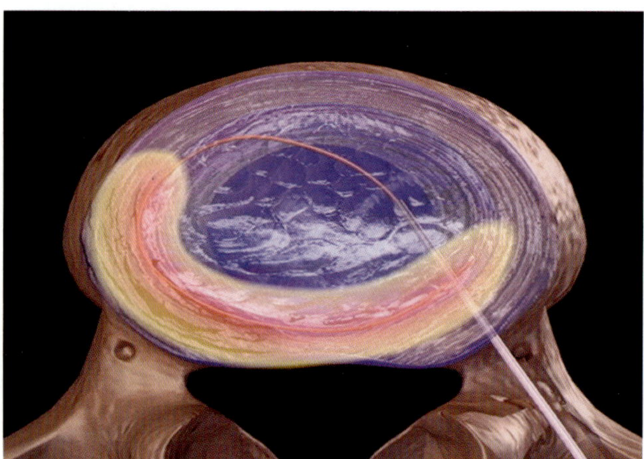

Figure 47–4   Artist's rendition of an intradiskal electrothermy (IDET) device inserted into the disk space, coiling so that the heating radiofrequency tip and heating area (gray zone) is located in the posterior annulus. (Figure courtesy of Smith & Nephew.)

demonstrated heating of the annulus to 40°C with concomitant biomechanical alterations.[10] Post-treatment nuclear pressures were decreased 6 to 13%, and annular stress concentrations were reduced by an average 0.28 MPa.

Initial clinical results by the innovators of IDET suggested excellent clinical results. In one study of 62 patients with chronic low back pain followed for an average of 16 months, visual analog scores improved an average of three points. Symptoms improved in 71% of patients.[11] However, subsequent studies have shown less efficacy.[10,12,13] Davis et al's study of 60 patients with positive diskography showed that at 1 year post-IDET, 97% continued to have back pain. Furthermore, six patients went on to have open surgery within 1 year. Fifty percent were dissatisfied with IDET, and only 53% would have the procedure again.[14]

An alternative method for energy delivery is the use of ultrasound. The Ultrazonix system (Ultrazonix, Malmö, Sweden) employs high-intensity focused ultrasound energy to the intervertebral disk. The procedure involves percutaneous insertion of a probe with a piezo-ceramic tip vibrating at high frequency. This technique also results in effective heating of the surrounding tissues to over 65°C.[15]

◆ Treatment after Placement of Intervertebral Prostheses

The development of motion-preservation devices for the spine has brought new concerns related to implant performance because continued motion leads to prolonged mechanical stresses in the functional spine unit (FSU). In this setting, the expectation is that disk arthroplasty and nuclear replacement devices will provide near-normal kinematics over many decades. Two concerns subsequently arise. First, the insertion of a large intradiskal prosthesis requires disruption of the annulus along with either the ALL or PLL. This disruption affects the biomechanical performance of the FSU. Although contemporary disk replacement techniques do not involve reconstruction of the annulus or ALL/PLL, future devices may benefit from such a repair because, biomechanically, the ALL and anterior annulus serve as an important tension band in spinal extension. Investigations are under way to apply porcine small intestinal submucosa (SIS) grafts to reconstruct the annulus/ALL following anterior disk arthroplasty. SIS has tremendous tensile durability and is beginning to find use in extremity joint ligament repair. Such an approach may serve to improve the biomechanical function of artificial disks.[16]

The second concern relates to intradiskal device extrusion. One of the major concerns over the first generation of nuclear replacement devices was the high extrusion rate. In one study of the PDN (prosthetic disk nucleus) (Raymedica, Inc., Minneapolis, MN), three of 33 patients had extrusions at 1-year follow-up.[17] For devices inserted posteriorly, dislodgment has led to compression of the cauda equina in select cases, and these concerns eventually resulted in withdrawal of the implants from the marketplace. In addition, the extrusion of polyethylene cores of certain arthroplasty implants has led to significant concerns over the safety of these devices.[18] In both instances, reconstruction of the annular rim and ALL/PLL could be beneficial to prevent these implant failures.

◆ Conclusion

Annular repair strategies are currently in their infancy. Critics would suggest that the treatment of annular disease is premature because our current understanding of annular biomechanics, nociception, and biology is inadequate. However, this emerging field holds great promise. The application of new implantable materials and devices coupled with biological strategies may prove more effective than contemporary approaches. As our understanding of the role of chemokines (such as fibroblast growth factors, transforming growth factor-b, and osteonectin) and disk matrix constituents (such as proteoglycans, collagen I, and collagen IX) advances, biological treatments for annular degeneration may be realized.[19–21] Ultimately, biological disk regeneration or replacement or both will have the potential to supplant our contemporary treatments for diskogenic low back pain.

References

1. MedMarket Diligence. Tissue engineering and transplantation: Products, technologies, and market opportunities, 2003–2013. Foothill Ranch, CA: Drug and Market Development Publishing; 2003

2. Wenger M, Mariani L, Kalbarczyk A, Groger U. Long-term outcome of 104 patients after lumbar sequestrectomy according to Williams. Neurosurgery 2001;49:329–335

3. Carragee EJ, Han MY, Suen PW, Kim D. Clinical outcomes after lumbar discectomy for sciatica: the effects of fragment type and annular competence. Spine 2003;28:2602–2608

4. U.S. Patent no. 6,592,625 B2. July 15, 2003

5. Saifuddin A, McSweeney E, Lehovsky J. Development of lumbar high intensity zone on axial loaded magnetic resonance imaging. Spine 2003;28:E449–E451

6. Lim CH, Jee WH, Son BC, Kim DH, Ha KY, Park CK. Discogenic lumbar pain: association with MR imaging and CT discography. Eur J Radiol 2005;54:431–437

7. Aprill C, Bogduk N. "High intensity zone": a diagnostic sign of painful lumbar disc on magnetic resonance imaging. Br J Radiol 1992;65:361–369

8. Freeman B, Walters R, Moore R, Fraser R. Does intradiscal electrothermal therapy denervate and repair experimentally induced posterolateral annular tears in an animal model? J Bone Joint Surg Am. 2003;85-A(1):102–108

9. Shah R, Lutz G, Lee J, Doty S, Rodeo S. Intradiskal electrothermal therapy: a preliminary histologic study. Arch Phys Med Rehabil 2001; 82:1230–1237

10. Pollintine P, Findlay G, Adams M. Intradiscal electrothermal therapy can alter compressive stress distributions inside degenerated intervertebral discs. Spine 2005;30:E134–E139

11. Saal J, Saal J. Intradiscal electrothermal treatment for chronic discogenic low back pain: a prospective outcome study with minimum 1-year follow-up. Spine 2000;25:2622–2627

12. Freeman BJ, Fraser RD, Cain CM, Hall DJ, Chapple DC. A randomized, double-blind, controlled trial: intradiscal electrothermal therapy versus placebo for the treatment of chronic discogenic low back pain. Spine 2005;30:2369–2377

13. Spruit M, Jacobs W. Pain and function after intradiscal electrothermal treatment (IDET) for symptomatic lumbar disc degeneration. Eur Spine J 2002;11:589–593

14. Davis T, Delamarter R, Sra P, Goldstein T. The IDET procedure for chronic discogenic low back pain. Spine 2004;29:752–756

15. Persson J, Strömqvist B, Zanoli G, McCarthy I, Lidgren L. Ultrasound nucleolysis: an in vitro study. Ultrasound Med Biol 2002;28:1189–1197

16. Ledet E, Carl A, DiRisio D, Tymeson MP, Andersen LB, Shee han CE, et al. A pilot study to evaluate the effectiveness of small intestinal submucosa used to repair spinal ligaments in the goat. Spine J 2002;2:188–196

17. Shim C, Park C, Lee H, Choi W, Choi W, Lee S. An early experience of prosthetic disc nucleus in Korea. Paper presented at: AANS/CNS Joint Spine Section Annual Meeting, March 5, 2003

18. van Ooij A, Oner FC, Verbout AJ. Complications of artificial disc replacement. J Spinal Disord 2003;16:369–383

19. Melrose J, Smith S, Little C, Kitson J, Hwa S, Ghosh P. Spatial and temporal localization of transforming growth factor-beta, fibroblast growth factor-2, and osteonectin, and identification of cells expressing alpha-smooth muscle actin in the injured anulus fibrosus: implications for extracellular matrix repair. Spine 2002;27:1756–1764

20. Melrose J, Ghosh P, Taylor T, Vernon-Roberts B, Latham J, Moore R. Elevated synthesis of biglycan and decorin in an ovine annular lesion model of experimental disc degeneration. Eur Spine J 1997;6: 376–384

21. Thompson J, Oegema T, Bradford D. Stimulation of mature canine intervertebral disc by growth factors. Spine 1991;16:253–260

Section IV

Future Biological Approaches to Disk Repair

48

Molecular Therapy of the Intervertebral Disk

S. Tim Yoon

◆ **Anticatabolics**

◆ **Mitogens**

◆ **Morphogens**

◆ **Intracellular Regulators**

◆ **Summary**

Biological treatment of disk degeneration encompasses a large diversity of different therapeutic approaches.[1–14] In broad categories, the therapeutic strategies under investigation involve the use of cells, matrix, or molecules. This chapter focuses on the molecular therapy approaches to treat disk degeneration. The term *therapeutic molecule* will be used as a broader way of encompassing all molecules that may be therapeutic but may not be classic "growth factors." This terminology is important because growth factors are defined by their effect on mitosis; however, effective therapeutic molecules may have therapeutic activity unrelated to cell replication. The therapeutic molecules can be categorized as anticatabolics, mitogens, chondrogenic morphogens, or intracellular regulatory molecules (**Table 48–1**). This chapter reviews key literature and defines each of these categories.

Table 48–1 Categories of Therapeutic Molecules

Category	Molecule
Anticatabolic	TIMP-1
	TIMP-2
Mitogens	IGF-1
	PDGF
	EGF
	FGF
Morphogen	TGF-b
	BMP-2
	BMP-7 (OP-1)
	BMP-13 (GDF-6 aka CDMP-2)
	GDF-5 (CDMP-1)
	Link N
Intracellular regulators	SMADs
	Sox9
	LMP-1

BMP, bone morphogenetic protein; CDMP, cartilage-derived morphogenetic protein; EGF, epidermal growth factor; FGF, fibroblast growth factor; GDF, growth and differentiation factors; IGF, insulin-like growth factor; LMP, LIM Mineralization protein-1; OP-1, osteogenic protein-1; PDGF, platelet-derived growth factor; SMAD, T/C; TGF-b, transforming growth factor-beta; TIMP, tissue inhibitors of matrix metalloproteinases.

To better understand molecular therapy strategies, it is important to understand the hallmarks of disk degeneration. These include loss of proteoglycan, water, and collagen II in the disk matrix in the nucleus pulposus. There are qualitative changes in the matrix that are less well defined, including loss of the higher molecular weight proteoglycans and other changes that are more difficult to quantify (collagen cross-linking, organization of the proteoglycan, etc.). An important change seems to be the loss of the differentiated chondrocyte phenotype from the nucleus pulposus into a more fibrotic phenotype. Changes in the annulus fibrosus include disorganization of the annular lamella layers and physical defects in the collagenous matrix. Typically, these matrix changes take many years to become apparent and are most likely a result of an imbalance between synthesis and degradation (**Fig. 48–1**). The goal of molecular therapy is to prevent or reverse these changes in the disk extracellular matrix by altering the balance of degradation to synthesis in favor of synthesis.

◆ Anticatabolics

Because matrix loss is a balance between matrix synthesis versus degradation, it is possible to increase disk matrix by increasing synthesis or by decreasing degradation. One approach is to prevent matrix loss by inhibiting the degradative enzymes. There are many different catabolic enzymes present in normal disk matrix, but the matrix metalloproteinases (MMPs) make up a particularly important group of catabolic enzymes.[15] MMPs play an important role in the normal turnover of matrix molecules and are probably important in disk degeneration.[16] Degenerated disks have elevated levels of MMPs, providing circumstantial evidence to support this hypothesis. Within the matrix, MMP activity is normally inhibited by tissue inhibitors of MMPs (TIMPs).[15,17] Wallach et al tested whether one of these anticatabolic molecules, TIMP-1, could increase the accumulation of matrix proteoglycans in in vitro experiments using an adenoviral gene therapy approach.[18] Wallach et al found that, indeed, TIMP-1 expression in disk

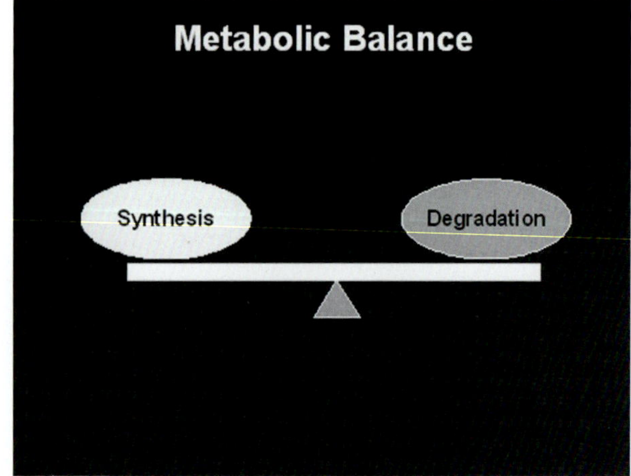

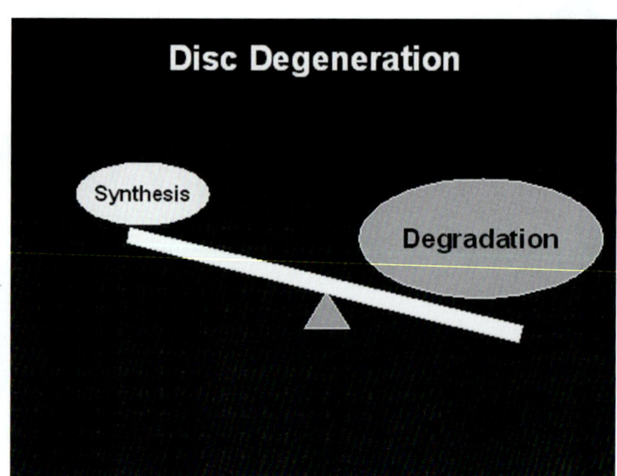

A

B

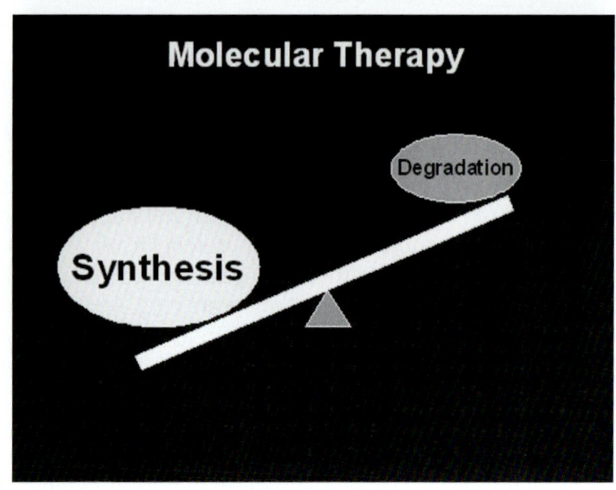

C

Figure 48–1   Disk matrix metabolism: balance of synthesis and degradation. **(A)** In the homeostatic state, the disk undergoes matrix synthesis and degradation in a balanced manner. **(B)** As the disk matrix undergoes turnover over the course of an individual's lifetime, any small imbalance between synthesis and degradation can lead to significant changes in overall disk matrix content. **(C)** One of the major goals of molecular therapy of the disk involves modulating this metabolic balance to the more favorable anabolic state. This can be accomplished by increasing synthesis or by decreasing catabolism.

cells increased accumulation and also increased the "measured synthesis rate" of proteoglycans. Another promising molecule is CPA-926 an esculetin prodrug that has a better pharmacokinetic profile than esculetin itself.[19] CPA-926 has been shown to be anti-inflammatory and antitumorigenic and to prevent degeneration in an osteoarthritic model of cartilage destruction.[19] Okuma et al showed that oral administration of CPA-926 can prevent or delay the onset of disk height loss and histological evidence of disk degeneration in an annulotomy model of disk degeneration in the rabbit.[19]

Along with the balance of synthesis and degradation, the rate of disk matrix metabolism may also be important. For example, the overall rate of disk metabolism in young disks may be much higher than in old disks. This may lead to qualitative changes in disk matrix such as the composition of degraded aggrecan versus newly synthesized aggrecan molecules. The overall metabolic rate may also dictate the nutritional requirements of the intradiskal cells. Cytokines such as interleukin (IL)-1 and tumor necrosis factor-alpha (TNF-a) may have critical roles in disk metabolism. Therefore, molecules such as IL-1Ra and infliximab, which can block IL-1 and TNF-a, respectively, may be useful.[20–22] Further research into anticatabolic molecules may yield important results.

◆ Mitogens

Mitogens are defined by the propensity of the molecule to increase the rate of mitosis. These molecules constitute the true growth factors, and for purposes of this review, we will differentiate mitogenic growth factors from the set of molecules that are highly chondrogenic (**Fig. 48–2**). These mitogenic molecules include insulin-like growth factor-1 (IGF-1), epidermal growth factor (EGF), and fibroblast growth factor (FGF).[23] Thompson et al[23] demonstrated in vitro experiments with mature canine disk cells that mitogenic molecules can increase the rate of mitosis and proteoglycan synthesis rates to various degrees depending on which region of the disk the cells were derived from. In general, EGF performed better than the other mitogens.[23] IGF-1 levels decrease in an age-dependent manner in rat disks.[24] Researchers have speculated that by restoring the IGF-1 in aging disks that perhaps matrix synthesis may be increased. In vivo experiments with growth factors using a mouse tail disk compression model for degeneration by Walsh et al[25] produced results that were consistent with in vitro experiments by Thompson et al.[23] IGF-1 had mild effects (especially in the inner annulus) and FGF had no effect. In a related but different potential mechanism of therapy, some growth factors may protect disk cells from death by apoptosis. Gruber et al[26] showed that disk

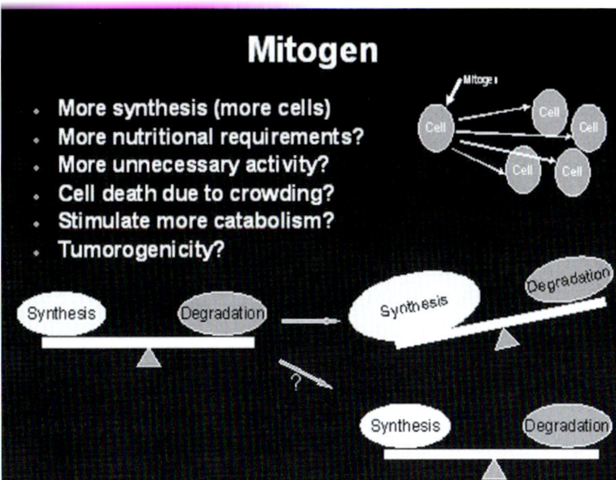

Figure 48–2 Mitogenic molecules are the true growth factors. They increase cell number without necessarily enhancing cell differentiation. The increase in cell number leads to increase in matrix synthesis. However, this may also increase the nutritional requirement in the disk due to higher overhead of keeping the cell alive and perhaps increase the overall catabolism as well as synthesis. Furthermore, very high cell density can lead to cell death with decreases in disk nutrition. Finally, mitogens may have a higher likelihood of causing tumors as opposed to morphogens, which increase cell differentiation.

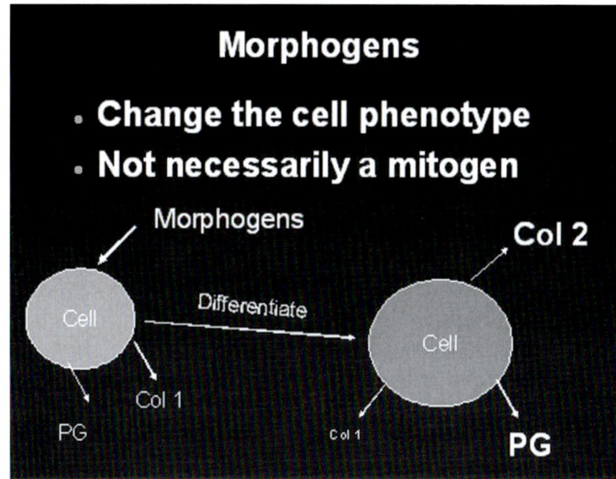

Figure 48–3 Morphogenic molecules change the phenotype of the cell as their major mechanism of action without necessarily increasing the cell number. In the disk, morphogens may be used to increase the chondrocytelike phenotype of the cells and enhance chondrocytic matrix synthesis.

cells in vitro placed in low serum conditions underwent apoptosis; however, this was prevented to a certain degree by the addition of insulinlike growth factor (IGF-1) or platelet-derived growth factor (PDGF). Although IGF-1 has some anabolic effects, it may also have an effect on catabolism because IGF-1 was shown to decrease the levels of active TIMP-2 in tissue culture experiments, indicating a complex effect on disk matrix metabolism by IGF-1.

◆ Morphogens

Chondrogenic morphogens are cytokines that may have mitogenic capability but are really characterized by their ability to increase the chondrocyte-specific phenotype of the cell (**Fig. 48–3**). Specifically, these chondrocyte-specific characteristics are the production of collagen II, Sox9, aggrecan, and sulfated-glycosaminoglycans. Most of the research in chondrogenic morphogens has been with transforming growth factor-beta (TGF-b), bone morphogenetic proteins (BMPs), or growth and differentiation factors (GDFs). Chondrogenic morphogens are particularly attractive because they may reverse the fibrotic phenotype of disk cells to the more chondrocytic phenotype of disk nucleus cells in younger and more "normal" disk. By definition, these molecules are secreted molecules and hence can potentially act in autocrine, paracrine, and endocrine fashion. The ability of cytokines to diffuse and affect many different cells makes cytokines very powerful. The activity of the prototypical chondrogenic morphogen is dependent on the presence of receptor molecules on the extracellular surface of the responding cells and the presence of a competent intracellular messenger system. Interestingly, disk cells have been shown to express TGF and BMP molecules and receptors, and the expression level and spatial distribution seem to change with the aging process.[27,28]

TGF-b1 is one of the first disk morphogenic molecules studied. Thompson et al reported that TGF-b1 was a mitogen but also showed that it was a highly anabolic molecule leading to significantly increased proteoglycan synthesis per cell.[23] Thompson et al reported that TGF-b1 was superior to growth factors such as EGF, IGF-1, PDGF, and FGF in increasing proteoglycan synthesis rate per cell.[23] Subsequently, Nishida et al demonstrated that an adenoviral vector containing the TGF-b1 gene can be directly injected into immunocompetent rabbit (normal) disks in vivo and lead to expression of TGF-b1 and increased rate of proteoglycan synthesis.[29] In vitro experiments with cells from degenerated human disks indicated that TGF-b1 can increase proteoglycan and collagen synthesis rates, suggesting that cells from even degenerated disks are capable of responding to TGF-b1.[30,31] In vivo experiments in mouse tail disks indicated that TGF-b1 had some effect on cell proliferation in the inner annulus, but TGF-b1 did not effect measurable change in the disk height.[25] Although TGF-b1 has potential, its efficacy in in vivo degeneration models has not yet been established.

BMP-2 is another prototypic chondrogenic morphogen. Hutton et al reported that recombinant human BMP-2 increased rat disk cell proteoglycan production and significantly increased the chondrocytic phenotype of the disk cells as demonstrated by increased aggrecan and collagen II gene expression while there was no change in collagen I gene expression.[32] Kim et al reported that BMP-2 can partially reverse the inhibitory effect of nicotine on disk cell proteoglycan synthesis.[33] Because BMP-2 is well known to promote the terminal differentiation of osteoblasts during bone formation, there was initially some concern that BMP-2 may also lead to disk cell differentiation along the osteoblastic lineage. However, in vitro experiments with human disk cells demonstrated that BMP-2 enhances the expression of chondrocytic genes but not osteogenic genes.[34] Further evidence of BMP-2 anabolic effects on disk cells have been reported with the use of a gene therapy approach within vitro human disk cells obtained during elective spinal surgery.[18] As of yet, there are no published reports on the BMP-2 efficacy of treating disk degeneration in in vivo models; however, this is currently a highly active area of research.

BMP-7, also known as osteogenic protein (OP-1), is another potent disk cell morphogen.[7–9] Masuda et al reported that rabbit disk cells from both the annulus fibrosus and the nucleus pulposus grown in vitro are stimulated by BMP-7 in a dose-dependent manner.[7] In response to BMP-7, the disk cells increased proteoglycan synthesis and increased the expression of chondrocytic genes aggrecan and collagen II. Takegami et al demonstrated that rabbit disk cells grown in alginate in the presence of the inflammatory cytokine IL-1 leads to loss of proteoglycan and collagen in the alginate as compared with controls.[9] However, adding BMP-7 at 200 ng/mL to the IL-1 culture led to increased synthesis of proteoglycan and collagen even compared with the controls without IL-1. Zhang et al reported that in vitro cultured bovine disk cells from three distinct spatial zones (outer annulus, inner annulus, and nucleus) all increased cellular proliferation in the presence of BMP-7.[8] However, only cells from the outer annulus and nucleus increased the rate of proteoglycan synthesis in the presence of BMP-7. Preliminary in vivo experiments with BMP-7 in rabbit models of disk degeneration have been presented and seem quite promising. These experiments show that direct intradiskal injection of BMP-7 increases disk height and proteoglycan content in rabbits.[35] Preliminary data also indicate that intradiskal injection of BMP-7 may be effective in treating an experimental rabbit disk degeneration model using a small annulotomy.[8,36]

BMP-13 is also known as GDF-6 or cartilage-derived morphogenetic protein-2 (CDMP-2).[37] Although BMP-13 is in the BMP family, BMP-13 has only 50% homology to BMP-2 in amino acid sequence.[38] Experiments with a cartilage cell line indicated that BMP-13 does increase proteoglycan synthesis rate and chondrocytic phenotype, but BMP-13 was much less potent than BMP-2. The effects of adding both BMP-2 and BMP-13 were additive, although there was no synergism between the two morphogens in proteoglycan production or chondrocytic gene expression.[38] BMP-13 is not a recombinant protein that is manufactured in large quantities such as BMP-2 or BMP-7, and therefore research that requires larger quantities of recombinant BMP-13 has been difficult to accomplish.

GDF-5 is also known as CDMP-1.[37] During embryogenesis, GDF-5 is predominantly found at the stage of precartilaginous mesenchymal condensation and throughout the cartilaginous cores of the developing long bones.[37] Walsh et al compared GDF-5, TGF-b1, IGF-1, and FGF in ability to treat a mouse tail disk degeneration model.[25] Of the four molecules tested, GDF-5 was the only molecule that increased the disk height as compared with saline controls. Furthermore, there seemed to be some increase in cellular proliferation in the middle and inner annulus and transitional zone as seen on histological sections. However, repeated injection induced an inflammatory response, which the authors speculate was due to the injury of the injections, not necessarily the GDF-5, because even the saline group had similar inflammatory changes. A gene therapy approach was used by Wang et al to demonstrate that GDF-5 delivered by an adenovirus promoted the growth of disk cells cultured in vitro.[39] GDF-5 is

being developed commercially for spinal fusion application; therefore, larger quantities of recombinant protein are available, making it easier to perform in vivo experiments.

Link N is an amino-terminal fragment of link protein that was shown by Mwale et al to have stimulatory activity on disk cells.[40] Pellet culture experiments indicated that Link N increased proteoglycan production modestly but did not increase cell number in a statistically significant fashion. More interestingly, collagen type II production was increased by 113% in cells derived from the nucleus pulposus and 25% in cells derived from the annulus fibrosus. The mechanism by which Link N induces the specific upregulation of an important chondrocyte marker (collagen II) without much effect on cell number is not yet clear. However, these findings allow categorization of Link N as a chondrogenic morphogen.

◆ Intracellular Regulators

Intracellular regulators are a class of molecules that are distinct because they are not secreted molecules and do not work through transmembrane receptors (**Fig. 48–4**). These molecules are neither cytokines nor growth factors in the classic sense, and yet they can have effects that are quite similar to the secreted molecules discussed earlier. This class of molecules typically controls one or more aspects of cellular differentiation. For instance, SMADs are intracellular molecules that mediate BMP-receptor signaling.[41,42] Although there are no specific published papers on the effect of SMADs on disk cells, SMADs such as SMAD-1 and SMAD-5 are predicted to induce similar effects on disk cells as BMP-2, such as increasing proteoglycan and collagen II synthesis.

Sox9 is a chondrocyte marker that is a positive regulator of collagen II messenger ribonucleic acid (mRNA) transcription.[6,43,44] Paul et al demonstrated that Sox9 delivered by adenovirus can increase Sox9 expression and disk cell collagen II production in vitro.[45] When injected in vivo, the adenovirus-Sox9 construct prevented histological evidence of degenerative changes in the disk in a rabbit

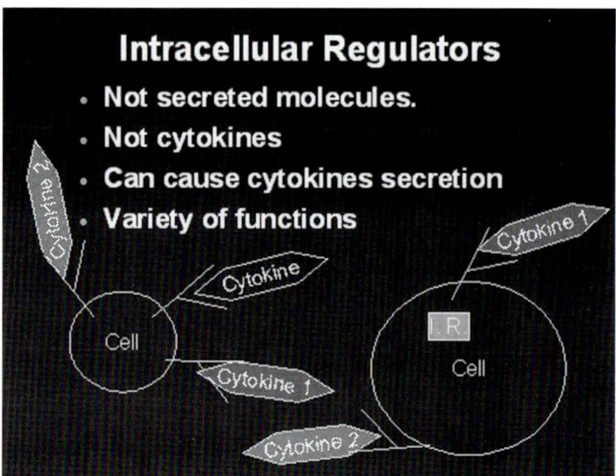

Figure 48–4 Intracellular regulatory molecules are differentiated from cytokines because intracellular molecules are not secreted molecules that act through a transmembrane receptor. Intracellular regulators, however, can induce the secretion of cytokines to act in autocrine or paracrine fashion or directly upregulate matrix production.

annulus puncture model. Of note, the disk degeneration model used consisted of a 27 gauge needle puncture, which is a very small injury to the disk and therefore may lead to mild or no disk degeneration. The main in vivo finding was that Sox9-treated disks had a more chondrocyte-like phenotype as compared with control virus-injected disks[45]; however, this paper did not present quantitative data on the effect on disk matrix quantity or composition from the in vivo experiment.

LIM mineralizaion protein-1 (LMP-1) is an intracellular molecule that was initially discovered by its positive effect on bone formation and osteoblast differentiation. Yoon et al found that in disk cells, LMP-1 upregulates the production of BMP-2, BMP-7, and proteoglycans both in short-term monolayer cultures and in longer (3-week) experiments in alginate cultures.[5] By showing that the upregulation of proteoglycan can be blocked with a specific inhibitor of BMPs (Noggin), Yoon et al demonstrated that the effect of LMP-1 involved a BMP-dependent mechanism. Subsequent in vivo work with rabbit disks showed that gene therapy with low doses of adenovirus-LMP-1 increased disk tissue mRNA levels of BMP-2, BMP-7, and aggrecan. Because LMP-1 stimulates

both BMP-2 and BMP-7, this was hypothesized to potentiate the formation of the BMP-2:BMP-7 heterodimers, which have been shown to be up to 20 times more effective than homodimers of BMP-2 and BMP-7.[46] It can be speculated that by inducing a more potent set of BMPs, it may be possible to reduce the dose of adenovirus that is necessary, minimizing any potential risks of adenovirus gene therapy.

◆ Summary

The molecules used to treat disk degeneration have expanded beyond the classic growth factor. There are at least four different classes of molecules that may be effective in disk repair. These include anticatabolics, nonchondrogenic mitogens, chondrogenic morphogens, and intracellular regulators. Although all of these molecules have some in vitro data, few have been tested in vivo with an animal model of disk degeneration. In the near future, the current screening experiments will be concluded. Then experiments with a realistic animal model of disk degeneration will be necessary prior to attempting human studies.

References

1. Sato M, Asazuma T, Ishihara M, et al. An experimental study of the regeneration of the intervertebral disc with an allograft of cultured annulus fibrosus cells using a tissue-engineering method. Spine 2003; 28:548–553

2. Luk KD, Ruan DK, Chow DH, Leong JC. Intervertebral disc autografting in a bipedal animal model. Clin Orthop Relat Res 1997;337:13–26

3. Luk KD, Ruan DK, Lu DS, Fei ZQ. Fresh frozen intervertebral disc allografting in a bipedal animal model. Spine 2003;28:864–869

4. Pfeiffer M, Boudriot U, Pfeiffer D, Ishaque N, Goetz W, Wilke A. Intradiscal application of hyaluronic acid in the non-human primate lumbar spine: radiological results. Eur Spine J 2003;12:76–83

5. Yoon ST, Park JS, Kim KS, et al. LMP-1 upregulates intervertebral disc cell production of proteoglycans and BMPs in vitro and in vivo. Spine 2004; In press

6. Yoon ST, Kim K, Li J, et al. The effect of bone morphogenetic protein-2 on rat intervertebral disc cells in vitro. Spine 2003;28:1773–1780

7. Masuda K, Takegami K, An H, et al. Recombinant osteogenic protein-1 upregulates extracellular matrix metabolism by rabbit annulus fibrosus and nucleus pulposus cells cultured in alginate beads. J Orthop Res 2003;21:922–930

8. Zhang Y, An HS, Song S, et al. Growth factor osteogenic protein-1: differing effects on cells from three distinct zones in the bovine intervertebral disc. Am J Phys Med Rehabil 2004;83:515–521

9. Takegami K, Thonar EJ, An HS, Kamada H, Masuda K. Osteogenic protein-1 enhances matrix replenishment by intervertebral disc cells previously exposed to interleukin-1. Spine 2002;27:1318–1325

10. Sakai D, Mochida J, Yamamoto Y, et al. Transplantation of mesenchymal stem cells embedded in Atelocollagen gel to the intervertebral disc: a potential therapeutic model for disc degeneration. Biomaterials 2003;24:3531–3541

11. Watanabe K, Mochida J, Nomura T, Okuma M, Sakabe K, Seiki K. Effect of reinsertion of activated nucleus pulposus on disc degeneration: an experimental study on various types of collagen in degenerative discs. Connect Tissue Res 2003;44:104–108

12. Brisby H, Tao H, Ma DD, Diwan AD. Cell therapy for disc degeneration: potentials and pitfalls. Orthop Clin North Am 2004;35:85–93

13. Gruber HE, Hanley EN Jr. Biologic strategies for the therapy of intervertebral disc degeneration. Expert Opin Biol Ther 2003;3:1209–1214

14. Alini M, Roughley PJ, Antoniou J, Stoll T, Aebi M. A biological approach to treating disc degeneration: not for today, but maybe for tomorrow. Eur Spine J 2002;11(Suppl 2):S215–S220

15. Roberts S, Caterson B, Menage J, Evans EH, Jaffray DC, Eisenstein SM. Matrix metalloproteinases and aggrecanase: their role in disorders of the human intervertebral disc. Spine 2000;25:3005–3013

16. Roberts S, Menage J, Duance V, Wotton S, Ayad S. 1991 Volvo Award in basic sciences: collagen types around the cells of the intervertebral disc and cartilage end plate: an immunolocalization study. Spine 1991;16:1030–1038

17. Nagase H, Woessner JF Jr. Matrix metalloproteinases. J Biol Chem 1999;274:21491–21494

18. Wallach CJ, Sobajima S, Watanabe Y, et al. Gene transfer of the catabolic inhibitor TIMP-1 increases measured proteoglycans in cells from degenerated human intervertebral discs. Spine 2003;28:2331–2337

19. Okuma M, An HS, Nakagawa K, Akeda K, Muehleman C, Masuda K. Oral Administration of Esculetin Prodrug Inhibits Intervertebral Disc Degeneration in The Rabbit Annular Needle Puncture Model. Mar 20, 2005

20. Muller-Ladner U, Roberts CR, Franklin BN, et al. Human IL-1Ra gene transfer into human synovial fibroblasts is chondroprotective. J Immunol 1997;158:3492–3498

21. Bandara G, Mueller GM, Galea-Lauri J, et al. Intraarticular expression of biologically active interleukin 1-receptor-antagonist protein by ex vivo gene transfer. Proc Natl Acad Sci U S A 1993;90:10764–10768

22. Olmarker K, Rydevik B. Selective inhibition of tumor necrosis factor-alpha prevents nucleus pulposus-induced thrombus formation, intraneural edema, and reduction of nerve conduction velocity: possible implications for future pharmacologic treatment strategies of sciatica. Spine 2001;26:863–869

23. Thompson JP, Oegema TR Jr, Bradford DS. Stimulation of mature canine intervertebral disc by growth factors. Spine 1991;16:253–260

24. Okuda S, Myoui A, Ariga K, Nakase T, Yonenobu K, Yoshikawa H. Mechanisms of age-related decline in insulin-like growth factor-I dependent proteoglycan synthesis in rat intervertebral disc cells. Spine 2001;26: 2421–2426

25. Walsh AJ, Bradford DS, Lotz JC. In vivo growth factor treatment of degenerated intervertebral discs. Spine 2004;29:156–163

26. Gruber HE, Norton HJ, Hanley EN Jr. Anti-apoptotic effects of IGF-1 and PDGF on human intervertebral disc cells in vitro. Spine 2000;25: 2153–2157

27. Matsunaga S, Nagano S, Onishi T, Morimoto N, Suzuki S, Komiya S. Age-related changes in expression of transforming growth factor-beta and receptors in cells of intervertebral discs. J Neurosurg 2003;98(Suppl 1): 63–67

28. Takae R, Matsunaga S, Origuchi N, et al. Immunolocalization of bone morphogenetic protein and its receptors in degeneration of intervertebral disc. Spine 1999;24:1397–1401

29. Nishida K, Kang JD, Gilbertson LG, et al. Modulation of the biologic activity of the rabbit intervertebral disc by gene therapy: an in vivo

study of adenovirus-mediated transfer of the human transforming growth factor beta 1 encoding gene. Spine 1999;24:2419–2425

30. Lee JY, Hall R, Pelinkovic D, et al. New use of a three-dimensional pellet culture system for human intervertebral disc cells: initial characterization and potential use for tissue engineering. Spine 2001;26:2316–2322

31. Tan Y, Hu Y, Tan J. Extracellular matrix synthesis and ultrastructural changes of degenerative disc cells transfected by Ad/CMV-hTGF-beta 1. Chin Med J (Engl) 2003;116:1399–1403

32. Hutton WC, Yoon ST, Elmer WA, et al. Effect of tail suspension (or simulated weightlessness) on the lumbar intervertebral disc: study of proteoglycans and collagen. Spine 2002;27:1286–1290

33. Kim KS, Yoon ST, Park JS, Li J, Park MS, Hutton WC. Inhibition of proteoglycan and type II collagen synthesis of disc nucleus cells by nicotine. J Neurosurg 2003;99(Suppl 3):291–297

34. Kim DJ, Moon SH, Kim H, et al. Bone morphogenetic protein-2 facilitates expression of chondrogenic, not osteogenic, phenotype of human intervertebral disc cells. Spine 2003;28:2679–2684

35. An HS, Takegami K, Kamada H, et al. Intradiscal administration of osteogenic protein-1 increases intervertebral disc height and proteoglycan content in the nucleus pulposus in normal adolescent rabbits. Spine 2005;30:25–31

36. Masuda K, Aota Y, Muehleman C, et al. A novel rabbit model of mild, reproducible disc degeneration by an annulus needle puncture: correlation between the degree of disc injury and radiological and histological appearances of disc degeneration. Spine 2005;30:5–14

37. Chang SC, Hoang B, Thomas JT, et al. Cartilage-derived morphogenetic proteins: new members of the transforming growth factor-beta superfamily predominantly expressed in long bones during human embryonic development. J Biol Chem 1994;269:28227–28234

38. Li J, Kim KS, Park JS, Elmer WA, Hutton WC, Yoon ST. BMP-2 and CDMP-2: stimulation of chondrocyte production of proteoglycan. J Orthop Sci 2003;8:829–835

39. Wang H, Kroeber M, Hanke M, et al. Release of active and depot GDF-5 after adenovirus-mediated overexpression stimulates rabbit and human intervertebral disc cells. J Mol Med 2004;82:126–134

40. Mwale F, Demers CN, Petit A, et al. A synthetic peptide of link protein stimulates the biosynthesis of collagens II, IX and proteoglycan by cells of the intervertebral disc. J Cell Biochem 2003;88:1202–1213

41. Nohe A, Keating E, Knaus P, Petersen NO. Signal transduction of bone morphogenetic protein receptors. Cell Signal 2004;16:291–299

42. Hatakeyama Y, Nguyen J, Wang X, Nuckolls GH, Shum L. SMAD signaling in mesenchymal and chondroprogenitor cells. J Bone Joint Surg Am 2003;85-A(Suppl 3):13–18

43. Li Y, Tew SR, Russell AM, Gonzalez KR, Hardingham TE, Hawkins RE. Transduction of passaged human articular chondrocytes with adenoviral, retroviral, and lentiviral vectors and the effects of enhanced expression of SOX9. Tissue Eng 2004;10:575–584

44. Aigner T, Gebhard PM, Schmid E, Bau B, Harley V, Poschl E. SOX9 expression does not correlate with type II collagen expression in adult articular chondrocytes. Matrix Biol 2003;22:363–372

45. Paul R, Haydon RC, Cheng H, et al. Potential use of sox9 gene therapy for intervertebral degenerative disc disease. Spine 2003;28:755–763

46. Israel DI, Nove J, Kerns KM, et al. Heterodimeric bone morphogenetic proteins show enhanced activity in vitro and in vivo. Growth Factors 1996;13:291–300

Index

Page numbers followed by "f" or "t" indicate figures and tables, respectively.

Abbot Spine Wallis Interspinous implant, dynamic stabilization procedures, 10, 11f
Acroflex device, total disk replacement, 6
Activ-L lumbar (Aesculap) total disk arthroplasty
  complications, 209–210
  design parameters, 204, 204f, 205t
  indications for, 204–205
  instrumentation, 205–206, 207f
  surgical techniques, 206–209
  system components, 205–206, 205f–207f
Acute Fixation Technology (AFT), Spinal Kinetics Cervical Disk, 56
Adjacent segment disease
  cervical total disk replacement and, 42–43
    Bryan cervical disk device, 59–66
    therapeutic role for, 45
  DIAM system applications for, 275–276, 278
  dynamic stabilization and avoidance of
    Coflex system, 268
    Cosmic stabilization system procedures, 333, 334f
    Isobar TTL dynamic instrumentation, 313–315, 314f–315f
    Wallis interspinous implant, 264–265
  ProDisc-C prosthesis and, 72–76
All-in-1 guide, Maverick artificial disk implants, 192
Allograft techniques, anterior cervical diskectomy with fusion, 18
Annular collapse
  annuloplasty for symptomatic tears, 376, 377f
  lumbar disks, 100–101, 100f–101f
  Prosthetic Disk Nucleus (PDN), 103
  total disk replacement and ablation of, 152
Annuloplasty
  annular anatomy and function, 375
  indications and techniques
    artifical disk prostheses, 378
    interventional strategies, 376–378, 377f
    microdiskectomy, 375–376
    outcome assessment, 378
    overview, 375
    symptomatic annular tears, 376, 377f
  surgical techniques, 376, 376f
Annulotomy defect, NUBAC artificial nucleus, 133
Annulus fibrosus, anatomy and function, 375
Anterior cervical diskectomy (ACD), 16
  complications of, 27

Anterior cervical diskectomy with fusion (ACDF)
  Bryan cervical disk device, 59–60
  cervical arthroplasty and, 20–21
  cervical total disk replacement with, 42
    comparisons of, 44–45
  decompression with, 17–18, 18f
  Porous Coated Motion arthroplasty vs., 83–84, 84t
  ProDisc-C prosthesis vs., 76
Anterior column support
  combined hybrid rigid and soft stabilization, 311
  Graf soft stabilization and ligamentoplasty, 308t, 309–311, 309f–310f
Anterior longitudinal ligament (ALL)
  annulus anatomy and function, 375
  CHARITÉ Artificial Disc implant, 165, 167–168
Anterior-posterior technique, Activ-L lumbar (Aesculap) total disk arthroplasty, 208, 208f
Anterior surgical technique
  CHARITÉ Artificial Disc, 165, 168f–169f
  Maverick artificial disk implants, 191–193, 191f–192f
  Mobidisc prosthesis, 199–200, 201f–202f
  Raymedica Prosthetic Disk Nucleus, 110, 110f
Anterolateral foraminotomy, Bryan cervical disk device, 59
Anteroposterior implantation, Mobidisc prosthesis, 197–198
Anticatabolics, molecular therapy with, 383–384
Aquacryl, NeuDisc device biocompatibility, 123
Aquarelle device, nucleus replacement techniques, 5–6
Arm pain management
  Bryan cervical disc device, assessment, 63–64, 64f, 64t
  Cervidisc device, 89
Arterial obstruction, total lumbar disk replacement complication, 223, 223f
Arthroplasty techniques, 4–10
  cervical, 20–21, 21f
    anterior cervical diskectomy with fusion, 20–21
    biomechanical aspects, 27–32
    biomechanical testing protocol, 33–40
    Bryan cervical disk device, 59–66
    design rationale, 27–28, 28t, 29f
    peer-reviewed literature on, 28–31, 30f–31f, 30t–31t
  DASCOR Disc system, 116–121
  facet replacement technology

Arthroplasty techniques (*Continued*)
as adjunct procedure, 350
indications for, 354–355, 355f
fusion *vs.* nonfusion, 20–22
historical review, 3
lumbar, 21, 21f
complications, 227–233
nucleus replacement, 4–6, 5f–6f
total disc replacement, 6–10
cervical disk, 8–10, 8f–9f
lumbar disk, 6–7, 6f–7f
Artificial disks
Activ-L Lumbar (Aesculap) arthroplasty, 204–210
annuloplasty and implants of, 378
Bryan cervical disc device, 59–66
cervical spinal arthroplasty, 21, 21f
cervical total disk replacement, 45–49
Bryan cervical disk, 47, 47f
CerviCore device, 49, 49f
Porous Coated Motion prosthesis, 47–48, 48f
Prestige ST device, 45–47, 45f–46f
ProDisc-C device, 48–49, 48f
CHARITÉ Artificial Disc, 160–178
clinical applications, 53
design parameters, 28, 28t
FlexiCore artificial disk, 7, 7f, 154–155, 161–162, 162f, 212–220
Maverick artificial disk, 186–192
nucleus replacement, 5, 5f
DASCOR system, 114–121
principles and expectations, 114–116
Porous Coated Motion disk, 78–84
Prestige cervical artificial disks, 67–71
ProDisc-C, 72–76
lumbar disk replacement, 179–185
Spinal Kinetics Cervical Disc, 52–58
total disk replacement, 6–7, 6f–7f, 9, 9f
historical background, 160–162
lumbar disk, 154–155
Mobidisc prosthesis, 196–203
Artificial ligaments
Graf ligament system, 238–239, 239f
tension band system biomechanics, 286
interspinous locker fixation, 287
tension band systems, 284–285, 285f
Axial rotation, TOPS system biomechanics, 357, 358f

"Ball joint" disk mechanism, nucleus replacement
techniques, 4–6, 5f–6f
Bench testing
Dynamic Stabilization System, 324–325, 325f–326f
Raymedica Prosthetic Disk Nucleus, 106–107
Bending moment distribution
cervical spine mechanics, 33, 34f
dynamic stabilization procedures, neutral angle modification,
238, 238f
NeuDisc device, 124, 124f
NUBAC artificial nucleus, 132–133
tension band system biomechanics, 286
TOPS system biomechanics, 357, 358f
Bertagnoli's criteria, ProDisc prostheses assessment,
182–183, 183f
Beta sheets, NuCore injectable nucleus, 143–144, 144f
Biocompatibility testing
NeuDisc device, 123
NUBAC artificial nucleus, 132
NuCore injectable nucleus, 144–145

Total Facet Arthroplasty System, 368–369, 368f–369f
Wallis interspinous implant, 260
BioDisc device, nucleus replacement techniques, 5
Biodurability properties, NUBAC artificial nucleus, 132
BioFlex spring rod pedicle screw system
basic components, 341–343, 341f–342f
biomechanical testing, 341, 343
case studies, 342f, 343, 344f
indications and contraindications, 340–341
outcome assessment, 344
overview, 340
surgical techniques, 343
Biomaterials
Cosmic stabilization system, 332
NuCore injectable nucleus, 143
Biomechanical testing
artificial nucleus replacement, 114–116
DASCOR artificial nucleus system, 118–121, 119f
NUBAC artificial nucleus, 132–133, 132f
SINUX system, 139–140, 139f–140f
Spinal Kinetics Cervical Disk, 56
BioFlex rod pedicle screw system, 341, 343
cervical arthroplasty, 28–31, 29t–30t, 30f–31f
displacement *vs.* load control, 37f–39f, 40
testing protocols, 33–40
dynamic stabilization techniques, 244–245
DIAM system, 274–275, 275f–276f
Dynesys Dynamic Stabilization System, 299–300,
299f–300f
Graf soft stabilization system, 306
Isobar TTL dynamic instrumentation, 315, 315f
lumbar disk mechanics
degenerative disks, 150–151
normal disk, 149–150, 150f
Mobidisc prosthesis, 198–199, 198f–199f
NeuDisc device, 123–126
partial disk replacments, 101–103
ProDisc-C prosthesis, 73, 179–180, 180f
SoftFlex flexible rod system, 245, 246f–248f
spine and intervertebral space, 196–197, 197f
of tension band systems, 285–286, 286f
TOPS system, 357, 358f
total disk replacement
artificial lumbar disks, 161–162
lumbar disk, 149–152
Total Facet Arthroplasty System, 365–366, 365f
Block copolymers, NuCore injectable nucleus, 144, 144f
Block diskectomy, Maverick artificial disk implants,
191–192, 191f
Blood loss, CERVIDISC opening, 88, 89t
Bone ingrowth, Porous Coated Motion arthroplasty,
implant-bone interface gaps, 84
Bone morphogenetic proteins (BMPs), molecular therapy
with, 385–386, 385f
Bryan cervical disc device
arthroplasty procedure, 61–63, 61f–63f
operating environment, 61
preoperative planning, 61
basic features, 60–61, 60f
cervical arthroplasty, 31
clinical experience with, 63–66, 64f–65f, 64t–65t
outcome assessment, 63
site preparation, 61–62, 61f
total disk replacement, 8, 9f
cervical disks, 47f
Bulk polymer nucleus, NUBAC artificial nucleus, 131, 131f

Cadaver study
  NeuDisc device, 126
  NUBAC artificial nucleus, 133–134
  NuCore injectable nucleus, 144–145
  ProDisc prostheses, 179–180, 180f
  Spinal Kinetics Cervical Disk, 56
  Wallis interspinous implant, 260
Center of rotation
  Charité artificial disk implant, 168, 170, 171f
  Maverick artificial disk, 187, 189f
  Mobidisc prosthesis, 199, 200f
  Prosthetic Disk Nucleus (PDN), 101–102
  spine and intervertebral space biomechanics, 196–197, 197f
Cerebrospinal fluid leakage, total lumbar disk replacement,
     231–232
Cervical disk
  radiculopathy
    Bryan cervical disk device, 59–66
    pathology of, 27
Cervical disks
  arthroplasty, 20–21, 21f
    biomechanical aspects, 27–32
    biomechanical testing protocol, 33–40
    Bryan device, 59–66
    design rationale, 27–28, 28t, 29f
    peer-reviewed literature on, 28–31, 30f–31f, 30t–31t
    Porous Coated Motion (PCM) prosthesis, 30
      bone ingrowth, implant-bone interface gaps, 84
      clinical outcomes, 81–82, 82f–83f
      complications, 82–84, 84t
      indications for, 78, 79t
    ProDisc-C prosthesis, 73–75, 74f–75f
  decompression techniques
    fusion, 17–18, 18f
    nonfusion, 16–17, 17f
  total disk replacement, 8–10, 8f–9f
    adjacent segment degeneration and disease prevention, 42–43
    design pros and cons, 49–50
    disadvantages, 44–45
    iliac crest bone graft donor site morbidity, 44
    indications for, 45
    postoperative dysphagia avoidance, 44
    prosthetic designs, 45–49
      Bryan cervical disk, 47, 47f
      CerviCore device, 49, 49f
      Porous Coated Motion prosthesis, 47–48, 48f
      Prestige ST device, 45–47, 45f–46f
      ProDisc-C device, 48–49, 48f
    pseudoarthrosis avoidance, 43–44
    rationale for, 42–44
    Spinal Kinetics Cervical Disc, 52–58
CerviCore disk prostheses
  clinical trials, 95
  design philosophy, 92, 93f–94f
  materials testing, 92
  preclinical testing, 95
  total cervical disk replacement, 49, 49f
Cervidiscs
  blood loss and operative time, 88, 90t
  complications, 88, 88t
  design parameters, 86–87, 86f
  outcome evaluation, 89–90, 90f
  patient demographics for, 87, 87t
  posterior longitudinal ligament opening, 88
  subsidence phenomena, 88, 89f–90f
  surgical techniques, 87, 87f–88f, 88

CHARITÉ Artificial Disc, 3, 3f
  artificial nucleus replacement and, 115–116
  clinical history, 164–165
  design criteria, 162–164, 162f–167f
  FDA IDE multicenter trial of, 172–173, 175f–176f
  historical background, 162–164, 162f–164f
  outcome assessment, 172–173, 175f–176f, 176, 177f
  revision techniques, 174, 176
  surgical techniques, 165, 167–171, 168f–173f
  total disk replacement, 6–7
    facet arthrosis complications, 232
    facet replacement technology as adjunct to, 350
    lumbar disk, 154–155
    migration, dislocation, or subluxation, 228
Chisel device
  Activ-L lumbar (Aesculap) total disk arthroplasty, 207–208, 208f
  Spinal Kinetics Cervical Disk, 54–55, 55f
Coflex dynamic stabilization system, 10, 11f
  complications, 271, 272f
  design parameters, 268, 269f
  indications/contraindications, 268–269
  intraoperative instability, 269
  outcome assessment, 269–273, 271f, 271t
  patient selection criteria, 269
  rigid fixation with, 269
  surgical technique, 269, 270f
Complications
  Activ-L lumbar (Aesculap) total disk arthroplasty, 209–210
  Cervidisc systems, 88, 88t
  Coflex system, 271, 272f
  Cosmic stabilization system, 337–338
  FlexiCore prosthesis implants, 219
  lumbar disk arthroplasty, 227–233
  Porous Coated Motion arthroplasty, 82–84, 84t
  ProDisc-C prosthesis implants, 76
  ProDisc prostheses, 185
  total disk replacement, lumbar disk, 221–226
  Wallis interspinous implant, 261–263, 262f–263f
Compression fractures, dynamic stabilization, BioFlex rod pedicle
    screw system, 343–344, 344f
Compression testing, Wallis interspinous implant, 260
Contact stress distribution, NUBAC artificial nucleus, 129–130,
    130f, 130t
Cosmic stabilization system, nonfusion stabilization, 330–338
  adjacent segment degeneration, 333, 334f
  basic components, 331–332, 331f–332f
  contraindications, 334
  disk herniation recurrence, 332
  diskogenic pain and facet syndrome, 332, 333f
  indications for, 331–333
  lumbar stenosis, 332, 333f
  multiple segment stabilization, 334
  outcome assessment, 336–338
  overview, 330–331
  spondylodeses procedures, 331, 333, 334f
  surgical techniques, 334–336, 335f–336f
CPA-926 molecule, molecular therapy with, 384
Creep testing, Wallis interspinous implant, 260
Cummins Bristol prosthesis, 67, 67f
  total disk replacement, cervical disks, 46–47
Cytokines, molecular therapy with, 384

Dallas pain scale (DPQ), posterior lumbar fusion,
    instrumentation, 20
Dampener element design, Isobar TTL system, 314–315,
    315f, 317

DASCOR device
  lumbar nucleus replacement, 116–121, 116f–118f
  nucleus replacement techniques, 5–6, 6f
Decompression techniques
  cervical
    fusion, 17–18, 18f
    neural element decompression, Bryan cervical disc
        device, 62–63
    nonfusion, 16–17, 17f
  facet replacement technology as adjunct to, 350–351
  laminotomy, tension band system, 287–288, 288f–289f
  lumbar, without fusion, 18–19, 19f
  lumbar neurogenic intermittent claudication, X STOP
      Interspinous Process Decompression system for,
      251–257
Deep venous thrombosis (DVT), total lumbar disk replacement
      complication, 223, 223f
Deformation mechanics, KIMPF-DI system, 296, 296f
Degenerative disk disease (DDD)
  basic principles of, 258–259
  Dynesys Dynamic Stabilization System, 300
  incidence and epidemiology, 122, 212
Degree of freedom (DOF) measurements, cervical arthroplasty
      biomechanical testing, 34
Denis's three-column theory, tension band system biomechanics,
      286
DePuy Spine prosthesis, total disc replacement, 6–7
Device for Intervertebral Assisted Motion (DIAM), dynamic
      stabilization procedures, 10, 10f
DIAM (Device for Intervertebral Assisted Motion) system,
      dynamic stabilization, 274–282
  biomechanics, 274–275, 275f–276f
  disk herniation applications, 275
  facet syndrome and disk dysfunction, 275, 277f
  flexion-extension range of motion assessment, 282, 282t
  indications for, 275–278
  inserter instrumentation, 279, 280f
  ligament fixation, 279, 280f
  outcome assessment, 279, 281f, 282, 282t
  stenosis, 275
  surgical techniques, 278–279, 278f–279f
  topping off applications, 275–276, 278
DISCOCERV device
  blood loss and operative time, 88, 90t
  complications, 88, 88t
  design parameters, 86–87, 86f
  goals of, 86–87
  outcome evaluation, 89–90, 90f
  posterior longitudinal ligament opening, 88
  subsidence phenomena, 88, 89f–90f
  surgical techniques, 87, 87f–88f, 88
Diskectomy, FlexiCore prosthesis, 217
Disk herniation
  annuloplasty for reherniation prevention, 375–376
  Cosmic stabilization system procedures, 332
  DIAM system applications, 275
Disk restoration
  DIAM system applications for, 275, 277f
  dynamic stabilization, Wallis interspinous implant, 265, 265f
Disk space height modification
  Activ-L lumbar (Aesculap) total disk arthroplasty, 207
  dynamic stabilization procedures, 238, 238f
Displacement testing, cervical arthroplasty biomechanical test-
      ing, 37f–39f, 40
Distraction components
  cervical arthroplasty, Bryan cervical disc device, 62, 62f
  CHARITÉ Artificial Disc implant, 170, 172f

DIAM system, 278–279, 278f–279f
Dynesys Dynamic Stabilization System, 301
FlexiCore prosthesis, 214–216, 214f–216f
  height restoration, 217
ProDisc prostheses, 181
Raymedica Prosthetic Disk Nucleus, posterior approach,
    108–109, 108f–109f
Durability testing
  Total Facet Arthroplasty System, 368–369, 368f–369f
  Wallis interspinous implant, 265–266
Dynamic characterization
  SINUX system, 139–140, 139f
  Spinal Kinetics Cervical Disk, 55–56
Dynamic instrumentation
  FlexiCore prosthesis, 214, 215f
  Isobar TTL system, 313–315, 314f–315f
Dynamic stabilization, 10–13. *See also* Instability management
  BioFlex rod pedicle screw system
    basic components, 341–343, 341f–342f
    biomechanical testing, 341, 343
    case studies, 342f, 343, 344f
    indications and contraindications, 340–341
    outcome assessment, 344
    overview, 340
    surgical techniques, 343
  Coflex system
    complications, 271, 272f
    design parameters, 268, 269f
    indications/contraindications, 268–269
    intraoperative instability, 269
    outcome assessment, 269–273, 271f, 271t
    patient selection criteria, 269
    rigid fixation with, 269
    surgical technique, 269, 270f
  Cosmic stabilization system, 330–338
    adjacent segment degeneration, 333, 334f
    basic components, 331–332, 331f–332f
    contraindications, 334
    disk herniation recurrence, 332
    diskogenic pain and facet syndrome, 332, 333f
    indications for, 331–333
    lumbar stenosis, 332, 333f
    multiple segment stabilization, 334
    outcome assessment, 336–338
    overview, 330–331
    spondylodeses procedures, 331, 333, 334f
    surgical techniques, 334–336, 335f–336f
  DIAM system, 274–282
    biomechanics, 274–275, 275f–276f
    disk herniation applications, 275
    facet syndrome and disk dysfunction, 275, 277f
    flexion-extension range of motion assessment, 282, 282t
    indications for, 275–278
    inserter instrumentation, 279, 280f
    ligament fixation, 279, 280f
    outcome assessment, 279, 281f, 282, 282t
    stenosis, 275
    surgical techniques, 278–279, 278f–279f
    topping off applications, 275–276, 278
  Dynesys Dynamic Stabilization system, 299–304
    benefits of, 299–300, 299f, 300f
    indications for, 300, 300f
    outcome assessment, 301–304, 301f–302f, 304f
    surgical techniques, 300–301
    technical aspects of, 299–300
  facet replacement, 12, 13f, 350–351
    Total Facet Arthroplasty System, 370–371

fusion vs. nonfusion techniques, 21–22
historical review, 3
indications for, 237
interspinous process spacers, 10, 10f–11f
intervertebral disk unloading, 239–240, 239f–240f
Isobar TTL dynamic instrumentation, 12, 12f
    biomechanical performance, 315, 315f
    finite element analysis, 315–317, 316f–317f
    indications for, 317–318, 318f–320f
    instrumentation and adjacent disk degeneration, 313–315,
        314f–315f
    isobar TTL rod placement, 318–321, 320f–321f
    overview, 312–313
KIMPF-DI fixing system shape memory implant, 292–298
    basic properties, 292–293, 292f, 293f
    case studies, 296–298
    components of, 294, 294f–295f
    deformation and installation, 296, 296f
    indications and contraindactions, 293f, 294
    loop fixings, surgical techniques, 294–296, 295f–296f
    surgical techniques, 294–296, 295f–296f, 298t
neutral angle and disk space height modification, 238,
    238f–239f
pedicle screw-based systems, 10–12, 12f
posterior stabilization devices, 237
sagittal plane bending control, 238–239, 239f
segment load distribution modification, 240–241, 242f
segment motion modification, 240, 241f
SoftFlex system, 244–249
    basic components, 244–245, 246f–248f
    outcome assessment, 245–246
    surgical techniques, 245, 249f
tension band system
    artificial ligament, 284–285, 285f
    basic principles, 284
    biomechanics, 285–286, 286f
    components of, 284–286
    decompressive laminotomy, 287–288, 288f–289f
    degenerative spondylolisthesis, 288, 290, 290f
    indications and contraindications, 286
    metal inerspinous locker, 285, 285f
    soft stabilization techniques, 290
    surgical techniques, 285f, 287–291, 288f
Wallis interspinous implant
    adjacent segment preservation, 264–265
    basic principles, 258–259
    biocompatibility testing, 260
    contraindications, 261
    duration of effects, 265–266, 266f
    fatigue testing, 260
    finite element analysis, 260
    first-generation implants, 261
    indications for, 258, 261
    motion preservation, 264, 264f
    outcome assessment, 263–266, 264f–266f
    pain relief, 264
    potential disk restoration, 265, 265f
    reversibility potential, 264
    safety issues, 263–264
    static testing, 260
    surgical technique, 261–263, 262t–263t
    system components, 259–260, 259f–260f
    in vitro cadaver testing, 260
X STOP interspinous process decompression system, lumbar
        neurogenic claudication, 251–257
Dynamic Stabilization System (DSS)
    clinical testing, 326–327

design principles, 323–326, 324f–326f
fatigue testing, 323
load sharing and motion restriction, 323
outcome assessment, 327, 329, 329f
surgical techniques, 327, 328f
Dynesys Dynamic Stabilization System (DDSS)
    Cosmic stabilization system comparisons, 337–338
    dynamic stabilization procedures, 11, 12f–13f, 21
    instability management, 299–304
        benefits of, 299–300, 299f, 300f
        indications for, 300, 300f
        outcome assessment, 301–304, 301f–302f, 304f
        surgical techniques, 300–301
        technical aspects of, 299–300
    neutral angle and disk space height modification, 238, 238f
    segment load distribution modification, 241

Elderly patients, Coflex dynamic stabilization in, 269
End mounting configurations
    Activ-L lumbar (Aesculap) total disk arthroplasty,
        206–207, 208f
    artificial nucleus replacement, lumbar disks, 115–116
    cervical arthroplasty biomechanical testing, 35, 35f
    CHARITÉ Artificial Disc, 164, 166f, 168, 170, 171f–172f
    FlexiCore prosthesis, 217
    Maverick artificial disk, 186–187, 188f
    Mobidisc prosthesis, 200, 201f–202f
    NUBAC artificial nucleus, 130
    Prestige LP artifical disk, 69–70, 69f–70f
    Spinal Kinetics Cervical Disk, 53–54
Endurance testing, NeuDisc device, 123–125, 124f
Epidermal growth factor (EGF), molecular therapy with,
        384–385, 385f
Equilibrium, total disk replacement and establishment of, 152
Expulsion test, Spinal Kinetics Cervical Disk, 56
Expulsion testing, NeuDisc device, 125–126
Extension motions
    NeuDisc device, 124
    SoftFlex flexible rod system, 245, 246f
Extractor components, FlexiCore prosthesis, 214, 215f
Extrusion characteristics
    annuloplasty and complications from, 378
    NUBAC artificial nucleus testing, 132–133, 132f

Facet replacement
    dynamic stabilization procedures, 12
    Prosthetic Disk Nucleus (PDN), 103
    technology overview, 347–351
        anatomy properties, 347, 348f
        current developments, 351, 351f
        outcome assessment, 351
        posterior dynamic reconstruction, post-decompression,
            350–351
        stand-alone devices for low-back pain, 347–349
        total disk replacement adjuncts, 349–350
    Total Facet Arthroplasty System
        clinical trials, 370
        design parameters, 366–368, 367f–368f
        development assessment, 351, 351f
        dynamic stabilization procedures, 12
            comparison of outcomes, 370
        facet biomechanics, 365–366, 365f
        outcome assessment, 370–371
        overview, 364, 364f
        performance evaluation, 368–369, 368f–369f
        spinal biomechanics restoration, 364–365
        surgical technique, 369–370, 369f–370f

Facet replacement (*Continued*)
  Total Posterior Facet Replacement and Dynamic Motion
      Segment Stabilization system
    biomechanical testing, 357, 358f
    design parameters, 355–356, 356f
    finite element analysis, 356–357, 357f
    indications for, 354–355, 355f
    outcome assessment, 362–363, 362f
    overview, 354
    pedicle screw loading, 357, 359f
    surgical technique, 357–358, 359f, 360–362, 360f–361f
Facet syndrome
  dynamic stabilization techniques
    Cosmic stabilization system procedures, 332, 333f
    DIAM system, 274–275, 277f
  total lumbar disk replacement, 232
Failed back surgery syndrome (FBSS), 137–138
Failure mode
  Dynamic Stabilization System, 323
  NUBAC artificial nucleus, 133–134
  Prosthetic Disk Nucleus (PDN), 103
Fatigue testing
  BioFlex rod pedicle screw system, 341, 343
  Dynamic Stabilization System, 323
    DSS-I *vs.* DSS-II results, 324–325, 326f
  NeuDisc device, 126
  NUBAC artificial nucleus, 132–133, 132f, 134–135, 134f
  SoftFlex flexible rod system, 245, 247f
  Spinal Kinetics Cervical Disk, 55
  Wallis interspinous implant, 260
Feasibility studies, Spinal Kinetics Cervical Disk, 57–58, 57f
Fernström ball, NUBAC artificial nucleus, 129–130, 131f
Fiber Annulus, Spinal Kinetics Cervical Disk, 53
Fibroblast growth factor (FGF), molecular therapy with,
      384–385, 385f
Finite element analysis
  Charité artificial disk, 164, 167f
  Isobar TTL dynamic instrumentation, 315–317, 316f–317f, 316t
  TOPS system, 356–357, 357f
  Wallis interspinous implant, 260–261
Fixation techniques
  Prosthetic Disk Nucleus (PDN), 102
  total cervical disk replacement, 49–50
  total disk replacement, 152
Flexibility testing
  DASCOR artificial nucleus system, 118–119
  NUBAC artificial nucleus, 133–134
FlexiCore prosthesis
  complications, 219
  contraindications, 213
  design parameters, 212–213
  historical background, 161–162, 162f
  indications for, 213
  surgical techniques, 216–219, 217f
  system components, 213–214, 213f–214f
  total disk replacement, 7, 7f
    lumbar disk, 154–155
Flexion motions
  dynamic stabilization procedures, neutral angle modification,
      238, 238f
  Graf soft stabilization system, 306
  NeuDisc device, 124
  SoftFlex flexible rod system, 245, 246f
  spine and intervertebral space biomechanics, 196–197, 197f
  TOPS system biomechanics, 357, 358f
Fluoroscopic techniques, cervical arthroplasty, Bryan cervical disc
      device, 62, 62f

Follower load concept, cervical arthroplasty biomechanical
      testing, 40
Fulcrum-Assisted Soft Stabilization (FASS) system
  design parameters, 323–324
  dynamic stabilization procedures, 10
Functional spinal units (FSUs)
  NUBAC artificial nucleus testing, 132–133
  Total Facet Arthroplasty System, 364–366, 365f
    product evaluation, 368–369, 368f–369f
Fusion techniques
  cervical arthroplasty, artificial disks *vs.*, 29–30, 29t
  cervical decompression, 17–18, 18f
  cervical total disk replacement, adjacent segment disease, 42–43
  instrumented laminectomy, 19
  nonfusion *vs.*, overview, 16
  posterior lumbar, 19–20
  spinal arthroplasty, historical review, 3
  total disk replacement *vs.*, 149

Geometry, Prosthetic Disk Nucleus (PDN), 101
Globular proteins, NuCore injectable nucleus, 144, 144f
Graf ligament system
  dynamic stabilization procedures
    sagittal plane balance, 238–239, 239f
  soft stabilization and ligamentoplasty, 305–311
    band placement, 307, 308f
    combined rigid and soft stabilization, 311
    concept and rationale behind, 305–306, 305f
    disease classification and indications for, 307–308, 308t
    indications and contraindications, 306
    outcome assessment, 307–311, 309f–310f
    surgical techniques, 306–307, 307f–308f
Growth and differentiation factors (GDFs), molecular therapy
      with, 385–386, 385f
Growth factors
  molecular therapy with, 384–385, 385f
  NuCore injectable nucleus, 143

Head-cup coupling, Cervidisc system, 87
Heterotopic ossification, total disk replacement, 232
Hybrid stabilization techniques, Graf soft stabilization and, 311
Hybrid testing method, cervical arthroplasty biomechanical testing,
      39f, 40
Hydrogels
  NeuDisc device, 122–127
  NuCore injectable nucleus, 143
Hydronephrosis, total lumbar disk replacement, 224–225, 225f
Hydrostatic pressure, lumbar disk degeneration, 151
Hydroxyapatite coating fixation
  Maverick artificial disk, 189, 189f
  TOPS system, 356, 356f

Iliac crest bone graft, donor site morbidity, cervical total disk
      replacement and avoidance of, 44
Iliolumbar vein, total lumbar disk replacement complications,
      222, 222f
Implant-bone interface gaps, Porous Coated Motion arthroplasty,
      bone ingrowth characteristics, 84
Implant Introducer device, Spinal Kinetics Cervical Disk, 54
Implant size
  BioFlex rod pedicle screw system, 341, 342f
  dynamic stabilization, DIAM system, 279, 279f
  FlexiCore prosthesis, 215f, 217–218
Infection, total lumbar disk replacement, 232
Inferior vena cava abnormalities, total lumbar disk replacement
      complications, 221–222, 222f
Injectable Disc Nucleus (IDN), nucleus replacement techniques, 5

Inserter/impactor
  DIAM system, 279, 280f
  FlexiCore prosthesis, 214, 215f
Instability management. *See also* Dynamic stabilization
  Coflex dynamic stabilization for, 269
  Cosmic stabilization system, 330–338
    adjacent segment degeneration, 333, 334f
    basic components, 331–332, 331f–332f
    contraindications, 334
    disk herniation recurrence, 332
    diskogenic pain and facet syndrome, 332, 333f
    indications for, 331–333
    lumbar stenosis, 332, 333f
    multiple segment stabilization, 334
    outcome assessment, 336–338
    overview, 330–331
    spondylodeses procedures, 331, 333, 334f
    surgical techniques, 334–336, 335f–336f
  dynamic stabilization, 244
  Dynesys system, 299–304
    benefits of, 299–300, 299f, 300f
    indications for, 300, 300f
    outcome assessment, 301–304, 301f–302f, 304f
    surgical techniques, 300–301
    technical aspects of, 299–300
  Graf ligamentoplasty, 305–311
    concept and rationale behind, 305–306, 305f
    disease classification and indications for, 307–308, 308t
    indications and contraindications, 306
    outcome assessment, 307–311, 309f–310f
    surgical techniques, 306–307, 307f–308f
  tension band system biomechanics, 286
Instantaneous centers of rotation (ICR)
  dynamic stabilization
    Isobar TTL system, 314–315, 314f–315f, 320–321
    neutral angle and disk space height modification, 238, 238f
    segment load distribution modification, 241, 242f
    segment motion modification, 240, 241f
  spine and intervertebral space biomechanics, 196–197, 197f
Instant axis of rotation (IAR), lumbar disk degeneration, 151
Instrumented fusions, debate concerning, 19–20
Insulin-like growth factor-1 (IGF-1), molecular therapy with, 384–385, 385f
Interleukin-1 (IL-1), molecular therapy with, 384
Interspinous locker, tension band system
  artificial ligament fixation, 285f, 287, 288f–289f
  biomechanics, 285, 285f
  decompressive laminotomy, 287–288, 288f–289f
Interspinous process spacers, dynamic stabilization procedures, 10, 10f–11f, 241–242
  DIAM system, 279, 281f
  mechanics of, 237
  Wallis interspinous implant
    adjacent segment preservation, 264–265
    basic principles, 258–259
    biocompatibility testing, 260
    contraindications, 261
    duration of effects, 265–266, 266f
    fatigue testing, 260
    finite element analysis, 260
    first-generation implants, 261
    indications for, 258, 261
    motion preservation, 264, 264f
    outcome assessment, 263–266, 264f–266f
    pain relief, 264
    potential disk restoration, 265, 265f
    reversibility potential, 264

safety issues, 263–264
    static testing, 260
    surgical technique, 261–263, 262f–263f
    system components, 259–260, 259f–260f
    in vitro cadaver testing, 260
Interventional strategies, annuloplasty for, 377–378, 377f
Intervertebral disk
  dynamic stabilization (*See* Dynamic stabilization)
  molecular therapy
    anticatabolics, 383–384
    intracellular regulators, 386–387, 386f
    mitogens, 384–385, 385f
    molecule categories, 383, 383t, 384f
    morphogens, 385–386, 385f
    outcome assessment, 387
  total disk replacement (*See* Total disk replacement)
Intervertebral space, biomechanics, 196–197, 197f
Intracellular regulators, molecular therapy with, 386–387, 386f
Intradiskal electrothermy (IDET), annuloplasty and, 377–378, 377f
Intraoperative instability, Coflex system, 269
In vitro testing
  NUBAC artificial nucleus, 133–134
  SINUX system, 139–140, 139f–140f
  Spinal Kinetics Cervical Disk, 55–56
  TOPS system biomechanics, 357, 358f
  Wallis interspinous implant, 260
In vivo motion studies, cervical spine mechanics, 33, 34f
Isobar TTL dynamic instrumentation
  biomechanical performance, 315, 315f
  dynamic stabilization procedures, 12, 12f
    instrumentation and adjacent disk degeneration, 313–315, 314f–315f
    isobar TTL rod placement, 318–321, 320f–321f
  finite element analysis, 315–317, 316f–317f
  indications for, 317–318, 318f–320f
  overview, 312–313

Joint decoupling, TOPS system facet replacement, 358, 360, 360f
Junghans biomechanics, spine and intervertebral space, 196–197, 197f

Keel osteotomy
  Maverick artificial disk, 189f, 192
  Spinal Kinetics Cervical Disk, 54
KIMPF-DI fixation system shape memory alloy, 292–298
  basic properties, 292–293, 292f, 293f
  case studies, 296–298
  components of, 294, 294f–295f
  deformation and installation, 296, 296f
  indications and contraindactions, 293f, 294
  loop fixings, surgical techniques, 294–296, 295f–296f
  surgical techniques, 294–296, 295f–296f, 298t
Kirkaldy-Willis cascade, basic principles, 312–313
Kyphosis, KIMPF-DI shape memory alloy, 297–298, 297f

Laminectomy
  cervical, historical review, 16, 17f
  Graf soft stabilization and ligamentoplasty vs., 307–308
  lumbar decompression, nonfusion techniques, 18–19, 19f
  posterior lumbar fusion, instrumentation, 19–20
  TOPS system facet replacement, 358, 359f
  vs. noninstrumented posterolateral fusion with, 19
Laminoforaminotomy, Bryan cervical disk device, 60
Laminoplasty, posterior cervical laminoplasty, 16–17, 17f
Laminotomy, tension band system, 287–288, 288f–289f
Lateral technique, Raymedica Prosthetic Disk Nucleus, 110, 110f

Leeds-Keio artificial ligament, dynamic stabilization procedures, 11
Leg pain assessment, Maverick artificial disk, 194
Leveling tools, FlexiCore prosthesis, 214, 215f
Ligament fixation, DIAM system, 279, 281f
LMP-1 molecule, molecular therapy with, 387
Load profile
    cervical arthroplasty biomechanical testing, 37f–39f, 40
    dynamic stabilization
        intervertebral disk unloading, 239–240
        outcome assessment, 241–242, 242f
        segment load distribution modification, 240–241, 242f
    Dynamic Stabilization System, 323–324, 325f–326f
    lumbar disk degeneration, 151
    SINUX system, 139–140
    TOPS pedicle screw system, 357, 359f
    Total Facet Arthroplasty System, 368–369, 368f–369f
Load to failure analysis, NUBAC artificial nucleus, 133–134
Loop fixing techniques
    indications for, 298, 298t
    KIMPF-DI system
        basic properties, 292, 293f
        surgical techniques, 294–296, 295f–296f, 298t
Lordosis
    dynamic stabilization techniques, SoftFlex system, 245, 246f
    ProDisc prostheses and, 180
Low back pain (LBP)
    facet replacement technology, stand-alone devices, 347–349
    Maverick artificial disk, 194
    total disk replacement complications, 231, 231f
Low back pain rating scale (LBPR), posterior lumbar fusion,
        instrumentation, 20
Lumbalgy recurrence, Cosmic stabilization system procedures,
        332, 333f
Lumbar disks
    arthroplasty, 21, 21f
        complications, 227–233
        subsidence, 227, 228f–229f
    artificial nucleus replacements
        DASCOR system, 114–121
        NUBAC artificial nucleus, 128–135
        NuCore injectable nucleus, 142–145
        prosthetic disks, 99–103
        Raymedica Prosthetic Disk Nucleus (PDN), 105–113
            anterior, lateral, and posterolateral approaches, 110, 110f
            materials and methods, 106–107
            outcome assessment, 110–112, 111f–112f
            patient selection, 107
            posterior approach, 108–109, 108f–109f
            postoperative care, 110
        SINUX system, 137–140
    biomechanical analysis
        degenerative disk, 150–151
        normal disk, 149–150, 150f
    decompression techniques, nonfusion, 18–19, 19f
    degeneration pathophysiology, 99–101, 100f–101f
    nonfusion decompression, 18–19, 19f
        Cosmic stabilization system, 330–338
    partial disk replacements, 101–103
    total disk replacement, 6–7, 6f–7f
        Activ-L Lumbar (Aesculap) arthroplasty, 204–210
        artificial disk prosthesis, 154–155
        biomechanical issues, 149–152
        case studies, 156–158, 156f–158f
        CHARITÉ Artificial Disc, 160–178
        complications, 221–226
        contraindications, 155–156
        FlexiCore artificial disk, 212–220
        historical background, 160–162
        indications, 154–159, 155t
        Maverick prosthesis, 186–194
        Mobidisc prosthesis, 196–203
        ProDisc prosthesis, 179–185
Lumbar neurogenic intermittent claudication, X STOP
        Interspinous Process Decompression system for,
        251–257

Material testing systems (MTS)
    cervical arthroplasty biomechanical testing, 33–34
    CerviCore disk prostheses, 92
    Isobar TTL dynamic instrumentation, 315–317, 316f–317f, 316t
    Prosthetic Disk Nucleus (PDN), 101
    Raymedica Prosthetic Disk Nucleus, 106–107, 106f–107f
Matrix metalloproteinases (MMPs), molecular therapy with,
        383–384
Maverick artificial disk
    basic components, 186, 187f–188f
    design parameters, 187
    historical background, 161–162, 162f
    hydroxyapatite coating fixation, 189, 189f
    metal-on-metal design, 187–188, 188f
    posterior center of rotation, 187, 189f
    Total Disc Replacement, 7, 7f, 186–194
        facet replacement technology as adjunct to, 350
        female end plate configuration, 186–187
        lumbar disk, 154–155
        male end plate configuration, 186
        outcomes assessment, 193–194, 193t, 194f
        patient selection, 190–191, 191f
        surgical techniques, 189–193, 190f–193f
Metal interspinous locker, tension band systems, 285, 285f
Metal-on-metal design, Maverick artificial disk, 187, 188f
Microdiskectomy, annuloplasty for reherniation prevention,
        375–376
Microendoscopic foraminotomy (MEF), 17
Migration test
    lumbar disk arthroplasty, 228
    Spinal Kinetics Cervical Disk, 56
Milling disk, Bryan cervical disc device, 62, 62f
Minimally invasive surgery, Dynamic Stabilization System,
        327, 328f
Mitogens, molecular therapy with, 384–385, 385f
Mobidisc prosthesis
    basic principles, 197
    biomechanical testing, 198–199, 198f–199f
    center of rotation, 199, 200f
    design parameters, 197–198, 198f
    outcome assessment, 202, 203f
    surgical techniques, 199–200, 201f–202f
Mobility properties
    Activ-L lumbar (Aesculap) total disk arthroplasty, 210, 210f
    Cervidisc devices, 89–90, 91f
Modular implant design, Cervidisc system, 87
Molecular architecture, NuCore injectable nucleus, 143–144
Molecular therapy, intervertebral disk
    anticatabolics, 383–384
    intracellular regulators, 386–387, 386f
    mitogens, 384–385, 385f
    molecule categories, 383, 383t, 384f
    morphogens, 385–386, 385f
    outcome assessment, 387
Morphogens, molecular therapy with, 385–386, 385f
Motion preservation and stabilization
    annuloplasty
        annular anatomy and function, 375

artifical disk prostheses, 378
  interventional strategies, 376–378, 377f
  microdiskectomy, 375–376
  outcome assessment, 378
  overview, 375
  surgical techniques, 376, 376f
  symptomatic annular tears, 376, 377f
dynamic stabilization, 10–13
  facet replacement, 12, 13f
  interspinous process spacers, 10, 10f–11f
  pedicle screw-based systems, 10–12, 12f
  segment motion modification, 240, 241f
  Wallis interspinous implant, 264, 264f
Dynamic Stabilization System, 323
facet replacement technology overview, 347–351
  anatomy properties, 347, 348f
  current developments, 351, 351f
  outcome assessment, 351
  posterior dynamic reconstruction, post-decompression,
      350–351
  stand-alone devices for low-back pain, 347–349
  total disk replacement adjuncts, 349–350
spinal arthroplasty, 4–10
  historical review, 3
  nucleus replacement, 4–6, 5f–6f
  total disc replacement, 6–10
    cervical disk, 8–10, 8f–9f
    lumbar disk, 6–7, 6f–7f
Total Facet Arthroplasty System
  clinical trials, 370
  design parameters, 366–368, 367f–368f
  development assessment, 351, 351f
  dynamic stabilization procedures, 12
    comparison of outcomes, 370
  facet biomechanics, 365–366, 365f
  outcome assessment, 370–371
  overview, 364, 364f
  performance evaluation, 368–369, 368f–369f
  spinal biomechanics restoration, 364–365
  surgical technique, 369–370, 369f–370f
Total Posterior Facet Replacement and Dynamic Motion
      Segment Stabilization (TOPS) system
  biomechanical testing, 357, 358f
  design parameters, 355–356, 356f
  finite element analysis, 356–357, 357f
  indications for, 354–355, 355f
  outcome assessment, 362–363, 362f
  overview, 354
  pedicle screw loading, 357, 359f
  surgical technique, 357–358, 359f, 360–362, 360f–361f
Motion segment unit rotations
  cervical arthroplasty, 30, 30f
    biomechanical testing protocols, 36–37, 36f–39f
  TOPS system biomechanics, 357, 358f
Multidirectional flexibility, NUBAC artificial nucleus, 133–134
Multiple segment stabilization, Cosmic stabilization system
      procedures, 334

Neck disability index (NDI), Porous Coated Motion (PCM)
      prosthesis, 81–82, 82f–83f
Neck pain, Bryan cervical disc device, assessment, 63–64, 65f
NeuDisc device
  basic principles, 122
  biocompatibility testing, 123
  cadaver fatigue testing, 126
  clinical studies, 126, 126f–127f
  design criteria, 123

endurance testing, 123–125, 124f
  expulsion testing, 125–126
  mechanical testing, 123–126
  range of motion testing, 125, 125f
NeuDisc SNI Hydrogel Polymer device, nucleus replacement
      techniques, 5, 5f
NeuDisc Spinal Nucleus Implant, 124–125
Neural element decompression, Bryan cervical disc device, 62–63
Neurogenic intermittent claudication
  Cosmic stabilization system procedures, 332, 333f
  DIAM system applications, 275
  X STOP Interspinous Process Decompression system for,
      251–257
Neurological assessment, Maverick artificial disk, 194
Neutral angle modification, dynamic stabilization procedures,
      238, 238f
Newcleus device, nucleus replacement techniques, 5–6
Nitinol shape memory alloys
  basic properties, 292, 292t
  BioFlex rod pedicle screw system, 340–343, 341f–342f
Nondestructive testing criteria, cervical arthroplasty biomechanical
      testing, 36
Nonfusion techniques
  cervical decompression, 16–17, 17f
  laminectomy vs., 19
  lumbar decompression, 18–19
    Cosmic system for, 330–338
Noninstrumented posterolateral fusion, laminectomy with, 19
NUBAC artificial nucleus
  basic principles of, 128–129
  biocompatibility and biodurability, 132
  biomechanical assessment and fatigue, 132–133, 132f
  clinical indications for, 135
  design criteria, 129–131, 130f–131f
  multidirectional flexibility and load failure analysis, 133,
      133f–134f
  wear and fatigue studies, 134–135, 134f
Nucleus replacement
  DASCOR system, 114–121
  NeuDisc device, 122–127
  NUBAC artificial nucleus, 128–135
  NuCore injectable nucleus, 142–145
  principles and expectations, 114–116
  SINUX system, 137–140
  spinal arthroplasty, 4–6, 5f–6f
NuCore injectable nucleus
  basic properties, 142
  biomaterial properties, 143
  structural elements, 143–145, 144f–145f

Oblique implant insertion, Activ-L lumbar (Aesculap) total disk
      arthroplasty, 208–209
Operative time estimates, CERVIDISC opening, 88, 90t
Ossification of posterior longitudinal ligament (OPLL), posterior
      cervical laminoplasty, 16–17, 17f
Osteolysis, total disk replacement, 232
Osteoporotic patients, Coflex dynamic stabilization in, 269
Oswestry Disability Index (ODI) score
  CHARITÉ Artificial Disc, 172, 177f
  Coflex dynamic stabilization assessment, 270
  Cosmic stabilization system, 336–338
  Dynamic Stabilization System, 327, 329, 329f
  Dynesys Dynamic Stabilization System, 303
  Maverick artificial disk, 193, 193t
  Mobidisc prosthesis, 202, 203f
  ProDisc prostheses assessment, 183–184
  TOPS posterior facet replacement, 362–363

Outcome assessment
    annuloplasty, 378
    Bryan cervical disc device, 63–64
    Charité artificial disk, 172–173, 175f–176f, 176, 177f
    DASCOR artificial nucleus system, 119, 120f
    dynamic stabilization
        BioFlex rod pedicle screw system, 344
        Coflex system, 269–273, 271f, 271t
        Cosmic system, 336–338
        DIAM system, 279, 281f, 282, 282t
        Dynamic Stabilization System, 327, 329, 329f
        Dynesys Dynamic Stabilization System, 301–304,
            301f–302f, 304f
        Graf soft stabilization and ligamentoplasty, 308–311,
            309f–310f
        Isobar TTL dynamic rod placement, 319–320
        SoftFlex flexible rod system, 245–246
        X STOP Interspinous Process Decompression system,
            254–257, 255f–256f
    facet replacement technology, 351
        stand-alone devices for low back pain, 349
        Total Facet Arthroplasty System, 370–371
    Maverick artificial disk, 193, 193t
    Mobidisc prosthesis, 202, 203f
    molecular therapy, 387
    NeuDisc device, 126, 126f–127f
    Porous Coated Motion prosthesis, 81–82, 82f–83f
    ProDisc-C prosthesis, 75–76
    ProDisc prostheses
        European data, 182–183, 183f
        U.S. data, 183–185, 183f, 184t
    Raymedica Prosthetic Disk Nucleus, 110–112, 111f–112f
    TOPS posterior facet replacement, 362–363, 362f
    Wallis interspinous implant, 261, 263–266, 264f–266f
Overdistraction complications, total disk replacement
        complications, 231, 231f

Pain intensity score, Mobidisc prosthesis, 202
Pain relief
    dynamic stabilization
        Cosmic stabilization system procedures, 332, 333f
        Isobar TTL system, 314, 314f
        Wallis interspinous implant, 264
    facet replacement technology, stand-alone devices for low back
        pain, 348–349
Parallel insertion distractor, FlexiCore prosthesis, 216
Partial disk replacement (PDR), lumbar disks, prosthetic disk
        nucleus, 99–104
Patient selection criteria
    Maverick artificial disk, 190–191, 191f
    Raymedica Prosthetic Disk Nucleus, 107
    total disk replacement complications, 231
PDN-SOLO implant, Raymedica Prosthetic Disk Nucleus, 106–107,
        106f–107f
Pedicle screw-based systems
    BioFlex rod pedicle screw system
        basic components, 341–343, 341f–342f
        biomechanical testing, 341, 343
        case studies, 342f, 343, 344f
        indications and contraindications, 340–341
        outcome assessment, 344
        overview, 340
        surgical techniques, 343
    CHARITÉ Artificial Disc implant, 168, 170, 172f
    Cosmic stabilization system, basic components, 331–332,
        331f–332f
    dynamic stabilization, SoftFlex flexible rod system, 245, 249f

dynamic stabilization procedures, 10–12
    mechanics of, 237
Dynamic Stabilization System, minimally invasive surgery,
        327, 328f
Graf soft stabilization system, basic principles, 305–306, 305f
TOPS system
    implant characteristics, 355–356, 356f
    load analysis, 357, 359f
    surgical techniques, 360–362, 360f–361f
total cervical disk replacement, 49–50
Total Facet Arthroplasty System
    clinical trials, 370
    design parameters, 366–368, 367f–368f
    development assessment, 351, 351f
    dynamic stabilization procedures, 12
        comparison of outcomes, 370
    facet biomechanics, 365–366, 365f
    outcome assessment, 370–371
    overview, 364, 364f
    performance evaluation, 368–369, 368f–369f
    spinal biomechanics restoration, 364–365
    surgical technique, 369–370, 369f–370f
PEEK-OPTIMA polymer, NUBAC artificial nucleus, 132
Peer-reviewed biomechanics literature, 28–31, 29t–30t, 30f–31f
Peripheral nerve complications, total lumbar disk replacement,
        225
Pinned-fixed (PF) mounting, cervical arthroplasty biomechanical
        testing, 34f, 35
    results, 36
Pinned-pinned (PP) mounting, cervical arthroplasty biomechanical
        testing, 34f, 35
    results, 36
Placement techniques, Bryan cervical disc device, 63, 63f
Poly-ether-ether-ketone (PEEK)
    anterior cervical diskectomy with fusion, 18, 18f
    NUBAC artificial nucleus, 129–130
    Wallis interspinous implant, 259
Polyethylene core migration, lumbar disk arthroplasty, 228
Polyethylene wear, total disk replacement, 232
Polymer Nucleus, Spinal Kinetics Cervical Disc, 53
Polymethyl methacrylate (PMMA), NUBAC artificial nucleus,
        128–129
Porous Coated Motion (PCM) prosthesis
    cervical arthroplasty, 30
        bone ingrowth, implant-bone interface gaps, 84
        clinical outcomes, 81–82, 82f–83f
        complications, 82–84, 84t
        indications for, 78, 79t
        single and multiple levels, 81–82
    cervical total disk replacement
        adjacent segment disease prevention, 43
        design characteristics, 47–48, 48f
    design parameters, 78–79, 80f, 81
    historical background, 79, 80f
    total disc replacement, 9, 9f
Postdiskectomy syndrome (PDS), 137–138
Posterior longitudinal ligament (PLL)
    annulus anatomy and function, 375
    Cervidisc opening, 88
    Porous Coated Motion implants and, 79, 80f
Posterior lumbar interbody fusion (PLIF), 149
    Dynesys Dynamic Stabilization System, 300
    Graf soft stabilization and ligamentoplasty, 308t, 309–310, 310f
Posterior osteophyte removal, CHARITÉ Artificial Disc implant,
        165, 167, 169f
Posterior surgical procedures
    cervical foraminotomy, 17

cervical laminoplasty, 16–17, 17f
Dynamic Stabilization System (DSS)
  clinical testing, 326–327
  design principles, 323–326, 324f–326f
  fatigue testing, 323
  load sharing and motion restriction, 323
  outcome assessment, 327, 329, 329f
  surgical techniques, 327, 328f
 facet replacement technology
  as adjunct procedure, 350–351
  indications for, 354–355, 355f
 lumbar fusion, instrumentation, 19–20
 mechanics of, 237
 Raymedica Prosthetic Disk Nucleus, 108–109, 108f–109f
Posterolateral approach, Raymedica Prosthetic Disk Nucleus, 110, 110f
Postkyphotic deformity, cervical laminectomy, 16, 17f
Postlaminectomy syndrome, Isobar TTL dynamic rod placement, 319–321, 320f
Postoperative care
 FlexiCore prosthesis implants, 218–219
 ProDisc prostheses implants, 181
 Raymedica Prosthetic Disk Nucleus, 110
 TOPS posterior facet replacement, 362
Postoperative dysphagia, cervical total disk replacement and avoidance of, 44
Postoperative radiculopathy, total disk replacement, 230–231, 231f
Preclinical studies, Spinal Kinetics Cervical Disk, 56, 56f
Prestige cervical artificial disks
 LP device, 69–70, 69f
 overview, 67–68, 67f
 performance evaluation, 70–71, 71f
 Prestige I device, 68
 Prestige II device, 68–69, 68f
 ST/STLP artificial disks, 69, 69f
  cervical arthroplasty, 30, 31t
  total disk replacement, 8, 8f
   cervical disks, 45–47, 45f–46f
ProDisc prostheses
 basic components, 72–73, 72f
 biomechanical effects, 29–31, 29t–30t, 30f–31f, 179–180, 180f
 clinical outcomes, 75–76
 complications, 76
 design parameters, 72–73, 72f, 179, 180f
 European outcome assessments, 182–183, 183f
 historical background, 161–162, 162f
 implantation technique, 180–181, 181f–182f
 overview, 72
 surgical technique, 73–75, 74f–75f
 total disk replacement, 6f, 7, 9
  cervical disks, 48–49, 48f
  facet replacement technology as adjunct to, 350
  migration, dislocation, or subluxation, 228
  vertical split fractures, 230, 230f
 U.S. outcome assessments, 183–185, 183f
Programmable single actuator biomechanical testing, cervical arthroplasty testing protocols, 34–35
Prostheses. See Artificial disks
 annuloplasty and, 378
Prosthetic Disk Nucleus (PDN)
 annuloplasty and complications from, 378
 complications, 22
 geometry, 101
 lumbar disk, partial disk replacement, 101–103
 NUBAC artificial nucleus vs., 131, 131f
 nucleus replacement techniques, 5, 5f

Raymedica device, 105–113
 anterior, lateral, and posterolateral approaches, 110, 110f
 materials and methods, 106–107
 outcome assessment, 110–112, 111f–112f
 patient selection, 107
 posterior approach, 108–109, 108f–109f
 postoperative care, 110
 tension band system repair with, 290
Pseudarthrosis, cervical total disk replacement and avoidance of, 43–44
Pseudosubluxation, Porous Coated Motion arthroplasty, 84
Pullout test, BioFlex rod pedicle screw system, 343

Rail cutting technique, Prestige LP artifical disk, 70, 70f
Range of motion data
 cervical arthroplasty, 27–28, 28t
  artificial, harvested, and fused spined procedures, 29–30, 29t
 cervical total disk replacement, adjacent segment disease prevention, 43
 Cervidisc design criteria and, 86–87
 CHARITÉ Artificial Disc, 162–164, 163f–167f
 dynamic stabilization, 244
  Coflex system, 271–273, 272f
 Dynamic Stabilization System, 324, 325f–326f
 NeuDisc device, 125, 125f
 NUBAC artificial nucleus, 133–134, 134f
 ProDisc prostheses, 180, 183–185
 Prosthetic Disk Nucleus (PDN), 101
Raymedica Prosthetic Disk Nucleus (PDN), 105–113
 anterior, lateral, and posterolateral approaches, 110, 110f
 materials and methods, 106–107
 outcome assessment, 110–112, 111f–112f
 patient selection, 107
 posterior approach, 108–109, 108f–109f
 postoperative care, 110
Recombinant human bone morphogenetic protein (rhBMP-2)
 anterior cervical diskectomy with fusion, 18
 NuCore injectable nucleus, 143
Reherniation prevention, annuloplasty for, 375–376
Repositioners, FlexiCore prosthesis, 214, 215f, 218, 219f
Retrolisthesis, tension band system biomechanics, 286
Retroperitoneal exposure technique, Charité Artificial Disc implant, 165, 168f
Reverse mutation assays, NeuDisc device biocompatibility, 123
Reversibility studies, dynamic stabilization, Wallis interspinous implant, 264
Revision techniques, CHARITÉ Artificial Disc, 174, 176
Rigid fixation
 Coflex dynamic stabilization with, 269
 combined hybrid rigid and soft stabilization, 311
Root injuries, total lumbar disk replacement, 231–232
Rotational displacement transducer (RDT), cervical arthroplasty biomechanical testing, 35, 35f

Saddle articulation, CerviCore disk prostheses, 92, 93f–94f
Safety issues, dynamic stabilization, Wallis interspinous implant, 263–264
Sagittal plane balance
 Bryan cervical disk device, 59–66
 dynamic stabilization procedures, 238–239, 239f
  total disk replacement and establishment of, 152
Satisfaction Index, Mobidisc prosthesis, 202
Scient'x titanium alloy
 biomechanical performance, 315, 315f
 dynamic stabilization procedures, 12, 12f
  instrumentation and adjacent disk degeneration, 313–315, 314f–315f

Scient'x titanium alloy (*Continued*)
  isobar TTL rod placement, 318–321, 320f–321f
  finite element analysis, 315–317, 316f–317f
  indications for, 317–318, 318f–320f
  overview, 312–313
Segmental instability, Coflex dynamic stabilization for, 269
Segmental Spinal Correction System (SSCS), Cosmic stabilization
    system *vs.*, 336
Sexual function testing, Mobidisc prosthesis, 202
Shape memory alloys (SMAs), KIMPF-DI fixation system shape
    memory alloy, 292–298
  basic properties, 292–293, 292f, 293f
  case studies, 296–298
  components of, 294, 294f–295f
  deformation and installation, 296, 296f
  indications and contraindactions, 293f, 294
  loop fixings, surgical techniques, 294–296, 295f–296f
  surgical techniques, 294–296, 295f–296f, 298t
Sheath structure, Spinal Kinetics Cervical Disk, 53
Short form (SF)-36 Health Survey
  dynamic stabilization outcomes, X STOP Interspinous Process
      Decompression system, 254–257
  Dynesys Dynamic Stabilization System, 303
  Mobidisc prosthesis, 202
SINUX system
  testing methodology, 138, 138f–139f
  in vitro investigation, 139–140, 139f–140f
Situs inversus abnormalities, total lumbar disk replacement
    complications, 221–222, 222f
SoftFlex system, dynamic stabilization, 244–249
  basic components, 244–245, 246f–248f
  outcome assessment, 245–246
  surgical techniques, 245, 249f
Soft stabilization
  Graf ligamentoplasty, 305–311
    concept and rationale behind, 305–306, 305f
    disease classification and indications for, 307–308, 308t
    indications and contraindications, 306
    outcome assessment, 307–311, 309f–310f
    surgical techniques, 306–307, 307f–308f
  tension band system repair, 290
Sox9 chondrocyte marker, molecular therapy with, 386–387
Specimen preparation, cervical arthroplasty biomechanical testing,
    36, 36f
Spinal biomechanics
  cervical arthroplasty biomechanical testing, 36, 36f
  Total Facet Arthroplasty System, 364–365
Spinal Kinetics Cervical Disc
  clinical feasibility, 57–58
  design parameters, 53–54, 53f
  instrumentation, 53, 53f
  preclinical studies, 56–57
  surgical technique for, 54–55
  total disk replacement, 9–10, 9f
  in vitro testing, 55–56
Spinal stenosis
  Cosmic stabilization system procedures, 332, 333f
  DIAM system applications, 275
  dynamic stabilization, BioFlex rod pedicle screw system,
      343–344
  KIMPF-DI shape memory alloy, 296–297, 296f
  tension band system repair, 288, 290, 290f
  X STOP Interspinous Process Decompression system for, 251–257
Spondylodesis, Cosmic stabilization system, 330–338
  adjacent segment degeneration, 333, 334f
  basic components, 331–332, 331f–332f
  contraindications, 334

disk herniation recurrence, 332
diskogenic pain and facet syndrome, 332, 333f
indications for, 331–333
lumbar stenosis, 332, 333f
multiple segment stabilization, 334
outcome assessment, 336–338
overview, 330–331
spondylodeses procedures, 331, 333, 334f
surgical techniques, 334–336, 335f–336f
Spondylolisthesis, tension band system repair, 288, 290, 290f
Stability of insertion, Bryan cervical disc device, 60
Static bending compression test, BioFlex rod pedicle screw
    system, 343
Static characterization
  Spinal Kinetics Cervical Disk, 55–56
  Wallis interspinous implant, 260
Static distractors, FlexiCore prosthesis, 214, 214f
Stiffness testing
  dynamic stabilization, intervertebral disk unloading,
      239–240
  Isobar TTL dynamic instrumentation, 315, 315f
  NUBAC artificial nucleus, 132–133
  Prosthetic Disk Nucleus (PDN), 101
Strain analysis, SINUX system, 139–140, 140f
Strength testing, Prosthetic Disk Nucleus (PDN), 101
Stress testing
  Isobar TTL dynamic instrumentation, 316–317, 317f
  SINUX system, 139–140
Subluxation complications, lumbar disk arthroplasty, 228
Subsidence
  Cervidisc systems, 88, 89f–91f
  lumbar disk arthroplasty, 227, 228f–229f
  NUBAC artificial nucleus, 130
  NuCore injectable nucleus augmentation, 142–145
  tension band system biomechanics, 286
  total disk replacement and, 151–152
Surgical techniques
  Activ-L lumbar (Aesculap) total disk arthroplasty, 206–209
  annuloplasty, 376, 376f
  BioFlex rod pedicle screw system, 343
  Cervidisc system, 87
  Coflex dynamic stabilization, 269, 270f
  dynamic stabilization
    Cosmic stabilization system procedures, 334–336, 334f–336f
    DIAM system, 278–279, 278f–279f
    Isobar TTL dynamic rod placement, 318–321, 320f–321f
    SoftFlex flexible rod system, 245, 249f
    tension band system, 285f, 287–291, 288f
    Wallis interspinous implant, 261–263, 262f–263f
    X STOP Interspinous Process Decompression system,
        253–254, 253f
  Dynamic Stabilization System, minimally invasive procedures,
      327, 328f
  FlexiCore prosthesis, 216–219, 217f
  Graf soft stabilization ligamentoplasty, 306–307,
      307f–308f
  KIMPF-DI system, loop fixing, 294–296, 295f–296f, 298t
  lumbar disks, artificial nucleus replacement, 115–116
  Maverick artificial disk, 189–193, 190f–193f
  Mobidisc prosthesis, 199–200, 201f–202f
  NUBAC artificial nucleus, 129–135
  Prestige LP artifical disk, 69–70, 69f–70f
  ProDisc-C prosthesis, 73–75, 74f–75f
  ProDisc prostheses, 180–181, 181f–182f
  Prosthetic Disk Nucleus (PDN), 103
  Raymedica Prosthetic Disk Nucleus, 108–109, 108f–109f
  Spinal Kinetics Cervical Disk, 54–55, 54f

TOPS posterior facet replacement implantation, 357–358, 359f, 360–362, 360f–361f

Total Facet Arthroplasty System, 369–370, 369f–370f

Tamp device, Spinal Kinetics Cervical Disk, 54–55

Tension Band system

dynamic stabilization

artificial ligament, 284–285, 285f

basic principles, 284

biomechanics, 285–286, 286f

components of, 284–286

decompressive laminotomy, 287–288, 288f–289f

degenerative spondylolisthesis, 288, 290, 290f

indications and contraindications, 286

metal inerspinous locker, 285, 285f

soft stabilization techniques, 290

surgical techniques, 285f, 287–291, 288f

dynamic stabilization procedures, 10, 11f

Tension testing, Wallis interspinous implant, 260

Therapeutic molecules, classification, 383, 383t, 384f

Three-dimensional analysis, SINUX system, 138, 138f

Tissue-based biomechanical studies, cervical anthroplasty, 33

Tissue inhibitors of matrix metalloproteinases (TIMPs), 383–384

Topping off technique

DIAM system applications for, 275–276, 278

KIMPF-DI shape memory alloy, 297, 297f

Total disk replacement (TDR)

cervical disks, 8–10, 8f–9f

design pros and cons, 49–50

disadvantages, 44–45

indications for, 45

prosthetic designs, 45–49

Bryan cervical disk, 47, 47f

CerviCore device, 49, 49f

Porous Coated Motion prosthesis, 47–48, 48f

Prestige ST device, 45–47, 45f–46f

ProDisc-C device, 48–49, 48f

rationale for, 42–44

Spinal Kinetics Cervical Disc, 52–58

facet replacement technology as adjunct to, 349–350

historical background, 160–162

lumbar disks, 6–7, 6f–7f

Activ-L Lumbar (Aesculap) arthroplasty, 204–210

artificial disk prosthesis, 154–155

biomechanical issues, 149–152

case studies, 156–158, 156f–158f

CHARITÉ Artificial Disc, 160–178

complications, 221–232

contraindications, 155–156

FlexiCore artificial disk, 212–220

indications, 154–159, 155t

indications for, 151–152

Maverick prosthesis, 186–194

Mobidisc prosthesis, 196–203

ProDisc prosthesis, 179–185

spinal arthroplasty, 6–10

cervical disk, 8–10, 8f–9f

lumbar disk, 6–7, 6f–7f

Total Facet Arthroplasty System (TFAS)

clinical trials, 370

design parameters, 366–368, 367f–368f

development assessment, 351, 351f

dynamic stabilization procedures, 12

comparison of outcomes, 370

facet biomechanics, 365–366, 365f

outcome assessment, 370–371

overview, 364, 364f

performance evaluation, 368–369, 368f–369f

spinal biomechanics restoration, 364–365

surgical technique, 369–370, 369f–370f

Total nucleus removal (TNR), development of, 117–118, 117f–118f

Total Posterior Facet Replacement and Dynamic Motion Segment Stabilization (TOPS) system

biomechanical testing, 357, 358f

design parameters, 355–356, 356f

finite element analysis, 356–357, 357f

indications for, 354–355, 355f

outcome assessment, 362–363, 362f

overview, 354

pedicle screw loading, 357, 359f

surgical technique, 357–358, 359f, 360–362, 360f–361f

Toxicity testing, NuCore injectable nucleus, 145

Transforaminal lumbar interbody fusion (TLIF), lumbar decompression, 18–19, 19f

Transforming growth factor-beta (TGF-β), molecular therapy with, 385–386, 385f

Translational displacement transducer (TDT), cervical arthroplasty biomechanical testing, 35, 35f

Translational/pinned-fixed (TPF) mounting, cervical arthroplasty biomechanical testing, 34f–35f, 35

results, 36–37, 36f–39f

Trial design, Spinal Kinetics Cervical Disk, 54

Trialing technique, Activ-L lumbar (Aesculap) total disk arthroplasty, 207–208, 208f

Tumor necrosis factor-alpha (TNF-α), molecular therapy with, 384

Ultrasound, annuloplasty and, 378

Unconstrained prostheses, design parameters, 28

Uncus drilling, CERVIDISC systems, 88

Urogenital complications, total lumbar disk replacement, 224–225, 225f

Vascular complications, total lumbar disk replacement, 221–226, 222f

arterial obstruction, 223, 223f

deep venous thrombosis, 224, 224f

venous tear and bleeding, 221–222, 221t

Vertebral body fracture, lumbar disk arthroplasty, 228, 230, 230f

Visceral complications, total lumbar disk replacement complication, 224

Visual analog scale (VAS)

Charité artificial disk, 172, 177f

Coflex dynamic stabilization assessment, 270

Cosmic stabilization system outcome assessment, 336–338

DASCOR artificial nucleus system, 119, 120f

Dynamic Stabilization System, 327, 329, 329f

iliac crest bone graft donor site morbidity, cervical total disk replacement, 44

Mobidisc prosthesis, 202

Porous Coated Motion (PCM) prosthesis, 81–82, 82f–83f

ProDisc prostheses assessment, 183–185

Von Mises stress test, Isobar TTL dynamic instrumentation, 317

Wallis interspinous implant, dynamic stabilization applications

adjacent segment preservation, 264–265

basic principles, 258–259

biocompatibility testing, 260

contraindications, 261

duration of effects, 265–266, 266f

fatigue testing, 260

finite element analysis, 260

first-generation implants, 261

indications for, 258, 261

motion preservation, 264, 264f

Wallis interspinous (*Continued*)
  outcome assessment, 263–266, 264f–266f
  pain relief, 264
  potential disk restoration, 265, 265f
  reversibility potential, 264
  safety issues, 263–264
  static testing, 260
  surgical technique, 261–263, 262f–263f
  system components, 259–260, 259f–260f
  in vitro cadaver testing, 260
Wear testing
  Bryan cervical disc device, 60–61
  Maverick artificial disk, 188
  NUBAC artificial nucleus, 134–135, 134f
  Spinal Kinetics Cervical Disk, 55
  total disk replacement, polyethylene wear, 232
  Total Facet Arthroplasty System, 368–369, 369f

Wedge-ramp distractor, FlexiCore prosthesis, 216, 216f
Williams sequestrectomy, annuloplasty for reherniation
      prevention, 376
Work status, Maverick artificial disk, 194
Wound complications, total lumbar disk replacement, 225–226f

X STOP Interspinous Process Decompression system
    design parameters, 252–253, 253f
    dynamic stabilization procedures, 10, 10f, 21–22
      lumbar neurogenic claudication, 251–257
        neutral angle and disk space height modification, 238, 239f
        sagittal plane balance, 239, 239f
      segment load distribution modification, 241

Zurich Claudication Questionnaire (ZCQ), lumbar neurogenic
      claudication treatment, X STOP Interspinous Process
      Decompression system outcomes, 254–257